The Radiotherapy of Malignant Disease

Edited by

Eric C. Easson and R. C. S. Pointon

With 324 Figures

Springer-Verlag
Berlin Heidelberg New York Tokyo 1985

Eric C. Easson, CBE, MD, FRCP, FRCR
Emeritus Professor of Radiotherapy, University of Manchester and formerly Director of Radiotherapy, Christie Hospital and Holt Radium Institute, Manchester, UK

R. C. S. Pointon, FRCP, FRCR
Director of Radiotherapy, Christie Hospital and Holt Radium Institute, Manchester, UK

ISBN 3-540-13104-3 Springer-Verlag Berlin Heidelberg New York Tokyo
ISBN 0-387-13104-3 Springer-Verlag New York Heidelberg Berlin Tokyo

Library of Congress Cataloguing in Publication Data
Main entry under title:
The radiotherapy of malignant disease.
Includes bibliographies and index.
1. Cancer – Radiotherapy. I. Easson, Eric C. II. Pointon, R.C.S. (Robert Charles Snow), 1923– . [DNLM: 1. Neoplasms – radiotherapy. QZ 269 R1325] RC271.R3R35 1984 616.99′40642 84 – 5581
ISBN 0-387-13104-3 (U.S.)

Printed in Great Britain

Filmset by Wilmaset Ltd, Birkenhead, Merseyside.
Printed by William Clowes Limited, Beccles, Suffolk.

2128/3916 543210

Preface

Radiotherapy or radiation therapeutics, as the name suggests, is a branch of general therapeutics. In this case the therapeutic agent is ionising radiation which induces specific and predictable biological changes. Radiotherapy is sometimes described as therapeutic radiology because historically the earliest X-ray machines were used both for diagnostic and therapeutic purposes. Diagnostic radiology has since become a very complex and time-consuming speciality requiring the undivided care and attention of the diagnostic radiologist. Similarly, radiotherapy now embraces both X-ray beams and the radiations from radium and various artificial radium substitutes. This too requires the full-time attention of the radiotherapist. In recent years radiotherapy has sometimes been described as radiotherapeutic oncology, to indicate the involvement of the radiotherapist in oncological management and indeed in all aspects of oncology from prevention and early detection to the treatment, after-care, and (for those who need it) terminal care of the patient. The radiotherapist, by total commitment to the cancer problem, is in truth the epitome of the oncologist.

In the same way as the medical physician or internist requires a proper understanding of the pharmacology of the therapeutic agents he or she employs—the nature, metabolic biochemistry, and biological effects of any administered drug—so also the radiotherapist needs to understand the nature, biological effects, and therapeutic potentialities of ionising radiations. The radiotherapist's "pharmacology" involves an understanding of the relevant physics and radiobiology. The first two chapters of this book therefore deal respectively with the physics and the radiobiology of specific relevance to radiotherapy and the radiotherapist's field of work. It might be added that the internist, whilst requiring a thorough understanding of pharmacology, is not expected to be a professional pharmacologist. Similarly a radiotherapist need not be a professional physicist or radiobiologist. An adequate understanding of the scientific basis of radiotherapy is, however, essential. Since radiation therapy is a branch of therapeutics we are concerned not only with the fundamental "mode of action" of ionising radiations but, as with digitalis, morphine, or penicillin, we are concerned with dosage. Dosage of ionising radiations is measured in precise physical terms, and sensitive physical instruments are employed to measure radiation dosage. However, the connotations of the word "dose" are much wider than the simple quantitative measurement of a centigray (the radiotherapist's equivalent of a milligram). Time is involved in all dosage systems whatever the nature of the therapeutic agent, but while the correct time interval between individual doses is vital, for example, in the case of insulin for the diabetic patient, it is clearly less vital when giving iron tablets for iron-deficient anaemia. The spacing or "fractionation" of radiation dosage is of considerable importance to the radiotherapist, and so also is the overall time in which a prescribed dose of radiation is given. The possible physical combinations and permutations of dosage (again, as with any drug) are infinite and thus we come to employ "courses" of treatment whose biological effects, at a clinical level, have become well-established and predictable.

Whereas physics and radiobiology are to the radiotherapist what pharmacology is to the physician, radiotherapeutic technique is the counterpart of the surgeon's operative surgery. The radiotherapist must ensure that the correct dose of radiation reaches the target tissue—usually a malignant tumour. The techniques for achieving this objective can be complex and always require a high degree of geometric precision. Different clinical situations present their own special technical problems, and the radiotherapist must be competent to overcome these problems, since to fail with a malignant lesion usually means the death of the patient. However, just as the surgeon may be compelled to accept that a lesion is technically inoperable, the radiotherapist may at times find a tumour equally beyond effective irradiation. As with all clinical medicine, such decisions are based on experience and clinical judgment. In this respect also the radiotherapist must be in every way as competent a clinician as the physician and the surgeon. Each must have wide general clinical experience as well as a profound knowledge and experience in his specialised field. Since so much of the radiotherapist's work (though not all of it) is concerned with cancer, he cannot know too much about its protean characteristics, its natural history and pathogenesis, its epidemiology, causation, prevention, detection, clinical care and treatment, after-care and rehabilitation, and finally, when necessary, the terminal care of cancer patients.

Medicine continues to become increasingly specialised, and this has led to the concept of multi-disciplinary teams concerned with the management and care of patients. However sensible this may seem, we feel it essential that once a decision is made about an appropriate line of treatment, the clinician concerned should then be solely responsible for that phase of the patient's management. So far as the radiotherapist is concerned, once the decision has been taken that irradiation is the appropriate method of treatment, the clinical care of the patient must remain firmly in the hands of the radiotherapist. It may be that surgery or chemotherapy has to precede or follow the irradiation and the patient may at that time pass into the care of a surgeon or a chemotherapist. It is important, therefore, that the radiotherapist must be not only competent but confident and self-reliant.

This book is aimed at the radiotherapist in training, but should be of value even to the more experienced radiotherapist by providing practical details of the technical approaches to specific clinical problems. Chapters 1 and 2 are concerned with the "pharmacology" or scientific basis of radiation therapy—physics and radiobiology respectively. It would clearly be out of place to attempt here an exhaustive account of these two subjects, and many complete textbooks are already available for the reader who requires them. Only the most clinically relevant and important aspects of physics and radiobiology are presented here, providing a background to what follows. Chapter 3 likewise provides a general outline of chemotherapy for malignant disease, concerned with principles rather than practice, though the latter is introduced where and when necessary in the subsequent chapters on practical radiotherapy. Many radiotherapists around the world are inescapably involved in adjuvant hormone treatment and chemotherapy, and an understanding of the scope and limitations of the agents involved is therefore essential. This, of course, is a rapidly changing field of medicine, characterised also by many extravagant claims of high success which further experience fails to confirm. We have, therefore, confined ourselves throughout this book to general commentaries and recommendations based on acceptable chemotherapeutic practice for the 1980s. In chapter 4 an account is given of the functions of a mould room, one of the nerve centres of a radiotherapy department. The technical staff of the mould room work in close collaboration with the radiotherapists in preparing a variety of precision-made applicators essential for the accurate treatment of many kinds of cancer. But the preparation of a surface mould or a beam-direction shell cannot be learned from the written word alone, however detailed and lucid the description. This is a practical task requiring much experience and meticulous care.

Before embarking on the main part of the text (chapters 6–18), some general principles of radiation therapy are discussed in chapter 5, to draw attention to what we regard as the fundamental clinical considerations in this field, some of which represent indeed the very essence of the Manchester school of thought.

The previous two textbooks from this hospital (Ralston Paterson, 1947 and 1963) were deliberately designed to discuss in detail how to treat, by X-rays and radium, malignant tumours in various anatomical sites. This third textbook has the same principal objective and we have endeavoured to provide practical guidance on how the radiotherapist can plan and execute a satisfactory technique for irradiating those lesions for which this kind of treatment is considered clinically appropriate. We have deliberately confined ourselves to describing "how it is done" at this hospital, and in a didactic fashion. We are, of course, conscious of widely differing practices around the world, and even surprisingly divergent opinions on basic principles. No one textbook could adequately present all these views, even in general terms, and ours is therefore unashamedly a Manchester book. We do, however, have statistical grounds for believing that our survival and cure rates are at least encouraging, at best excellent, and this book tries to show how these results can be achieved.

Some readers may be surprised that we do not discuss the treatment of some tumours which they are themselves called upon to treat. Examples of this are cancer of the stomach or of the pancreas. It has been our experience over five decades that these tumours (and others) do not lend themselves to curative irradiation, and palliative radiotherapy is in our view likely to create more problems than it solves. This does not mean that were some new, as yet unforeseen development to present itself we would not eagerly re-examine our established attitudes. At the moment, however, the contributions presented in chapters 6–18 must remain our testament of faith.

Acknowledgments

The editors would like first to acknowledge their profound indebtedness to Mrs. Elsa Hughes and Miss Joan Moores for their labours, over many months, to prepare the typescripts for this book. They are also indebted to Mr. Richard Schofield and the staff of the Department of Medical Illustration for their painstaking work to provide the many illustrations, graphs, and photographs. They are grateful, too, to those colleagues who, in spite of heavy clinical commitments, were willing to burn the midnight oil in order to contribute their chapters to this work. Finally, the editors are acutely aware of the vital collaborative involvement of many colleagues in other disciplines, all contributing in their special ways to the dynamic life of the hospital. They are too numerous to mention by name but to all of them we owe a deep debt of gratitude.

Manchester, 1984

Eric C. Easson
R. C. S. Pointon

Contents

Contributors

M. P. Cole, MSc, MD, FRCR
(Late Consultant Radiotherapist, Christie Hospital and Holt Radium Institute)

D. Crowther, MSc, PhD, MA, MB, BCh, FRCP
(Professor of Medical Oncology, Christie Hospital and Holt Radium Institute)

D. P. Deakin, MB, ChB, FRCR
(Consultant Radiotherapist, Christie Hospital and Holt Radium Institute)

M. B. Duthie, BSc, MB, ChB, FRCR
(Consultant Radiotherapist, Christie Hospital and Holt Radium Institute)

E. C. Easson, CBE, MSc, MD, FRCP, FRCR
(Late Emeritus Professor of Radiotherapy in the University of Manchester)

B. W. Fox, BSc, PhD, FLS
(Professor of Experimental Chemotherapy, Department of Oncology, University of Manchester)

R. Gibb, MB, ChB, FRCR
(Late Director of Radiotherapy, Christie Hospital and Holt Radium Institute)

D. Greene, PhD, FInstP
(Asst. Director, Physics Department, Christie Hospital and Holt Radium Institute)

N. K. Gupta, MB, BS, FRCR
(Consultant Radiotherapist, Christie Hospital and Holt Radium Institute)

J. H. Hendry, BSc, MSc, PhD
(Head of Radiobiology Section, Paterson Laboratory, Christie Hospital and Holt Radium Institute)

R. D. Hunter, MB, ChB, MRCP, FRCR
(Consultant Radiotherapist, Christie Hospital and Holt Radium Institute)

R. D. James, MA, MB, ChB, MRCP, FRCR
(Consultant Radiotherapist, Christie Hospital and Holt Radium Institute)

M. K. Palmer, FSS, PhD
(Principal Medical Statistician, Christie Hospital and Holt Radium Institute)

D. Pearson, MB, ChB, FRCR
(Consultant Radiotherapist, Christie Hospital and Holt Radium Institute)

R. C. S. Pointon, MA, FRCP, FRCR
(Director of Radiotherapy, Christie Hospital and Holt Radium Institute)

G. Read, MA, MRCP, FRCR
(Consultant Radiotherapist, Christie Hospital and Holt Radium Institute)

G. G. Ribeiro, MB, ChB, FRCR
(Consultant Radiotherapist, Christie Hospital and Holt Radium Institute)

E. Sherrah-Davies, MA, FRCS, FRCR
(Consultant Radiotherapist, Christie Hospital and Holt Radium Institute)

S. K. Stephenson, BScTech, FInstP
(Deputy Director, Physics Department, Christie Hospital and Holt Radium Institute)

D. Studd, FBIST
(Chief Mould Room Technician, Christie Hospital and Holt Radium Institute)

M. L. Sutton, MA, MRCP, FRCR
(Consultant Radiotherapist, Christie Hospital and Holt Radium Institute)

I. D. H. Todd, FRCP, FRCR
(Deputy Director of Radiotherapy, Christie Hospital and Holt Radium Institute)

P. M. Wilkinson, MSc, MB, ChB, MRCP
(Consultant Physician/Clinical Pharmacologist, Christie Hospital and Holt Radium Institute)

1 Physics

D. Greene and S. K. Stephenson

This chapter provides some background about the physical aspects of radiotherapy. The provision of a treatment by ionising radiation is very much a team effort by the radiotherapist, the physicist, and the radiographer, but we shall concentrate here on the basic technology and will not discuss who does what.

Radiation Sources

The radiation sources used in radiotherapy may be classified into (1) beam sources, where the radiation is delivered to the patient in the form of beams of X-rays, gamma rays, electrons, or neutrons; (2) brachytherapy sources, where a radionuclide emitting gamma or beta rays is contained in sealed needles, tubes, or plaques which may then be applied on the body surface, interstitially, or into a natural body cavity; and (3) radionuclides used in a liquid form and administered orally or by injection.

Beam Sources

The desirable properties of a beam for radiotherapy are (1) that the penetrating properties of the beam should be suited to the depth of the lesion to be treated; (2) the dose distribution across the beam should be uniform, or, by the use of a "wedge filter", be non-uniform in a prescribed way; (3) the beam should be well-defined, that is, the "penumbra region" at the beam edge should be as narrow as possible (ideally the dose level would fall to zero, though in practice it falls to something like 1% of the level inside the beam); (4) the beam should be stable, that is, the dose distribution inside the beam should remain constant; and (5) the beam should be movable so that it can be directed accurately at the patient.

Choice of Equipment and Facilities

In choosing equipment to meet the above requirements it is necessary to consider a large number of additional factors some of which are listed below:

1) Are the mechanical movements of the radiotherapy generator and the patient support system, which serve to direct the radiation beam at the patient in the prescribed way, reliable and convenient?
2) Are the available field sizes and collimator systems appropriate?
3) Is the machine stable and reliable in operation?
4) Is the accessory equipment (e.g. front and back pointers) satisfactory?
5) Is the dose-monitoring system adequate?
6) What are the relative advantages between tele-isotope and X-ray machines?
7) Are replacement parts readily available at acceptable cost and can the machine be maintained properly without unacceptable interruptions?

Choice of equipment will, of course, also be

influenced by personal experience, by the opinions of others and by financial considerations. It is necessary to bear in mind that radiotherapy equipment is often expected to be used for 15–20 years and that although the capital and operational costs are very high, the cost per patient compares very favourably with the costs of surgery and chemotherapy.

Surveillance of Equipment

Very high reliability is essential in radiotherapy equipment, to ensure that treatment for the patient is available as required, that fractionation schedules are adhered to and that all the systems necessary to deliver the correct dose to the patient are operating. For these reasons it is essential to carry out regular preventive maintenance on the electrical and mechanical systems which make up the treatment unit. It is also essential to carry out regular checks on the properties of the radiation beam, e.g. on radiation quality and dose distribution and on the dose-monitoring systems.

Production of Physical Data

All treatment prescriptions, whether prepared manually or by computer, require detailed knowledge of the patterns of radiation (e.g. isodose charts) and the quantity of radiation (beam output) generated by a particular treatment machine. It is the responsibility of the physicist to provide adequate data for these purposes and it is a matter for local judgement whether these data need to be measured individually, or whether published information or information provided by the manufacturer is used. If either of the latter courses is adopted it would be necessary to carry out some checks to ensure that the radiation beam from a particular machine conforms to the published data. Moreover, as already indicated in the previous section, these checks need to be repeated at regular intervals during the lifetime of the equipment.

Characteristics of Radiotherapy Beams

The penetrating properties of an X-ray or gamma-ray beam depend on the photon energy, on the field size, and on the source-to-skin distance (SSD). X-ray beams have a continuous photon energy spectrum extending up to the energy of the electrons which generate the photons at the X-ray target. As a rough rule, the mean photon energy is about one third that of the accelerated electrons. In practice, the quality of the X-rays is often described in terms of the energy of the accelerated electrons. For example, the term "4 MV X-rays" is a shorthand way of saying "that photon spectrum which is generated when 4-MeV electrons collide with an X-ray target". The effect of passing the beam through a metal filter is differentially to attenuate the lower photon energy component, thus increasing the mean photon energy and the penetrating properties of the beam in tissue. For X-rays generated in the range up to about 300 kV, filtration makes a substantial difference to the mean photon energy, and for this reason it is necessary to add to the description of the beam. It is usual to add a statement about the penetrating properties of the radiation in a specified metal, usually aluminium or copper, by stating the thickness of the metal required to reduce the beam intensity by a factor of 2. This thickness is called the "half value thickness" (HVT). An example would be "250 kV radiation, HVT 2.5 mm Cu", which means that radiation quality produced when 250-kV X-rays are filtered to produce a photon beam whose intensity is halved by passing through a 2.5-mm thickness of copper.

Megavoltage X-rays are usually heavily filtered owing to the need for a "beam-flattening filter" (as discussed in the next section) and additional filtration makes only a minor difference to their penetrating properties in tissue. For this reason the previous description in terms of the energy of the accelerated electrons is adequate for the radiation beams in the megavoltage range of quality discussed in this volume.

The only radionuclide used extensively as a beam therapy (teletherapy) source is cobalt-60, which emits photons of energy 1.2 and 1.3 MeV. "Cobalt-60 gamma rays" is an unambiguous description of this radiation source.

The penetration properties of radiation beams in tissue are most simply expressed by means of relative depth-dose curves, which show dose as a function of depth, in relation to the maximum dose, which is normalised to 100%. Some examples are shown in Fig. 1.1a for radiation qualities referred to in subsequent sections of this book. It

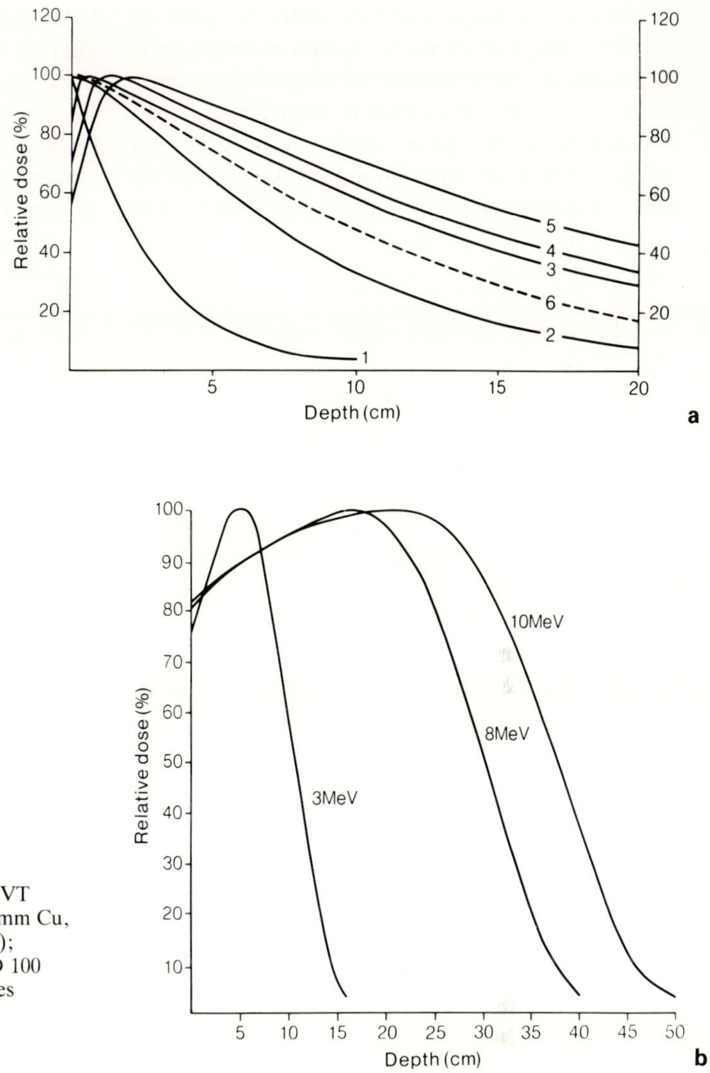

Fig. 1.1. **a** Depth-dose curves: *1* 100-kV X-rays (HVT 2 mm Al, SSD 30 cm); *2* 250-kV X-rays (HVT 2.5 mm Cu, SSD 50 cm); *3* Cobalt-60 gamma rays (SSD 100 cm); *4* 4-MV X-rays (SSD 100 cm); *5* 8-MV X-rays (SSD 100 cm); *6* 15-MV neutrons (SSD 100 cm). All these curves are for a 10 cm × 10 cm field at the source-to-skin distance (SSD) most commonly used. **b** Depth-dose curves for 3-, 8-, and 10-MeV electron beams.

can be seen that for the lower energy radiations (curves 1 and 2) the maximum dose occurs at the surface, while at higher energies the maximum dose occurs at increasing depths below the surface.

Electron beams have penetrating properties which depend mainly on the energy of the electrons, and examples of depth-dose curves are given in Fig. 1.1b, for the electron energies discussed in the clinical section of this book.

Neutron beams have very similar penetrating properties to photon beams and can be best described in terms of the mean neutron energy generated by a particular source. Figure 1.1a shows a depth-dose curve for 15-MeV neutrons, as an example.

Isodose Charts

The dose distribution given by the various types of radiation beam is described by an isodose chart which shows the dose distributions, in water, in a longitudinal plane through the central axis of the beam. Figure 1.2a shows an isodose chart for 4-MV X-rays for the normal beam, that is, where a cone-shaped "beam-flattening filter" is incorporated to create a uniform dose distribution across the beam. It should be noted that the dose distribution can be uniform, i.e. the field can be "flat", at only one depth. At increasing depths the effect of radiation scattered inside the beam is to increase the relative dose at the beam centre, that is, to make the isodose curves more rounded. As can be seen from Fig. 1.2a, this is not a very significant effect for megavoltage X-ray beams. The width of the penumbra is determined by the size of the radiation source (the focal spot), by the design of the beam-defining system, and by scattered radiation from inside the beam. The beam definition given by most linear accelerators is very satisfactory.

Figure 1.2b shows a wedged-field isodose chart for 4-MV X-rays, where the dose distribution has been made non-uniform by the use of a wedge-shaped metal filter. It is a major advantage of megavoltage radiation that very satisfactory wedge

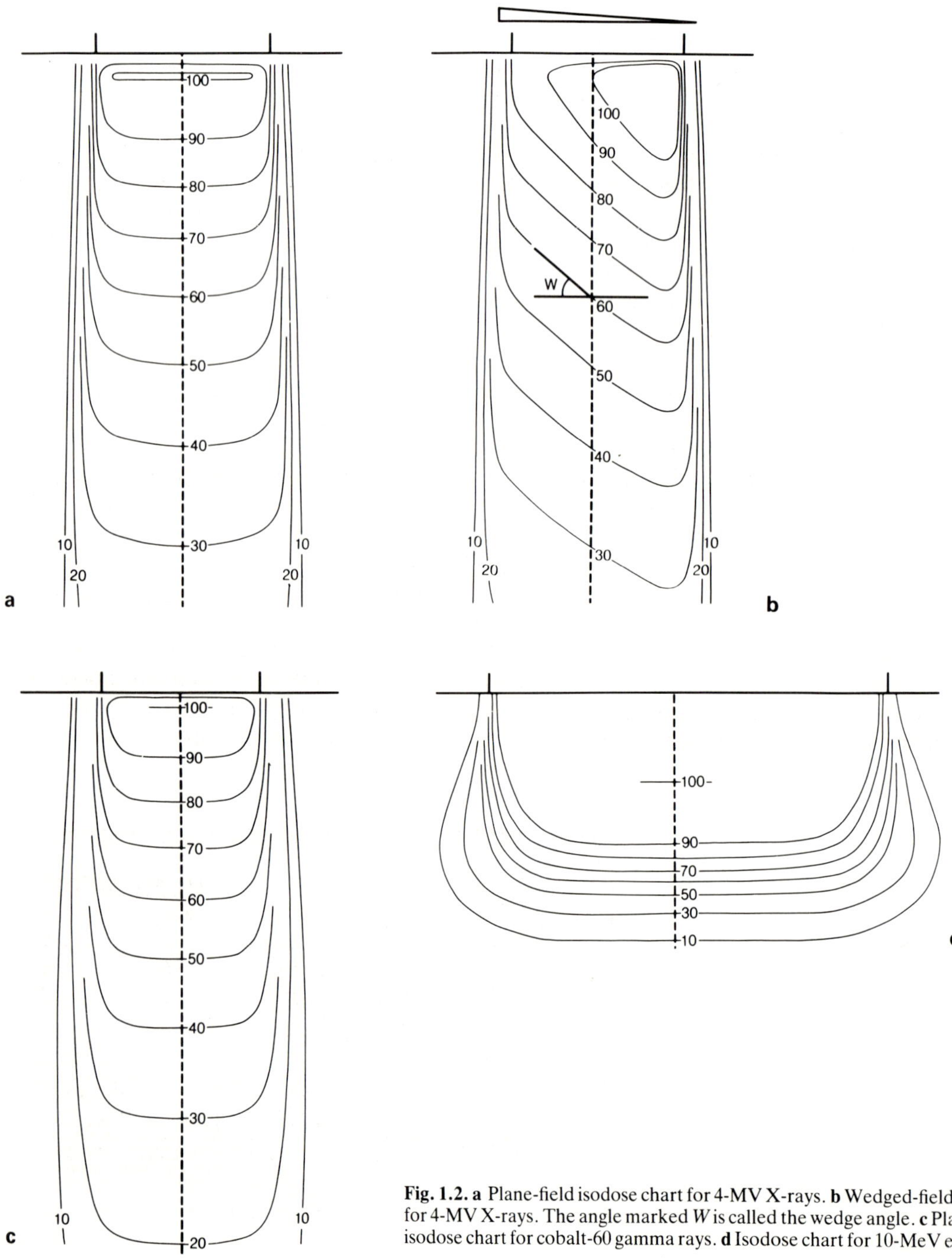

Fig. 1.2. a Plane-field isodose chart for 4-MV X-rays. **b** Wedged-field isodose chart for 4-MV X-rays. The angle marked *W* is called the wedge angle. **c** Plane-field isodose chart for cobalt-60 gamma rays. **d** Isodose chart for 10-MeV electron beam.

filters can be designed and that the "wedging" of the beam changes very little with depth. It is convenient to call the angle marked *W* on Fig. 1.2b the "wedge angle".

Figure 1.2c shows a cobalt-60 beam isodose chart. The main difference between this and the chart for an X-ray beam of comparable mean photon energy is an increased penumbra width, resulting from the larger radiation source required.

Figure 1.2d shows an isodose chart for a 10-MeV electron beam. The notable features here are the limited range of the beam and the bulging penumbra due to scattering of the electrons.

Since the edges of a radiation beam are not perfectly sharp (see Fig. 1.2), there has to be a convention about the meaning of the term "field size". In this volume, the convention for megavoltage X-ray fields is the distance between the 80% isodose lines at the build-up depth. For electron treatments the field is defined by an aluminium applicator extending onto the patient's skin. The field size is then given as the internal size of the applicator at the surface of the patient. For X-rays in the kilovoltage range, the beam-defining applicator also extends to within a few centimetres of the surface of the patient and field size is given as the size of the applicator at the surface of the patient.

Radiotherapy Generators

The types of radiotherapy generators referred to in the clinical sections are briefly described below.

For the treatment of skin cancer, X-ray units operating at voltages between 10 and 100 kV are used. These give depth doses adequate for treatments to a depth of a few millimetres, while sparing deeper tissue. In theory, this type of treatment would be better done using electrons with an energy of about 1 MeV, but for small-field treatments the superficial X-ray units give excellent results and, of course, they are simpler and cheaper machines than a corresponding electron source. For large-field treatments, up to and including the whole skin surface, 3-MeV electrons have the advantage of delivering an adequate skin dose while producing a negligible bone marrow dose and are used for this reason.

Conventional X-ray units operating in the range 250–300 kV, with filtration to give a radiation quality of HVT 2.5 mm Cu, are used for the treatment of less superficial lesions, and in particular for postoperative chest wall treatments for cancer of the breast.

For small-field treatments of the head and neck, 4-MV X-rays from linear accelerators are used. One of these machines is illustrated in Fig. 1.3. It is our considered view that the optimum radiation quality for these treatments is in the range of 4–6 MV X-rays. Higher energy X-rays are at a disadvantage for these treatments mainly because of the increased depth of the maximum dose (see Fig. 1.1a). X-rays of this energy are also useful for regional and mantle treatments.

For treatments of the larger body sections, in particular the pelvic region, it is an advantage to have higher energy X-rays, and an 8-MV linear accelerator is appropriate for this purpose. This

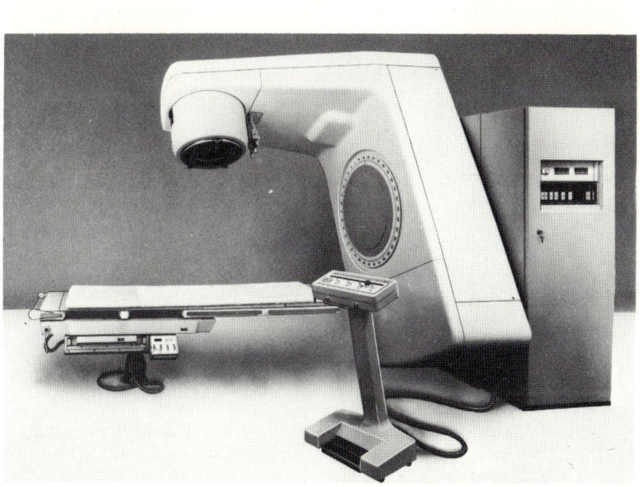

Fig. 1.3. A 4-MV linear accelerator.

machine can also be used as a source of 3-, 8-, and 10-MeV electrons.

Radiological Protection for Beam Therapy Units

For radiotherapy generators operating above 50 kV the patient must be alone in the treatment room during radiation exposures, so that staff and the general public will be protected from the radiation by the construction of the room. For superficial X-ray treatments, the operator may be protected by a suitable screen inside the room.

X-ray and gamma-ray therapy equipment can usually be rotated through 360° about a horizontal axis and those parts of the walls, floor, and ceiling which may be irradiated by the direct beam must be of adequate thickness to attenuate the primary beam sufficiently. These sections of the protective structure are called "the primary protective barrier" and have to be wide enough to intercept the largest beam available for the equipment, at the position of the barrier. The other parts of the walls, ceiling, and floor of the treatment room will receive radiation from three sources—radiation scattered from the patient, radiation scattered from the primary barriers, and leakage radiation penetrating the protective housing of the machine. These parts of the structure are called "secondary protective barriers" and have to be of adequate thickness to attenuate these radiations sufficiently.

Access to the treatment room will be through a protective door or maze, either of which should be located in a secondary protective barrier. For radiation qualities up to about 300 kV it is practicable to use lead-lined doors. For higher energy radiations the necessary doors become ponderous structures which need to be operated mechanically and it is therefore more convenient to use a maze.

As examples of protective structures for radiotherapy rooms, Fig. 1.4 shows the plan view

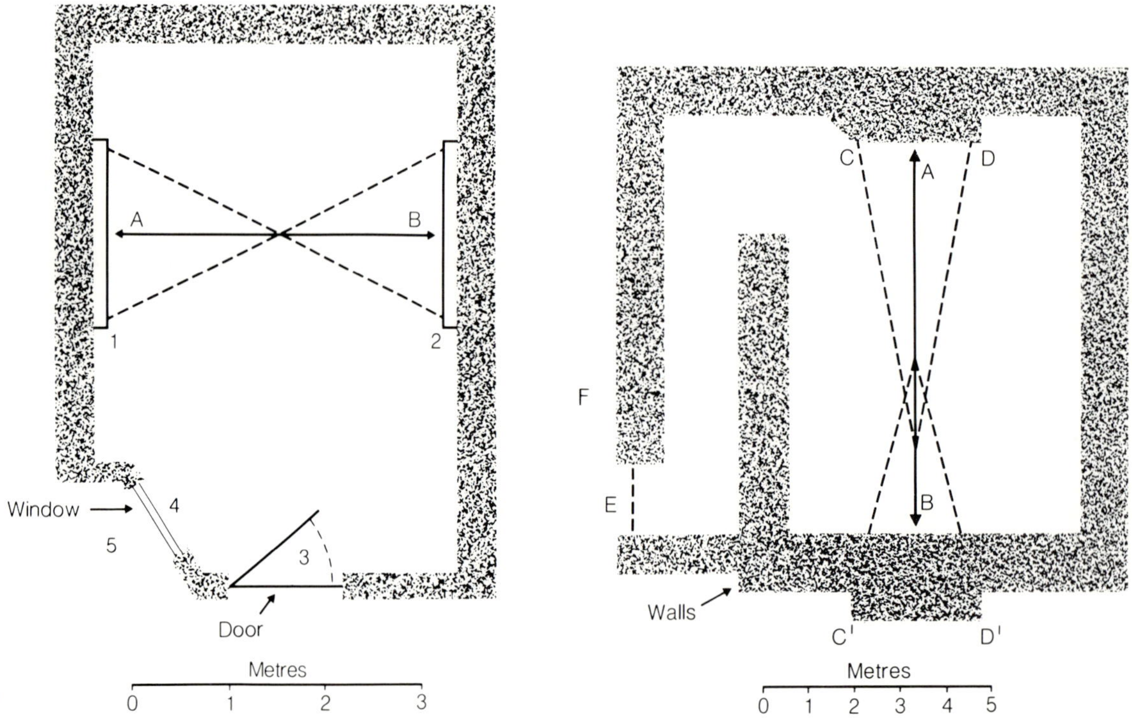

a b

Fig. 1.4. **a** Plan of 300-kV X-ray therapy room. The line *AB* is the central axis of the X-ray beam. *1, 2* Additional protective material on walls to intercept the primary beam; *3* lead-lined door; *4* lead glass window; *5* operator's position during treatments. The divergent lines show the maximum size of the X-ray beam.
b Plan of 4-MV X-ray room. *AB*, line of central axis of the X-ray beam. The divergent lines show the maximum size of the X-ray beams. *CD* and C^1D^1, primary barriers; *E*, light-beam interlock; *F*, operator's position during treatments. The walls of both rooms are made of ordinary concrete.

of a 300-kV treatment room and a 4-MV room. In the former case it is practicable to use a lead glass window to observe the patient during treatment. For megavoltage installations it is now common practice to use closed-circuit television to keep the patient under observation.

Radiation warning signs must be displayed at the entrance to treatment rooms, as well as warning lights to indicate when radiation is being produced. The door in Fig. 1.4a is fitted with an interlock switch to prevent the production of radiation when the door is open. In Fig. 1.4b a light-beam is used as the interlock. Interruption of the light-beam will prevent the production of radiation, and the interlock circuit should require a deliberate action to reset it after interruption before it is possible to switch on the radiation.

Provided adequate resources are allocated to the construction of beam therapy rooms, a high degree of safety for patients, staff, and the public can be achieved. Implementation is, however, very dependent on adequate staff training, on well-thought-out working procedures and well-defined allocation of responsibility.

Brachytherapy Sources

Radiotherapy treatments may be carried out using the radiations from relatively weak, sealed radioactive sources which may be placed in, or within a few centimetres of, the tissues to be treated. This branch of radiotherapy is called "brachytherapy".

The properties of some of the radionuclides used for brachytherapy are summarised in Table 1.1. These radionuclides have to be sealed in suitable containers which serve three main purposes:

1) To contain the radioactive material. This includes:
   a) Holding the radioactive material in a desirable geometrical shape.
   b) Stopping the radioactive material from contaminating the tissues or, indeed, any other material when it is to be handled or stored.
2) To filter out unwanted radiation coming from the source. For example, if the source is being used as a gamma-ray emitter, then the material of the container may be chosen so that any associated alpha and beta rays are absorbed in the walls.
3) To facilitate the clinical use of the source. For example, the container is fabricated in the form of a needle so that it can be inserted into tissues and subsequently withdrawn with the aid of a silk thread through the eyelet.

Figure 1.5 shows the form of the types of brachytherapy source listed in Table 1.1.

Historically, brachytherapy was based on the use of radium or its derivative radon, which has a half-life of 3.8 days. The long half-life of radium is a great advantage, since treatment times for any particular type of source can be kept unchanged throughout the working life of the source. The

Table 1.1. Brachytherapy sources. Some of these radionuclides, e.g. radium-226, are accompanied by an equilibrium amount of one or more radioactive daughter products, which have different half-lives and emit different radiations. The half-life given is the half-life of the parent radionuclide and the energy is the mean photon energy for what may be a complex spectrum of gamma-ray lines.

Radionuclide	Radiation emitted	Energy	Half-life	Form
Radium-226	Gamma rays	1 MeV	1620 years	Needles, tubes
Caesium-137	Gamma rays	0.66 MeV	30 years	Tubes, needles, pellets
Cobalt-60	Gamma rays	1.25 MeV	5.26 years	Rods
Iridium-192	Gamma rays	0.4 MeV	74 days	Wires
Gold-198	Gamma rays	0.41 MeV	2.7 days	Seeds
Strontium-90	Beta rays	2.27 MeV max	28.5 years	Plaques
Yttrium-90	Beta rays	2.27 MeV max	64 hours	Rods

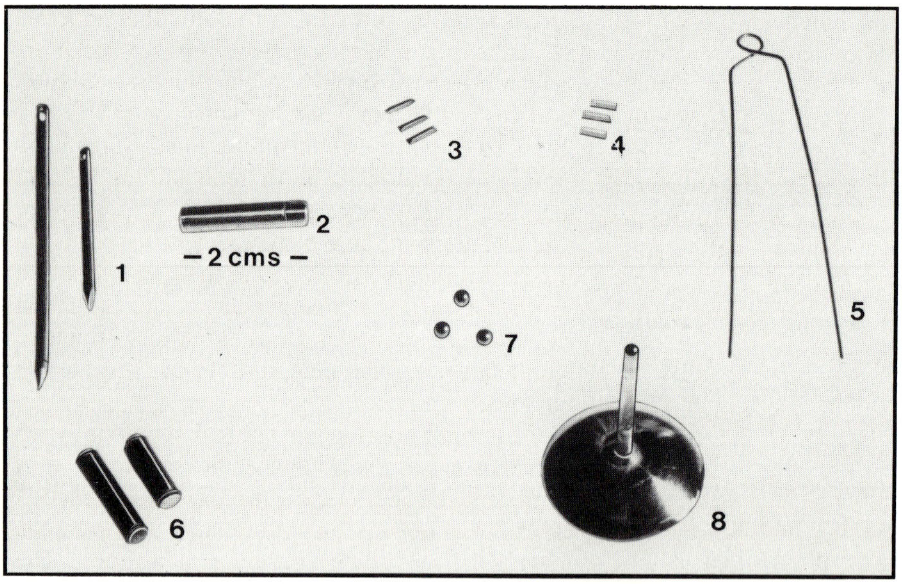

Fig. 1.5. Photograph showing the brachytherapy sources listed in Table 1.1: *1* radium needles, *2* radium tube, *3* gold seeds, *4* yttrium rods, *5* iridium wire, *6* cobalt rods, *7* caesium pellets, *8* strontium plaque.

working life is limited in this case mainly by mechanical wear and tear on the containers, but with careful handling sources may be used for about 20 years.

Caesium-137 sources are now more commonly used and are available in needles and tubes of similar construction and strength to radium sources. The main advantages of caesium are lower radiotoxicity of the radioactive material in the event of an accidental leakage from the source, and the fact that it emits lower energy gamma rays, which makes for simpler shielding and storage systems. The 30-year half-life corresponds to a loss of source strength of about 2% per year and allowance must be made for this. Caesium sources can be regarded as of constant strength throughout any single treatment. They can also be fabricated in suitable forms for afterloading equipment.

Cobalt-60 sources can be prepared in a very wide range of source strengths and are cheap and convenient. The relatively short half-life of 5.26 years corresponds to a decay rate of about 1% per month, so that the source strength can still be regarded as constant throughout any individual treatment. Amendments to nominal source strength, however, should be made every 3 months, and a stock-holding and replacement system is required to cater for the appreciable decay of the sources over several years.

Iridium-192 is used as a gamma-ray source because it is available in the form of flexible wires, which may be drawn into previously implanted nylon tubes.

Gold-198 is used for permanent gold seed implants. The activity of these seeds has decayed to about one eighth after 8 days and after 27 days to one thousandth.

The only radionuclides utilised as beta-ray emitters are strontium-90, which can be fabricated into suitably shaped plaques for surface and ophthalmic applications, and yttrium-90, rods of which are used for permanent implantation in the pituitary gland.

Handling of Brachytherapy Sources

In the wrong place, or in the wrong hands, these are quite dangerous devices, but they can be used without serious hazard with adequate facilities and trained staff. The essential features of a system for this purpose are:

1) Adequate shielding of the storage facilities to keep the radiation levels in adjoining spaces within recognised limits.
2) Shielded bench space for preparation and cleaning of sources.

3) A book-keeping system by which the location and current usage of every source is accounted for, at all times.
4) Well-thought-out procedures in theatre where the sources are inserted and in the wards where patients receiving brachytherapy are nursed. These procedures are based on two principles, namely quick handling and use of the inverse square law, to limit doses to staff.
5) Regular inspection of sources for mechanical damage.

Source Strength

In the SI system of units, the activity of a radionuclide source is given in becquerels (Bq), where one becquerel is defined as one disintegration per second. The old unit, the curie, was defined as 3.7×10^{10} disintegrations per second. Sources for brachytherapy have activities more conveniently expressed in megabecquerels (MBq), i.e. in units of 10^6 Bq. The activity of a source is sometimes referred to as the source strength.

For a brachytherapy source it is necessary to distinguish between source strength and effective source strength. Some of the radiation generated in the source will be absorbed in the material of the source itself and in its container, so that a radiation measurement made from outside the container will correspond to a smaller amount of activity than that actually present. In principle, this type of measurement gives the effective source strength, which is that activity of a point source (with no self-absorption) which corresponds to the measured radiation. As brachytherapy systems have been evolved from radium treatments, it is often convenient to express effective source strength in terms of milligrams of radium equivalent for sources which do not decay appreciably during a treatment.

Afterloading Equipment

The radiation from brachytherapy sources represents a significant radiation protection problem for theatre and ward staff, especially in relation to the relatively strong sources used for intracavitary treatments of the cervix. Afterloading equipment is designed to solve this problem, the principle being to place in the patient suitable catheters which are subsequently to contain the radiation sources and facilitate quick placing and removal of these sources. In *manual* afterloading systems the sources are mounted on the end of long flexible handles, so that they can be pushed into position in the catheters and thus reduce exposure to theatre staff. In *automatic* systems the catheters are connected to a machine which can quickly insert the sources or withdraw them into a shielded container to reduce the exposure of both theatre and ward staff.

Automatic afterloading equipment falls into two main categories: (1) where the sources are of sufficient strength to deliver a prescribed fraction of the required dose in minutes and, (2) where the dose is delivered over a period of many hours. The choice between these high or low dose-rate alternatives is essentially clinical and involves judgements about the biological significance of dose rate.

The afterloading techniques described in this book involve the use of a low dose-rate system, which uses caesium-137 pellets of the type illus-

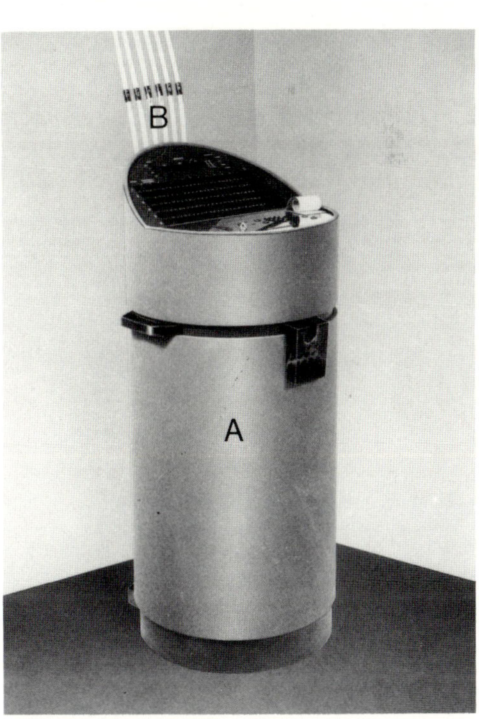

Fig. 1.6. Selectron afterloading unit. *A*, control unit and shielded containers for sources. *B*, source tranfer tubes.

trated in Fig. 1.5. The machine, the "Selectron" (see Fig. 1.6), is kept in a modestly shielded room on the ward and transfers "trains" of pellets in and out of catheters which have been placed in the patient in theatre. The pellets are transferred between patient and safe pneumatically. Radiation exposures to the nursing and other staff are then eliminated by transferring the sources from the patient into the safe at any time when it is necessary to approach the patient. The detailed properties of the source to go in each catheter are controlled by making up a train of active and inactive pellets. A relatively complex system (based on a microprocessor) is required (1) to control the selection and make-up of source trains; (2) to time the exposures given to the patient, allowing for the fact that the sources may be withdrawn from time to time; and (3) to ensure that the sources are correctly placed in the catheters, or in the safe, as required.

Unsealed Radionuclide Sources

The ideal radionuclide for radiotherapy treatments with an unsealed source would have the following properties:

1) It could be concentrated or retained in a particular organ or volume of the body.
2) It should be a beta-ray emitter, so that the radiation dose would be limited to the tissues in which the radionuclide is incorporated, beta rays having a range of only a few millimetres in tissue. With gamma-ray emitters, most of the radiation will extend beyond the organ containing the radionuclide and deposit energy elsewhere in the body.
3) It should have a half-life of a few days. If the half-life is too short, very high activities would have to be given to the patient to deliver an adequate dose and this would pose radiation protection problems for the staff. On the other hand, too long a half-life would extend the period when radiation from the patient is a potential hazard to other individuals.

The half-life in the present context is not necessarily the physical half-life of the radionuclide, but is also dependent on the biological half-life associated with removal or excretion of the radioactive material. The effective half-life is a combination of these two and will depend on their relative values.

There are very few radionuclides which meet these criteria, and those referred to in this book are listed in Table 1.2. There is no isotope of iodine which is a pure beta emitter and it can be seen from the table that iodine-131 emits both beta and gamma rays. When this material is used to treat the thyroid gland, about 85% of the absorbed dose is delivered by the beta particles.

The calculations of the dose delivered by a radionuclide which is uniformly distributed throughout an organ or volume of the body have to be done separately for the beta and gamma ray components.

1) Since beta rays are absorbed locally, the mean dose is obtained by dividing the energy emitted by the radionuclide as beta rays by the mass of the organ. The energy depends on (a) the total activity, (b) the effective half-life, and (c) the mean beta-ray energy per disintegration.
2) The dose delivered by gamma rays is not limited to the volume in which the radionuclide is concentrated. It is therefore necessary to estimate the fraction of the emitted energy that is absorbed within the volume of interest.

Table 1.2. Radionuclides suitable for unsealed use.

Radionuclide	Form in which used	Half-life	Radiation emitted	Method of administration
Iodine-131	Sodium iodide solution	8 days	Beta rays Gamma rays	Oral
Phosphorus-32	Sodium orthophosphate solution	14.3 days	Beta rays	Intravenous injection
Yttrium-90	Colloidal liquid	64 hours	Beta rays	Intracavitary injection

Handling of Unsealed Radionuclide Sources

The radionuclides used for therapy are chosen to deliver short-range radiation, so that it is not difficult to protect staff from external irradiation by these materials. The main requirement is therefore to prevent spills of the solutions used and to protect staff from skin exposure or ingestion or inhalation of the radioactive materials. The scale of this problem arises from the high activities required for therapy doses. For example, the occupational annual limit of intake for iodine-131 is only about one ten-thousandth of the activity which may be administered to a thyroid cancer patient in a single drink.

These radionuclide solutions should be prepared and administered in rooms which are used only for these purposes. All surface finishes in these rooms, bench tops, floors and other furnishings should be of impervious material and should be regularly checked for surface contamination. Staff at risk from iodine-131 should be periodically measured for thyroid radioactivity.

There should be well-thought-out schemes for dealing with spills of radioactive material, or coping with possible emergencies such as fire. Spills in this context include the possibility of a patient vomiting just after receiving a high-activity drink or of the patient being incontinent.

Transport within the hospital site of radioactive materials and of patients who have received radioactive treatments requires careful consideration and methods of disposal of radioactive residues, excreta, and other contaminated wastes must be organised and implemented according to statutory requirements.

Perhaps the most important aspect of the safe handling of unsealed radionuclide sources is staff training, and only trained staff should be involved in the preparation and administration of such materials.

Dosimetry

The technical aspects of radiotherapy are mainly concerned with delivering the correct dose distribution to the patient; thus it is clear that the determination of dose, or more correctly, absorbed dose, is of prime importance. Absorbed dose is defined as the energy absorbed in unit mass of material when it is irradiated and for radiotherapy purposes would be ideally stated as absorbed dose in a particular tissue. In practice, absorbed dose in soft tissue is usually given. It is, of course, much easier to measure absorbed dose in water rather than in tissue, and to make a subsequent correction to dose in soft tissue.

The SI unit of absorbed dose is the gray (Gy) which is defined as one joule per kilogram. The older unit, the rad, was defined as 100 ergs per gram, so we can say that 100 rad is equal to 1 Gy, or 1 rad is equal to 1 centigray (cGy).

The dose prescribed by the radiotherapist for any treatment is based on previous clinical experience. To establish this experience and make future use of it requires that radiation doses be delivered and measured at a sufficient level of consistency over very long periods. To establish this level of consistency within one treatment centre and to extend it between centres, it is important to have access to the national radiation standards, which are themselves related to the standards in other countries.

There is no national standard for the unit of absorbed dose, the only standards available being for the quantity "exposure", which is defined as the ionisation produced in a specific mass of air by X or gamma radiations. The SI unit of exposure is one coulomb of charge of either sign per kilogram of air. No name has so far been given to this unit. The historical unit of exposure, the röntgen, is equal to 2.58×10^{-4} coulombs per kilogram. This rather odd number arises from the original definition of the röntgen as "that amount of radiation which will liberate 1 electrostatic unit of charge of either sign in 1 cc of dry air at NTP (0.001293 g of dry air)".

The röntgen can be related to the unit of absorbed dose in air because the production of one electrostatic unit of charge requires the expenditure of a known amount of energy in a specified mass of air, and it turns out that an exposure of 1 röntgen corresponds to an absorbed dose of 0.869 cGy in air.

Dosemeters

Although many physical and chemical systems are available and are used as radiation dosemeters, the most commonly used device is the ionisation chamber. This is illustrated in Fig. 1.7, where the

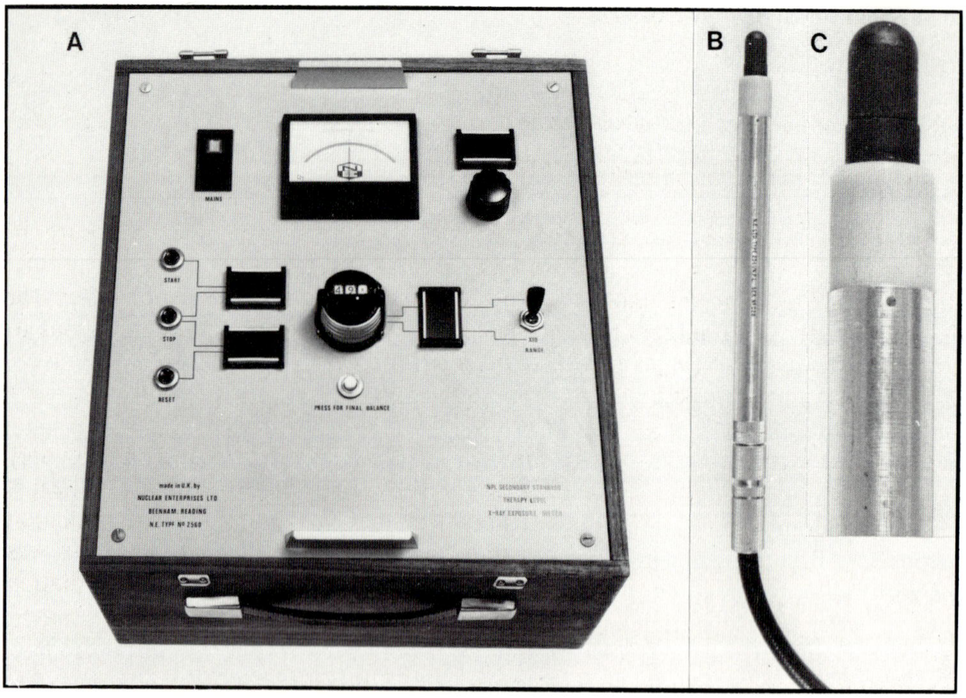

Fig. 1.7. A radiation dosemeter.
A Control box, **B** dosemeter probe showing cable which connects it to the control box, **C** ionization chamber.

air cavity in which the ionisation is to be measured is defined by a thimble-shaped graphite cap. The charge collected in this cavity is carried via the coaxial cable to the control box which contains a voltage supply, to produce the electric field in the chamber to collect the charge, and an electrometer, to measure the amount of charge produced in the air cavity when it is irradiated.

At the national standardising laboratory the chamber is given a known exposure, and a calibration factor N is determined such that

$$\text{Exposure in röntgens} = RN$$

where R is the reading given by the electrometer when the chamber is irradiated. The reading R depends on the mass of air in the chamber, and if the graphite cap defining the volume is not air-tight (and this is usually the case), the mass of air will depend on the temperature and atmospheric pressure. The reading R has then to be corrected to that which would be obtained at standard temperature and pressure (20 °C and 760 mm Hg). The multiplying correction factor is

$$\frac{T+273}{293} \times \frac{760}{P}$$

where T and P are the temperature and pressure at which the reading R was obtained.

Ideally, the value of the calibration factor N would be independent of radiation quality, so that the dosemeter could be used at all radiation qualities, or indeed, where the radiation quality is not known. In practice, with the best available ionisation chambers, N will vary 5%–10% over the kilovoltage to megavoltage range.

In the United Kingdom the National Physical Laboratory can offer calibrations for a range of radiation qualities up to 250 kV and for 2-MV X-rays. Many other national standardising laboratories provided an exposure calibration for cobalt-60 radiation.

From the previous discussion, we can then say that when the calibrated ionisation chamber is irradiated,

$$\text{Absorbed dose in air in cGy} = 0.869\ RN$$

where R is the reading given by the dosemeter, corrected to standard temperature and pressure, and N is the calibration factor for the radiation quality involved.

The quantity of interest is not dose in air, but

dose in tissue, and this can be determined by the equation:

Absorbed dose in tissue in cGy

$$= \text{dose in air} \times \frac{\text{dose absorbed in a small sample of tissue}}{\text{dose absorbed in a small sample of air}}$$

where the two small samples of these materials are given the same exposure.

This ratio is equal to the ratio of the mass attenuation coefficients for the two materials, which are denoted by $(\mu_{en}/\rho)_{tissue}$ and $(\mu_{en}/\rho)_{air}$. These attenuation coefficients are a function of radiation quality.

The equation can then be rewritten:

Absorbed dose in tissue in cGy

$$= 0.869\, RN \frac{(\mu_{en}/\rho)_{tissue}}{(\mu_{en}/\rho)_{air}}$$

$$= f_c RN \qquad (1)$$

where

$$f_c = 0.869 \frac{(\mu_{en}/\rho)_{tissue}}{(\mu_{en}/\rho)_{air}}$$

The quantity f_c is a function of radiation quality. Tabulated values for this are available and are given in Table 1.3.

Table 1.3. Values of the quantity f_c.

Radiation quality	f_c
45 kV, HVT 0.5 mm Al	0.89
100 kV, HVT 2 mm Al	0.87
300 kV, HVT 2.5 mm Cu	0.95

For the 2-MV calibration, the ionisation chamber has to be fitted with a plastic cap 5 mm thick to establish "electronic equilibrium" in the chamber. If the chamber is given a series of constant exposures in air, starting with no plastic cap, and then successively using plastic caps of increasing thickness, the readings obtained will increase up to a thickness of 5 mm and then decrease again for greater thicknesses. Only for the thickness where the reading is a maximum can it be said to be proportional to the exposure. To utilise the calibration factor N for 2-MV X-rays, the chamber must always be used with its 5-mm-thick plastic cap, in which case the equation, exposure in röntgens=RN, will still apply.

To determine absorbed dose in water for megavoltage radiation an equation analogous to Eq. (1) may be used:

$$\text{Absorbed dose in water in cGy} = RNC_\lambda$$

where C_λ is a quantity which takes account not only of the "röntgens to cGy" factor, but also of the fact that the chamber may be used for radiation qualities different from that at which it was calibrated. Values of C_λ as a function of radiation quality are given in Table 1.4.

Table 1.4. Values of the quantity C_λ.

Radiation quality	C_λ
Cobalt-60 gamma rays	0.951
4-MV X-rays	0.952
8-MV X-rays	0.946

Practical Dosimetry

The arrangement for measuring the output from an X-ray generator is shown in Fig. 1.8. The ionisation chamber is being used to determine the dose at a point in a water phantom and for this purpose it must be placed in a water-tight tube. For this it is convenient to use a Perspex tube since it also serves as a rigid support to place the chamber at the desired position. For megavoltage radiation this Perspex tube will incorporate the build-up cap previously mentioned, while for kilovoltage quality a thin-walled tube should be used.

In accordance with the previous discussion, the dose delivered to the point in the water phantom coincident with the centre of the ionisation chamber cavity is given by:

$$\text{Dose in cGy} = RNf_c$$

where R, N, and f_c have already been defined, the latter two being the values relevant to the radiation qualities used.

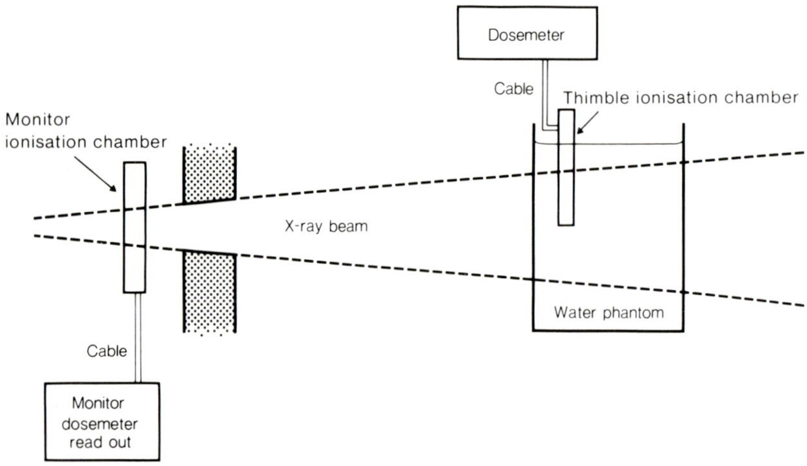

Fig. 1.8. Arrangement for measuring dose delivered in a radiation beam. The reading obtained at a specified point in the phantom is used to calibrate the dose-monitoring system.

For megavoltage quality radiation, the absorbed dose at the position of the centre of the chamber is given by:

$$\text{Dose in cGy} = RNC_\lambda$$

where R is the reading, N is the röntgen calibration factor for 2-MV X-rays, and C_λ is the value for the radiation quality concerned.

This process will then measure the dose at one point in the water phantom. It is conventional to measure the dose at a depth of 5 cm on the central axis of the beam. The doses at other points in the radiation field are determined by relative measurements, expressed in the form of an isodose chart.

Dose Monitoring

Figure 1.8 shows a monitor ionisation chamber in the radiation beam. This chamber is usually formed by a pair of thin aluminium plates which extend right across the largest field to be used; the plates are connected to a monitor read-out system at the control position of the X-ray generator. Essentially the same process as described in the previous section is used to calibrate the monitor system, and it is our practice to adjust the monitor scale so that its reading will give the dose in centigrays at a known position in a water phantom, usually at the maximum of the depth-dose curve. This monitor reading can directly give the dose at only one position, for one particular field size, and one SSD. For other conditions the monitor reading can be corrected to give the dose at a reference point in the phantom by the use of a table of multiplying factors. These factors are determined by a series of measurements, as described in the previous paragraph, for a wide range of field sizes and SSD values. For routine calibrations of the beam monitor it is then only necessary to make a measurement for one field size and SSD.

A failure of the dose-monitoring system during a treatment may result in underdosing or overdosing of the patient, with serious clinical consequences. To guard against this risk, X-ray machines should be fitted with two independent monitor ionisation chambers and associated electronics. In the United Kingdom it is further required that the readings from the two monitor systems should be automatically compared with each other, and that a circuit be incorporated to switch off the X-rays if the two systems disagree by more than a specified amount. In other words, the X-rays will automatically switch off in the event of a failure of one of the monitoring circuits.

For a cobalt-60 teletherapy unit, the dose rate is constant during the period of the treatment, so that a dose-monitoring system is not required. The procedures illustrated in Fig. 1.8 may therefore be used to measure the dose rate, and the dose delivered to a patient can be controlled by a timing device. Again, a failure of the timer during a treatment has to be guarded against. This can be done by using a dual timer system. The dose rate from this type of unit falls continuously as a result of the decay of the source, but it is sufficient to adjust the stated value of the dose rate once a month.

Radiotherapy Simulators

A radiotherapy simulator (Fig. 1.9) consists of a diagnostic X-ray source mounted so that its movements are the same as the therapy unit being simulated. Its function is to facilitate the marking out of patients for treatment, to investigate the feasibility of a proposed treatment set-up, and to check that the proposed treatment fields will irradiate the required treatment volume.

The detailed functions required are:

1) To move the X-ray source with respect to the patient in the same way as that of the therapy machine being simulated. This normally requires that the diagnostic X-ray head can be rotated through 360° in a vertical plane about a horizontal axis. The radius between the centre of rotation and the X-ray focal spot is 100 cm for most radiotherapy units, but provision is made on most simulators for varying this distance, so that the movements of more than one therapy machine may be simulated.
2) The size of the treatment field is indicated by two pairs of parallel wires whose separation can be controlled and which can be rotated about the central axis in the same way as the beam-defining system of the therapy machine. The X-ray image then shows the treatment field and the surrounding anatomy.
3) A light source is so aligned that it can cast an optical beam which indicates the position of the X-ray beam and also of the field-defining wires.
4) The head unit is fitted with beam position indicators, either optical or mechanical pointers which show the position of the central axis of the X-ray field.

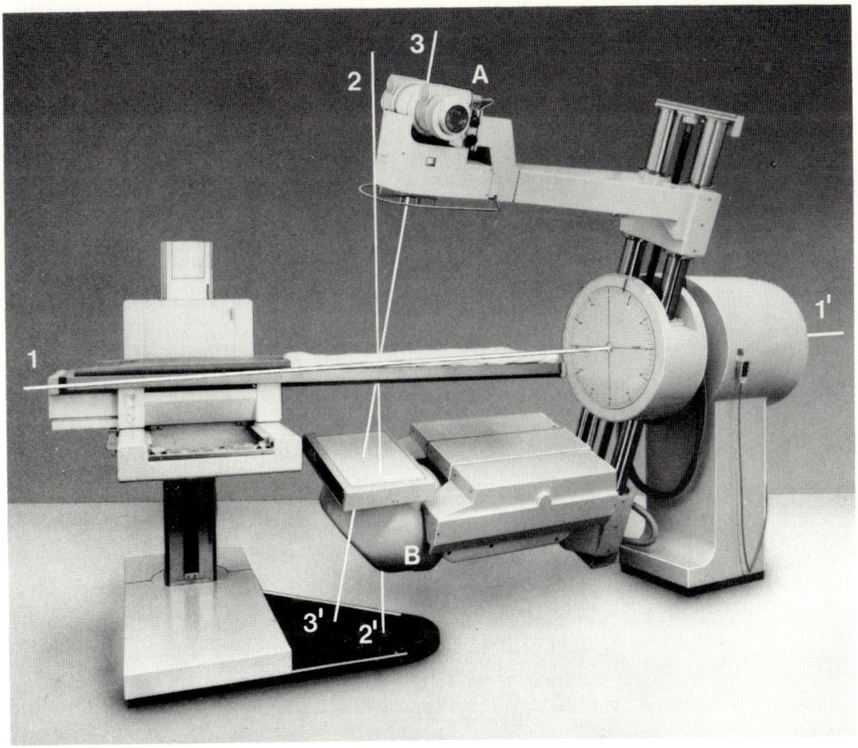

Fig. 1.9. A radiotherapy simulator. *Line 1 1*^{1}, horizontal axis of rotation of gantry. *Line 2 2*^{1}, vertical axis of rotation of couch. *Line 3 3*^{1}, central axis of X-ray beam. *A*, X-ray source and beam-defining system. *B*, image intensifier.

5) The patient support system (the simulator couch) can be continuously moved in a vertical direction, rotated about a vertical axis and adjusted longitudinally and laterally with respect to the long axis of the couch. To simulate most radiotherapy generators, the horizontal axis of rotation of the X-ray source, the vertical axis of the patient support system, and the central axis of the X-ray beam should all pass through the same point in space to give a so-called "isocentric mounting".
6) An image intensifier is mounted so that it is always opposite the X-ray source and produces an image of the treatment field and surrounding anatomy. For regional treatments the field size required may be larger than the largest available image intensifier. It may therefore be necessary to move the intensifier by remote control so that the whole field can be explored.
7) Facilities to take X-ray films are required.
8) All the variables in the system, such as field size, couch position, and gantry angle, need to be indicated, to facilitate transfer of information to the radiotherapy machine.
9) It is convenient to be able to control all these variables, as well as the X-ray unit itself, from behind an X-ray protective screen.

Radiotherapy Treatment Planning

The planning of a radiotherapy treatment requires decisions on the following:

1) Selection of the volume and location of the region to be treated (subsequently referred to as the target volume)
2) The dose to be delivered to the target volume (dose and volume being interrelated variables)
3) How this volume is to be treated, that is, whether by radiation beams or by brachytherapy
4) Detailed planning of the beam therapy or brachytherapy

The first two of these decisions are essentially clinical and outside the scope of this chapter, which will deal mainly with item (4). The planning of beam therapy and brachytherapy treatments are very different processes and are considered separately.

Planning of Beam Treatments

Radiation beam treatments fall into four categories: (1) regional treatments, where a large fraction of the patient's trunk is to be uniformly irradiated; (2) mantle treatments, where fields of complex cross-section are used to deliver a uniform dose to a selected region of the patient's anatomy; (3) small-field treatments, where a small volume of the body is to be given a radiation dose while sparing adjoining tissues; and (4) special treatments, e.g. irradiation of the whole central nervous system as a treatment for medulla-blastoma, or where the whole of the skin surface is to be irradiated as a treatment for mycosis fungoides. This discussion is intended mainly to deal with the third category, small-field treatment planning. Categories 1, 2, and 4 are dealt with in the appropriate clinical chapters.

It is convenient, and conventional, to think of radiotherapy treatment planning in terms of cross-section anatomy, usually in a right section of the patient through the centre of the volume to be treated. Ideally, one would think in three dimensions, or in a series of sections parallel to the one just mentioned, so that the total volume treated could be examined in detail. In practice, for small-field treatments the body is often sufficiently uniform in cross section, over the volume of interest, for a treatment plan in the central plane to be adequate. The present discussion, therefore, is limited to this plane and it is assumed that all necessary anatomical information about this plane and the region to be treated is available.

The object of treatment planning is to achieve a dose distribution inside the volume to be treated (the target volume) which is uniform within ±5% of the prescribed dose, while limiting the dose to adjacent regions to below tolerance levels. It is immediately obvious that, except for very superficial lesions, this object cannot be achieved by the use of a single beam of radiation and that multiple beams, crossing in the target volume, will usually be required. In general, the radiation fields should take the shortest route between the skin and the target volume, although this condition has often to be relaxed to spare critical tissues, to achieve the necessary dose uniformity in the target volume, or to achieve the necessary shape for the target volume.

Use of Beam Data

Depth-dose data and isodose charts are usually obtained by measurements made in a rectangular-section water phantom, with the beam axis at right angles to the entrance surface. To use these data to examine the dose distribution in a patient it may be necessary to correct (1) for changes in SSD, (2) for oblique incidence on the skin surface, (3) for tissue heterogeneity, and (4) for the shape of the field.

1) The relative dose along the central axis decreases partly because of attenuation of the radiation and partly because of increase in distance from source, according to the inverse square law. The rate of fall-off because of the inverse square law depends on the SSD, which results in practice in the percentage dose at a particular depth increasing as the SSD is increased. Megavoltage radiation depth-dose curves can be corrected for changes in SSD by the inverse square law formula

$$P(S^1,d) = P(S,d) \times \left(\frac{S + d}{S + b}\right)^2 \times \left(\frac{S^1 + b}{S^1 + d}\right)^2$$

where $P(S^1,d)$ is the percentage dose at depth d for SSD=S^1, $P(S,d)$ is the percentage dose at depth d for SSD=S, and b is the depth for maximum dose.

2) The effect of oblique incidence is illustrated in Fig. 1.10 where XX^1 is the central axis of the beam and CD is the oblique surface of the patient. To keep the diagram simple only the 80% and 50% isodose lines are shown. The dotted lines are the usual ones for normal incidence on the surface AB while the solid ones are those resulting from the beam's oblique incidence on CD. The position of the oblique incidence isodose lines can be determined from the normal incidence isodose chart by the "isodose shift method". For example, to find the positions where the oblique incidence isodose lines will cross the line RR^1, the normal incidence isodose chart is displaced to put the surface at position E, half way between the lines AB and CD, the central axis of the isodose chart being kept on the line XX^1. To find the positions for the oblique incidence along the line LL^1 the normal incidence isodose chart is placed with its surface at the point F. By repeating this process for a set of lines parallel to RR^1 it is then possible to draw the oblique incidence isodose lines as shown. This half-way shift method works for 4- and 8-MV X-rays. For cobalt-60 radiation a two-thirds shift in the forward direction is required.

Alternatively, the depth dose values along a line like LL^1 may be calculated by the inverse square law formula for the SSD where LL^1 crosses the line CD.

The isodose shift method is convenient for manual calculations, while the inverse square law method of correction lends itself to computer techniques. Although the illustration in Fig. 1.10 refers to oblique incidence on a plane surface, the correction methods work equally well for curved surfaces.

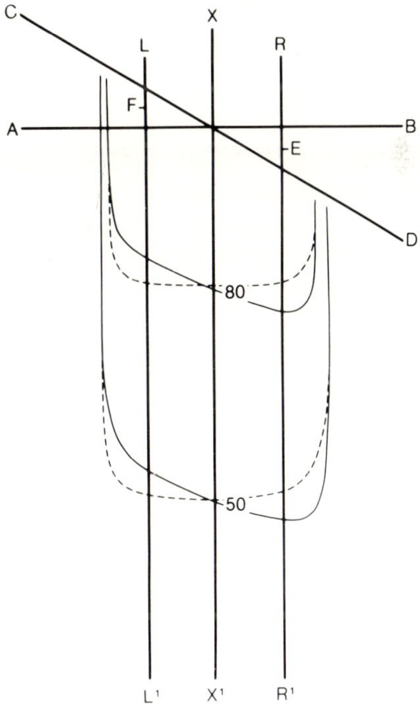

Fig. 1.10. Correction of isodose lines for oblique incidence. Dotted isodose lines for normal incidence on surface AB, solid isodose lines for oblique incidence on surface CD.

3) The depth doses in a patient have to be corrected for tissue heterogeneity, mainly to allow for increased penetration in air-filled volumes and lung, and also for decreased penetration through bone. In practice, air-filled volumes in the body (e.g. the larynx) are sufficiently small for the disturbance they produce not to be significant. Similarly, only the large bone sections, such as the head of the femur, are likely to produce significant changes from uniform tissue dose calculations, so that in most practical cases a tissue heterogeneity correction is required only when the radiation is penetrating lung tissue.

   Corrections for tissue heterogeneity can be made by the use of isodose shift methods, but where computer calculations are being made it is more common to determine water-equivalent depths for the attenuation components of the depth-dose data. Another alternative for allowing for increased penetration of radiation through lung is to increase the depth dose by a small percentage for each centimetre of lung in the path of the beam (e.g. $2\frac{1}{2}$%/cm at 4 MV).

   All these methods for correcting depth-dose and isodose data are approximations which have been shown to agree within 2%–3% of measured data for megavoltage radiation.

4) The beam-defining system of most megavoltage X-ray generators will give a continuous range of rectangular fields from about 4×4 cm up to 35×35 cm at 100 cm SSD. Larger field sizes may be obtained if necessary by employing larger SSD values. Within these limits it is necessary to consider the effect of field shape on two factors, namely the machine output (as measured in a phantom as previously described) and the depth-dose values. Both these quantities are normally listed for square fields. As a general rule it can be stated that both output and relative depth-dose values are reduced for a long narrow field in comparison with a square field of the same area, because less scattered radiation will reach any point in the phantom for the long narrow field. The effect is less than 3% for rectangular shapes where the ratio of the length of the long side to the length of the short side is less than 3:1. For an extreme case of, say, 35×4 cm, the output may be 5% lower than for a square field of the same area.

   Fields of more complex shape may be produced by blocking off the appropriate parts of a rectangular field with lead, or a low-melting-point heavy alloy. The actual thickness of the lead or alloy blocks is a compromise between the need to reduce X-ray transmission through the block and a reasonable weight to be handled or supported. The thickness used for 4- and 8-MV X-rays is 5 cm, which will allow a radiation transmission of only a few percent. The block or blocks may be supported on a Perspex tray 5 mm thick, which should be at least 20 cm from the patient's skin to minimise the skin dose.

   Again, for shaped fields (i.e. fields with parts blocked off as described), the machine output and the depth-dose values will be less than for the area of the unblocked field. If the actual field area irradiated is estimated, the error in using data for a square field of the same area is not likely to exceed 5%. It is possible, on the basis of fairly complex manual or computer calculations, to estimate output and depth-dose values for complex shaped fields to an accuracy of about 2%, but whether it is useful to do these calculations is a matter for clinical judgement.

Production of Beam Treatment Plans

Manual Methods

For these methods, isodose charts drawn on transparent plastic are required, from which the dose may be read off at any point on a full-sized body section. As already explained, these values may need to be modified to correct for oblique incidence or tissue heterogeneity.

Production of a treatment plan then falls into two phases: (1) selection of field sizes, beam directions, and wedge filters, and (2) detailed calculation of the treatment plan.

1) For any body site, experience shows that the number of possible treatment plans is limited and this will become clear in the clinical chapters. Having decided on the basic arrangement of the treatment fields, the choice of wedge filters and the relative dose to be delivered by the different fields can be made by looking at the doses at the centre of the target volume and also at four symmetrically placed

points towards the edge of that volume. This process will be discussed in more detail later in this chapter.

2) Detailed calculation of the treatment plan then requires that the contributions from each field at a suitable array of points on the body section be read off, summed, and normalised to 100% at the field centre, followed by the drawing of the isodose lines. This is a fairly tedious process and requires several hours' work for the production of one plan.

These two processes interact, because it is possible that the plan produced by the second procedure may show that the choices made by the first were not adequate.

Computer Methods

Many radiotherapy departments now use computers for producing treatment plans. A number of systems designed specifically for this purpose are commercially available and Fig. 1.11 shows the Emiplan system.

A system of this type has to be able to handle five main functions:

1) It has to be able to store and "call up" the necessary beam data. In many systems this information is stored on a magnetic disc.
2) It has to be able to "accept" the necessary information about the individual patient. In the system shown, this information may be in the form of a computerised tomography (CT) scan, and is transferred from the scanner to the treatment planning computer on a magnetic disc. Alternatively, the outline of the patient and any other necessary anatomical information may be fed into the system by drawing on a "graphic input device".
3) The operator can interact with the system through the keyboard, or by using a light pen on the monitor showing the treatment plan (see Fig. 1.11). With the keyboard he can "tell" the system which radiation beams are to be used for the treatment plan, while he can use the light pen on the image on the monitor to place them in the desired positions to treat the tumour.
4) The system can then carry out the necessary arithmetical procedures to generate a treatment plan, showing the result in the conventional way as a set of isodose lines, normalised to 100% at a point selected by the operator.
5) A paper copy of the treatment plan is printed out.

The actual computing time involved in stage 4 of this procedure is only a few seconds, the total time for stages 1 to 5 being determined mainly by the

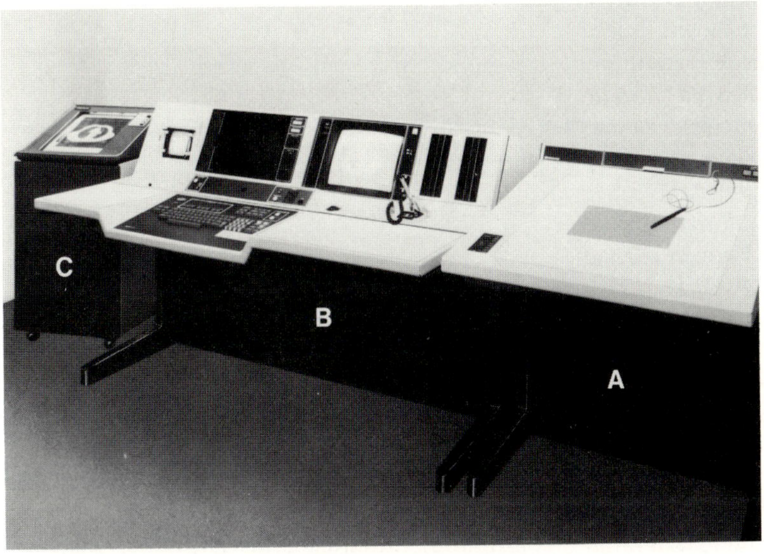

Fig. 1.11. The Emiplan treatment planning computer.
A Graphic input device. Lines drawn on this with special digitiser pen are recorded in the system, and displayed on the monitor.
B Console, which includes keyboard and monitor showing patient section with superimposed treatment plan. It is also possible to "draw" on the monitor using a light pen.
C Printer to give paper copy of treatment plan.

operator interactions. It will take 10–15 min to generate a treatment plan, but the acceptability of the plan is still, of course, a matter of clinical judgement.

The combination of CT scan information with the treatment plan superimposed on it gives the radiotherapist very precise information about all the anatomical structures which will be irradiated.

Some Examples of Beam Treatment Planning

Although many treatment plans are shown and discussed in the clinical chapters, it may be helpful to show some examples of how treatment plans may be developed to meet the criteria mentioned earlier in this chapter.

Pelvic Treatments

Figure 1.12a shows a single field (4-MV X-rays, 8×8 cm at 100 cm SSD) superimposed on a pelvic body section. It can be seen that if the volume to be treated is as marked, this field will not provide a suitable treatment plan because (1) the dose gradient across the tumour is unacceptably high and (2) the dose anterior to the treatment volume is actually higher than the tumour dose.

If two parallel opposing beams of the same field size as before are applied to the same pelvic area, the resulting dose distribution is as shown in Fig. 1.12b, where the dose at the centre of the volume to be treated has been normalised to 100%. The isodose lines shown on this diagram are drawn to the convention used for treatment plans elsewhere in this book. The area between the 95% and 105% lines is regarded as the volume being treated, the regions receiving in excess of 105% are receiving excessive dose, the area between 95% and 85% lines get a mean dose of 90% of the tumour dose, while the areas between the 85% and 65% lines and the 65% and 35% lines are receiving mean doses of 75% and 50% of the tumour dose, respectively.

The treatment plan in Fig. 1.12b fails to meet the basic criteria in that the treatment volume is large compared with the target volume and in that large volumes are being given excessive dose (referred to as hot spots). These comments only apply if the target is relatively small. Where a large volume of tissue is to be treated, the use of two parallel opposed fields may be an acceptable treatment.

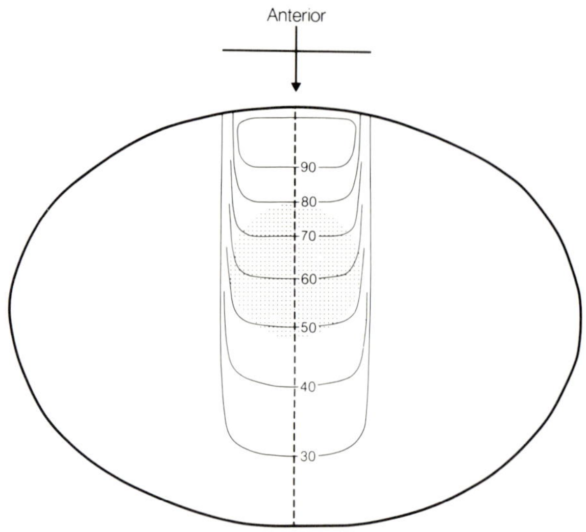

a

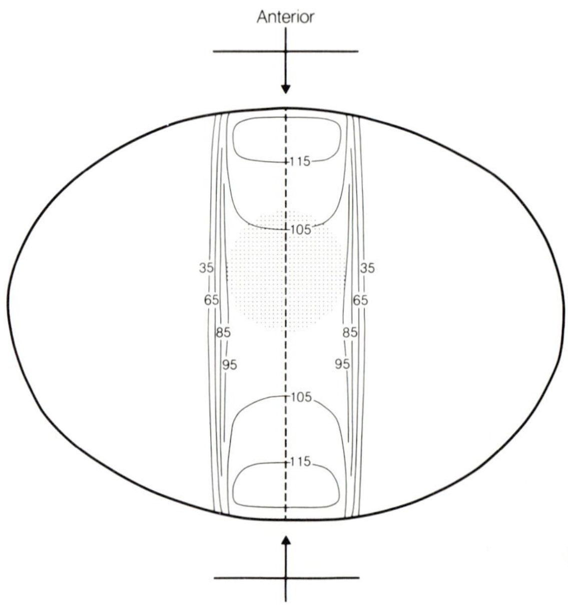

b

Two pairs of parallel beams (four fields) may be used to restrict the high dose to a smaller volume as in Fig. 1.12c. The lateral fields have to penetrate a greater depth of tissue than the anterior and posterior fields, so that to give equal dose contributions from each field at the tumour, it is necessary to deliver more "given dose" to the lateral fields. The dose delivered to each field is normally stated as the dose at the maximum of the depth-dose curve for that field and normally

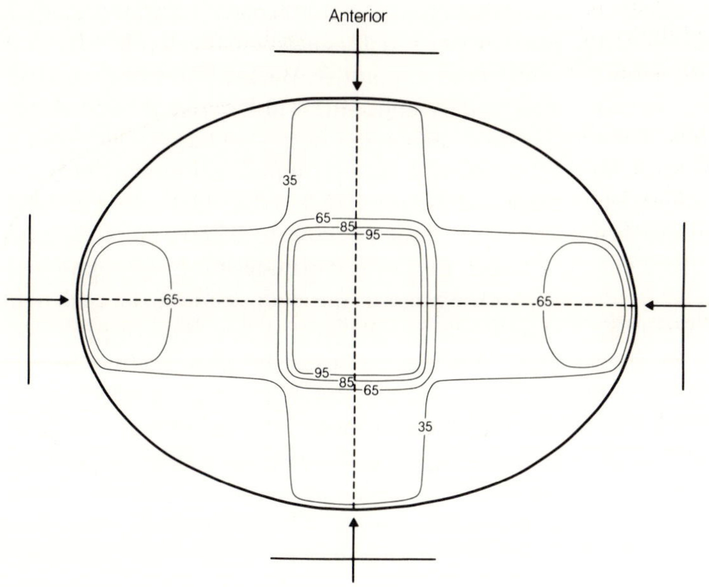

c

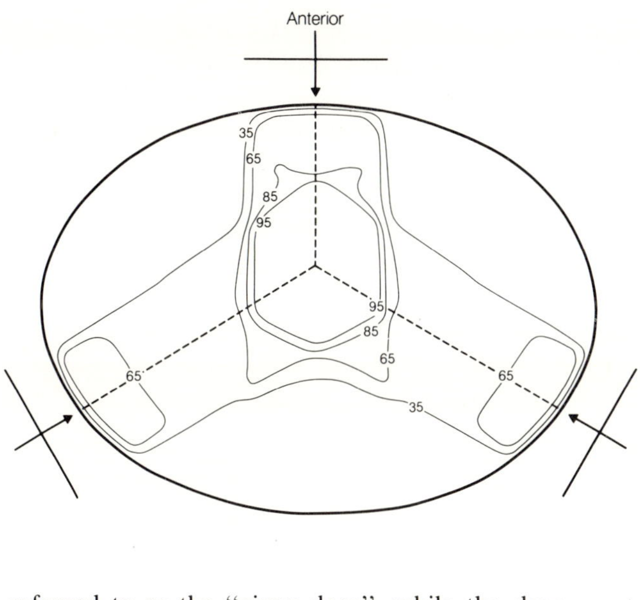

d

Fig. 1.12a–d Treatment plans for a pelvic body section: **a** Using a single field of 4-MV X-rays. The target volume is stippled.
b Using two parallel opposed fields.
c Using four fields (two parallel opposed pairs).
d Using three symmetrically placed fields.

referred to as the "given dose", while the dose delivered to the treatment volume is referred to as the "tumour dose", or the "prescribed dose". In Fig. 1.12c the depths to the point at which the fields intersect are 12.5 cm for the anterior and posterior fields and 17.5 cm for the lateral fields, corresponding to percentage depth doses of 52% and 38% for the 4-MV radiation used. If the prescribed dose is 4000 cGy, and equal contributions are to be delivered by each field at the centre of the treatment volume, then the contribution from each field is 1000 cGy. The given dose to the lateral fields is then 1000×100/38=2630 cGy, while for the anterior and posterior the given dose is 1000×100/52=1920 cGy.

This arrangement of four fields is used for some pelvic treatments where a square or rectangular high-dose zone is required.

The use of three symmetrically placed fields gives a treatment plan as shown in Fig. 1.12d, where the high-dose zone is approximately hexagonal in shape. This may be advantageous in some cases in giving a better approximation to the shape of the volume to be treated. This plan delivers equal given doses to each field and gives a high-dose zone (defined by the 95% isodose lines) which meets the criterion of uniformity to ±5% of the prescribed dose.

If the tumour dose required for the treatment described by the plan in Fig. 1.12d is 4000 cGy, and equal given doses are to be used for each field, then the value of the given dose is calculated as follows. The dose at the centre of the target volume from the anterior field is 61% of the given dose from that field, while the contribution from each of the posterior fields is 38% of the given dose. The target volume will thus receive 2×38+61=137% of the given dose from each field, which is therefore given by:

$$4000 \times \frac{100}{137} = 2920 \text{ cGy}$$

Head and Neck Treatments

Many head and neck treatments are required for lesions which are sufficiently near the surface to achieve adequate dose in the target volume, in relation to adjacent regions, by the use of only two crossed fields. In this situation it is necessary to use wedge filters to achieve uniformity of dose in the target volume.

Figure 1.13 shows a simplified outline comparable to a section through the larynx (this outline could be achieved in practice using wax bolus) where two fields can give a high-dose zone of the required shape. If two plane fields were used, it is

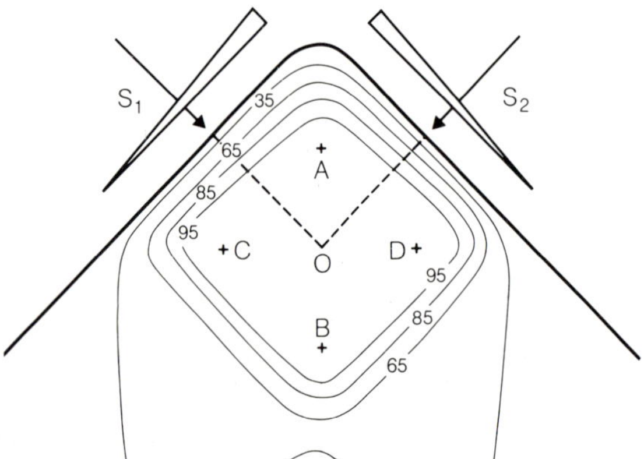

Fig. 1.13. Treatment plan showing the use of two wedged fields to treat a section through the larynx. The orientation of the wedge filters is shown.

clear that point A would receive a higher dose than point B, because for each field the depth to point A is less than to point B. Wedge filters in each field, designed to reduce the relative dose at the A side of the field, can remedy this situation. The wedge filters should be orientated as shown, with the thick end of each wedge reducing the dose at the A side of the field. Further, to achieve equal doses at A and B, thus avoiding undesirable dose gradients across the tumour, the isodose lines from each field should run parallel to the line AB. In principle, then, this treatment can be planned by having a family of wedged isodose charts, and selecting the one which has isodose lines parallel to AB when placed with its central axis along either of the lines S_1O or S_2O. In addition, field S_1O will give a higher dose at point C than at point D, while field S_2O will give a higher dose at D than at C, so that if equal doses are delivered from each field the sums of the doses at C and D will be equal. This again avoids a dose gradient across the CD axis and ensures that the whole target volume receives a remarkably uniform dose.

Figure 1.13 also shows the complete treatment plan, while Table 5 shows the doses at points A, B, C, D, and O.

Table 1.5. Doses at points in Fig. 1.13.

Points	A	B	C	D	O
Contribution from S_1O	89	89	104	76	90
Contribution from S_2O	89	89	76	104	90
Combined contribution	178	178	180	180	180

The principles involved here may be stated in a different way. Referring again to Fig. 1.13, if we call the angle S_1OS_2 (the angle between the two central axes) the *hinge angle*, we can say that the wedge angle required is equal to 90° minus half the hinge angle. This can be regarded as a general rule for selecting wedge filters, provided (as in Fig. 1.13) the entrance surface is perpendicular to the central axis, avoiding the distorting effect of oblique incidence.

In this example the wedge filters are being used to achieve uniformity of dose where two fields are meeting at an angle.

A different use of a wedge filter is illustrated in Fig. 1.14, where a parallel pair of beams is being used to irradiate a larger volume around the larynx than is required in Fig. 1.13. If plane fields were used the dose at *A* would be much higher than at *B* because the radiation arriving at *A* has to penetrate much less tissue (Fig. 1.14a). Saying the same thing in another way, the dose at *A* is higher than at *B* because of the oblique incidence of the beams on the skin surface. One way to equalise the doses at *A* and *B* would be to use bolus material as in Fig. 1.14b to give normal incidence for both beams, but this would result in the skin on the entrance surfaces receiving full tumour dosage. There may, of course, be clinical circumstances where this would be an acceptable treatment plan.

The bolus material in Fig. 1.14b is in the form of "wedges" and could, therefore, be replaced by equivalent metal wedge filters placed sufficiently far from the skin surface to restore skin-sparing. The metal wedges could be individually designed "compensators", but in practice it is possible to use one of a limited set of standard wedge filters. Two choices then arise. We could use wedge filters in both fields with their thick ends on the *A* side of the field, or, alternatively, we could use a plane field and a wedge field as in Fig. 1.14c, where the wedge will have to be approximately twice as thick at the thick end as the wedges used if both fields were wedged. To choose a suitable wedge filter involves the following steps:

1) Determine the dose contribution from the plane field, using a standard isodose chart and the isodose shift method to correct for oblique incidence.

2) It is now necessary to select a wedge filter to give a smaller dose at *A* than at *B*, after correcting for oblique incidence for the wedge field. In principle this can be done by having a family of isodose charts and selecting one which will give suitable doses at *A* and *B* to balance those from the plane field, again after correction for oblique incidence.

There is a useful approximation to facilitate the choice of wedge filters to correct for oblique incidence, which can be illustrated with Fig. 1.14. In this diagram the effect of oblique incidence for either field is to increase the dose at *A* in relation to that at *B*, while the effect of the wedge filter is to decrease the dose at *A* in relation to that at *B*. In other words, the effect of oblique incidence is to reduce the effect of the wedge filters; oblique incidence "unwedges" the beam. From the isodose shift method we can say that the effect of oblique

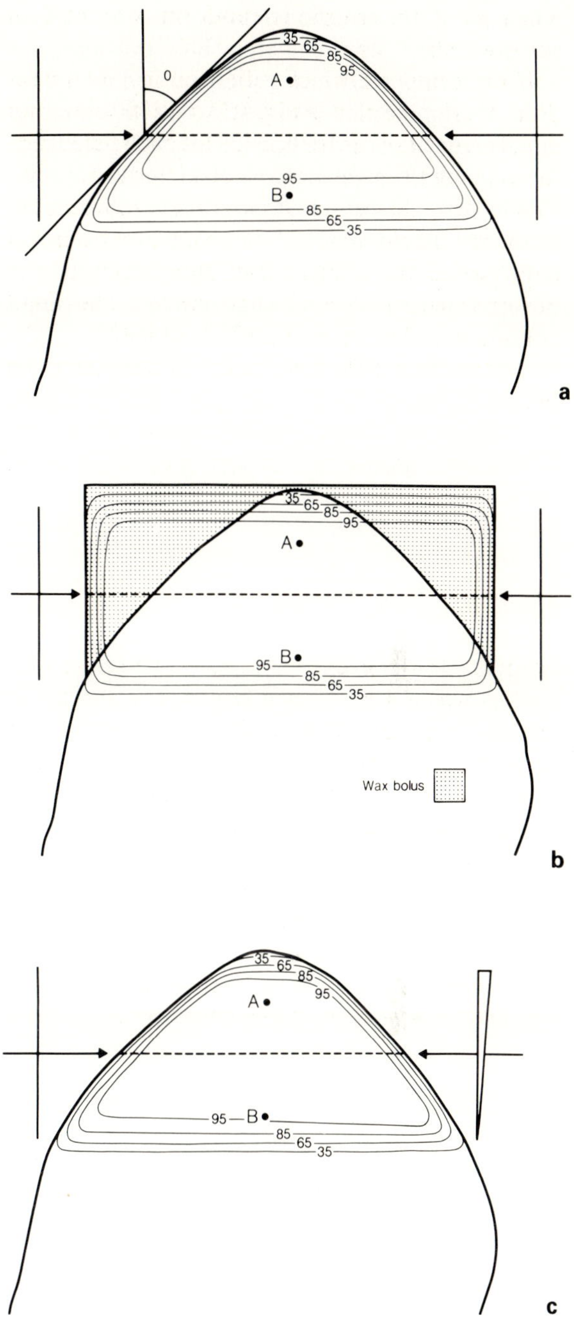

Fig. 1.14a–c Treatment plans using two parallel fields to treat a volume around the larynx.
a Using two plane fields. This gives an unacceptable dose gradient in the direction *AB*. *O* is defined as the angle of oblique incidence.
b Using two plane fields and wax bolus to give normal incidence.
c Using a plane field and a wedged field to achieve uniform dose in the direction *AB*.

incidence is to turn the isodose lines through an angle which is approximately half the angle of oblique incidence, which is defined in Fig. 1.14a. This rule applies to 4- and 8-MV X-rays. It follows that for Fig. 1.14, if both fields are to be wedged, then the wedge angle of the isodose charts required should be equal to half the angle of oblique incidence. Alternatively, if only one of the fields is to be wedged, as in Fig. 1.14c, the wedge angle of the appropriate isodose chart is equal to the angle of oblique incidence for the wedged field.

The example shown in Fig. 1.13 demonstrates the use of wedge filters to achieve a uniform dose distribution for crossed angled beams, while Fig. 1.14 shows the use of a wedge filter as a tissue compensator. Quite often wedges are used to serve these two functions at the same time, and an example of this is shown in Fig. 1.15. Here the

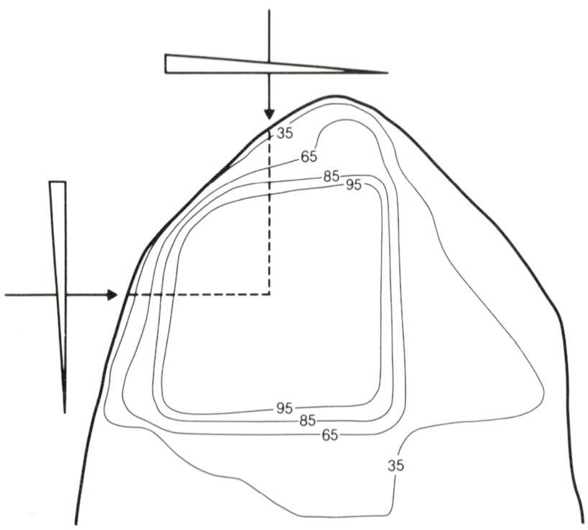

Fig. 1.15. Use of two wedged fields to treat a tumour of the antrum.

shape of the treatment volume required can be provided by using two fields at right angles, that is using a hinge angle of 90°. If the fields were at normal incidence to the skin, each field would require a wedge filter which implies a wedge angle of 45°. However, it can be seen that there is a considerable amount of oblique incidence for both fields, which will "unwedge" them, so that steeper wedge angles than 45° are required. The wedge angle required is then 45° plus half the angle of oblique incidence, and in fact in Fig. 1.15, 55° wedges are used.

Figure 1.16 is an example of the use of three fields using wedge filters for the treatment of a brain tumour. The required uniformity of dose in

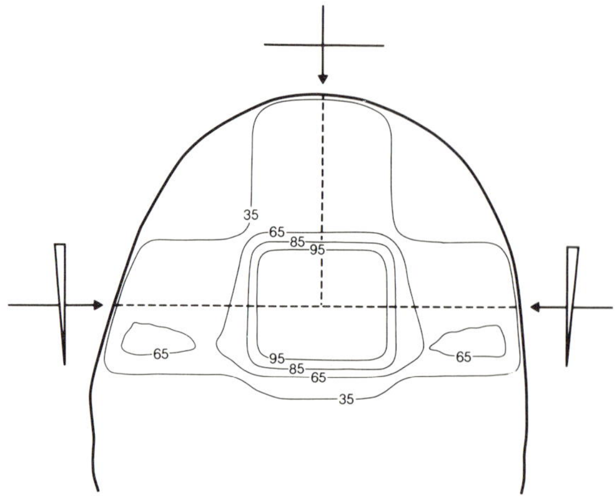

Fig. 1.16. Use of one plane and two wedged fields to achieve a uniform dose in the target volume.

the treatment volume could be achieved by the use of three symmetrically placed plane fields in the right transverse plane, but this would involve irradiating the eyes, which is avoided by the field arrangement shown. This plan is in the coronal plane. The contribution from the superior field gives a higher dose at the superior side of the treatment volume, so that the wedged fields have to be applied in such a way that they deliver a higher dose at the inferior side. This then determines the direction of the wedges, the thick end placed as shown in Fig. 1.16, and the dose gradient across the wedged fields has to be equal to that along the superior field.

Rotation Treatments

In rotation therapy the X-ray source is rotated around the patient who is set up so that the geometric centre of the target volume is on the centre of rotation (the isocentre). The dose delivered at the centre can then be determined by the use of "tissue-phantom ratios".

The basic dose measurement is carried out by setting an ionisation chamber 10 cm deep in a phantom (Fig. 1.17a), with the chamber at the isocentre. If the chamber is kept at the same position but its depth in the phantom is varied (Fig. 1.17b), the ratio of the reading in Fig. 1.17b to that in Fig. 1.17a is called the tissue-phantom ratio and is a function of the depth d, and of the field size. Tissue-phantom ratios can be tabulated for a particular X-ray generator and a specified reference depth r as in Fig. 1.17a.

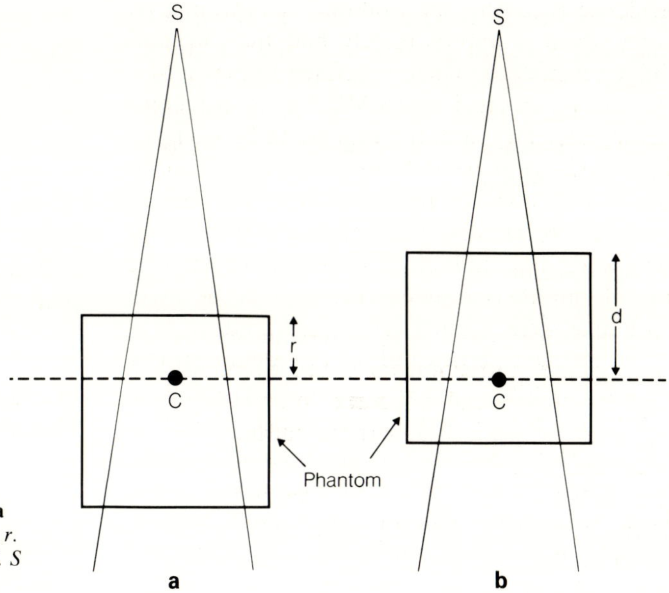

Fig. 1.17. Measurement of "tissue-phantom ratio". **a** Ionisation chamber *C* at isocentre at reference depth *r*. **b** Ionisation chamber at isocentre at another depth *d*. *S* is the radiation source.

For the patient whose body section is shown in Fig. 1.18, the mean tissue-phantom ratio, when the X-ray source is rotated through 360°, can be determined by measuring the centre-to-skin distance at frequent angular intervals, say 10°, applying the appropriate tissue-phantom ratio for each of these distances and calculating the mean value. If this mean value is multiplied by the measured dose rate at the reference depth (Fig. 1.17a), this gives the mean dose rate at the centre of rotation. The dose delivered to the centre is then given by this mean dose rate multiplied by the time to rotate the system round the patient (360°). Calculation of the dose at other points in the patient is a very complex procedure and gives a treatment plan as shown in Fig. 1.18a, where the high-dose volume is approximately cylindrical in shape.

Figure 1.18b shows an example where the rotation is restricted to two arcs of 140° from the vertical line through the isocentre, in order to reduce the dose to the posterior segment. If wedge

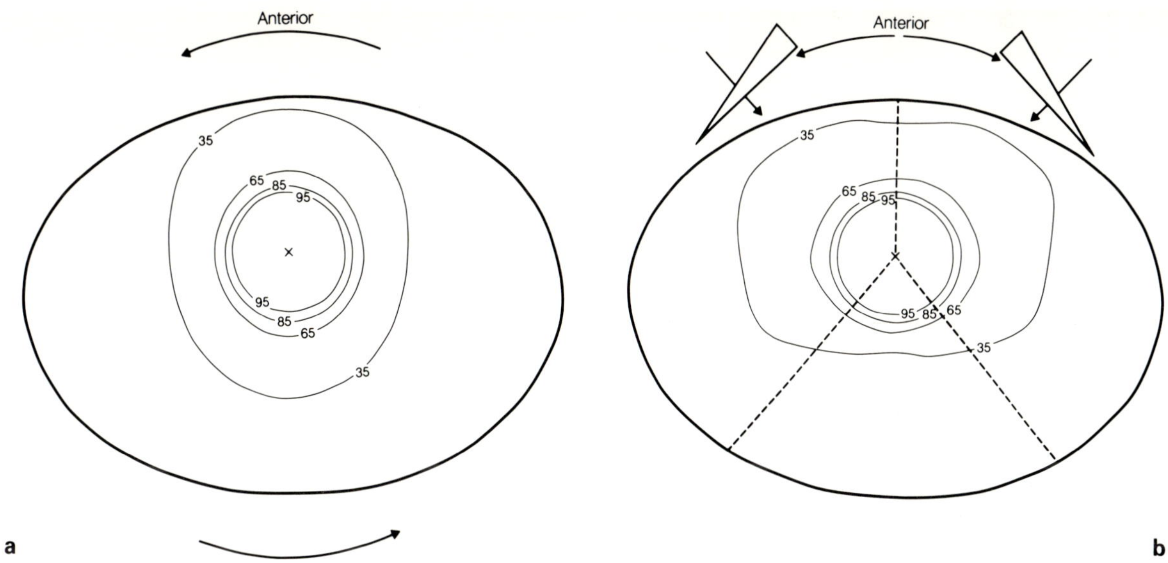

Fig. 1.18. **a** Rotation therapy treatment for a bladder tumour, where the X-ray generator is rotated through 360°. **b** Rotation therapy plan, where the X-ray source is rotated through two arcs of 140° from the vertical, and wedge filters are orientated as shown.

filters are used during each arc, as shown in the diagram, it is still possible to maintain uniform dosage over the target volume. Without the use of wedge filters there would be an unacceptable gradient in dose from anterior to posterior inside the target volume.

Lung Treatments

As previously stated, lung treatments are the only ones where correction for tissue inhomogeneity makes a substantial difference to the relationship between the given dose and the tumour dose. An example of a symmetrical three-field treatment of the chest is shown in Fig. 1.19. This has been done (quite artificially) for the same body outline as used for the examples of pelvic treatments (Fig. 1.12), so that the effect of the lung correction can be shown. In fact, the shape of the high-dose zone is not much changed when the lung corrections are applied. The reason for this is that for the posterior fields, which penetrate a large volume of lung, the boundaries of the lung sections are approximately parallel to each other. The effect of the increased penetration in lung tissue is then to displace the isodose lines for the posterior fields to a greater depth than for unit density tissue, but because the lung sections have parallel boundaries, the displaced isodose lines are still parallel to their original positions and will give nearly the same shape to the high-dose zone. (Compare Figs. 1.19 and 1.12.) The relationship between the tumour dose and the given dose is, however, significantly changed by about $2\frac{1}{2}\%$ for every centimetre of lung transversed by the X-ray beam. The two posterior fields each pass through 10 cm of lung tissue, which increases the tumour dose from each field relative to the given dose by 25%. This shows up in Fig. 1.19 by the absence of 75% zones near the surface of the posterior fields (again compare with Fig. 1.12).

Peripheral lung tumours are often treated with a pair of wedged fields, using the "short way in".

Wedge Filters Required for Treatment Planning

As was stated earlier, wedge filters are described in terms of the wedge angle, that is, the angle through which the isodose lines are turned by the presence of the wedge filter. For example, a 45° wedge is one which turns the isodose lines inside the beam from their normal position, at right angles to the central axis, to 45° from that position.

The methods for choosing wedge filters for particular treatment plans, outlined in the previous section, allow some latitude in wedge angle for three reasons: (1) the condition that the dose in the treatment volume should be uniform to ±5% allows, for example, that the wedge angle does not have to be exactly equal to 90° minus half the hinge angle (see Fig. 1.13); (2) it is often possible to adjust the hinge angle slightly so that it can be matched to one of the available wedge filters; (3) it is often possible to compromise between the hinge angle and the angle of oblique incidence, to make

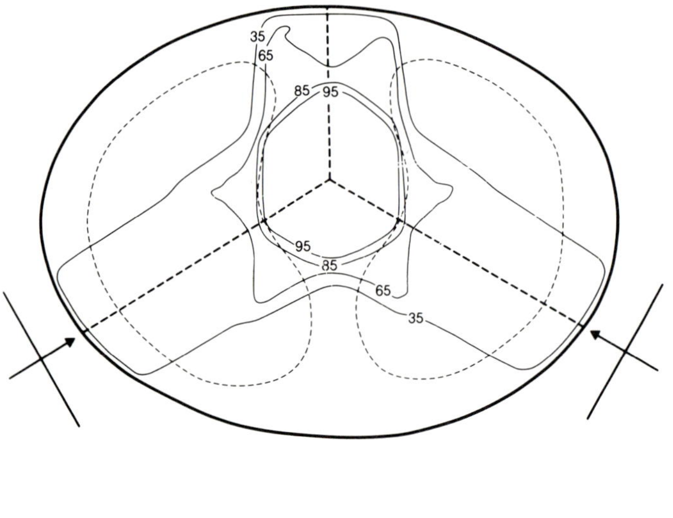

Fig. 1.19. Use of three symmetrical fields for a chest treatment where the treatment plan has been corrected for increased penetration through lung tissue.

use of one of a limited range of wedge filters.

All the treatment plans in this book make use of six wedge filters, giving wedge angles of 12°, 35°, 40°, 45°, 55°, and 80°, and of these, those for 35° and 45° are used for more than half of the number of wedge filter treatments. The 12° wedge is used basically as a compensator for oblique incidence.

Conclusion

At first sight the processes involved in the planning of radiation beam treatments seem to be very complex, and indeed they are. As with other complex processes, however, the only way to become proficient in their use is by practice and, even where a computer system is available, some practice of the manual methods is recommended as valuable training. Some discussions in the radiotherapy literature about computerised treatment planning seem to imply that the production of each treatment plan is an "ab initio" exercise. This is not the case. For any particular tumour an experienced radiotherapist will be able to narrow the possibilities down to one or two basic plans before the detailed calculations are started.

Planning of Brachytherapy Treatments

The techniques for the use of sealed gamma-ray emitting radioactive sources to be described in this book may be divided into three groups: interstitial implants, mould treatments and intracavity treatments. For interstitial treatments the sealed sources are inserted directly into the tissues to be treated. In mould treatments the sources are mounted on a plastic mould which is then applied to the surface of the patient, while in intracavity treatments the source or array of sources is placed in a natural body cavity. All these techniques are based on the dosimetry system initiated by Paterson and Parker in 1934 and subsequently developed to form what is known as the Manchester radium dosage system.

The Manchester Radium Dosage System

In respect of mould and implantation techniques, the system provides two related groups of data to facilitate treatment design:

1) Rules for the patterns of arrangements of radioactive sources ("distribution rules") so as to produce dose distributions over treated surfaces, or throughout treated volumes, which are uniform (within limits of $\pm 10\%$) except in close proximity to implanted sources.
2) Tables or graphs of numerical data from which dosimetry calculations for every arrangement of sources prescribed by the distribution rules can be quickly performed without the need for more than simple arithmetic. These data were originally expressed as the total number of milligram-hours of radium required to deliver a "uniform" exposure of 1000 röntgens. More recently, the data have been converted to the form "radium milligram-hours per 1000 centigrays" and will be employed in this form in this book.

The Manchester radium dosage system may be implemented not only with sealed sources of radium-226 but also with other gamma-emitting radionuclides such as caesium-137, cobalt-60, iridium-192, and gold-198. (See section entitled "Brachytherapy Sources" above.) For sources which do not decay appreciably during an individual treatment, it is convenient to express their strengths in "milligrams radium equivalent with 0.5 mm platinum filtration" and to design the treatments as if they were, in fact, radium sources. With some of these sources it may be necessary, rarely, to make some special allowances for small differences, as compared with radium, resulting from the effects of oblique filtration in the wall of the source. The advice of an experienced physicist should be obtained. For these slowly decaying sources, the dose rate, expressed in centigrays per hour, is numerically equal to 1000 times the total milligrams radium equivalent employed, divided by the figure for radium milligram-hours per 1000 cGy, for the particular treatment, obtained from the dosage system data:

$$\text{cGy per hour} = \frac{1000 \times \text{total mg Ra equivalent}}{\text{mg-hours per 1000 cGy}}$$

If *radium* sources filtered by other than 0.5 mm platinum are employed, it is usually most convenient to express their strengths also in "milligrams of radium equivalent with 0.5 mm platinum filtration". This is done by deducting 2% from their radium content for each 0.1 mm of platinum filtration greater than 0.5 mm. For radium sources, gold filtration may be treated as platinum, silver and lead as half their thickness in platinum, and monel, brass, steel, etc. as one third their thickness in platinum.

Table 1.6. Data for short half-life sources for different treatment times.

Treatment time (h)	Radium milligram-hours (at 0.5 mm platinum filtration) per initial equivalent MBq of gold-198
96	0.46
120	0.52
168	0.60
240	0.66
Complete decay	0.72

With *short half-life sources* such as gold-198, source strengths may be expressed in equivalent megabecquerels of gold-198 and a table of radium milligram-hours (at 0.5 mm platinum filtration) per initial equivalent megabecquerel of gold-198, for various treatment times, will then enable these sources to be employed in the Manchester radium dosage system (Table 1.6). In this case, the dose delivered, expressed in centigrays, is equal to 1000 times the total initial equivalent megabecquerels multiplied by the radium milligram-hours per initial megabecquerel for the treatment time employed, and divided by the radium milligram-hours per 1000 cGy for the particular treatment, as shown in the equation below:

When moulds are used to treat relatively superficial conditions, the value of the percentage depth dose achieved at relevant depths beneath the surface is determined mainly by the "treating distance" employed, i.e. the distance between the treated surface and the plane above that surface in which the sources are mounted. To a lesser extent, depth dose is influenced also by the size of the area treated and by whether the treated surface has a convex curvature. Treating distances for moulds are usually in the range 0.5 cm to 2.5 cm. Higher percentage depth doses are attained with the larger treating distances and are enhanced when the area treated is large and when the surface has a convex curvature. For example, the percentage depth dose (DD) at 0.5 cm deep to the surface for a simple, flat mould varies as follows:

Area 10 cm^2
- Treating distance 0.5 cm: DD=54%
- Treating distance 1.5 cm: DD=71%
- Treating distance 2.5 cm: DD=78%

Area 100 cm^2
- Treating distance 0.5 cm: DD=67%
- Treating distance 1.5 cm: DD=77%
- Treating distance 2.5 cm: DD=86%

If there is very substantial convex curvature, the corresponding depth dose for a 100 cm^2 area with treating distance 1.5 cm might be increased to something like 85% and with a 2.5-cm treating distance to about 94%. For any individual case, the percentage of the surface dose received at a particular depth of clinical interest is numerically equal to 100 times the ratio of the milligram-hours per 1000 cGy applicable to the surface and to the particular depth, respectively.

$$\text{cGy} = \frac{1000 \times \text{total initial equivalent MBq} \times \text{radium mg-hours per initial equivalent MBq}}{\text{mg-hours per 1000 cGy}}$$

Sandwich moulds are sometimes employed to irradiate a slab of tissue one or two centimetres thick when it is practicable to apply moulds to both sides of the slab. This is the brachytherapy counterpart of a parallel opposed pair of X-ray fields. Each mould is designed to give "uniform" irradiation of the tissue surface nearest to it and, if the treating distances chosen are about the same as the thickness of the slab of tissue, the combined dose in the centre of the slab will typically be in the region of 90% of the doses on the surfaces.

A cylinder mould is a means of treating the whole (or large percentage of) a cylindrical body surface. The arrangement of sources on the larger concentric cylinder, at the chosen treating distance, is usually a series of coaxial rings separated by a distance equal to twice this treating distance. Detailed distribution rules are provided by the dosage system, which also supplies data for radium milligram-hours per 1000 cGy.

A line source may be used to treat the inside surface of a cylindrical body cavity. A line of similar sources, such as radium or caesium tubes, is carried axially in an intracavitary applicator such as a rubber cylinder. The depth dose beyond the treated surface falls quite rapidly, especially when the radius of the cylinder is small. For example, with a cylinder of radius 1.0 cm and length 7.0 cm the dose at 0.5 cm beyond the surface is only about 61% of the surface dose.

Single-plane implants (see Fig. 1.20a) are intended to treat a slab of tissue 1 cm thick, conceived as containing all the tissues to be effectively treated, by implanting radioactive sources in the mid-plane of the slab. The arrangement of these sources should be such as to give "uniform" irradiation of the outer surfaces of the slab (as for a mould with a treating distance of 0.5 cm) and the "stated dose" for the treatment is this dose on these surfaces. Within the slab, the dose is everywhere greater than the surface dose, rising to very high values in close proximity to individual sources and typically to about 130% of the surface dose midway between sources in the central plane. For practical radiotherapy, tissue tolerance dosage levels for this type of implant have been determined, from long experience, in terms of the stated dose on the surfaces of the 1-cm-thick slab, for different body sites and different sizes (areas) of

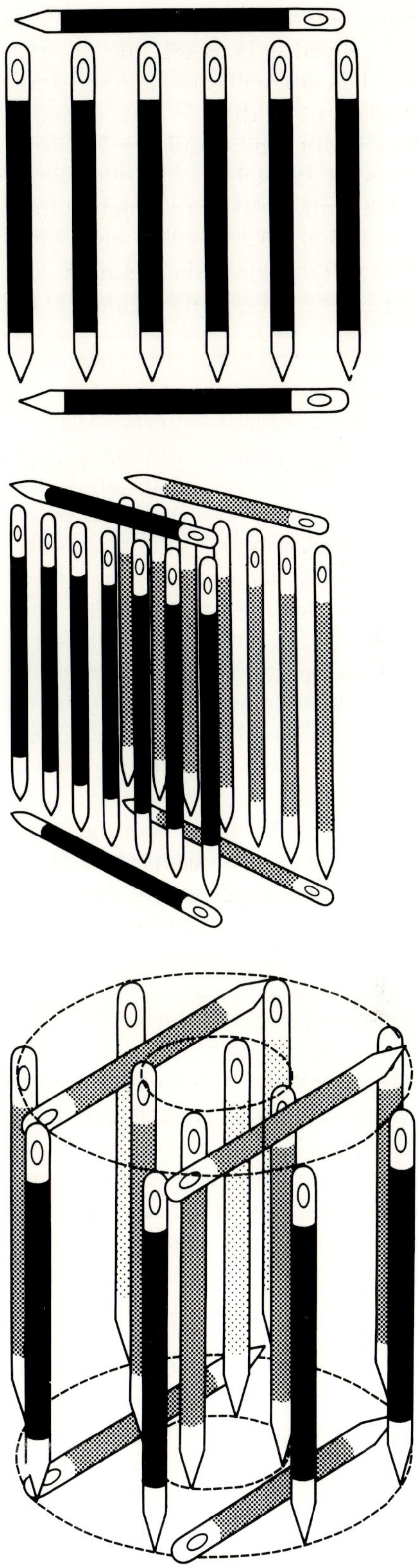
a
b
c

Fig. 1.20a–c. Arrangement of needles for: **a** a single-plane implant; **b** a two-plane implant; **c** a volume implant.

implant. Not infrequently, it is impracticable to implant sources along one edge (usually that deepest in tissue) of the desired area, i.e. there is an "uncrossed end". This inevitably means that this end of the implant will receive a substantially lower dose than the remainder, but the implant may still be clinically satisfactory if the tumour is confined to the part of the implant at least about 7–10 mm away from the uncrossed end. F r routine dosimetry calculation purposes (only) the area of the implant is then taken to be 10% less than that actually carrying radioactive sources.

Two-plane implants (see Fig. 1.20b) are an extension of the single-plane implant concept to treat somewhat thicker slabs of tissue, typically 1.5 cm or 2.0 cm thick. In this case, the radioactive sources are implanted in both of the main outer faces of the slab and, ideally, the patterns of distribution of these sources are such that each array of sources produces "uniform" irradiation of the plane 0.5 cm distant from it, i.e. 0.5 cm inside the slab of tissue. The combined dose from the two arrays of sources at each of these inside planes has been taken to be the stated dose for this class of implant. Dose midway between sources, in a plane of sources, is 10% to 20% higher than the stated dose. In the mid-plane of an implant 1.5 cm thick, the dose is less than the stated dose by about 10% when the implant area is about 10 cm^2 and by about 5% for 30 cm^2. The corresponding figures for an implant 2.0 cm thick are about 20% and 10%, respectively, and for 2.5 cm thickness, 30% and 20%, respectively. In the latter case the dose may well be unacceptably low. Uncrossed ends are dealt with in the same way as for single-plane implants.

Volume implants (see Fig. 1.20c) are the type conceived for dealing with blocks of tissue for which the smallest dimension is greater than about 2.0–2.5 cm. By far the commonest shape of these implants nowadays is a cylinder. In this case, following the appropriate source distribution rules, a minimum of eight needles are implanted in the curved outer wall of the cylinder, after the manner of a palisade, to enclose the treatment volume, while a further four needles (at least) are introduced as evenly as possible throughout the volume and two or three more placed across each flat end. With this kind of distribution of sources there are, of course, very high doses in close proximity to needles while doses fall to minima in regions roughly midway between adjacent needles. When the system's distribution rules for volume implants are obeyed, all these minima—at many places throughout the implant—are approximately equal, and the stated dose is a value 10% above this common minimum value. Hence, except for the high local doses relatively close to needles, the dose throughout the treated volume deviates by not more than about ±10% from the stated value. As with planar implants, it is frequently not practicable to place crossing needles at both ends of the implanted volume but the treatment will still be clinically satisfactory if the uncrossed end extends well beyond the limits of tumour. For dosage calculation purposes (only), $7\frac{1}{2}$% should be deducted from the volume containing radioactive sources to allow for an "uncrossed end".

Gynaecological Brachytherapy

For gynaecological brachytherapy, special systems have been developed whereby radium, caesium-137, or equivalent sources of pre-determined strengths are mounted in intracavitary applicators positioned along the uterine axis and in the vagina near to the cervix. These applicators are packed securely in position so that they will not move appreciably during a treatment period of up to about 3 days. The packing also serves to maintain as big a distance as possible between the sources and the rectal wall and bladder, thereby reducing the probability of high-dose effects at these vulnerable sites. Details of these treatments are presented in Chap. 11. It may be noted here that source arrangements prescribed for cancer of the cervix uteri by the Manchester system produce "concentric" isodose surfaces which are roughly pear-shaped, though somewhat flattened in the anteroposterior direction, and the treatment dose is commonly stated at the special "Point A", which is defined in Chap. 11.

However, it must be emphasised that, compared with the multiple-field dose distributions attained in external-beam photon therapy, the dose gradients across isodose surfaces in intracavitary therapy are very much steeper and doses will commonly vary by 50% or more when moving distances of only a few millimetres perpendicularly to isodose surfaces. It is essential that these steeply falling dose gradients be always kept in mind when discussing the dosimetry of intracavitary treatments and its clinical implications, and that the doses delivered to Point A are not studied in isolation from other dosimetric information.

Afterloading Techniques

These are an important means whereby staff radiation exposure resulting from brachytherapy may be significantly reduced. Very considerable care with practical technique and sophistication of equipment are, however, almost always required if the use of afterloading techniques is not to lead to less accurate and potentially inferior treatments. On the other hand, when technically reliable equipment and consistently successful techniques for afterloading have become an established part of regular clinical practice, the way would appear to be opened for the application of certain refinements of radiotherapeutic technique which may be advantageous to the patient.

For interstitial implantation work, staff exposure (particularly to the fingers of the implanter) may be reduced by the use of afterloading systems such as those described by Paine, Pierquin, and others which employ iridium-192 wires introduced into pre-inserted nylon tubes. At Manchester, however, it has been felt that the potential advantages of this class of afterloading are outweighed by the simplicity of use of rigid needles and by the consequent closer approximation to the patterns of source distributions prescribed by the Manchester radium dosage system which such needles facilitate in the hands of a skilled and experienced operator.

Intracavitary treatments in gynaecological radiotherapy present one of the last remaining major problems of staff exposure to ionising radiations in the medical field. With preloaded applicators, careful attention to working procedures and the use, where applicable, of appropriate handling and shielding devices can limit the exposure of all workers concerned to levels less than the internationally accepted occupational dose limit. When, however, the work load is heavy with this common class of treatment, a moderate number of involved individuals are likely to be exposed in the range 30%–90% of the permissible dose limits, and a larger number in the range 20%–30%. This situation has to be seen in the context that in all other radiation work in the medical field, including diagnostic radiology, radiotherapy of non-gynaecological conditions, and nuclear medicine, workers' exposures have now been reduced to levels which are rarely more than 10%, and frequently only about 1%, of the permissible dose limits. Moreover, this position is accentuated by the emphasis from the International Commission on Radiological Protection in recent years that all workers' exposures must be not only less than the permissible dose limits but also "as low as reasonably achievable". There is therefore almost irresistible pressure for the use of afterloading techniques such as those mentioned earlier in this chapter to reduce workers' exposures in gynaecological brachytherapy.

Comparison of Brachytherapy and Beam Therapy

In order to compare the physical aspects of these two types of treatment, it is useful to summarise their essential features.

Brachytherapy

1) By placing the radiation source or sources inside, or immediately adjacent to, the volume of tissue to be treated, the dose to other tissues can be minimised. This is so because the radiation does not have to pass through any other tissue before arriving at the treatment volume.
2) Inside the treatment volume, the dose is necessarily non-uniform and dose gradients are often high. For treatment such as a needle implant the dose level must always be relatively high for tissues near the sources. The rules for the Manchester system are designed to achieve a specified level of uniformity of dose at points situated in a specified plane or throughout a specified volume.
3) Brachytherapy is normally limited to accessible sites, either near the surface of the body or near natural body cavities.
4) Within the limitations imposed by (3), any volume may, in theory, be treated by using a

sufficiently complex array of sources. In practice the size of the array may be limited by anatomical barriers, and also by radiation protection considerations. The larger the total activity employed, the greater the potential hazard to ward and theatre staff.

5) Dose rates are usually relatively low.

Beam Therapy

1) Any volume of the body is accessible to beam therapy, but the relative dose to tissues outside the treatment volume will in general be greater than with brachytherapy. If the treatment volume is deep in the body, the radiation beams will have to pass through normal tissue on the way in, and they will also irradiate tissue beyond the treatment volume.
2) By suitable design, any required degree of dose uniformity can in principle be achieved inside the treatment volume.
3) There is no physical limitation to the size of the volume that can be treated.
4) Dose rates are usually relatively high.

Choice of Brachytherapy or Beam Therapy

From the foregoing summaries it can be seen that on physical grounds brachytherapy is the treatment of choice for small volumes which are accessible to this type of treatment. In practice the limitations mentioned restrict brachytherapy to volumes of dimensions less than about 10 cm.

The choice of brachytherapy or beam therapy also involves other considerations, such as the comfort and convenience of the patient and the availability of appropriate equipment and skills. The effects of brachytherapy or beam therapy may also be influenced by the very different dose rates involved, and these matters are further considered in later chapters.

Suggestions for Further Reading

This chapter was intended to give only an outline of what is involved in the physics of radiotherapy and associated radiological protection. More detailed information may be found in the following publications:

Meredith WJ, Massey JB (1977) Fundamental physics of radiology. Wright, Bristol.

Code of Practice for the Protection of Persons against Ionizing Radiations from Medical and Dental Use. HMSO 1972.

Reports of the International Commission on Radiation Units and Measurements.

Reports of the International Commission on Radiological Protection.

2 Applied Radiobiology

M. L. Sutton and J. H. Hendry

Introduction

The most satisfactory therapeutic regimens for local tumour control have been derived empirically, but the empiricism fails to explain why the best available regimens do not succeed in every case. Not only does empiricism fail to explain failures, it also fails to explain successes. Radiobiological explanations of treatment failure offer, in principle, suggestions for the design of novel regimes of radiotherapy, alone or in combination with other physical and chemical agents, which may reduce the incidence of treatment failures. This is the "predictive" role of radiobiology as opposed to its "interpretive" role. To date, benefits of predictive radiobiology have not been striking, leading to the attitude that radiobiology is an expensive irrelevance.

The experience of courses in radiobiology suggests a very widespread failure to relate the phenomena of "classical" radiobiology to what is observed, or ought to be observed, in the clinic. This chapter will describe the changes that occur in normal and malignant tissues during and after therapeutic irradiation as exemplified by treatments at the Christie Hospital. It is in no way intended as a substitute for the more comprehensive introductions to radiobiology which are to be found elsewhere (see the recommended reading at the end of this chapter). This chapter is intended to be interpretive with respect to current Christie Hospital clinical practice. For example, in the past, we chose not to participate in the evaluation of certain alleged advances in radiotherapy (most notably the use of the hyperbaric oxygen tank) though for some years a neutron generator was in clinical use at the Christie Hospital. Some of the radiobiological considerations behind these decisions will also be discussed.

Most accounts of radiobiological phenomena start with submolecular events and go on to describe their consequences at molecular, subcellular, cellular, and tissue levels, in the expectation that the reader will comprehend such a logically developed sequence of events. As mentioned above, this expectation is not always realised. This fact and our clinically interpretive intentions have dictated the structure of this chapter. Clinically apparent responses of tissues to irradiation will first be described, followed by explanations of those responses in terms of currently accepted radiobiological and histopathological concepts.

Philosophy and Empiricism Behind Current Christie Hospital Practice

The first prospective randomised clinical trials in malignant disease were carried out at this Institute, and the evolution of most of the treatment policies to be advocated in later chapters has been dominated by such clinical trials. Whenever two or more different radiation treatments have been compared it has been our intention to fulfil the following criteria:

1) A stated dose is given to the target volume in a stated number of fractions in a finite overall treatment time. Partly for historical reasons,

this overall time is commonly shorter than that employed at other centres. The treatment course is regarded as virtually sacrosanct, deviations from it being permitted only in exceptional circumstances.

2) Whenever possible, the trial results should lead to a more precise definition of the "optimum dose" for a given situation.

There is a fundamental difference in the aims of therapeutic radiation in normal and malignant tissues. In the former case, the intention is to deliver to the normal tissue a dose of ionising radiation which will deplete the number of those cells capable of regenerating that tissue (clonogenic cells, see below) to levels at or above that necessary for continued function of the tissue, and which will be consistent with the *long-term* integrity of its associated stroma and vasculature. In the case of the irradiation of malignant tissues the aim is quite different, being the total eradication of the tumour clonogenic cells in as many instances as possible. The latter cells may constitute as little as 1% of the total tumour cell mass. On the one hand is the need to preserve a proportion of one cell population (or populations), and on the other hand is the imperative need for the frequent complete annihilation of another population of cells, bearing in mind that all populations share the same physical territory.

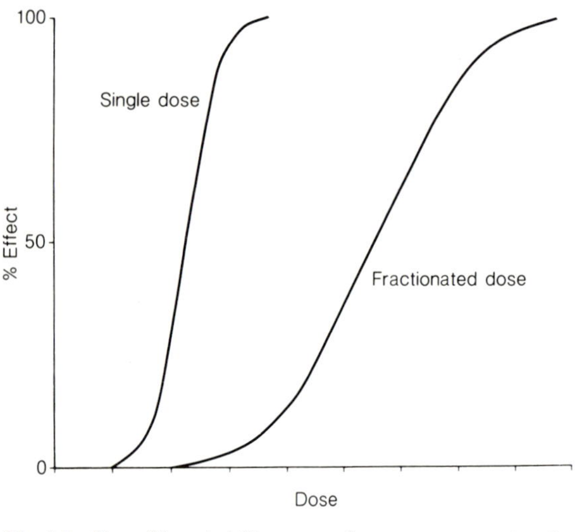

Fig. 2.1. Sigmoid probability curves for tumour control or for normal tissue necrosis, using single doses (*left curve*) or fractionated doses (*right curve*). Note that the curve for fractionated doses is less steep than the curve for single doses. Equally important, it can be seen in this example that the criticality of dose to be prescribed is less for fractionated doses than for single doses, i.e. when the steepness is expressed as a fraction of the given dose. Thus, at 5% necrosis on the two curves, the ratio of doses is 2.0, whereas at 50% necrosis the ratio is 2.3. This is because the curve for fractionated doses reflects the steepness for low doses per fraction, where threshold doses per fraction are proportionately also lower.

The relationship between the dose and the incidence of a given effect can be described by a dose-response curve. These curves are usually sigmoidal (S-shaped) and demonstrate a threshold region followed by a region where the incidence changes sharply with increasing dose, and finally a plateau at the full incidence (Fig. 2.1). The sigmoid nature of dose-response curves has been experimentally confirmed for a wide range of tissues, both normal and malignant, and for an equally wide variety of effects or end points. For example, the curves illustrated in Fig. 2.1 could equally well describe (with appropriately scaled axes), the relationship between increasing doses of irradiation and the production of necrosis in normal tissue, or the local eradication of tumours. The general applicability of the sigmoid relationships is increasingly well established and accepted in laboratory situations, yet the few *clinical* reports on dose-effect relationships in tumour control virtually all show what are evidently straight-line curves. This apparent paradox may be satisfactorily resolved by the following two considerations:

1) Most patients in reported series received something approximating to the alleged opti-

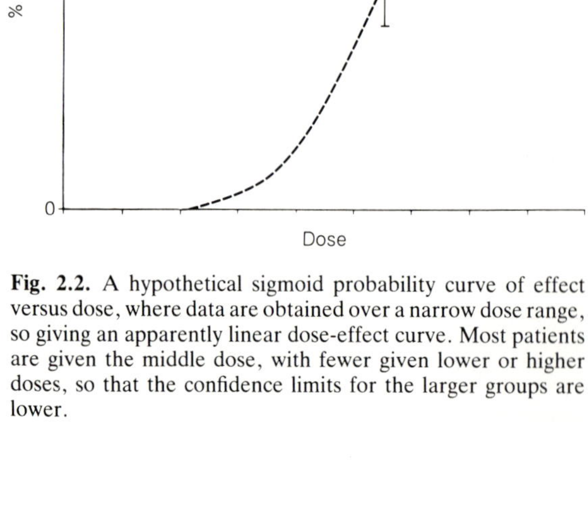

Fig. 2.2. A hypothetical sigmoid probability curve of effect versus dose, where data are obtained over a narrow dose range, so giving an apparently linear dose-effect curve. Most patients are given the middle dose, with fewer given lower or higher doses, so that the confidence limits for the larger groups are lower.

mum dose and patients who received higher and lower doses are usually smaller in number, hence statistical vagaries may obscure the curvilinear nature of the relationship (see Fig. 2.2).

2) The middle of the dose range quoted is (usually) close to the considered optimum for the regimen being reported, and the lower and higher doses on either side of this optimum dose rarely differ from it by more than 7.5%, often by as little as 5%. This means that only a small portion of the dose-response curve is demonstrated. This is entirely proper, since doses much higher than the optimum would result in an unacceptably high incidence of severe radiation damage in the normal tissues, whereas doses much lower than the alleged optimum would be expected to result in unacceptably low tumour control rates.

One consequence of therapeutic irradiation is the complete and permanent local disappearance of the tumour. Depending on the site and size of the tumour, this is frequently achieved with adequate subsequent restoration of the irradiated normal tissues. When this situation (i.e. cure with healing) occurs, the "necrosis" dose-response curve must lie to the higher-dose side of the tumour cure dose-effect curve, and since in such situations a small proportion of patients do unfortunately develop necrosis, the two curves must be sufficiently close together to overlap to some extent (Fig. 2.3). In the model illustrated in Fig. 2.3, dose D_2 gives a high percentage of cures without incurring a high penalty in necrosis. A relatively small increase in dose, to D_3, secures a small increase in cure, but at the expense of a numerically much larger increase in necrosis. Reduction of dose to D_1 gives no necroses but the tumour cure rate is greatly reduced because of the steepness of the tumour cure curve.

By subtracting the necrosis curve from the cure curve at each dose, a new curve representing "complication-free tumour cure" can be con-

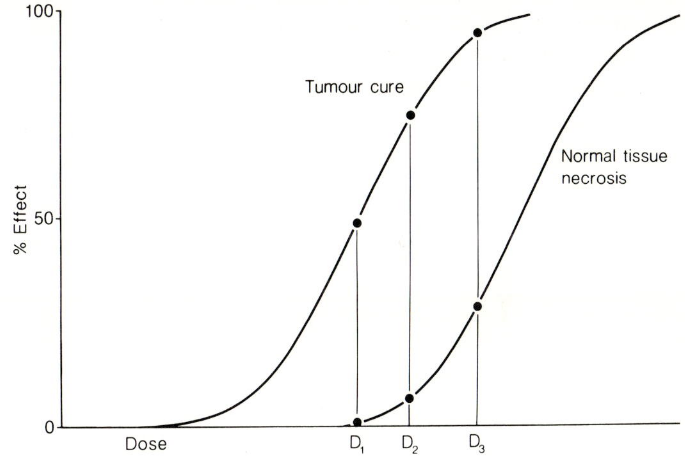

Fig. 2.3. Sigmoid dose-effect curves for tumour cure and for normal tissue necrosis. For convenience, curves of the same shape have been drawn separated by a shift in the dose.

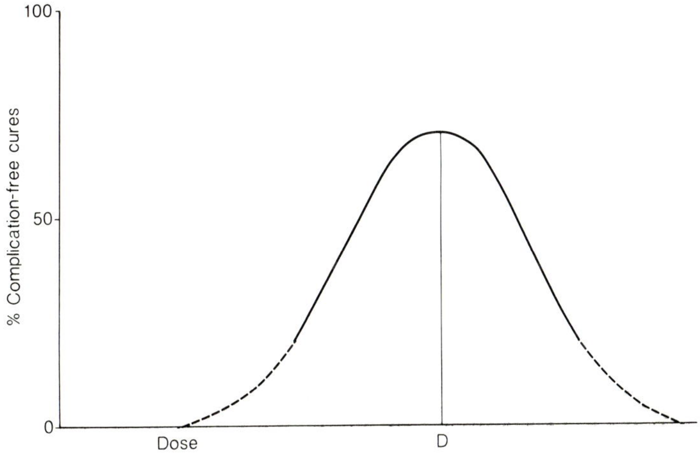

Fig. 2.4. Complication-free cures versus dose. This curve was calculated from the similar-shaped curves shown in Fig. 2.3, and hence the resultant curve is symmetrical about dose D.

structed (Fig. 2.4). Dose *D* in Fig. 2.4 offers the most complication-free cures, but this dose should not necessarily be considered as the optimum dose, nor is the dose at which tumour treatment failures are equally matched with late complications necessarily the optimum dose. Amongst the factors which may influence the final choice of dose are the acceptability and functional consequences of the necrosis, and its amenability to conservative management or surgical correction. The acceptability of the late radiation effect may be influenced by age, sex, and cultural considerations. Unsightly late radiation stigmata on the facial skin of a septuagenarian male may be acceptable, but radiation myelitis or encephalopathy are unacceptable for any patient at any time.

The ability of surgery to rescue patients from untoward consequences of their irradiation varies from site to site whether those consequences be late radiation damage or persistence or recurrence of tumour. In general, surgery is much more effective in achieving long-term survival when the surgical specimen shows late radiation effects rather than the anticipated persistence of recurrence of malignant disease. Therefore, at certain sites and stages of disease the dose used may be justifiably higher than the dose at which the necroses are numerically balanced by the failed cures.

The Christie Hospital concept of optimum dose clearly implies that adequate treatment is certain to be associated with the occasional occurrence of late complications. The acceptable level of incidence of late radiation effects is determined by the same factors that influence the acceptability of the necrosis itself, namely, site, stage of disease, age, and sometimes sex and culture. Some malignant tumours, by the time of presentation, have already caused considerable erosion of the structures in which they have arisen, and sometimes of adjacent structures also. The successful eradication of such tumours by irradiation may leave a substantial anatomical and functional defect in the surviving normal tissues, and when such a defect fails to heal, as it may indeed fail to do, the result is frequently loosely described as a "radiation necrosis". It is more proper to call such results "tumour-related necroses". Unless distinction between devitalisation of tissues by radiation and the disruption of tissues by destructive malignancy is clear, there is an obvious temptation to give less than the optimum dose, with predictable results on tumour control.

In summary, the optimum dose is that which results in a balance between high cure rates and low rates of incidence of late high-dose effects. This optimum dose varies with the site and the extent of disease, but in all events will be a dose which is destined to be administered in a stated number of fractions in a stated overall time.

This Institute exploits a relatively small number of fractionation schedules (in all of which the fractions are given daily, five times a week):

Single exposure 4 fractions in 3 days (inclusive) 8 fractions in 9 or 11 days	Often used in radical treatment but more commonly palliative
15 fractions in 20 days 16 fractions in 21 days 20 fractions in 25 or 27 days	Always given with radical intent

The optimum doses employed are discussed, site by site, in subsequent chapters. The effects of doses different from the optimum dose can be directly compared only when the number of fractions and the overall treatment time remain constant, that is, within any one regimen. Thus the cure and necrosis rates for a 16-fraction, 21-day treatment can be plotted directly on dose-effect coordinates for say, doses of 4750, 5000, and 5500 cGy (as in Fig. 2.3). The result of, say, treatment at 6500 cGy given in 30 fractions over 40 days cannot be plotted on the same graph unless the value assigned to "dose" is reduced in an empirical fashion to account for the fact that the radiation has been delivered in a larger number of smaller fractions over a longer period. This can be done either by using nomograms (Fig. 2.5) or by using a formula to reduce the total dose (in this case 6500 cGy) to a nominal standard dose (NSD), and then converting the NSD to a new total dose appropriate to 16 fractions over 21 days. The most widely adopted formula for this manoeuvre is the relationship $D=\text{NSD}\times N^{0.24}\times T^{0.11}$ where D=total cumulative dose in cGy, N=number of fractions, and T=overall time. The NSD is the single dose *calculated* to be tolerated by the tissue, and equivalent in its effect to the fractionated tolerance dose. It should be noted that the NSD is not necessarily the *actual* single dose required, as predictions using the equation tend to be less accurate outside the range of about 4 to about 30

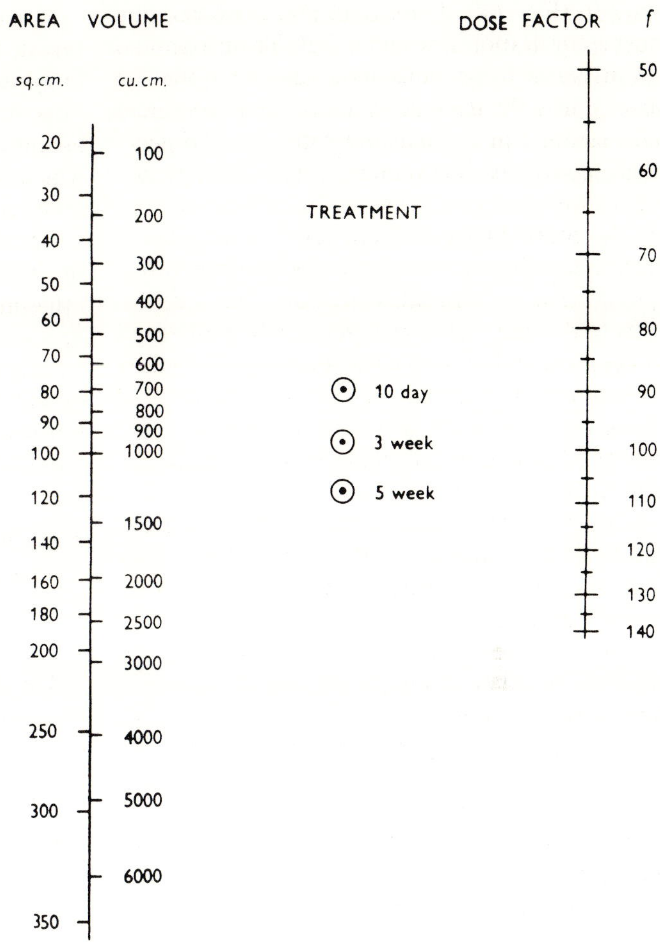

Fig. 2.5. Equivalent dose nomogram for area, volume, and time. The nomogram relates a dose factor to treatment time and area of field or treatment volume. The dose factor is proportional to treatment dose for all generally similar treatments. The dose is arrived at by laying a ruler through the appropriate area or volume and treatment time and reading off the factor on the right-hand scale. For treatments under similar conditions, the ratio of the prescribed dose for one treatment to that for a known prescription with different time and field size is the ratio of the dose factors given by the nomogram. Example: Let us accept 4000 cGy as a known satisfactory dose for a 10×10 cm parallel field treatment to the neck over 3 weeks. What would be the equivalent dose for a 10×15 pair of fields over a 10-day treatment?
Factor for 10×10 cm at 3 weeks=97
Factor for 10×15 cm at 10 days=76
The equivalent dose will therefore be 4000×76/97=3150 cGy. Taken from: The treatment of malignant disease by radiotherapy, 2nd edition. 1963. R. Paterson. p. 35. (Edward Arnold Ltd. London).

daily fractions. Also, despite the widespread acceptance of this relationship (but see below), the conviction evidently persists that treatment regimens giving much higher cumulative doses are somehow inherently superior to those giving lower cumulative doses. For example, visitors to the Christie Hospital commonly express surprise at the very "low" 3750 cGy dose for adult cerebral gliomas, compared to their own "high" dose of 6000 cGy. The former, however, is given in 16 fractions over 3 weeks, whereas the latter is given in 30 fractions over 6 weeks. The two regimens result in strikingly similar survival curves, in spite of the fact that the NSD for the shorter regimen is 78% of that for the longer regimen.

Equivalence of morbidity should be achieved in clinical trials. The morbidity referred to here is the late morbidity, to which the severity of the acute radiation reaction is at best a poor guide. When an established radiation regimen is compared to a new regimen, one regimen may appear superior to another in terms of cure rate, but if this is accompanied by a higher incidence of unacceptable late effects, there may be no true superiority. The "inferior" regimen may be capable of the same results as the "superior" regimen simply by increasing its total dose. Clinical trials should be carried out at two dose levels in the novel arms of the trial. These two dose levels should be close to the anticipated optimum dose for the new regimen; it should be noted that differences less than ±3% are below detectability in most situations, while differences greater than ±7.5% are usually unacceptable, because of the steepness of the dose-response curves in the region of the optimum dose (see Fig. 2.3). The adoption of two dose levels permits the relevant portions of the dose-response curves for both cure and late complications to be constructed. In the example illustrated in Fig. 2.6, the known 5% complication rate of treatment *A* corresponds to a dose in treatment *B* which is associated with a higher cure rate than that of treatment *A*. If treatment *B* had been carried out at one dose only, no firm conclusion could be drawn about the relative merits of the two treatments except in the fortuitous event that the dose chosen happened to be dose D_3. The employment of two dose levels in a regimen removes the element of chance, and ensures that a trial will be able to answer the questions asked of it. There is another most important advantage in that the method of equivalent morbidity obviates the need for the doses in the arms of the trial to be adjusted to account precisely for differences in fractionation and overall time, or for exact differences in relative biological effectiveness, which may be imprecisely known.

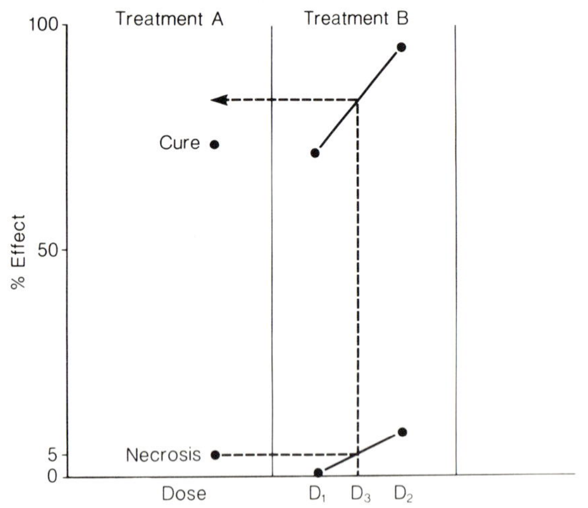

Fig. 2.6. A comparison of the optimum dose in treatment *A* with a trial of two doses (D_1 and D_2) in treatment *B*. The optimum dose in treatment *B* would be D_3. This could truly improve the cure rate, whereas dose D_1 would not, and dose D_2 would spuriously increase the cure rate at the expense of a higher incidence of necrosis.

Gross Response of Tissues—General Considerations

The effects of radiation on tissues are manifested in several ways, and all effects are mediated by the response of the cells constituting the tissue. Some tissue effects are transient, for example the temporary initial erythema in skin and the early rise in intracranial pressure that can arise during cerebral irradiation. These are associated with changes in cellular membrane permeability, and they are reversible. The metabolic processes of cells are radioresistant, and hence tissue function is generally radioresistant (i.e. largely unaffected) in the short-term, until cell loss occurs. However, the genetic apparatus of the cell is much more susceptible to radiation injury. Unless two almost perfect copies of the genetic apparatus are produced, cell division cannot result in viable daughter cells. The first division of irradiated cells can be successfully accomplished in most instances, and the use of this ability to undergo one mitosis as an end point of radiation damage would lead to a dose-response curve characteristic of resistant cells. Such a curve describes the decreasing proportion of cells achieving the end point after increasing doses. The second, third, and fourth mitoses result in the deaths of more and more of the irradiated cells, leaving progressively fewer survivors, and this expresses a greater *sensitivity* for the initial complement of cells. A maximum sensitivity is expressed after about five divisions, and cells which have accomplished these five divisions successfully are then the true survivors capable of a further large amount of repopulation to form *clones* of cells and hence they can regenerate the tissue. The *rate* of division of cells after radiation will govern the *responsiveness* of a tissue. Tissues will *respond early* if the cells accomplish several divisions quite soon after irradiation, as in intestinal epithelium, but will respond *late* where the parenchymal cells divide only occasionally, as in liver and in thyroid. These are the basic phenomena determining the response of all normal and malignant tissues, but they are influenced by other factors. All irradiated volumes consist of several types of tissue, which usually differ from one another in respect of the normal rates of division of their constituent cells, their inherent radio-sensitivities, and their *apparent* sensitivities depending on the number of divisions that they are called upon to undergo, as described above. The early phases of a tissue response depend first on that component of the tissue in which the cells are dividing most rapidly, and on the radiosensitivity of those cells. Epithelia such as the epidermis and gastrointestinal mucosa are tissue components, in skin and gut respectively, which are constantly and rapidly being eroded and replaced, and these are classic examples of renewing and hence radioresponsive components of tissues.

Tissues can be classified broadly into two categories:

1) Those which have to produce a population of mature cells with a rather limited life-span, as for example in the surface epithelia, and in the haemopoietic and spermatogenic systems. Such tissues generally contain a small population of progenitor (stem) cells, amounting to sometimes less than 1% of the total cell population, which consists mainly of the mature cells. The stem cells give rise to the mature cells by a series of amplifying cell divisions of intermediate precursor cells. The sequence of cells from stem cell to mature cell forms a hierarchy of developmental stages—a cell lineage. The stem cells can be identified by their ability to form colonies of daughter cells in a tissue in which the stem cells are distributed much more sparsely than normal. This can be achieved with many tissues by a dose of irradiation which sterilises most of the stem cells, i.e. prevents all but a few from forming clones, or by transplanting a few viable cells into a heavily irradiated tissue.
2) Those which consist of well-differentiated but long-lived cells, for example, muscle, liver, and thyroid. Such tissues are not known at present to arise from a series of amplifying cell divisions from a relatively small number of progenitor cells. They are generally considered to represent a more homogeneous population of cells, *all* of which are capable of dividing occasionally to maintain the complement of functional cells.

These two types of tissue should respond very differently to radiation, exemplified by the time course of the responses seen after high radiation doses. The category 2 homogeneous cell populations will not manifest their response until late after radiation, when the reduction in the rate of successful cell replacement (which is dependent on dose) begins to show as impaired function. There may be a regenerative response to this reduced function, and this may reveal faster the latent injury in the cells called upon to divide. Hence tissue function decreases gradually and often imperceptibly to start with, but later may decrease rapidly. The overall time course can be over many months or years, and would be expected to be dose-dependent.

This relationship of dose to latent period is shown clearly for limb paralysis in rats resulting from spinal cord irradiation.

Tissues of type 1 above, which are renewed from precursor cells, should show little appreciable change until the production of new mature cells ceases. The time at which this occurs will correspond to the normal turnover time of the proliferative and maturing component of the tissue if the stem cell component is sensitive to irradiation and is ablated, if the intermediate amplifying cell divisions are few in number and hence expected to be relatively resistant, and if the processes of differentiation, maturation, and migration are also resistant. When the production of new mature cells ceases, the size of the mature cell population should decrease at a rate which is governed by the normal rate of loss of the mature cells. This of course equals their rate of production in the normal steady state. The mature cell population should be totally depleted when the initial mature population and that derived after irradiation from the resistant transit cells have both been used and lost from the tissue. Very high doses do not usually cause a more rapid depletion of the mature population (in contrast to tissues of type 2), and cannot of course increase its completeness. These principles are demonstrated quite well by the epithelial components of skin and gut.

The later phases of the responses of tissues containing rapidly renewing components can be governed by two mechanisms. The first is that of the slowly dividing supportive tissues, where damage may be enhanced by indirect effects caused by early damage to the fast-renewing components, e.g. dermal injury after epidermal denudation. The second is damage to the rapidly renewing components, which is expressed after the initial recovery phase. This can be caused by persistent radiation injury, leading to a prolonged increased turnover rate and amplification from a reduced complement of stem cells, but only for a limited time, as demonstrated by late marrow hypoplasia. The sigmoid dose-response curve, described empirically above, expresses the incidence of a severe (lethal) tissue effect, e.g. tumour control or necrosis of normal tissue, after various doses. The induced effect in a cell population or a tissue can be described as a level of depopulation which is below the level consistent with regeneration of that cell population. If that level of depopulation was achieved in all cases by the same dose, the dose-response curve would not be sigmoidal. It would demonstrate a threshold region where increasing doses did not produce the effect at all, until a critical dose was reached where the effect would be produced in all instances. However, this hypothetical situation involving such a very sharp change is not observed in any treatment of the type considered here, because of heterogeneity in the response of different samples.

There are three causes of this heterogeneity. The first is the mechanism of the killing of cells in tissues by radiation. The killing is initiated by the random deposition of energy in discrete microscopic subcellular volumes. Consequently, the spatial distribution of killed cells in a tissue, or the distribution of numbers of killed cells between samples, can be described by statistical probability theory. Therefore, at dose levels which bracket the lethal dose for a tissue, there will be no dose at which the tissue *just* manages to regenerate in *every* instance, and also no dose at which it just fails to regenerate in all cases. At each dose there will be a certain incidence of the lethal effect among the sample of tissues given that dose; for example a 5% incidence is usually accepted as a tolerance level. The change in incidence with increasing dose is governed by the average proportion of the initial number of target cells (clonogenic cells) which survive after each dose in a series of increasing doses. As already discussed above, these proportions are determined directly by the *sensitivity* of the cells, and hence their sensitivity governs the steepness of the sigmoidal dose-response curve.

The second cause of heterogeneity is a true variation between samples in the initial content or in the sensitivity of the clonogenic cells. The third possible cause would involve different types of (clonogenic) cells being responsible for tissue failure after different doses. However, as dose-response curves are usually steep, the likelihood is rare that two types of tissue would contribute to the slope of the dose-response curve which covers only a narrow range of dose, and no clear examples of a biphasic dose-response curve have been reported. Both the second and third causes would make the dose-response curve less steep. These general features will be illustrated by the response of skin and other normal tissues and of tumours.

Skin

Although injury to skin is no longer a major problem in radiotherapy, since the epidermis is spared by the build-up of dose with megavoltage beams, skin effects are still a reliable biological dosimeter when treatments are modified. The response of skin will be described first for single doses, as this situation is the simplest to analyse, followed by the response to fractionated doses and low dose rates of the type discussed in subsequent chapters.

Early Effects

Acute doses of up to 600 cGy produce few gross effects in skin, apart from the hyperpigmentation in hair follicles which can be seen sometimes as a dark mottled line surrounding the field in the penumbra region of dose. The reason for this effect is still uncertain but it is considered likely to be due to a diffusible factor released from the irradiated melanocytes in the follicle which stimulates the production of melanin in neighbouring cells in the follicle germ that do not normally synthesise it. After single doses above 600 cGy the effects are more marked. There is sometimes an erythema, a loss of pigment as the melanocytes are killed, and dysplasia and epilation due to the killing of germ cells in the follicles. There will be some sterilisation of cells in the basal layer of the epidermis, so that there may be a delay in the continued production of keratinised cells leading to the exposure of immature cells at the surface. At doses approaching 2000 cGy the effects are severe. Following the initial transient erythema there is a delay period before the erythema reappears more noticeably. This is followed by a gradual breakdown of the epidermis starting from gross changes seen at about the ninth day, and leading to ulceration and epithelial necrosis unless regeneration intervenes to restore the complement of keratinised layers. The sequence of events at these doses results from the sterilisation of progenitor cells in the basal layer, so that the normal input of maturing cells into the stratum corneum is reduced. As the surface keratinised cells are continuously lost at a normal rate, but are no longer being replaced at this rate, the epithelium becomes thinner and eventually the deeper layers are exposed at the surface. The processes of the last cell division, migration, and maturation are very resistant, so that even at doses well over 2000 cGy the same pattern of response is seen. If the dose is such as to leave a small proportion of surviving progenitor cells in the basal layer of the epidermis and in the appended follicles, these will gradually repopulate the irradiated surface.

The new epithelium normally functions quite well but is commonly devoid of pigment and hair. (See also the remarks on cellular depletion under "Late Effects" below.) The new epithelium is also more easily damaged by further radiation or by other cytotoxic agents and physicochemical trauma. The dermis is largely unresponsive to radiation in the short term because of the slow turnover of the constituent cells in its tissue components. The severity of the epidermal reaction with increasing dose has been quantified in several ways. The erythema can be given a score depending on its severity, either seen by eye or measured with a spectrophotometer, but this is subject to quite marked variability and is rather insensitive to small changes in dose. At higher doses the severity of the skin reaction can be scored on an arbitrary numerical scale, with the numbers relating to effects such as erythema, dry desquamation, moist desquamation, and scar formation. The effects are reproducible and quantitative, and this method is able to resolve doses which are different by about 3%. The method is also applicable to all species. With increasing dose the time course of the skin reactions is similar, even for those which proceed to necrosis, and this is characteristic of a renewing hierarchical cell population, as discussed earlier.

Dosage Modifications

The dose necessary to produce a skin reaction can be modified in various ways. The skin reaction is modified by field size, so that higher doses can be tolerated with small fields. With fields smaller than a 2-cm-diameter circle much higher doses can be given, largely because of migration from the edges of unirradiated epidermal cells across the substratum. The reason for the field-size effect for larger areas is not fully understood. *Area for area*, field shapes which have greater circumferences, e.g. squares, heal more readily in general than those which have lower circumferences, e.g. ellipses or circles. The shape with the minimum circumference is the circle, and circular lead cut-outs are frequently used in the treatment of skin lesions. The field size is determined by the dimensions of the lesion and the need to include a circumferential margin of apparently uninvolved normal skin and, although a square has a bigger circumference, the total area treated would be greater than if a circle were used. (However, square fields are employed where multiple skin malignancies exist, to facilitate the matching-on of fields that may subsequently be required.)

Oxygen

Even with a constant field size, the effectiveness of radiation can be changed in many cases by changing the oxygen tension directly or indirectly. Oxygen is involved in the initial radiochemical stages of radiation action, and cells and tissues lacking oxygen are more radioresistant, so that doses have to be increased by up to three times for equivalent biological effects. Doses to the skin can be increased by cooling or compressing the skin and increased by up to two times when a tourniquet is applied to limbs. Also, an environment of hyperbaric oxygen at 3 atmospheres necessitates, for the same end point, a reduction in dose to the skin by up to 40% at high single doses.

Although there are exceptions, many observations in animals have indicated that these changes due to oxygen are virtually dose-modifying, e.g. for 5% necrosis and 10% necrosis, doses would be changed by the same factor. Figure 2.7 shows hypothetical dose-response curves in air, hyperbaric oxygen, and when a tourniquet is applied. Each effect point on the hyperbaric curve occurs at 60% (100% minus 40%) of the dose for the same level of effect in air (or 90% of that in the case of laryngeal cartilage, as will be explained under "Tumour Radiation Response" below) and each effect point on the tourniquet curve occurs at 200% of the dose in air. The steepness of the hyperbaric oxygen and tourniquet curves is expected to differ from that of the air curve. Whereas in hyperbaric oxygen the dose-response curve is steeper, lower radiation doses are required for each level of effect, so that the criticality of dose relative to treatments in air is expected to remain approximately the same. This does *not* imply that doses are changed in the same proportion for different effects in a composite tissue,

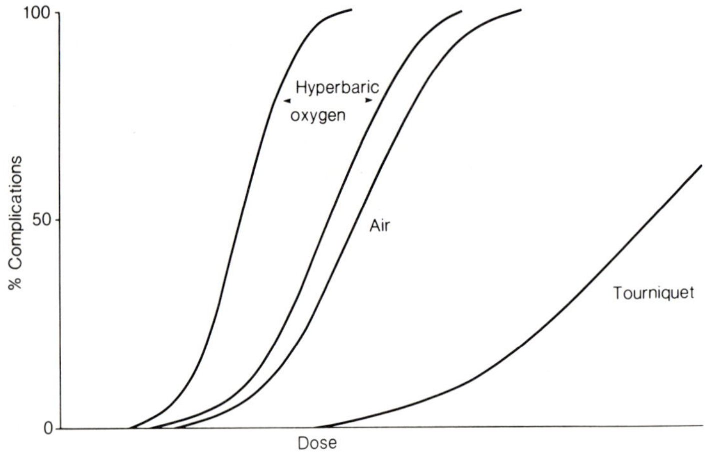

Fig. 2.7. Hypothetical sigmoid probability curves of complications versus dose, assuming a dose-modifying effect of oxygen. The hyperbaric oxygen curves are separated from the air curve by 40% in dose at all doses (left curve, skin) and by 10% (second curve from left, laryngeal cartilage). The curve obtained using a tourniquet is moved to the right by a factor of 2 in dose at all doses.

since tissue components responsible for different effects may be at different oxygen tensions. For example, there are some reports of larger dosage changes required in skin for moist desquamation than for erythema.

Dose Rate

Responses to single doses can also be modified by changing dose rate. At rates less than about 10 cGy/min, doses are less effective than at the commonly used rates of 100–1000 cGy/min. The reason for this is that some of the radiation injury to cells is sublethal and is repairable during the radiation exposure. For near-homogeneous irradiation of skin, as in external beam or interstitial therapy, the relationship of overall time T to dose rate R in man and mouse is given approximately by the empirical expression $T=AR^{-1.35}$ where A is a constant dependent on the site. This relationship describes an effect mainly due to dose rate rather than to overall time, as discussed further below. Ultra-high dose rates are also less effective, but for a very different reason. At such dose rates the rate of deposition of energy is faster than the rate of diffusion and usage of the available oxygen, so that a state effectively equivalent to one lacking in oxygen is achieved. However, this effect occurs at dose rates above 10^5 cGy/min and is not usually encountered in radiotherapy. Fortuitously, the generators and isotopes available to the early clinicians provided dose rates sufficiently high to exceed the rates at which cells in human tissues can repair sublethal damage. Had the dose rates available been lower, the effects of radiation on normal and malignant tissues would very probably have gone unrecognised for some time.

Fractionation

The majority of tissues are affected less by a dose of radiation when it is fractionated. This lesser response is due to the same phenomenon which is responsible for the dose-rate effects, namely repair of sublethal cellular damage. After an acute exposure the half-time of this repair effect is about $1\frac{1}{2}$ h so that the majority of the repair is completed in 4–5 h. More sublethal injury is inflicted with increasing dose, and similarly more repair can be demonstrated until saturation is reached after high doses. Hence, the proportion of dose which is effectively "wasted" due to this cellular recovery is dependent on the dose. An example of this is a single skin dose of 2000 cGy, close to tolerance for a 2-cm-diameter circle. If this treatment is split into two fractions of equal size given 4 h or more apart, to produce the same effect on normal skin each fraction must be about 1250 cGy, or 2500 cGy total dose. Thus 500 cGy, or 25% of the original dose is wasted when two doses are given instead of one. In comparison, if a 20-fraction treatment were to be changed to a 40-fraction treatment over the same overall time, such that each small fraction would be split into two equal parts, somewhat less than 25% extra total dose would need to be given for equal normal tissue effect. In practice, the extra fractions would be given over a longer interval, and repopulation (see below) would become a major factor, requiring *more* total dose for equal effect (see Fig. 2.8). Although radiation induces a

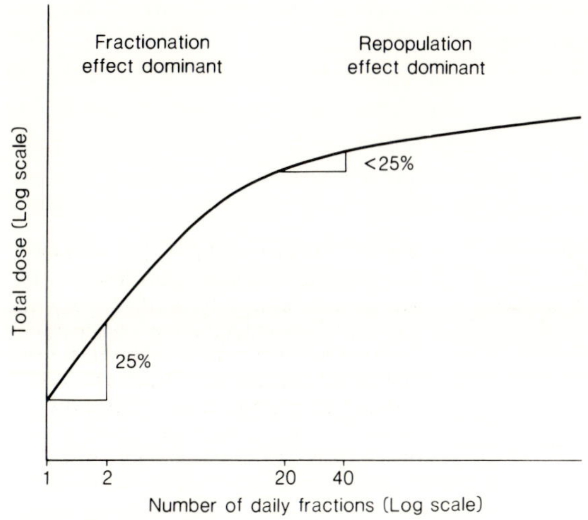

Fig. 2.8. Log total dose versus log number of daily fractions for equal biological effect. There is a greater effect of fractionation when a few large fractions are used than with a large number of small fractions. Hence relative increases in total dose with increasing numbers of small fractions are less than with increasing numbers of large dose fractions.

transient mitotic delay in cells (about 1 h for every 100 cGy for rapidly proliferating cells, or one tenth of a cell cycle per 100 cGy even for slowly cycling cells) this is a minor restriction on growth when dose fractions are commonly 200–400 cGy, spaced 1 day apart. Moreover, cell multiplication in renewing tissues will often quicken during the first part of treatment, and will reach a maximum rate towards the end. This comes about by the normal homeostatic response of renewing tissues to cellular depletion, and is termed *repopulation*. For early skin reactions this time effect corresponds to about 30 cGy per day in many species, including man. The relationship of total dose D to number of fractions N and to overall time T is given approximately by the empirical relationship $D=\text{NSD}\times N^{0.24}\times T^{0.11}$ (as mentioned earlier), where the NSD is dependent on the site, and is 1800–2000 cGy for skin. The NSD may not be equivalent to the actual single dose required, as the relationship is considered to be applicable only between about 4 and about 30 daily fractions (five fractions per week). This relationship should be considered as only a guide to doses required when changing schedules, since as little as 5% change in dose is detectable in some situations because the dose-response curves are steep (see discussion of dose-response curves above). The above formula was derived using clinical observations on squamous cell carcinoma and early skin reactions, and it assumes a common exponent of N for both normal tissue and tumour, and an exponent of T for the skin, but none for the tumour. These assumptions are unlikely to hold for the wide range of normal tissues and tumours encountered in therapy, but they are sufficient to establish such a guide to required changes in dose. If the empirical expression relating overall time to dose rate (see above) is re-arranged to relate total dose to overall time in keeping with our clinical practice at the Christie Hospital, the exponent of time is 0.26. This is much larger than the value of 0.11 in the expression for fractionated, high dose rate treatments, and it indicates that for prolonged low dose rate treatment, the irradiation dose rate is much more important than overall time per se. These considerations of course apply to homogeneous irradiations of tissues, and not necessarily to point sources, where the dose rate at the unknown position of the true target cells is difficult to define.

As mentioned above, the steepness of dose-response curves for fractionated treatments is an important consideration. Dose-response curves for fractionated treatments can be generated in two distinct ways. With longer fractionation schedules of 5–7 weeks, dose fractions are usually 200 cGy, and hence the dose-response curve (of complications or of tumour control) will be determined by the response to the last few fractions of 200 cGy. With short schedules of, say, 8 days for palliation or 3 weeks for short radical treatments, the dose per fraction is commonly varied with the same overall time and number of fractions. Thus the dose-response curve will reflect the steepness over a very narrow range of dose per fraction, say 300–350 cGy, and the steepness or the "criticality" of the total dose in the treatment will be greater than for a treatment consisting of increased numbers of 200 cGy fractions.

At this Institute, within a given regimen, the number of fractions and the overall treatment time are kept fixed, whereas the total cumulative dose may be modified under certain circumstances. This contrasts with the approach in many centres in Europe and the United States, where radiotherapists exploit the relatively lower criticality of total dose when 200 cGy increments are delivered daily, five fractions per week, over a longer but relatively indeterminate period of time. We believe that a major disadvantage of this more flexible approach is that in radical treatment situations, it fails to generate true dose-response curves, because (1) at 200 cGy per day the decision to terminate treatment appears often to be made on the "acceptability" of the acute radiation reaction towards the end of the treatment, and (2) proponents of the flexible approach commonly "rest" patients towards the end of their treatments for one or more days on one or more occasions; this extends the overall treatment time. Doses have to be adjusted, when results are reported, using a formula such as the NSD statement. The aim of these adjustments to total dose and overall time is to result in a uniform level of acute reaction which the individual clinician finds acceptable. The severity of the acute radiation reaction is an imperfect predictor of the late radiation changes, but when the same normal tissue response is aimed at in all patients, the late effects are likely to be similar. Thus, in the absence of dose-response curves, for tumour and normal tissue, few convincing conclusions can be made about the optimum dose. A totally inflexible approach to dose is undesirable, but we believe that dose adjustments during treatment should be avoided; when adjustments are necessary, they are best achieved by reducing the dose per fraction in the last few treatments, keeping the overall treatment time and number of fractions constant.

Late Effects in Skin

Knowledge of the processes which result in the observed late effects of irradiation in skin is incomplete. None the less, the late changes in skin can be considered as the outcome of three processes:

1) Cellular depletion
2) Vascular changes
3) Alteration of connective tissue

These three processes occur in all heavily irradiated tissues and the degree to which they variously contribute to the ultimate radiopathological picture is dependent on the physiological functions of the tissue and its consequent proliferative dynamics.

Radiation-induced carcinogenesis is not here considered, since it is a rare consequence of therapeutic irradiation alone. At present, the late consequences of relatively small-field irradiation in close association with high-dose single- and multiple-agent chemotherapy are largely unknown; our own practice, at least in solid tumours, is too recent for analysis. In the case of advanced head and neck tumours treated by combined modalities, it may reasonably be predicted that no great increase in induced second malignancies will be seen, since the radiotherapy administered is of relatively small volume and to a high dose. In general, radiation shows its oncogenic capabilities best when large volumes are treated to relatively low doses. It is probable that when radiation treatments are given, many cells become altered in such a way as to make them likely precursors of potentially malignant clones. But when radiotherapy is given to the high doses commonly prescribed, the great majority of these cells are so damaged genetically that their proliferative capacity peters out before the development of recognisable malignancy.

Cellular Depletion

The reduced cellularity in irradiated skin affects both the epidermis and the dermis, as well as the specialised organs which are derived from the latter. Irradiated skin is hairless, sweatless, virtually bereft of sebum, and is thin. Cells responsible for the production and storage of pigment are often depleted, so that the irradiated area is pale, sometimes having a surrounding halo of pigmentation at the junction of irradiated and unirradiated tissues. This is due mainly to the induced production of pigment in other cells after low doses in the margin (discussed under "Early Effects" above). The atrophy and paucity of sweat glands is not normally of significance, but may become so when very large areas of the integument are irradiated, for instance in the treatment of mycosis fungoides by electrons. The more aggressive forms of this disease sometimes require repeated treatments, and imperfect control of body temperature, resulting from an impaired ability to sweat, has occasionally been reported. Epilation is never of more than cosmetic significance. The ability of radiation to abolish hair growth has been exploited in the management of pilonidal sinus. When the cumulative radiation dose to the dermis is sufficiently low to permit regrowth of hair, the new hair is more sparsely distributed than before irradiation, the individual strands are finer than previously, and pigment formation in the follicle is often disturbed. This usually takes the form of a depigmentation, but in elderly subjects the irradiated skin may support the growth of hair carrying pigment reflecting the patient's genotypic constitution at an earlier age. The sebaceous glands are more easily damaged by radiation than the sweat glands and the reduction of sebum secretion has noticeable functional consequences, predisposing the skin to dryness, fissuring, and slow healing. In spite of the thinness of the overlying epidermis, irradiated skin in the long term is not unduly sensitive to ordinary stimuli and although the relevant sensory organs are closer to the external environment, they are reduced in number and possibly in sensitivity also. Whether or not this is a result of a direct depletion effect or irradiation on a cell renewal system is unclear; like the changes in the epidermis, the dermis, and the latter's associated organelles, it may partly be a reflection of chronic underperfusion of blood.

Vascular Effects

Blood flow in irradiated skin is significantly reduced, although to the naked eye the area may seem to be unduly richly supplied with blood vessels. Telangiectatic capillaries have wider lumina and are closer to the surface than normal capillaries. Telangiectasis may result from the regenerative attempts of isolated clones of endothelial cells (there may here be an analogy with posthepatitic cirrhosis of the liver). When only a few endothelial survivors are left in an irradiated area they become subject to proliferative stimuli and their disorderly multiplication results in the formation of irregular vessels, some of which are occluded by these regenerative attempts, and others of which may compensate by acquiring wide lumina. Because of the overall depletion of endothelial cells, the richness of the capillary network in the irradiated skin is considerably reduced, so that the area is generally pale and yet has a few very prominent superficial blood vessels irregularly disposed throughout it. The striking histological change in irradiated arterioles is the accumulation of fibrinous material deep to the intima, which may greatly reduce the lumen of the vessels. The overall appearance differs from that seen in the arterioles of severely hypertensive patients, in that medial muscle hypertrophy does not occur, and "onion skin" endothelial proliferation is absent. The origin of the lumen-reducing fibrinoid material under the epithelium is not known, but it is possibly precipitated fibrin which has leaked across the endothelium under the hydrostatic influence of the intra-arteriolar blood pressure. Radiation causes alteration in the normal selective permeability of the endothelium, so that larger molecules such as fibrinogen can cross it; once the fibrinogen is under the endothelium, it is in a metabolically rather inert position, so that it is removed only very slowly, if at all. Carbon monoxide has a similar effect on endothelial permeability, and the chronic leakage and retention of macromolecules is thought to be in part responsible for the high prevalence of vascular occlusive disease in heavy smokers.

Alteration of Connective Tissue

The heavily irradiated dermis often undergoes both fibrosis and contraction. The former is clinically manifest as thickening and induration, most easily felt along the junction of irradiated and unirradiated skin. This change is most commonly seen in the dermis overlying the mandible, the upper neck, and the lower anterior abdominal wall, including the inguinal regions, but it is not clear if this represents a peculiar locally determined susceptibility, or is merely the reflection of the fact that in clinical practice these areas of dermis are the ones most frequently given high radiation dose. Certainly, at other sites the density of this fibrosis is related to dose. For example, the incidence of non-malignant "frozen pelvis" following external irradiation rises with increasing dose, and the radiologically evident contraction that is seen in irradiated volumes of lung is similarly related. Contraction of the irradiated dermis is usually less obvious on casual inspection. In certain clinical situations it is often considered prudent to tattoo the skin at the corners of rectangular treatment fields in order to avoid overlap with a possible later adjacent treatment field. If the dimensions of the rectangle as defined by its four tattooed corners are measured 12–18 months after treatment, it is often found that they are 5%–10% less than the dimensions of the original field. Contraction is rarely of clinical significance where the dose to the dermis is not high, for instance following high-volume irradiation for seminoma or lymphoma. However, following treatments giving high dose to the skin (over 5000 cGy in 16 fractions over 20 days or its equivalent) care is needed in the application of a later closely adjacent field. Although skin will tolerate a second somewhat smaller treatment after a suitably long interval, beam divergence may lead to serious over-irradiation of subjacent structures. In practice the potential hazards of applying a closely adjacent field are often avoided.

Skin which has recovered from radiation injury appears to function quite well for long periods of time. Defects can be detected at a cell kinetic level in the epidermis, as a slight chronic hyperplasia in the non-keratinised layers. Also, the epidermis will withstand a second radiation treatment quite well although the dose has to be reduced. It is likely that the tissue elements responsible for the *late* effects in skin will not withstand such a large retreatment dose, since tissue repair is in general greatest in those tissues where the stem cells are rapidly renewed. After a tolerance treatment (i.e. a treatment leading to a 5% necrosis rate) with gamma or X-rays to rodent skin, the healed skin will commonly withstand a further 90% of the original dose. Skin recovered after a first dose also responds more severely to other cytotoxic agents, particularly actinomycin D and adriamycin, which are noted for this "recall" phenomenon. These agents (and radiation) express a latent residual injury present even in renewing tissues, so that even when the stem cells are renewed they are still partly defective.

Other Normal Tissues

Other renewing tissues than epidermis respond to radiation in a basically similar fashion.

In *gut epithelium* the stem cells are situated in the crypts of Lieberkühn near the basement membrane. After acute radiation injury, severe denudation of the epithelium is seen in mice by day 4 due to the rapid normal turnover of the epithelium. During fractionated treatments the turnover of the stem cells is substantially and quickly increased, more so than in epidermis, so that a very marked sparing effect is seen in gut epithelium with dose protraction. Late effects in gut, such as constriction and fistulae, are the expression of injury in slowly replaced stromal elements, which are not expected therefore to show the sparing effect resulting from regeneration during the treatment.

Mucosal reactions, where these can be readily observed as in the mouth and larynx, can be seen to pursue a similar sequence to that of the epidermis, but the time course is shorter. The transit time of mucosal cells is shorter than that of epidermal cells, and following an erythema like that found in skin, the submucosa is denuded several days earlier. A fractionated treatment with sufficiently large daily increments can result in a confluent mucosal pseudomembrane within 10–14 days of the commencement of treatment. This pseudomembrane consists of a layer of precipitated fibrin, and its yellow-white appearance is due to the entrapment of large numbers of leucocytes. It is fairly adherent to the submucosa, and to some extent protects it from bacterial invasion and chemical insult. Since mucosae are constantly moist, a crust does not ordinarily form, and the membrane retains some flexibility. Mucosal fibrinous reactions develop at different times at different sites, reflecting the normal wear and tear at each particular site. For example, hypopharyngeal membranous reactions develop days before those in the supraglottis.

Haemopoietic tissue, the classical tissue dependent on less than 1% complement of stem cells, is notably sensitive to radiation. This is due primarily to the high sensitivity of the stem cells, such that a large proportion are killed by quite moderate doses. This contrasts with the lower sensitivity of stem cells demonstrated in other tissues in mice, and the reason for this is unknown. The time course of the expression of damage is again dependent on the normal turnover of maturing cells. All three critical blood cell populations—erythrocytes, leucocytes, and platelets—are derived from the common ancestral stem cell, and their numbers will be depleted at different rates depending on their turnover time and on secondary factors such as haemorrhage. Lymphocytes are an exception to this; these mature cells are very sensitive to radiation and die in interphase, not by mitotic death. After high doses, death of the animal ensues variously from the depletion of one or more of the cell lineages among different species, usually within 3 weeks. There is little dose-rate effect with haemopoietic tissue, largely because of the high sensitivity of the stem cells at low doses. The effect of fractionation is substantial, but this is due mainly to a time factor, since the stem cells are capable of rapid repopulation after depletion. Late effects, seen as marrow hypoplasia, can result from environmental defects such as late vascular lesions after high local doses, or from a defect in the stem cells manifested by a reduced ability to renew themselves after whole-body irradiation. The stem cell defects are manifested to a larger extent following protracted injury, e.g. chronic or repeated irradiations, than after single doses. The stroma appears more radioresistant than the marrow it supports, partly owing to the radiosensitivity of its progenitor cells and partly owing to the slow rate of turnover of the stromal cell populations. Late damage does, however, occur following high doses to the stroma, as shown by its inability fully to support the growth of injected marrow stem cells.

Testis, very responsive to radiation, possesses spermatogenic stem cells on the periphery of the tubules, some of which in the mouse are as resistant as those in gastric or jejunal epithelium. The responsiveness of the testis rests largely on the fact that the Type A and B transit spermatogenic stages are particularly radiosensitive. Moreover, during fractionation the stem cells move into more sensitive phases of the cell cycle and do not multiply during most treatments.

It has been our practice to irradiate the remaining testis in the postoperative treatment of seminomas. After 3000 cGy in 20 fractions over 25 days, sterility is ultimately universal, although for many weeks the ejaculate may contain spermatozoa formed before irradiation was given. In addition, there is evidence of late Leydig cell failure, manifested by loss of libido and elevated luteinising hormone levels. Leydig cell failure may not occur till many years after irradiation.

The ovary, in contrast to the testis, has a germ cell population which is fixed at birth, and normally decays thereafter without replenishment. It has a spectrum of radiosensitivity dependent on the stage of follicular development. The oocyte is one of the most radiosensitive cells known, and like the lymphocyte, it undergoes interphase death. Therefore, in females, permanent sterility is produced by lower doses than in the male. Furthermore, hormonal deficiency is seen much sooner, often within 3 months, because no or very few oestrogen-producing corpora lutea are formed after irradiation. This latter circumstance is exploited in the management of dysfunctional uterine bleeding and in some cases of advanced breast cancer. In women over 40 years, a single dose of 500 cGy is usually adequate to abolish menstruation permanently within 2–3 months. In women under 40 years, 1500 cGy in four consecutive daily fractions is required.

Slowly proliferating tissues, such as *lung, thyroid, liver*, and the central nervous system, may not show striking early signs of injury, but later the defect in function becomes apparent and progressive. The response of lung to fractionated doses has been investigated in detail in the mouse. There is an effect of overall time for treatments up to about 14 days, with a time exponent of 0.07 (less than the 0.11 for skin). Whether this represents repopulation of target cells or an induced resistance is unknown. Many organs show a fractionation effect which is not precisely the same as for skin. Spinal cord, investigated in detail in the rat, shows a fractionation effect ($N^{0.4}$) greater than for skin, and a negligible effect of overall time until the latter is greater than 2 months (in the rat), after which proliferation of Schwann cells in the lumbosacral region participates in the recovery phenomenon. Severe injury to the spinal cord expressed as paralysis can originate from different lesions depending on the dose levels. After single doses in the range 2000–4000 cGy to the cervical cord, the latency period decreases with increasing dose (expected for a non-hierarchical cell population), and the primary lesion observed is demyelination and necrosis of the white matter, which is mainly attributed to damage to the oligodendrocytes. After lower doses which do not induce these changes, paralysis can develop after very long latency periods (similar to those in humans) probably as a result of vascular lesions. The vascular type of lesion in the central nervous system is dependent on blood pressure. Induced hypertension in rodents causes the vascular lesions to be more common, more severe, and of earlier onset than is the case in normotensive animals. In the lumbosacral region, the type of damage is different from that seen in the cervical cord, and the nerve roots are implicated. At high doses the nerve roots show demyelination and necrosis, attributed to damage to Schwann cells.

The *lens* is formed physiologically by the migration to its posterior pole of fibre-forming cells which arise in the anterior equatorial region, which is the only region of the lens to show mitotic activity, and which persists throughout life. Since it is not known what mechanism, if any, disposes of effete cells, the mechanism of cataract formation is also unknown. When the equatorial cells are irradiated, their progeny follow the normal migratory path, and if the radiation damage is sufficiently severe, the resulting fibres are opaque. The congregation of opaque material at the posterior pole results in a cataract. At low radiation doses, this opacity may regress, suggesting that there is indeed some mechanism for the removal of redundant material from the lens (see above). When only a sector of the equator has received radiation, the resultant cataract may be restricted to the corresponding segment of the lens. Human radiation cataracts may take months or many years to appear, reflecting the slow cell turnover in the avascular lens tissue. Below single doses of 200 cGy, cataracts do not form, but as the dose increases above this threshold, the likelihood of cataract formation increases, the latency decreases, and the cataracts themselves become more severe with a greater tendency to progression. Fractionation has a sparing effect, but when the total cumulative dose exceeds 1500 cGy, progressive cataract formation which seriously impairs vision is very likely. Total body irradiation can cause cataracts, implying that cataractogenesis can occur at the relatively low doses compatible with long-term human survival; most of the evidence for this comes from atomic bomb survivors, and in this situation the known high efficiency of neutrons for cataract formation may partly be responsible.

Tumours

Introduction

The clinically observed results of the radical X-ray treatment of tumours are as follows:

1) Complete and permanent disappearance, which may occur quickly or slowly.
2) Apparently complete disappearance with subsequent local recurrence.
3) Incomplete disappearance, i.e. residual tumour, or no discernible change in tumour volume. (Occasionally increase in tumour volume occurs during radiation treatment.)

All three outcomes are regularly observed at radiation dose levels compatible with acceptable structural and functional recovery in the unavoidably irradiated surrounding normal tissues, but equally, all three are seen at dose levels too high to be consistent with the survival of normal tissues.

Outcomes 2 and 3 above represent failure of treatment, for which radiobiological explanations are legitimately sought; other causes of failure, for instance "topographic miss" and inadequate or inhomogeneous dosage, are discussed in Chap. 5.

A tumour is a mixture of tissues, and although the presence of a tumour can be an acute discomfort, not all the tissue elements in the tumour tissue constitute a fatal threat to the patient. Indeed, in many commonly occurring curable tumours only a small percentage of the tumour's bulk consists of cells which can ultimately result in the patient's death. These cells are the clonogenic cells of the tumour, which are analogous to the clonogenic cells of normal tissues but which differ from them in certain very important respects. The potentially clonogenic cell population of a normal tissue responds in an orderly and controlled fashion to the demands placed upon it, whether this be the steady-state maintenance of dynamic equilibrium between cell loss and cell replacement, or the acutely accelerated activity following induction of unexpected high cell loss. Such order and control appear to be lacking in the clonogenic populations of tumours; whereas they certainly are subject to constraints on their proliferative behaviour, these constraints appear to operate in an almost exclusively passive manner. It is not known what purely tumour-related factors influence the proportion of potentially clonogenic cells that are actually in cycle, but it does appear that nutritional deprivation in parts of a tumour is associated with low or absent expression of proliferative capacity.

Tumour Vasculature

Stromate tumours produce angiogenic factors which induce the formation of a capillary vasculature within the tumour and its immediate vicinity. This vascular bed is derived from the pre-existing capillary network of the normal tissues in which the tumour arises, and therefore the blood supply to the tumour capillaries is delivered not at high pressure from the arteriolar end, as in the case of normal tissue capillaries, but from the low pressure capillary system of the pre-existing normal tissues.

However efficient the tumour angiogenesis factor is in producing new capillaries, and however luxuriant the provision of the new capillaries is, the *rate* of blood flow is determined and limited by the poor perfusion pressure available from the network from which the new vessels have arisen. The tumour capillary system is analogous to the portal systems found for example in the normal liver and pituitary; these normal portal capillary systems exist for physiological purposes, but are themselves inadequate to supply the nutritional requirements of the tissues that they perfuse, so that second additional capillary networks exist, which are fed from arteriolar supplies, thereby providing an alternative supply of adequately oxygenated blood. Tumours lack such an independent supplementary supply of blood, so that their perfusion rates (volume of blood/volume of tumour/time) depend almost exclusively on the ability of the pre-existing normal tissue capillary bed to dilate passively to accommodate the increased "run-off" presented by the new tumour capillary circulation. Occasionally this accommodation is striking, leading ultimately to recognisable hypertrophy and dilatation of the normal arteries and arterioles supplying the volume of tissue or organ in which the malignancy has arisen, as seen, for instance, in angiographic studies of osteogenic sarcomas. More usually, the accommodation is seriously inadequate, causing marked overall underperfusion of the tumour capillary network. This general underperfusion may be exaggerated by transient arteriovenous shunting in the tumour, producing a population of acutely hypoxic cells, and by local anatomical features in the capillary bed itself. For example, some tumour capillaries have a cross-sectional area many times that of a normal capillary. When dilation occurs, the volume of flow may increase whilst the linear rate is diminished. This situation becomes very inefficient in terms of extraction of molecules from within the blood stream of dilated capillaries. Also, the combination of low perfusion pressure and local dilatation of particular vessels leads to a low linear rate of flow. Accordingly, the almost stagnant blood in giant capillaries is soon rendered anoxic and after an interval, large populations of tumour cells in the immediate vicinity undergo irreversible changes leading to cell death.

Necrosis

Focal microscopic necrosis occurs when several capillaries surround and supply an increasing volume of tumour. When the separation of the capillaries becomes greater than 300–400 μm, necrosis will appear in the centre. The necrotic focus will then increase in size as cell proliferation proceeds around the capillaries and more cells move subsequently into the necrotic centre but the thickness of the viable tumour shell does not exceed 150–200 μm. Focal necrosis can also be seen with invasive tumours at the tumour/normal tissue interface, where microscopic fingerlike extensions from the bulk of the tumour project into and invade the well-vascularised surrounding normal tissue. In this case the focal necrosis can appear as a central core of necrosis.

Cylindrical microscopic necrosis is observed as the classical tumour cord, where tumour cells are growing around a capillary which forms the central axis of the cord. Necrosis appears around the periphery when the radius of the cord is again 150–200 μm. Capillaries deep inside tumours may have a low blood flow, and hence in these cases the thickness of viable tumour from the capillary could be reduced. The growth rate of tumours varies considerably. The two main factors determining growth rate are the rate of division of the clonogenic cells and the proportion of the progeny of cell division which continue to proliferate. This proportion is reduced by differentiation, by aberrant divisions due to chromosomal defects, and to malnutrition mediated by the environment. There is evidence in some tumours of an origin from a single cell and that growth rate is approximately exponential, i.e. the volume doubles sequentially in equal times, over much of the early growth of a tumour. During this period the tumour develops its own vascular network. When tumours become large, their growth rate slows down, largely because of an inability of the new vascular supply to support the large volumes of such tissue, as already discussed.

Radiation Response

The *responsiveness* of a tumour to radiation depends, as does that of a normal tissue, on the normal kinetics of cell turnover (see "Gross Response of Tissues—General Considerations" above). The responsiveness is different from the *radiosensitivity* of a tumour, which can be measured by the dose required to control it almost permanently. The latter depends on the number and sensitivity of the target cells, i.e. those cells which can reproduce themselves almost indefinitely and from which the tumour can regrow. Many responsive tumours are of epithelial origin, e.g. seminomas and carcinomas, and these are tumours which shrink more rapidly than others after, and often during, treatment. It should be noted that the word sensitivity was used instead of responsiveness in the early era of radiotherapy. The present terminology is used to conform to current convention, which has largely been instigated through experimental work. Tumour sensitivity can be assessed in the short term by growth delay and in the long term by tumour control or cure. The rate of regression of a tumour is not a measure of sensitivity since it is determined by the cell kinetics in a particular tumour. However, the later regeneration is caused by a repopulation of surviving cells and hence the time delay in the regrowth of the tumour to its original size is largely a measure of the initial sensitivity of the clonogenic cells. The rate of regrowth of a tumour is often slower after irradiation, particularly after high doses, and this has been shown in mouse tumours to be due variously to a residual effect in the surviving clonogenic cells and also to a "tumour bed effect" where the stroma and vasculature are also damaged by the treatment. In addition, the dose necessary to control or cure a tumour is a measure both of clonogenic cell number and clonogenic cell sensitivity. The sensitivity can also be estimated using xenografts, i.e. grafts in different species, usually human tumour explants growing in immune-suppressed mice. Some tumours, particularly melanomas and osteosarcomas, are often described as being inherently radioresistant. Moreover, there is evidence for a considerable effect of fractionation with human melanoma, more marked than for skin. The resistance and fractionation effect have been claimed by some, but not all, to be mirrored by the striking resistance of these tumour cells to low doses, and other factors probably contribute.

The question of whether clonogenic cells in tumours are inherently more sensitive than their normal tissue counterparts is still not answered satisfactorily, because of the difficulty in making comparable measurements. There is evidence that clonogenic cells in some solid tumours in mice are more sensitive at low doses than are the stem cells responsible for skin reactions, but more evidence is required for other tumours and normal tissues. At the high single doses which are needed to cure tumours there is considerable evidence that higher doses are required than would be expected on theoretical grounds to sterilise all the clonogenic cells. The nature of tumour resistance has been under study for 50 years, and effective methods for dealing with it have not yet been found. One feature of solid tumours which has dominated the study of tumour resistance is the presence of the severely hypoxic cells described above. Such cells are known to require up to three times as much dose to kill them. Cells on the periphery of tumour cords, normally doomed in the kinetic growth pattern, are moving into the necrotic zone, and will be some of the most resistant cells in the tumour. Although these cells would be of no consequence after radiation if the oxygen supply through the cell layers was unchanged before the hypoxic but viable cells had moved into the dead necrotic zone, unfortunately this does not seem to occur completely. It is considered that the ultimately sterilised but still metabolically competent oxygenated cells cease using oxygen at the same rate, thus releasing some oxygen which diffuses further through the layers and "reoxygenates" and rescues the resistant hypoxic cells. Many experiments with murine tumours have demonstrated the presence of about 10% severely hypoxic cells, but the actual percentage varies widely between tumour types. The failure of single doses to cure all but the smallest human tumours supports the hypothesis that hypoxic cells are an important determinant of the outcome of treatment. At present, the most convincing demonstration of the presence of radiotherapeutically important hypoxic cells in human tumours has been the ability of oxygen-mimicking electron-affinic compounds to reduce substantially the single radiation dose required for delay of tumour regrowth of subcutaneous metastatic nodules. Average intra-tumour oxygen tensions can be measured and these rise during fractionated treatments, so that the predicted phenomenon of reoxygenation does indeed occur during fractionation. This has been used as an argument in favour of prolonged treatments, but in practice a rise in intra-tumour oxygen tension throughout treatment is a poor predictor of ultimate local tumour control, and short treatments (2–3 weeks) are capable of achieving tumour control rates at least equal to those obtained with more protracted regimens (5–7 weeks). The reason for the poor correlation between tumour oxygen tension and tumour control is likely to be that the important factor is the oxygen tension in the microenvironment of the clonogenic cells, rather than the average oxygen tension in the tumour as a whole. It has been suggested that reoxygenation is linked to the rate of regression of tumour volume during treatment, implying that it is related to the dynamic histology of the tumour. It is true that in some situations a rapid reduction in tumour bulk is associated with superior local tumour control, but conversely, excellent results are regularly achieved in other situations in which the primary tumour appears to alter little or not at all during the course of treatment. For example, many easily observed oral and oropharyngeal tumours seemingly change little in size from the commencement to the conclusion of their course of irradiation, yet their ultimate total disappearance is commonplace. This appears to disprove the view that reoxygenation caused by cell removal is a major determinant of radiocurability. However, comparatively trivial or unnoticed reduction in the dimensions of a tumour can be associated with substantial reduction in its volume. For example, a 2-cm-diameter spherical tumour which shrinks to a 1.8-cm-diameter sphere has lost no less than 27% of its volume. Clinically, the detection of such a small change in tumour diameter is rarely possible, particularly in the presence of a fibrinous mucosal reaction, so that quite large changes in tumour volume frequently go unrecognised. In larger tumours, shrinkage can be obvious to the naked eye, and in Stages IIB and III of cancer of the cervix, when good resolution has occurred following external irradiation, the ultimate results are better than when tumour resolution has been poor. This is cited as evidence that reoxygenation is important in radiotherapy, but it is equally arguable that only those cervical tumours which have shrunken considerably have the volume and configuration which make them vulnerable to the nearly ideal dose distribution that their subsequent intracavitary treatment provides (see Chap. 11). At present there remains a real possibility that temporarily hypoxic tumour cells may be an important cause of local failure of treatment, but past clinical attempts to demonstrate this (i.e. hyperbaric oxygen and fast neutron therapy) have failed to provide convincing evidence, and hypoxic cell sensitisers have yet to do so. (See the section entitled "Adjuvants" below.) Hyperbaric oxygen failed to fulfil its promise for four main reasons:

1) Only a relatively small amount of "extra" oxygen can be carried in a simple solution in the blood, haemoglobin being virtually saturated at normal temperature and pressure.
2) Even luxuriantly vascular tumours usually have regions of feeble perfusion, which the little extra available oxygen cannot reach.
3) The toxicity of hyperbaric oxygen prevents sufficiently prolonged saturation of the patient's tumour.
4) Several normal tissues are slightly hypoxic, including laryngeal cartilage which is avascular. Accordingly, normal tissue reactions were enhanced with hyperbaric oxygen, and tumour doses to the larynx had to be reduced by 10%. A reduction in tumour dose might not have been disadvantageous were reasons 1, 2, and 3 above not true, but unfortunately they are.

The failure of hyperbaric oxygen may appear to be an example of the limited value of "predictive" radiobiology (see beginning of chapter), but this may not be so. Hyperbaric oxygen failed possibly because it did not achieve its primary objective, that is, the delivery of substantially increased amounts of oxygen to the clonogenic cells in tumours before irradiation.

Guides to tumour prognosis have not been widely used, but one technique involved tumour histology during treatment. In well-differentiated tumours, an increase in the proportion of differentiated cells was seen for the majority of tumours that responded well to radiotherapy. Whether this reflects a direct effect of radiation on the rate of differentiation and hence effectively an induced death of tumour cells, or whether differentiation is simply the course normally taken by such a sterilised cell, is still unknown.

Special Situations

Changes in Dose Rate

The early and continuing success from the use of radium and its substitutes in intracavitary and interstitial treatments suggests that the low-dose-rate treatments (i.e. of the order of 1–5 cGy/min) may confer special benefits in terms of tumour control. Equally, in this Institute we believe that under certain circumstances low-dose-rate treatments can be very advantageous in terms of the sparing of normal tissues. For example, although lip cancer can be equally well controlled by a radioactive cobalt mould (lose dose rate) and by fractionated orthovoltage treatment (high dose rate), the late cosmetic and functional results of the former treatment are unarguably superior. The previously described cellular dose-rate effects do not themselves adequately explain the apparent advantages of low-dose-rate treatment. In the case of early carcinoma of the cervix or carcinoma of the tongue, it may be that the physical distribution of dose between malignant and adjacent normal tissues is so favourable that higher doses can be given to the tumour than would be possible with external photon-beam treatments. Since high-precision beam-directed megavoltage X-ray treatments can reproduce almost identical distributions of radiation reactions to those resulting from interstitial implants, and since the time course of the healing of these reactions is not dissimilar, dose distribution advantages are unlikely to be the important explanation of the apparent superiority of low-dose-rate treatments. Nor do dose distribution considerations explain the superiority, in terms of normal tissue sparing, of low-dose-rate treatments of the skin; the dose distribution from a radioactive lip mould (see Chap. 7) is in fact somewhat inferior to that achieved by a well-planned lead-shielded orthovoltage treatment. The efficacy of low-dose-rate treatments in sterilising malignancies and in sparing normal tissues is very probably an expression of several phenomena: (1) Dormant normal tissue stem cells have a capacity to respond to the need for recruitment into an actively dividing role within the time-span of the period of irradiation, while the malignant clonogenic cells are unable to respond in a similar fashion. (2) Some phases of the cell cycle are relatively insensitive to radiation. For cells in late S phase the mean lethal dose can be nearly three times that for cells in M and late G1. This cell-cycle-dependent radiosensitivity is not known to be consistently different for normal and malignant cells, but in a protracted (168-h) treatment at low dose rate, it is likely that some malignant clonogenic cells will be exposed to radiation during their most sensitive phases of the cell-cycle which otherwise would have escaped such exposure during intermittent short-duration high-dose-rate treatments. This may also be true of the normal tissue stem cells, but as noted in (1) above, there are other normal tissue reparative responses which influence the ultimate effect. (3) Some evidence suggests that at low dose rates hypoxic cells are less protected from lethal effects than at high dose rates because repair of radiation damage is a metabolic process which is abolished by prolonged anoxia. (4) There may be a difference in the repair capability of normal cells compared with their malignant neighbours.

Afterloading techniques are increasingly employed for intracavitary treatments in gynaecological malignancy, and the design of the apparatus used for non-manual afterloading often dictates that an increase in dose rate occurs. The increase may be relatively small ("low-dose-rate" techniques, e.g. the Selectron) or quite large ("high-dose-rate" techniques, e.g. the Cathetron). The application of dose corrections for changes in dose rate is uncertain. Experimental evidence suggests that bigger reductions in dose are required than seem to be necessary clinically, and this may be a reflection of the fact that the conventional radium system doses were and are comfortably within the upper limits of tolerance. Certainly, low dose rates should be more effective in sparing small-bowel mucosa, because of the notable ability of its constituent clonogenic cells to repair radiation damage. (See also Chap. 11.)

Fast Neutron Therapy

Patients were first treated with fast neutrons in the United States in the late 1930s, but the treatment was abandoned because the late normal tissue effects were severe and seemingly out of proportion to the severity of the early effects. In the mid 1960s fast neutrons were tried again in London, because it was by then known that cell killing by densely ionising radiations is less dependent on the presence of oxygen than is the case with sparsely ionising radiation, i.e. gamma rays or X-rays. This is because the primary reactions occur within the dense tracks and oxygen has insufficient access to enhance the reactive radiation products in the short time available. Accordingly, if hypoxic tumour cells were a real therapeutic problem, they would be less so with neutrons. Moreover, it was realised that the fractionated doses given in the original treatments had been too high, because they were based on X-ray/neutron comparisons carried out mainly after single doses. Densely ionising radiations cause relatively less sublethal damage than X-rays, so that less repair can take place, and the effects of fractionation on dose (see section on fractionation in the discussion of skin response above) are reduced. For example, the exponent of N in the formula given is reduced from 0.24 to 0.04. Hence, with increasing fractionation the total X-ray dose required for a given effect increases much more than does the total neutron dose. One consequence of this is that once a tolerance dose has been established for a fractionated course of neutrons, it can be used reasonably safely for other fractionation schedules, say from 2 to 16 fractions. At this Institute the 14.7-MeV neutron beam (deuterium/tritium reaction) has not been employed in schedules of more than 15 or 16 fractions, because apart from the direct comparison with similar X-ray schedules, there is some advantage in limiting both the number of fractions and the overall treatment time, since intracellular repair is minimal and fast neutron treatments are less dependent on reoxygenation during fractionation. Fast neutrons deposit most of their energy by displacing protons from hydrogen nuclei, and the absorbed dose in different tissues depends on the relative abundance of hydrogen within these tissues. Substantially higher ionisation occurs in subcutaneous fat and in tissue of the central nervous system tissue than in skin or lean muscle, whereas ionisation in bone is much lower. This means that tolerance doses determined at one site cannot necessarily be applied safely to different sites. The only safe course is to determine the tolerance dose for the late effects site by site, bearing in mind that if the results of treatment are to be compared with other forms of radiation treatment, equivalence of morbidity must be assured by the use of two neutron dose levels. Cells which have a high capacity to repair sublethal damage, such as some melanoma cells and the epithelial clonogenic cells in the small bowel, are relatively resistant to fast neutrons. Neutrons are reputed to be relatively efficient at controlling deposits of human malignant melanoma, but the long-term effects of high-dose neutron irradiation on human small bowel are not yet known, and could prove to be more severe than expected.

Re-irradiation of previously irradiated tumour-bearing volumes is unusual at this Institute. Such retreatments should certainly not be given following neutron therapy, because long-term recovery of radiation tolerance is less than with photons.

Adjuvants

Many drugs used in protocols with radiation are in principle simply additive, so that more cells are killed. Other drugs, such as actinomycin D and adriamycin, interact with the radiation injury and have a greater effect than expected from the sum of the effects of each agent. Such effects are due largely to the interaction with the DNA and associated repair mechanisms when treatments are at tolerance levels, and these adjuvants can only be of benefit if they differentially affect tumour and normal tissue. That may arise for example from differences in drug access or cellular repair capability, but this is only partly established empirically in practice. Many adjuvants perturb the cell cycle, inducing varying degrees of synchrony, and the eventual outcome can markedly depend on the sequence and time intervals in combined treatments. This is very clearly demonstrated in many experimental systems, and although there is as yet no clinical evidence for the importance of those factors, combined modality treatments should always be standardised with respect to sequence and timing.

Another class of drug adjuvants has been designed specifically to interact with radiation effects on hypoxic cells, and these agents are known as radiosensitisers. They act in a broad sense like oxygen, but none is as efficient as oxygen. They probably act slightly differently in the primary stages of radiation action, and these mechanisms are currently under study. Radiosensitisers are designed to replace the techniques of limb tourniquets and hyperbaric oxygen, which were both designed to equalise the oxygen tension in the clonogenic cells in tumours and in normal tissues, i.e. effectively to remove the potential problem of resistant hypoxic cells in tumours. Chemical sensitisers are considered better than oxygen because they are not metabolised by the tumour tissue between the capillary and the hypoxic cells. The two sensitisers which, at the time of writing, have been tried clinically, metronidazole and the more efficient misonidazole, both have toxicity which has limited their dosage (in particular neurotoxicity after misonidazole) and hence limited the anticipated benefits.

Particular attention must be paid, when these agents are used, to any sensitisation of normal tissues, particularly for radiation treatments truly at tolerance dose levels. A 10% reduction in dose was considered necessary with hyperbaric oxygen treatments when laryngeal cartilage was irradiated, and a smaller but not insignificant reduction in dose may similarly be necessary with efficient chemical sensitisers. An old modality now receiving considerable attention experimentally is heat or hyperthermia. A temperature of 43–44 °C (6–7 °C above body core temperature) is severely lethal to cells, and moderately elevated temperatures of 41–43 °C are sufficient to increase markedly the radiation response of cells. Tumours with a relatively poor blood supply will be heated more than their neighbouring normal tissues. Also, cells synthesising their genetic components and cells nutritionally deprived are more sensitive to heat, in contrast to their greater resistance to radiation, and hence hyperthermia is a promising adjuvant for the future. Unfortunately, the temperature is critical, and only 0.5 °C at lethal temperatures can make a vast difference to the response. Hence the problem of heat deliverance, blood flow, and temperature measurement, make the application difficult, but optimistically not insuperable with developing technology.

Whole-Body Irradiation

There are three classical modes of death from whole-body irradiation. At very high doses in excess of 10 000 cGy, death occurs within hours as a result of cerebrovascular disturbances. At lower doses not inducing death within 36 h, down to about 1000 cGy, death occurs at 4–10 days owing to a denudation of the intestinal mucosa. Death results from a massive loss of fluid, electrolytes, and proteins into the gastrointestinal tract, causing circulatory failure. At lower doses not inducing this effect, down to about 400 cGy in man, death ensues between the third and eighth weeks from bone marrow failure. The whole-body radiation dose which leads to the deaths of 50% of humans within 60 days following an acute exposure of X-rays or gamma rays is thought to be in the range of 400–450 cGy. This dose is called the LD 50/60. Survival is more likely if the individual is female, in the middle period of life, and is allowed to recover at rest in a hospital environment.

In therapeutic whole-body irradiation designed to ablate the marrow before grafting, doses considerably in excess of the LD 50/60 are required. In order to spare the other sensitive tissues at risk, i.e. the lung and the intestine, low-dose-rate treatments are given. This approach exploits the lower dose-rate effect demonstrated by marrow compared with most other tissues. The differential sparing effect arises from the different properties of the stem cells in these tissues. Other effects of whole-body irradiation, such as life shortening, oncogenesis, cataractogenesis, and genetic effects, are long-term problems of secondary importance when dealing with patients with malignant disease.

Further Reading

For deeper understanding of the general aspects covered in this chapter, the reader is referred to the following brief bibliography.

General Radiobiology for the Radiotherapist

Hall EJ (1978) Radiobiology for the radiologist. Harper and Row, New York

The Radiobiology of Tissues

Selected chapters in: Potten CS, Hendry JH (eds) (1983) Cytotoxic insult to tissues: effects on cell lineages. Churchill Livingstone, Edinburgh

Tumours

Kallman RF, Rockwell S (1977) Effects of radiation on animal tumour models. In: Becker FF (ed) Cancer, vol 6, p 225. Plenum, New York

New Treatments

Neutrons

Catterall M, Bewley DK (1979) Fast neutrons in the treatment of cancer. Academic Press, and Grune and Stratton, New York

Hyperthermia

Hahn GM (1982) Hyperthermia and cancer. Plenum Press, New York.

Radiosensitisers

Adams GE (1977) Hypoxic cell sensitisers for radiotherapy. In: Becker FF (ed) Cancer, vol 6, p 181. Plenum, New York

3 Principles of Chemotherapy

P. M. Wilkinson and B. W. Fox

Introduction

The principles underlying the administration of cytotoxic drugs for the treatment of malignant disease differ fundamentally from those of bacterial, fungal, or antiviral infections in that it is not possible to administer a drug that is toxic only to the tumour and therefore some adverse affects on the host are inevitable. The therapeutic ratio is often close to unity and in such circumstances treatment must produce some toxicity in order to induce a worthwhile regression of the tumour. Similarly, the difference between successful therapy and severe or even fatal iatrogenic effects may depend on only minor dose adjustments. It is of the utmost importance therefore to understand those factors which influence response to therapy.

Cell Cycle

The phases of the cell cycle are shown in Fig. 3.1. Two aspects are of direct relevance to therapy: (1) the individual stages and (2) doubling time of individual tumours.

Individual Stages of Cell Cycle

The majority of cytotoxic drugs act on the S phase only, that is the period of DNA synthesis, and for this reason they are often referred to as cycle phase specific drugs. The response to an S phase drug is directly related to the number of cells in S at any moment of time. Thus, if a 10-cm mass in log-phase growth contains 90% of cells in S, considerable tumour regression will be observed after the

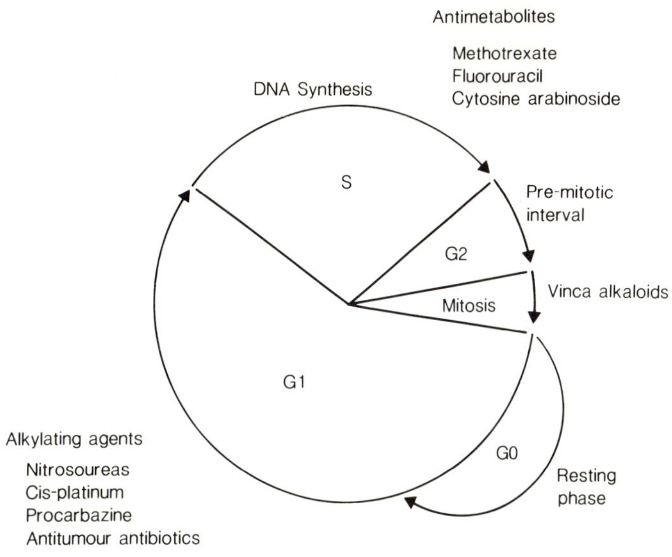

Fig. 3.1. The cell cycle.

administration of a single course of treatment, with possible disappearance of the mass after two courses. However, there will always be a proportion of cells not in S phase and therefore it is theoretically impossible to achieve total resolution with this particular type of drug. Conversely, in a tumour containing only 5% of cells in S, treatment will produce virtually no resolution as at any time only 5% of cells are capable of response. Thus, other drugs must be given if substantial tumour reduction is to be achieved. It is therefore important to know in any particular tumour what fraction of cells are in the S phase as this will clearly help in selecting the type of drug or drug combination to be administered. Until recently this has largely been an empirical choice but the introduction of new techniques has allowed a more objective assessment of the cycle characteristics of any tumour. The cytofluorograph will produce a visual display of the proportion of cells in each phase. An example is shown in Fig. 3.2 and by computational analysis this can be improved to provide a 3D image. Using these techniques it is now possible to plan a more logical treatment and critically to assess the response obtained. This is important because a drug treatment which is capable of inducing a remission will require modification to achieve long-term control and possibly cure.

An alternative approach is to interrupt the cell cycle at a particular stage so that, when released, a substantially greater fraction of the tumour will contain an increased proportion of S-phase cells thereby allowing an S-phase-specific drug to be more effective. For example, the administration of bleomycin by continuous infusion is one means of arresting the cell at the G2 interphase and when this treatment is discontinued a greater proportion of cells will enter the S phase. There are, however, difficulties with this technique, the most important being that synchronisation of normal host cells also occurs, notably in the bone marrow and gastrointestinal tract, and this therefore potentiates drug toxicity. Current research is being directed towards better means of synchronising the tumour but not normal host tissues.

Whilst there is some debate as to whether a resting phase exists, the G0 or resting cell offers a plausible explanation for late relapses and apparent resistance. Such cells are analogous to spore-forming bacteria, being far more resistant to drug action when in this phase of the cycle. The factors that ultimately influence cells to resume cycling are not known, but current thought might suggest an immunological mechanism.

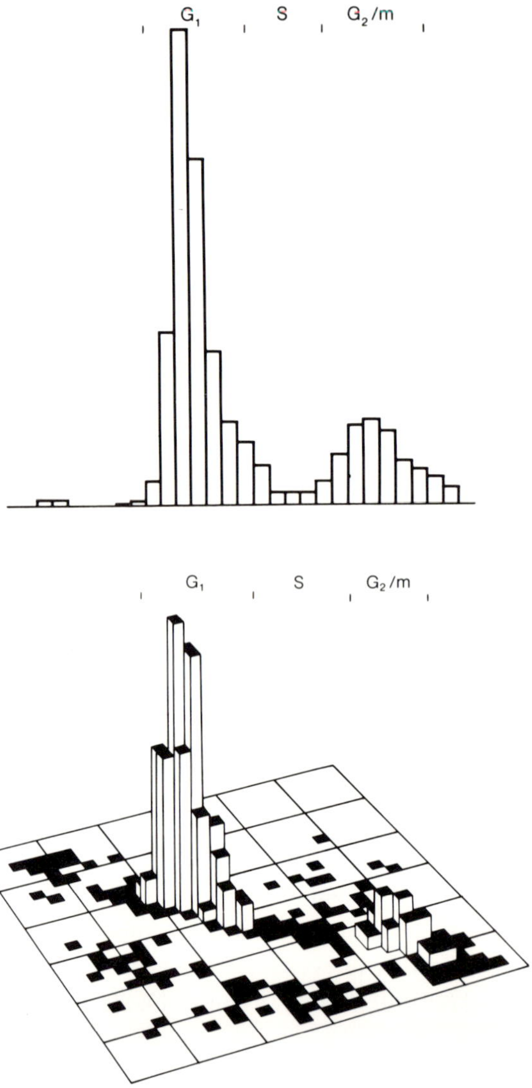

Fig. 3.2. Computational enhancement of cytofluorographic analysis. The upper figure illustrates the conventional histogram illustrating the proportion of cells in the respective stages of the cell cycle; the lower figure is a 3D enhancement showing that the majority of cells are in G1 with none present in S.

Doubling Time

In general terms tumours with a fast doubling time have a greater proportion of cells in S and slow-growing tumours substantially less. The doubling time of Burkett's lymphoma, for example, is 1 day and this is reflected in its rapid response to therapy. Conversely, relapse, when it does occur, is equally rapid. Slow-growing tumours may show initially no response to therapy, but with perseverance gradual resolution of the tumour will occur and it may be some time before a relapse develops. Whilst it would be useful therefore to know the doubling time of any tumour before commencing therapy, it is generally not possible to achieve this because the majority of human tumours cannot be grown in tissue culture, and for those that can, the necessary techniques and equipment are out of reach of all except the most highly specialised centres.

The mass doubling time of a tumour depends upon the number of dividing cells in a tumour mass and both human and animal tumours have a Gompertzian growth (Fig. 3.3). The initial period

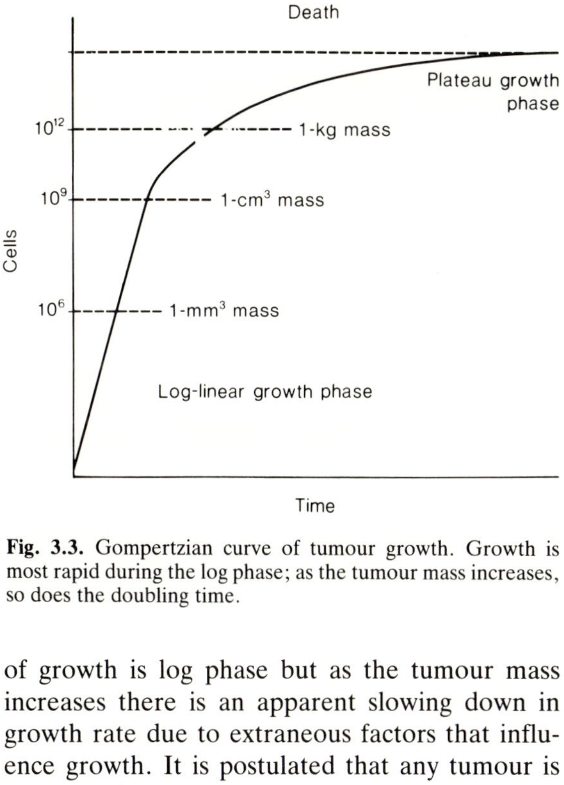

Fig. 3.3. Gompertzian curve of tumour growth. Growth is most rapid during the log phase; as the tumour mass increases, so does the doubling time.

of growth is log phase but as the tumour mass increases there is an apparent slowing down in growth rate due to extraneous factors that influence growth. It is postulated that any tumour is most sensitive to drug therapy during the initial phase of growth and this certainly holds true for animal tumours. In animal systems small numbers of cells can be successfully eradicated with drug combinations that are unsuccessful if a more substantial mass is present. For any given tumour, the clinical stage at presentation is important, therapy being most effective when the tumour burden is minimal.

Tumour Burden

Substantial claims have been made in recent years relating to the problem of tumour burden versus response. The situation in acute leukaemia is illustrated in diagrammatic form in Fig. 3.4. It is

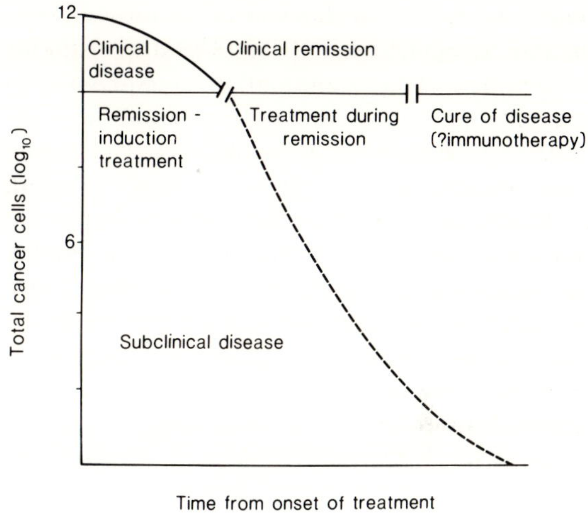

Fig. 3.4. Course of successful treatment of acute leukaemia. (Adapted from Frei 1972).

generally accepted that a minimal tumour burden of 10^{10} cells must be present before the patient experiences symptoms of sufficient severity to urge him to seek medical advice, and indeed, the majority of patients have a burden of 10^{12} cells before advice is sought. After successful therapy, the patient enters complete remission and at this stage there is no clinical evidence of disease, all previous abnormal radiological, haematological, and biochemical parameters having returned to normal. However, when this stage is reached, there may still remain in the body a residue of 10^9 cells and clearly these must be completely eradicated if there is to be any hope of cure. Herein lies the dilemma facing the chemotherapist, since it is not known how many courses are required completely to eradicate all tumour cells. Also, if S-phase-specific drugs are used alone or in combination, a complete cure can never result. It is assumed but not proven that if the cell population could be reduced to less than 10^4 then a different drug combination would thereafter be necessary to eradicate disease. It was hoped that immune stimulants would be capable of eradicating small tumour burdens of 10^4 or less, but regrettably the initial promise of early trials of immunotherapy in acute leukaemia has not been substantiated. In animal experiments it is possible to eradicate many solid tumours completely when small numbers of cells are present but not when this number is exceeded. This evidence is put forward by the proponents of adjuvant therapy as a rationale for giving treatment early rather than waiting until overt recurrence declares itself. However, this cannot be applied to all tumours since patients presenting with substantial lymphomatous tumours may show dramatic response to chemotherapy while with other solid tumours a small, 5-mm metastasis can often prove totally resistant to treatment. Clearly, other equally important biological factors must be taken into consideration to explain these wide variations in response. As a general rule, however, for one particular tumour type the most favourable response and prognosis is seen in those patients who present with small tumour burdens.

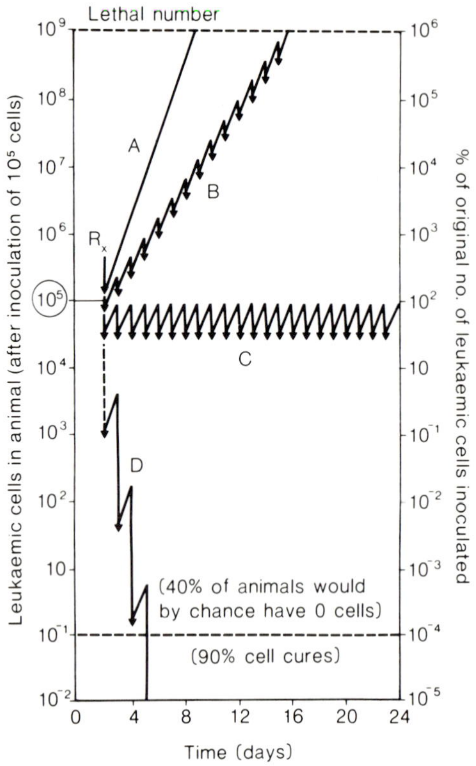

Fig. 3.5. Differential response of experimental leukaemia to chemotherapy. Mice inoculated on day 0 with 10^5 leukaemia cells and different treatment schedules administered on day 2. Treatment D represents curative therapy. (From Skipper 1965)

Theoretical Response to Drugs

Whatever the type of tumour requiring treatment there are three possible responses to therapy, which are illustrated in Fig. 3.5. Here mice have been inoculated with 10^5 leukaemic cells and the response to treatment has been measured. Untreated animals (group A) die on day 8 because the lethal tumour burden is reached; this is the situation also with a tumour that is totally resistant to the drug therapy. Animals in group B have received a treatment which only partly reduces the tumour burden, and by the time a further dose is given, the tumour has already increased to beyond its pretreatment size. Cell proliferation increases and the lethal number in this particular experiment is reached on day 16 when the animals die. This, however, represents a doubling of the survival time which, if translated to a slow-growing tumour with a doubling time of, for example, 150–200 days (commonly seen in breast cancer), may represent an increase in useful life of 2–3 years. Group C illustrates stable disease where the tumour burden is constant and therapy holds the disease for an indeterminate time. This situation is common in the chronic leukaemias and some lymphomas. Eventually escape from therapy occurs due to the emergence of a drug-resistant strain, or the disease transforms to a more malignant type. Treatment D is clearly the most effective but unfortunately is seen only in the rare human malignancies such as acute lymphoblastic leukaemia, lymphomas, and Hodgkin's disease. Here each course of treatment results in a substantial reduction in tumour mass and ultimately a cure is achieved. It is probable, even in this situation, that when only 1–10 cells remain the residue is removed by an alternative, probably immune, mechanism.

Drug Resistance

Even with successful treatment, relapses are unfortunately all too common and this is due to the emergence of drug-resistant strains. Drug resistance develops in tumour cells in a very similar manner to that in bacteria, for example, by emergence of new biochemical pathways, changes in the permeability of the cell wall, or increased synthesis of a new enzyme. Some cells are resistant from the outset and therapy simply eradicates the sensitive cells and leaves the resistant strain to multiply. The introduction of combination chemotherapy by administering different drugs with different mechanisms of action is one means of overcoming the problem of drug resistance.

Pharmacological Factors

Assuming that the tumour is chemosensitive, a number of pharmacological factors can influence the response to therapy.

Dose Response

In many situations the pharmacologist is able to evaluate scientifically the dose-response relationship that exists between the drug and the effector cell. An example is shown in Fig. 3.6. No response is seen with small doses, but as the dose is increased in a logarithmic manner there exists a

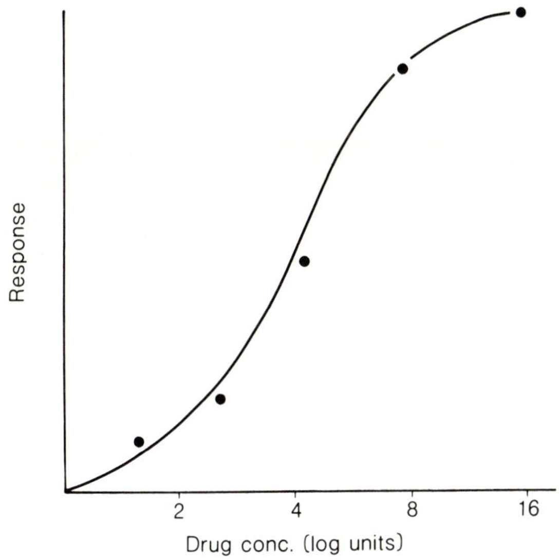

Fig. 3.6. The dose-response curve.

period when there is a direct relationship between the dose and the end organ response. Finally, when all receptor sites are saturated no further dose increase alters the response. The slope of the response curve may be steep or shallow and this is directly related to the sensitivity of the cells to the drug. Animal experiments in vivo, whilst seeking to establish a dose-response relationship for cytotoxic drugs, do not generally result in the type of curve illustrated. The top portion cannot be reached because animals die of toxicity before the optimal tumour response can be observed. It is possible, however, with such systems to evaluate whether the curve is steep or shallow, and from this, useful practical information can be applied to the treatment of disease in man. Figure 3.7 shows

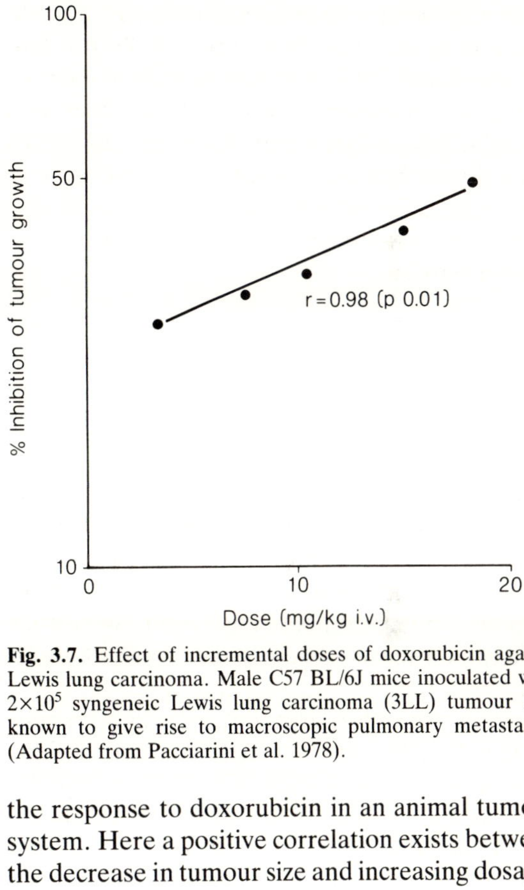

Fig. 3.7. Effect of incremental doses of doxorubicin against Lewis lung carcinoma. Male C57 BL/6J mice inoculated with 2×10^5 syngeneic Lewis lung carcinoma (3LL) tumour line known to give rise to macroscopic pulmonary metastases. (Adapted from Pacciarini et al. 1978).

the response to doxorubicin in an animal tumour system. Here a positive correlation exists between the decrease in tumour size and increasing dosage. The curve is shallow, which implies that dose increments must be large to produce substantial increases in the response. Thus, in this example a 10-fold dose increase was necessary to increase the response from 30% to 50%. If this were translated to, for example, human breast cancer, then a 10-fold dose increment would be necessary to increase the response by 20%. Clearly this could not be introduced in clinical practice as this increase would produce fatal toxicity. Therefore, for breast cancer an alternative means must be sought to improve the response. On the other hand if a steep dose-response relationship exists then doubling the dose may have a very real advantage by increasing the response and in some instances converting a partial to a complete response.

Drug Distribution

A finite intracellular concentration of drug is necessary to bring about the intracellular effects which result in cell death, which implies that drug must reach the cell in an adequate concentration. For practical purposes the body can be divided into two compartments: a central compartment representing blood and extracellular fluid and a peripheral or tissue compartment. Drug must gain access to the central compartment before it can reach the tissues, and there are a number of physiological parameters that then determine the proportion of drug that reaches the peripheral compartment.

A drug can be administered to the central compartment either by mouth or parenterally. Oral administration is obviously preferable for the patient, but one must consider patient compliance and the degree of absorption before concluding that a drug may be ineffective. Assuming that the patient is taking the drug, then absorption may be dose-dependent, as illustrated in Fig. 3.8. With small doses, absorption is complete since methotrexate is absorbed by an active transport process. If the dose is increased then this process becomes saturated, so that further dose increments do not increase the proportion of drug absorbed, and the concentration in the central and therefore in the peripheral compartment cannot increase. Any protocol therefore which includes methotrexate in a dose that requires administration by mouth could be invalidated by failing to have reliable evidence that the drug is absorbed satisfactorily. Fortunately, from a pharmacological point of view, the majority of cytotoxic drugs are administered intravenously, either because they are not absorbed from the gastrointestinal tract or because they are so irritant that administration by mouth is not tolerated. Therefore, one is certain that the drug reaches at least the central compartment. However, the ultimate processes that result in drug reaching the peripheral compartment are complex. Drug metabolism, cell permeability, the size of the drug molecule, and the degree of ionisation all influence the passage of the drug into the cell. Although much information on intracellular transport can be obtained from tissue and animal experiments, the transport of drug into a tumour in humans is a neglected area and there is little if any information as to which are the most important factors that influence drug transport in man.

Protein Binding

A drug that is bound to protein is inactive. In the protein-bound state it cannot be metabolised or excreted, nor can it diffuse into another compart-

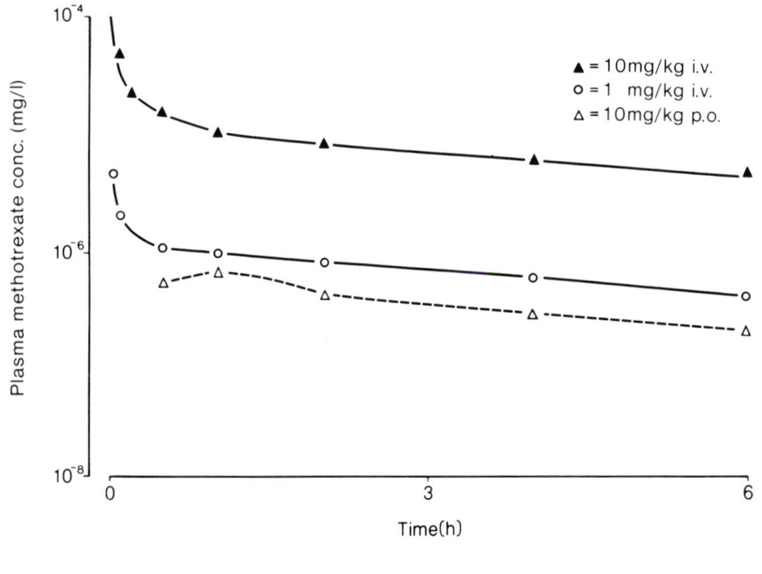

Fig. 3.8. Plasma methotrexate concentration contrasting the administration of 1 and 10 mg/kg p.o. or i.v. 10 mg/kg p.o. results in the same concentration/time curve as 1 mg/kg i.v. (From Henderson et al. 1965).

ment. The weakly acidic drugs, for example methotrexate, are most affected. The concurrent administration of a similar class of drug (for example, salicylates, sulphonamides, anticoagulants), result in a situation where one drug competes with the other for the binding site and will result in displacement of one drug in favour of another. Methotrexate is displaced by sulphonamides, and therefore the concurrent administration of methotrexate with cotrimoxazole increases the free concentration of methotrexate within the central compartment and this results in increased toxicity. A similar situation exists if the serum albumin level falls, as is commonly seen in patients with disseminated malignancies. Often patients in a malnourished state exhibit increased toxicity with a drug dose that is considered safe for patients with a normal serum albumin level.

Elimination

Drugs are eliminated by the kidney, liver, skin, or lungs. The last two are largely unimportant in cytotoxic therapy, but the renal and hepatic routes are clearly of importance.

Renal Excretion

Drugs may be eliminated from the kidney either by glomerular filtration or renal tubular secretion. Any drug that is eliminated entirely by filtration at the glomerulus will produce increased toxicity if the kidney is damaged and glomerular function is reduced. The best guide is the serum creatinine and creatinine clearance; caution is necessary if the creatinine clearance falls below 40 ml/min. Most cytotoxic drugs in current use, however, are metabolised or excreted by other routes and therefore renal elimination is unimportant. Renal tubular secretion is rarely impaired to such an extent that drug will accumulate and produce increased toxicity. The renal tubules have a vast capacity to excrete drugs and this cannot be exceeded with conventional doses. However, when large doses of drug are administered then toxicity may develop. This is seen with the administration of high-dose methotrexate (>3 g). A guide to dose modification when renal function is compromised is given in Table 3.1.

Table 3.1. Dose modification for patients with renal dysfunction.

No change	Decrease
Doxorubicin	Methotrexate
Bleomycin	Cis-platinum
Cyclophosphamide	
5-Fluorouracil	
Vinca alkaloids	

Hepatic Elimination

The liver is responsible for the metabolism of a large number of cytotoxic drugs. Normally the enzyme systems involved can adequately deal with the dose administered, but a guide to dose modification is given in Table 3.2. Should the hepatic route be the prime route of elimination, then toxicity will be seen in the presence of obstructive jaundice. This is best illustrated by the drug doxorubicin: Fig. 3.9 illustrates the increased drug exposure seen in patients with cholestasis compared with those with normal hepatic function. Here the product of concentration and time is increased by a factor of almost 2 with a corresponding increase in toxicity. Appropriate dose reduction will however lessen toxicity. Recommended reductions are shown in Table 3.3.

Table 3.2. Dose modification for patients with liver dysfunction.

No change	Decrease
Cyclophosphamide	Vinca alkaloids
5-Fluorouracil	Methotrexate
Melphalan	Etoposide
	6-Mercaptopurine

Table 3.3. Recommended dose reduction for doxorubicin.

Serum bilirubin mmol/l	Liver enzymes normal (N) or raised (↑)	Recommended dose (% of normal)
<20	N	100
<20	↑	100
20–40	N or ↑	75
40–60	N or ↑	50
60–90	N or ↑	25
90	N or ↑	None

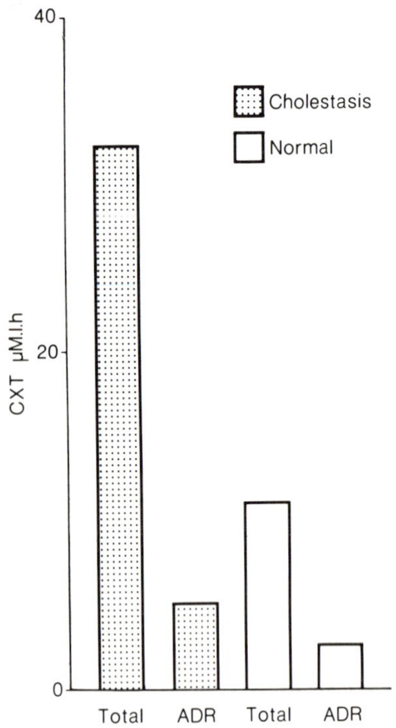

Fig. 3.9. Concentration/time product (CXT) (μmol $l^{-1}\cdot h$) following i.v. administration of doxorubicin (ADR) to patients with normal hepatic function and in the presence of obstructive jaundice. (Adapted from Benjamin et al. 1974).

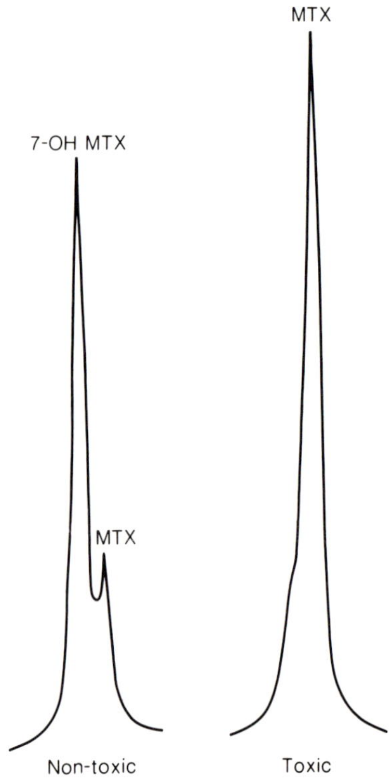

Fig. 3.10. Chromatographic analysis of serum samples obtained at 24 h from two patients who received methotrexate (MTX) 100 mg/m^2 i.v. In the patient who experienced lethal toxicity (*right-hand curve*) only unchanged drug was identified, in contrast to the non-toxic patient (*left-hand curve*), where a substantial proportion has been converted to the metabolite 7-OH methotrexate.

Metabolism

The ultimate fate of many drugs involves metabolic breakdown by the liver and it is now becoming clear that variation in this metabolic process has a direct bearing on toxicity and almost certainly on tumour response.

By way of illustration, Fig. 3.10 relates to two patients of the same age and body weight with normal liver and renal function who received the same dose of methotrexate. Patient A experienced no toxicity and there is clear evidence of substantial biotransformation to the inactive metabolite 7-OH-methotrexate. In patient B no evidence of biotransformation was seen and fatal toxicity ensued. This observation explains in part the sudden and unexpected toxicity sometimes associated with this drug. It has also been observed that with repeated courses of methotrexate there is increased metabolism due to enzyme induction; this implies that repeated fixed doses may ultimately be ineffective. Cyclophosphamide metabolism also varies with increasing doses and this has a direct relationship to toxicity and probably also to response. Both examples illustrate the dangers of administering standard doses of cytotoxic drugs to heterogenous patient groups and the pitfalls inherent in evaluating response. It is only from more detailed investigation of individual drug-treatments that we can learn how best to achieve worthwhile tumour control with confidence. This continued approach is even more essential with the various combinations of cytotoxic agents commonly employed today. Many drugs will influence the degree of metabolism by a process of either enzyme induction or inhibition and there are several examples of this that can readily be demonstrated in animal experiments. However, as regards clinical oncological practice, this does not appear to affect substantially the response for the vast majority of drug combinations used. Thus for cyclophosphamide, which requires activation by the mixed-function oxidase system, the rate of activation is not influenced by the concurrent administration of steroids or immune stimulants, both of which are powerful enzyme inducers in animal systems. Probably the most important determinant of an abnormal reaction is genetic and this cannot be readily ascertained before treatment.

Drug Distribution Within the Peripheral Compartment

Once drug has reached the cellular tissues it should not be assumed that distribution is uniform. Intracellular distribution cannot be determined for cytotoxic drugs in man as it is not possible to sample relevant tissues, and distribution can only be inferred indirectly from animal experiments. An example is given in Fig. 3.11 which shows the distribution of doxorubicin in the rat, 3 h and 24 h after administration of radiolabelled drug. There is preferential accumulation of the drug in the lung, liver, spleen, and bone marrow and relatively

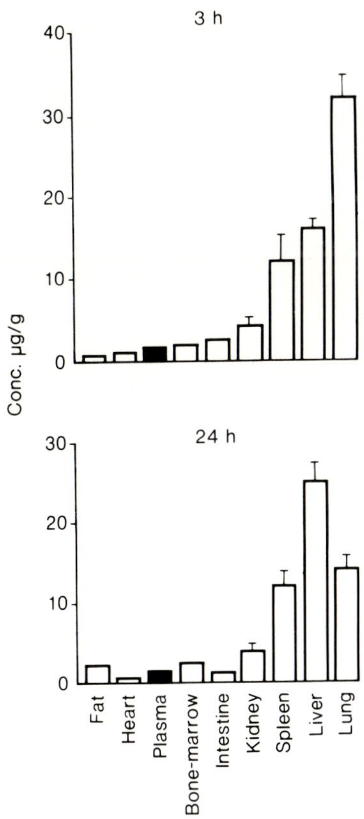

Fig. 3.11. Tissue concentration of ^{3}H-doxorubicin (mean±SEM) in the rat 3 and 24 h after the administration of 2 mg/kg i.v.

little, if any, drug present in other tissues. Clearly, inequalities in drug distribution of this type must explain the differential response in tumours at some sites in favour of others.

Note on Complex Drug Combinations

The various physiological and pharmacological factors outlined above give the physician an indication of the complexity of drug handling in man. As a general concept, when treating patients with malignant disease with cytotoxic drugs, it is better to gain experience with one or possibly two drugs in depth rather than to ring the changes, using an ever increasing number of drugs. When one considers the factors that can influence the effect of one drug, one can see how with combinations of two, three, four, and indeed sometimes six drugs, it becomes almost impossible to separate out what is producing what. It is quite probable that many patients have been exposed to toxic and ineffective combinations when the judicious selection of a more simple drug combination would have been adequate.

Mechanism of Action and Properties of Cytotoxic Drugs in Current Use

Alkylating Agents

This group contains a number of active drugs that have been in clinical use for the past 30 years. The original observation that mustard gas, in addition to causing irritation of the respiratory tract produced myelosuppression, led eventually to the synthesis of nitrogen mustard which was used successfully to treat a patient with generalised lymphoma. Following this a number of compounds were synthesised chemically that are now used to treat a wide variety of malignant neoplasms.

The alkylating agents have in common the property of interfering with the separation of DNA strands after initially cross-linking them. This interferes with the expression of the DNA both in its transcription and as messenger RNA required for essential protein enzyme production. In contrast to many other drugs, alkylating agents are not cell cycle specific and can act at all stages of the cell cycle. Maximal activity, however, is seen during the S phase. There is marked similarity between the biological effect of the alkylating agents and that of ionising radiation; alkylating agents have therefore sometimes been referred to in the past as radiomimetic drugs.

Mechlorethamine (nitrogen mustard, mustine, HN_2)

This is the most active member and was the first to be introduced in clinical practice. It is highly reactive and can only be administered safely as an i.v. injection either as a bolus or via the tubing of a fast-running saline drip. Accidental extravasation results in severe tissue necrosis. Biodegradation within the plasma is rapid and the parent drug cannot be identified 3–5 min after administration. Distribution within the tissues is not uniform and there is preferential accumulation within the lymphoreticular system. Although this drug possesses a wide clinical spectrum of activity it is now used only for the treatment of Hodgkin's disease and occasionally non-Hodgkin's lymphoma.

DOSE

6 mg/m^2 i.v. on days 1 and 8 when used in combination for Hodgkin's disease
10–15 mg/m^2 i.v. bolus as a single agent

TOXICITY

Mustine is highly reactive and therefore severe tissue necrosis will ensue if accidental extravasation occurs. Myelosuppression is common and thrombocytopenia may occasionally occur. Some epilation is usual. Central nervous system effects are rare but occasionally a toxic reaction can occur.

Cyclophosphamide (Endoxana, Cytoxan, CTX)

This is probably the most widely used of all cytotoxic drugs. As a *pro-drug* it requires activation by the mixed-function oxidase system within the liver, with the formation of the active principle *phosphoramide mustard* and a variety of toxic and non-toxic metabolites. Originally it was postulated that the enzyme responsible for the production of phosphoramide mustard occurred in greater concentrations in the tumour and this would therefore selectively permit anti-tumour action. However, it was subsequently shown that the enzyme responsible has a ubiquitous distribution throughout the body with high concentrations in the liver, which is the principal site of activation. Administration is either by mouth or parenterally. It has been accepted practice to give the drug orally, commonly in a dose of 100 mg/m^2 daily for a variety of tumours. The efficacy of this route has, however, been questioned and many regimes now employ a larger dose given intravenously, alone or in combination with other drugs. Following i.v. administration, the plasma decay is biphasic and the half-life of the terminal phase ranges from 2 to 10 h. The drug is metabolised principally within the liver, and the metabolites are eliminated via the kidney. One such metabolite, acrolein, is responsible for the production of sterile cystitis, which occurs in 5%–10% of patients.

Although animal studies indicate that other drugs given concurrently with CTX alter the proportion converted to phosphoramide mustard, in man there is no convincing evidence that a similar effect occurs. Indeed it is almost impossible to saturate the enzyme system required for activation, even with doses as high as 3.5 g/m^2 (Fig. 3.12). Clinically the drug is used for the treatment of many solid tumours and also tumours of the lymphoreticular system, given either alone or in combination.

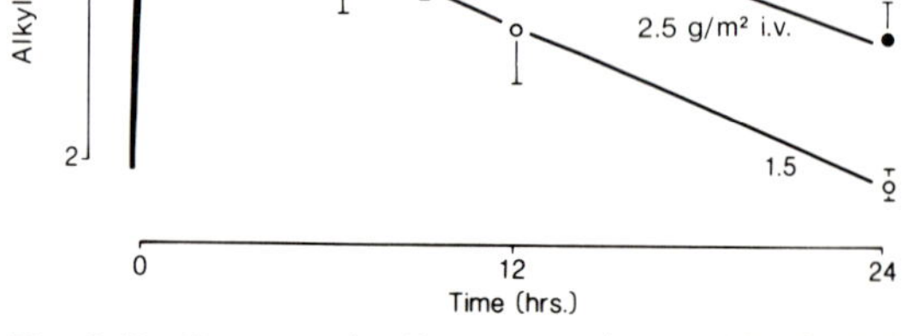

Fig. 3.12. Concentration/time curve (mean±SEM) of total alkylating activity in eight patients with bronchial carcinoma who received incremental doses of cyclophosphamide i.v.

DOSE

By mouth—100 mg/m^2 continuous
Intravenously—1–4 g/m^2; it is essential to give adequate i.v. hydration to avoid cystitis.

TOXICITY

The toxicities of the commonly used alkylating agents are summarised in Table 3.4. Mention

Table 3.4. Toxicity of the alkylating agents.

	Nausea and vomiting	Epilation	Myelosuppression	Bladder irritation	Thrombocytopenia	Delayed pancytopenia
Busulphan	−	+	+	−	+	+++
Cyclophosphamide	+++	+++	+	++	−	−
Mechlorethamine	+++	+	++	−	−	−
Chlorambucil	+	−	+	−	++	+
Melphalan	−	+	+	−	+	+

must, however, be made of certain specific side effects of CTX. Sterile cystitis with haematuria occurs in 5%–10% of patients and in such cases treatment must be withdrawn otherwise intractable cystitis and bladder fibrosis will result. Treatment is often unsatisfactory and occasionally cystectomy is required. In children an increased incidence of bladder carcinoma has been noticed several years after successful therapy in those children who have experienced cystitis. Other side effects include interstitial pneumonitis, inappropriate antidiuretic hormone secretion, amenorrhoea, and sterility. Cardiomyopathy may develop, particularly if CTX is given concurrently with anthracyclines.

Melphalan (L-phenylalanine mustard)

This drug was synthesised on the hypothesis that the inclusion of an essential amino acid (phenylalanine) would lead to selective concentration of drug in dividing cells that require large amounts of amino acids for protein synthesis prior to mitosis. There is no evidence, however, that selective distribution does occur. The drug has a wide spectrum of activity, but in current clinical practice it is reserved principally for the treatment of myeloma and cancer of the breast and ovary.

Although generally administered by mouth, melphalan is often incompletely absorbed. Thus, the intermittent daily administration of fixed doses to a patient-population with one disease must result in some patients receiving inadequate therapy. Attention should be directed to the white cell count and the dose adjusted until an acceptable level of myelosuppression has been obtained. Intravenous preparations are available but have not yet become standard therapy.

DOSE

6 mg/m^2 daily for 5–7 days as single agent. The dose is modified if used in combination.

TOXICITY

Occasionally nausea and vomiting occur. Moderate myelosuppression develops with delayed white cell and platelet count nadir at day 28. Cycles of treatment can therefore only be given at *6-week intervals*.

Chlorambucil

This combines chemically the reactive *bis*-(2-chloroethyl)-amino group with an aromatic carboxylic acid. The rationale for this combination was to facilitate the passage of the alkylating function through cell membranes and thus selectively increase drug concentration within proliferating cells. Although it is now recognised that selective toxicity has not been achieved, chlorambucil is still widely used in the management of lymphoreticular disorders and certain solid tumours such as carcinoma of the breast and ovary. Chlorambucil is too unstable for i.v. use and is therefore always given orally. Absorption is rapid and peak concentrations are achieved approximately 1 h after administration. Parent drug is metabolised by a process of beta-oxidation to metabolites which may have some therapeutic activity.

It is the drug of choice for generalised lymphoma of favourable prognostic type and for chronic lymphocytic leukaemia.

DOSE

The preferred method of administration when used as a single agent is 5–10 mg daily for 14 days repeated at monthly intervals. In this way irreversible thrombocytopenia and occasional fatal marrow aplasia is avoided. Thrombocytopenia particularly is likely to occur if the drug is given continuously by mouth.

TOXICITY

The principal toxicities are thrombocytopenia and marrow aplasia. Epilation is uncommon.

Prednimustine

This is a prednisolone ester of chlorambucil, synthesised in the hope that selectivity of action could be achieved by preferential uptake of the drug by cells that possess suitable steroid receptors. Thereafter, intracellular hydrolysis would independently produce prednisolone and chlorambucil and these would act to produce therapeutic activity against the appropriate tumour. Although introduced into clinical trial there is no direct evidence that the combination is superior to the administration of prednisolone and chlorambucil separately.

Busulphan (Myleran)

This is a methane sulphonate ester whose chemical reactivity is considerably less than that of mechlorethamine. Absorption from the gastrointestinal tract is satisfactory and therefore the oral route is the preferred method of administration. The drug is generally reserved for the treatment of chronic granulocytic leukaemia and is capable of inducing long-term control of disease. It is, however, of no value in the management of the blastic crisis of this disease or indeed in the management of acute granulocytic leukaemia.

DOSE

Generally 2–10 mg daily—the dose titrated according to the blood count and response.

TOXICITY

Busulphan is generally well tolerated. However, continuous daily administration can induce marrow hypoplasia which can progress to irreversible and fatal aplastic anaemia. Continuous monitoring of the blood count is therefore necessary and patients on continuous therapy should be seen at least every 6–8 weeks to check the white cell and platelet counts.

Nitrosoureas

The general structure is shown in Fig. 3.13. The presence of a chloroethyl group in position *R* bestows alkylating activity which is responsible for

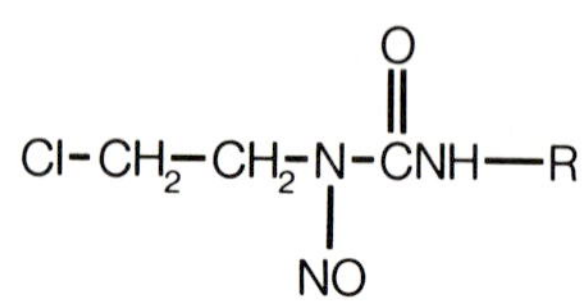

Fig. 3.13. Structure of the nitrosoureas.

the anti-tumour action. The precise mechanism of action is unknown but there is evidence that nitrosoureas undergo both alkylation and carbamoylation in vivo. They are lipid-soluble and are widely distributed throughout the body, including the central nervous system. Kinetic information is scanty in view of the rapid plasma decay. Some metabolism does occur and one product is isocyanate which undergoes hydrolysis to carbamic acid, the formation of which is responsible for the severe marrow toxicity that can occur with this group. The nitrosoureas in clinical use are CCNU, BCNU, and streptozotocin.

CCNU (*cis*-chloronitrosourea; Lomustine) is administered by mouth at intervals of 6 weeks. It is used principally as second-line therapy for lymphoreticular disorders and for brain tumours. Its initial promise in successfully treating gastrointestinal cancer, superseded by its close relative methyl-CCNU, has not been fulfilled.

BCNU (*bis*-chloronitrosourea; carmustine) must be given intravenously, again at intervals of 6 weeks. Its clinical use is similar to CCNU although it has been used with some success in the treatment of myeloma.

Streptozotocin is similar to BCNU but has glucozamine in the *R* position and is diabetogenic.

Carbamic acid is not a product of in vivo metabolism and severe myelotoxicity is therefore uncommon. It is used principally for the treatment of islet cell tumours.

DOSE

CCNU 100–130 mg/m^2 every 6 weeks by mouth
BCNU up to 200 mg/m^2 i.v. bolus every 6 weeks

TOXICITY

Nausea and vomiting are common during the first 24 h after administration. The principal toxicity affects the bone marrow, where both resting and proliferating cells are equally damaged. The effect on the bone marrow is cumulative and affects all three formed elements: erythrocytes, leucocytes, and platelets. At least 4 weeks are required for recovery so that the drug can only be repeated at intervals of 6 weeks. With repetitive treatments myelosuppression may become severe and recovery can be delayed for several weeks. This makes clinical usage somewhat difficult and probably accounts for the drug's restricted clinical use.

Other toxic effects include pulmonary fibrosis (carmustine), which may be fatal, optic neuroretinitis, and gynaecomastia.

Platinum Compounds

Although a number of platinum analogues have been synthesised only one is currently in clinical use, namely *cis*, diamminodichloroplatinum II (cisplatinum). This is a complex formed by a central atom of platinum surrounded by chlorine and ammonium atoms in a *cis* position in the horizontal plane as shown in Fig. 3.14. The *trans* isomer is less active.

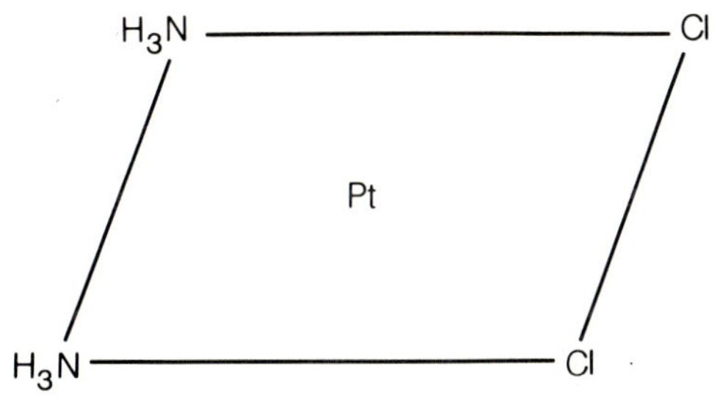

Fig. 3.14. Structure of *cis*-diamminodichloroplatinum (II).

The mechanism of action is unknown but it is thought to be one of alkylation. It is a mustard-like substance that causes damage to the DNA molecule, producing cross-links. The drug must be administered intravenously. Plasma decay is biphasic with a terminal half-life of up to several days. Approximately half of the administered dose is excreted in the urine, some via the biliary tract. However, metabolic studies have failed to account for the total dose administered and there is probably long-term accumulation in the bones and possibly kidney. There is no penetration of the intact blood-brain barrier but in patients with intracerebral tumours appreciable concentrations have been demonstrated.

Cis-platinum has a wide spectrum of clinical activity. Combined with other drugs it forms part of the curative combination for testicular cancer. It is considerably more active in ovarian cancer than standard alkylating agents and also has comparable activity in head and neck cancer to both bleomycin and methotrexate. The next decade should identify its precise role since its use is always associated with considerable toxicity.

DOSE

Single agent 100 mg/m^2 bolus i.v. with hydration $\pm$ frusemide or mannitol
100 mg/m^2 as 24-h infusion with hydration
20 mg/m^2 i.v. days 1–5 with i.v. hydration

TOXICITY

Nausea and vomiting are universal; they occur in all patients whatever the route of administration, and control with standard emetic therapy is difficult. The other principal toxic effect is renal tubular damage and *all* patients receiving cisplatinum require close monitoring of renal function. The administration of this drug is best controlled by those with experience in special centres. The principal damage is to the renal tubules and renal failure will occur if inadequate hydration is given with repetitive doses.

Other toxicities are given in Table 3.5. Should severe myelosuppression occur requiring antibiotics, then aminoglycosides and cephalosporins *should be avoided* since fatal acute renal failure may follow.

Table 3.5. Toxicity of cis-platinum.

Common	Less common
Myelosuppression	
High-tone deafness	Late demyelination syndrome
Peripheral neuropathy	Seizures
Hypomagnesaemia	Platinum gum line
Haemolytic anaemia	Optic neuritis
	Allergic reactions, including anaphylaxis

Anti-tumour Antibiotics

Actinomycin D

This high-molecular-weight anti-tumour antibiotic is isolated from *Streptomyces parvullus*. On a molar basis it is one of the most potent cytotoxic drugs available. Actinomycin D binds to double helical DNA, resulting in selective inhibition of DNA-dependent RNA synthesis. The drug also has a hypocalcaemic effect similar to but less evident than that with mithramycin. Absorption from the gastrointestinal tract is incomplete and variable and the drug is therefore given parenterally. The half-time of the terminal phase is 36 h, distribution is uniform, but penetration of the cerebrospinal fluid is poor. There is no evidence of metabolism and unchanged drug is eliminated via both bile and urine.

DOSE

500 μg daily for 5 days as i.v. injection
2–2.5 $\mu g/m^2$ as i.v. bolus

TOXICITY

Gastrointestinal effects are common and vomiting in particular can be severe; mucositis and diarrhoea occurs in 30% of patients. Bone marrow suppression is common and there is a delayed white cell and platelet count nadir at 3 weeks. Other toxic effects include skin pigmentation, alopecia, and recall skin reaction with irradiation. Actinomycin D exhibits little anti-tumour activity against the common solid tumours, e.g. those of breast, gastrointestinal tract, lung, head, and neck. In contrast it is active against the rarer tumours such as rhabdomyosarcoma, Ewing's sarcoma, choriocarcinoma, and teratoma of the testis.

Bleomycin

Bleomycin is the generic name for a group of antibiotics isolated from *Streptomyces verticillus* and contains a number of sulpha-containing polypeptides, the principal component being bleomycin A_2. Commercial preparations vary in the ratio of the differing compounds, a fact which is reflected in differing degrees of toxicity.

MECHANISM OF ACTION

Bleomycin inhibits cell proliferation and prevents DNA replication by selective DNA inhibition so that progression of cells through the S phase of the cell cycle is inhibited. In addition, progression out of G2 phase is inhibited and this property has been used to synchronise cells kinetically before the administration of other cytotoxic drugs.

SPECTRUM OF ACTIVITY

Bleomycin is active against squamous cell carcinoma, for example in the head and neck, cervix, and lung. It is also active against lymphomas and Hodgkin's disease, and against testicular cancer. However, remissions are rarely complete and tend to be of short duration, and its main use now is generally in combination for the treatment of lymphomas, restricted to second-line therapy. It does, however, form part of the curative therapy for testicular cancer.

DOSE

As a single agent bleomycin is administered in a dose of 10–20 mg/m^2 intramuscularly or subcutaneously twice weekly. The dose and frequency of administration depend on the precise regime.

The drug has a terminal half-life of 2.5 h and there is some metabolism in vivo. Approximately half of the administered dose can be recovered in the urine. In patients with renal impairment there is evidence of drug accumulation with conventional doses and this can be associated with increased toxicity. The drug can also be instilled into the pleural or peritoneal cavities; the former presents no difficulties but anaphylactic reactions and sudden deaths have followed intraperitoneal administration and this route should therefore be avoided.

TOXICITY

Although relatively non-myelosuppressive, bleomycin administration is associated with a number of toxic reactions. Fifty percent of patients experience chills and fever up to 40 °C within 6 h of administration and this can be associated with hypertension. Occasionally a fatal anaphylactic reaction may occur. These reactions can readily be prevented by the simultaneous administration of hydrocortisone succinate 100 mg i.v. Nausea and vomiting are rare.

There is selective concentration in the skin so that cutaneous toxicities are common and will occur in all patients eventually. Pigmentation is the commonest and may be general or restricted to exposed areas. The pulp of the terminal phalanges may become tender and quite painful. General ichthyosis and alopecia may also occur.

Apart from the rare anaphylactic reaction, none of the above is life-threatening. Pulmonary toxicity is, however, more serious. Clinically the patient presents with an unproductive cough and progressive exertional dyspnoea. Pulmonary function tests reveal a decrease in the carbon monoxide diffusing capacity with a low PaO_2. The incidence of this side effect is directly related to total dose, i.e. with doses totalling less than 300 mg the incidence is less than 5%; with a dose of 280 mg/m^2 it is 55%, rising to 66% at 400 mg/m^2. The incidence increases if there has been previous pulmonary irradiation. The side effects are irreversible and indeed in some patients when the drug is withdrawn progressive changes continue to occur with a fatal outcome. Therapy, therefore, should be directed at administering no more than *300 mg in total*, particularly to elderly patients.

Mithramycin

This antibiotic is isolated from *Streptomyces plicatus*. Although it is active in some solid tumours, its principal use is in the treatment of hypercalcaemia and it is reserved for this condition in the United Kingdom. Mithramycin inhibits the action of parathyroid hormone peripherally thereby preventing bone reabsorption. It also blocks the hypercalcaemic effect of large doses of vitamin D and inhibits the action of that vitamin on the intestinal absorption of calcium. A fall in serum calcium occurs about 12–18 h after administration, with maximum activity at 24–48 h, but this effect may last up to 10 days. Only a fraction of the dose required to produce a tumoricidal effect is required to lower the serum calcium, but even so toxicity may occur.

DOSE

25 μg/kg i.v. (for the treatment of hypercalcaemia)

TOXICITY

Nausea is common and thrombocytopenia may occur with repetitive treatments. Impaired coagulation due to inhibition of factors II, IV, VII, and X may also occur.

Mitomycin

Mitomycin is a purple antibiotic isolated from *Streptomyces caespitosus*. It inhibits DNA synthesis by a combination of intercalation and alkylation. Analogues deficient in the aziridine ring are capable of inhibiting DNA but have no antitumour activity. The drug is active against adenocarcinoma, including that of stomach and breast. In the United Kingdom its use is restricted because of its toxicity. Myelosuppression is cumulative and dose-limiting. This usually appears as thrombocytopenia, but there is also an associated neutropenia. The most serious side effect is progressive renal damage, which can culminate in irreversible renal failure; this is dose-related but may also arise idiosyncratically. The haemolytic uraemic syndrome may also occur.

DOSE

10–20 mg/m^2

Ideally this should be given in combination with other drugs, therefore permitting mitomycin to be given every 2 months to a maximum total dose of 100 mg. In this way the incidence of renal damage is considerably reduced.

Anthracycline Antibiotics

The anthracycline antibiotics constitute an important group of anti-cancer drugs and have made a considerable contribution to cancer therapy. The original member, daunomycin, was later superseded by doxorubicin (adriamycin, ADR). Daunomycin is now reserved solely for the treatment of acute myeloid leukaemia as doxorubicin has a much wider spectrum of activity.

Doxorubicin was isolated from *Streptomyces peucetius*, but can now be synthesised chemically. It consists of the tetracyclic aglycone, adriamycinone, linked to the amino sugar daunosamine. Doxorubicin binds to DNA, thereby inhibiting synthesis. The binding is tight (but not irreversible) and by elongation of the DNA chain, replication is inhibited. RNA synthesis is also affected, particularly that involved in ribosomal DNA synthesis. There has been recent interest in free radical formation as a separate mechanism of action; this is mediated by NADPH-dependent one-electron reduction with the formation of hydrogen peroxide and cell death. This mechanism is considered to be involved in the production of cardiac damage.

Doxorubicin has a wide spectrum of activity. It is the drug of choice, alone or in combination, for acute leukaemias and generalised lymphomas of poor prognostic type. Amongst solid tumours it is used in combination for treatment of carcinoma of the breast, ovary, lung, and stomach. It is not absorbed from the gastrointestinal tract and can only be administered i.v. usually as a bolus. The serum decay is biphasic with a terminal half-life of 30 h. Distribution in the tissues is rapid and extensive and there is preferential accumulation in the lymphoreticular system. Considerable metabolism occurs within the liver to a number of inactive but probably toxic metabolites. The principal active metabolite is daunorubicinol. The main route of elimination is via the bile and only a small proportion is excreted in the urine. The major fraction of the urinary excretion takes place in the first 6 h and this explains the red discoloration of the urine commonly noted by patients. As the liver is the main excretory organ the dose must be reduced in the presence of obstructive jaundice, since impaired hepatic excretion produces increased drug exposure with resultant increase in toxicity.

DOSE

As a single agent 60–80 mg/m^2 i.v.

TOXICITY

In common with other cytotoxic drugs anthracyclines will produce gastrointestinal upset, bone marrow depression, and epilation. Gastrointestinal upset consists principally of nausea and vomiting in association with lethargy that may be profound and of such severity that patients may refuse further therapy. Bone marrow depression is not normally a problem. Epilation is universal and complete. The most serious side effect is cardiotoxic damage. This is seen clinically as congestive cardiomyopathy with symptoms of progressive dyspnoea and oedema. There are unfortunately no reliable tests (apart from endomyocardial biopsy) that will predict the development of this side effect, and once clinical signs have developed there is no successful treatment.

The incidence of cardiotoxicity is related to total dose. It is less than 5% with a total dose of 550 mg/m^2, but increases progressively and is nearly 100% with a total dose of 1000 mg/m^2. Current practice, therefore, restricts the total dose of doxorubicin, whether alone or in combination, to a maximum of 500 mg/m^2. In this way cardiac damage is unlikely to occur. There are, however, predisposing factors and it is sensible practice to reduce the total dose to 350 mg/m^2 in patients who have had concurrent mediastinal irradiation, in those who are also receiving cyclophosphamide, and in those with a history of cardiac damage from ischaemia.

Antimetabolites

Methotrexate

Methotrexate was first used for the treatment of acute lymphocytic leukaemia following the observation that folates aggravated the disease process. Although superseded by other drugs for this disease it is still used extensively for a variety of solid tumours, in particular choriocarcinoma and head and neck cancer. Methotrexate is an S-phase-specific drug which acts by preventing the conversion of folic acid to tetrahydrofolate by stoichiometric inhibition of the enzyme dihydrofolate reductase (DHFR). The binding to DHFR is both reversible and competitive, but complete inhibition of DNA synthesis requires the presence of free intracellular drug as well as the proportion bound to DHFR. The concentration necessary to produce inhibition is specific for each tissue and is directly related to plasma concentration. Thus for each target organ a critical minimal extracellular concentration threshold exists which must be exceeded if toxicity is to be avoided. The degree of toxicity is a function of both concentration and duration of exposure during the initial period of rapid cell-kill.

Methotrexate is absorbed from the gastrointestinal tract, but the absorption is complete only with small doses. Both methotrexate and folic acid are absorbed by an active transport process and this is saturated with doses of 30 mg/m^2 so that doses in excess of this must be given intravenously. An oral dose of 30 mg/m^2 will produce in serum a peak concentration of 1 μM that decays with a terminal half-life of 25 h. This is greater than the threshold required to produce inhibition of DNA systems in the bone marrow and explains why frequent oral doses produce cumulative toxicity in both marrow and the gastrointestinal tract. It is questionable whether the concentrations achieved are sufficient to achieve cytotoxic activity.

Intravenous administration is the preferred route as this, in particular, avoids problems with patient compliance. The serum decay is triphasic with a terminal half-life of 27 h. Methotrexate is a weakly acidic drug and therefore is bound to albumin, and will be displaced by other drugs of a similar class. Thus, concurrent administration of sulphonamides, acetylsalicylic acid, or the warfarin group of anticoagulants may produce a serious drug interaction. Caution should therefore be exercised if the patient is currently taking these drugs and indeed it is probably wiser to discontinue other therapy altogether.

The distribution of methotrexate within the tissues is not uniform; there is some diffusion into the cerebrospinal fluid, though the doses achieved with conventional therapy are suboptimal. Ascitic or pleural fluid acts as a reservoir for the drug and will result in increased toxicity. Therefore patients in whom third spaces are present require appropriate dose reduction.

A small proportion of methotrexate is metabolised by enzymes within the liver and excretion is principally by the urine, although a small proportion is excreted by the biliary tract. There is some evidence of an enterohepatic circulation and this is responsible for a number of metabolites being formed. There is also evidence of accumulation within the lacrimal gland with continual recycling of drug. This phenomenon is responsible for the ocular irritation commonly seen in patients who receive repeated doses of methotrexate.

Although the renal route is the predominant route of elimination there is a very poor correlation between excretion of methotrexate and the creatinine clearance. A patient with a normal clearance may excrete very little drug and conversely patients with a low clearance may eliminate up to 95% of the administered dose. This variability is probably accounted for by varying degrees of tubular secretion and urine pH.

Methotrexate is currently used in combination with other drugs for the treatment of acute leukaemia and lymphomas of poor prognostic type. It is also a useful second-line drug for Hodgkin's disease. For solid tumours it is probably the drug of choice when given singly for the treatment of head and neck cancer, and there is some evidence that when administered synchronously with irradiation the effects of the latter are considerably enhanced. It is also active in carcinoma of the bladder and squamous cell carcinoma of the bronchus. It is commonly employed in combination with other drugs in the treatment of breast cancer, but has little activity against gastrointestinal tumours, ovarian malignancy, and tumours of the central nervous system.

DOSE

Although methotrexate has been used in clinical practice for over 30 years there is still considerable confusion concerning the optimum dose. It is recommended, therefore, that users of this drug consult appropriate journals or pharmacopoeias for a dose regimen for the particular disease that is under consideration.

TOXICITY

The single dose of methotrexate required to produce bone marrow toxicity is extremely variable and in man varies by a factor of 18. It is an unpredictable drug and small doses that in the majority of patients will not produce toxicity can produce severe and indeed fatal toxicity in a sensitive patient. For this reason, therefore, it is wise when giving methotrexate to have facilities to monitor the 24-h serum concentration as in this way patients with potentially toxic concentrations can be rescued by the administration of citrovorum factor. In some centres there is still enthusiasm for administering methotrexate in very high doses followed routinely by rescue. Doses of up to 20 g can be administered in this way, but it is strongly recommended that this type of therapy should only be undertaken in specialist centres by clinicians with considerable experience. These regimes are complicated, potentially lethal, and moreover there is little scientific evidence that they do increase the response.

Fluorouracil

5-Fluorouracil (5-FU) is a fluorine-substituted analogue of uracil differing from the normal DNA substrate by a fluorine atom at the number five position of the uracil ring. It is still one of the most effective agents for the palliative treatment of carcinoma of the stomach, colon, and pancreas and is active also in carcinoma of the breast and ovary.

5-FU is not active by itself but must be converted to the nucleotide 5-fluoro-2′-deoxyuridine-5′-monophosphate (5dUMP). This inhibits the enzyme thymidylate synthetase by displacing the natural substrate uracil deoxyribonucleotide. In this way the incorporation of the methyl group into thymidine is prevented and the cell dies in what is known as "thymineless death". Because the principal role is to deplete the system of thymidine, the cytotoxic activity of 5-FU can be reversed by the simultaneous administration of thymidine, but as yet this particular approach has not been successfully exploited therapeutically. 5-FU can be administered by mouth but absorption is erratic and unpredictable and also is inhibited by acidity and certain foods. Thus, it is recommended that only the i.v. route be used. Following i.v. administration 5-FU undergoes rapid conversion to a number of metabolites, one by an anabolic process which results in 5dUMP, and the second by a catabolic process which results in subsequent enzymic degradation to carbon dioxide, urea, and ammonia. The degraded enzymes for this are ubiquitous but are found in particularly high concentration in gastrointestinal epithelium and this therefore is an additional reason for not administering the drug by mouth. Interestingly, these enzymes are present in low concentrations only in colonic carcinomas, a finding that may in part explain the susceptibility of this tumour to 5-FU.

Many different schedules of administration of 5-FU have been subjected to clinical trials. Two schemes most commonly used are i.v. administration once a week, or daily for 5 days every 4–6 weeks. For both schedules the optimum dose is 10–15 mg/kg and this dose will produce peak plasma concentration of 10^{-3} to 10^{-4}M. The plasma decay is rapid and it is impossible to detect the drug 3 h after administration.

The major metabolic route is via the liver and 80% of the dose is eliminated through hepatic metabolic degradation. The remainder is excreted via the urine. In view of this, no alteration of drug dosage is necessary in those patients with compromised renal function. Studies on distribution are scant and uninformative.

There is some suggestive evidence that continued infusion of 5-FU is more efficacious than the methods of administration suggested above. However, the clinical trials of prolonged infusion have not clearly substantiated this claim and it is far simpler to administer the drug as a single intravenous push.

The principal toxicities seen with 5-FU are myelosuppression and stomatitis, which are dose-related. In patients given large doses intravenously or where there have been cumulative doses over a period of time, cerebellar ataxia may occur and in some patients myocardial ischaemia due to the metabolite fluorocitrate.

A number of important interactions may occur with other drugs administered concurrently with 5-FU. The principal one is the interaction of 5-FU with methotrexate, which is important particularly as this combination is currently used widely in the treatment of breast cancer. Methotrexate administered prior to 5-FU blocks purine synthesis and increases 5-FU activation, whereas in the reverse situation 5-FU blocks thymidylate synthesis, prevents consumption of the reduced folate pool, and therefore antagonises the antipurine effect of methotrexate. There appears to be no disadvantage in administering the two drugs simultaneously.

Two purine analogues are currently in clincial use, 6-mercaptopurine and 6-thioguanine.

6-Mercaptopurine

6-Mercaptopurine must be converted to the corresponding ribonucleotide before it is active as a cytotoxic drug. It is a substrate for the enzyme hypoxanthine-guanine phosphoribosyltransferase. The corresponding nucleotide is the active form and as such acts by inhibiting purine biosynthesis, interfering with the formation of glutamines. The drug is administered by mouth, but again there is evidence of incomplete and occasionally erratic absorption. It is widely distributed in the body but only a small fraction of the dose is present in the cerebrospinal fluid. It is used principally in the treatment of acute leukaemia, usually in maintenance schedules, and also for the maintenance treatment of generalised lymphomas of poor prognostic type.

The principal toxicities are nausea and vomiting, but occasional bone marrow depression will occur with prolonged usage. In some patients liver damage may also occur. The simultaneous administration of allopurinol blocks the metabolism of 6-mercaptopurine and thereby potentiates the action of this drug. Therefore, the two should not be given simultaneously unless there is a prima facie case for this, when the dose of 6-mercaptopurine must be reduced by one third.

6-Thioguanine

6-Thioguanine must also be converted to the corresponding nucleotide before it is active and this blocks the conversion of inosinic acid to guanylic acid by inhibiting the enzyme inosinate dehydrogenase. It is also administered by mouth but there is little evidence available on bioavailability. Again it is used principally for maintenance treatment of the leukaemias and occasionally generalised lymphoma. Its toxicity is similar to that of 6-mercaptopurine, being occasional nausea and vomiting with bone marrow depression. There are no specific side effects.

Cytosine Arabinoside

This is a pyrimidine nucleotide similar in structure to cytosine differing only in that the sugar moiety is arabinose rather than deoxyribose. On administration there are two main metabolic pathways, one which converts the drug to an inactive compound and the second to the active nucleotide which inhibits the enzyme DNA polymerase.

The drug is ineffective when administered by mouth, being rapidly inactivated by passage through the liver. Following intravenous administration, deamination again is also rapid, principally by the liver but to a certain extent by the kidney. The serum decay is rapid and parent drug cannot be detected 30 min after administration. It is administered either as a bolus or as a continuous infusion and there is some evidence that the latter may be more effective. It is possible to prolong serum concentrations by the concurrent administration of tetrahydrouridine, an inhibitor of cytosine deaminase, but this particular approach has not yet been used in routine clinical practice.

TOXICITY

Cytosine is a potent myelosuppressive drug and the principal toxicity is therefore seen on all formed elements of the haemopoietic system. Severe bone marrow hypoplasia will occur with therapeutic doses and during this period septic episodes and bleeding may occur which require appropriate antibiotic therapy and supportive care. These effects are, however, reversible and recovery generally occurs within 10–20 days. Occasional hepatic dysfunction has been noted and chromosome abnormalities have been observed in patients on long-term treatment.

Vinca Alkaloids

Vinblastine (Velbe) and vincristine (Oncovin) are two naturally occurring plant alkaloids isolated from *Vinca rosea* and they have an established place in the management of lymphoreticular disease. Both are cell cycle specific agents and act by binding to tubulin, which disrupts the microtubules of the mitotic spindle. Higher concentrations inhibit RNA synthesis through effects on the DNA-dependent RNA polymerase system. Although their structure is similar the small difference in structure between the two drugs results in differing side effects and therapeutic activity.

Both must be administered intravenously and the plasma decay is triphasic, with a terminal half-life of 30 h for vinblastine and up to 44 h for vincristine. Tissue concentrations are comparable to those obtained in serum, although penetration of the blood-brain barrier is poor. A number of intermediate metabolites have been identified, but none possesses cytotoxic activity. Excretion is via both urine and bile and increased toxicity has been noted in patients with obstructive jaundice.

The principal use of both drugs is in the treatment of Hodgkin's disease, the lymphomas and acute leukaemia. Vinblastine is used in combination with other drugs in testicular cancer.

DOSE

Velbe 6 mg/m^2 given in combination; as a single agent, 12 mg/m^2 in divided doses
Oncovin 1.2 mg/m^2 (maximum 2 mg) whether used as a single agent or in combination

TOXICITY

Vinblastine is more myelosuppressive than vincristine and the latter can be given when the bone marrow is compromised as a result of previous radiotherapy or chemotherapy. Peripheral neuropathy is common and occurs most with vincristine. This is manifested as a mixed sensorimotor neuropathy. Patients complain of paraesthesia of the fingers and toes with some associated muscle weakness. Examination reveals loss of deep tendon reflexes with impaired proprioception and loss of touch. Autonomic neuropathy may also occur, giving rise to vasovagal attacks, constipation, and paralytic ileus.

Vindesine (desacetyl vinblastine amide sulphate) is a new alkaloid derived from vinblastine. The anti-tumour spectrum is close to that of vincristine, however, but it is less neurotoxic. Its precise role in the management of malignant disease is uncertain at the time of writing.

Miscellaneous Drugs

Hydroxyurea

Hydroxyurea is a specific inhibitor of DNA synthesis and blocks the cell cycle at G1. It is well absorbed from the gastrointestinal tract; the plasma decay is biphasic, with a terminal half-life of approximately 3 h. Elimination is principally from the kidney. There is very little hepatic elimination.

Its clinical use is restricted to the treatment of the chronic leukaemias, principally that of alkylating agent resistant chronic granulocytic leukaemia. It is also used experimentally to synchronise cells, in a similar way to bleomycin, to try to increase the proportion of cells in the S phase.

Etoposide

Etoposide is a semi-synthetic derivative of podophyllotoxin, a natural extract from certain plants of the genus *Podophyllum*. The natural products were unacceptable for human use because of excessive toxicity and the derivation of this drug represents a major advance in treatment. It is a mitotic inhibitor acting in the cell cycle at or before the initiation of mitosis, but by a mechanism of action different from the classical mitotic inhibitors, the vinca alkaloids. As such, it is cell cycle dependent and phase specific.

Clinical trials suggest that the drug has a wide spectrum of activity and indeed it is active in a number of solid tumours, principally oat cell carcinoma of the bronchus, testis, hepatoma, and neuroblastoma. In the lymphoreticular malignancies, evidence of activity is seen in the whole spectrum of disease, including Hodgkin's disease, poor-prognosis lymphoma, and acute leukaemia. The precise place of this drug has not yet been decided at the time of going to press, but there is no doubt that during the next decade this drug will figure prominently in a number of drug combinations for a wide spectrum of tumours.

Administration is either by mouth or intravenously. The optimum intravenous schedule has not been derived but there are two common methods of administration:

1) 100 mg/m^2 i.v. daily for 5 days
2) 600 mg/m^2 i.v. bolus

The drug is also available as a capsule, but there is evidence of variable absorption from the gastrointestinal tract, ranging from 30% to 70% of the administered dose. The recommended oral dose is twice that of the fractionated intravenous dose, namely 200 mg/m^2 daily for 5 days.

The principal toxic effects are nausea and vomiting and myelosuppression which is similar in degree to that seen with intravenous cyclophosphamide. Alopecia is common and often complete, but it is reversible. In some patients allergic reactions may occur, with fever, chills, hypotension, and bronchospasm. After repetitive doses a peripheral neuropathy may develop. This is mild and less severe than with the vinca alkaloids. However, there is a potential serious interaction with concurrently administered vinca alkaloids in that a severe peripheral neuropathy may ensue and therefore it is recommended that these two drugs are not given simultaneously.

Procarbazine

Procarbazine was discovered during the search for an alternative monoamine oxidase inhibitor. It was noted that procarbazine had activity against a number of tumours in animals and it was later introduced into clinical practice. The mechanism of action is uncertain but the principal one is inhibition of RNA-dependent DNA synthesis. Its use now is restricted solely to combination treatment for Hodgkin's disease.

DOSE

50 mg three times a day for 14 days, given in combination with mechlorethamine, vinblastine, and prednisolone

TOXICITY

Toxicity with this drug is minimal. The occasional allergic skin rash may occur and this necessitates withdrawal of the drug. Marrow suppression can occur but the other two cytotoxic agents employed in the combination treatment of Hodgkin's disease contribute mainly to the myelosuppression experienced with this particular therapy. Being a weak monoamine oxidase inhibitor the same precautions apply to the prescribing of this drug as to any other of that class. Thus patients should avoid alcohol and foods containing tyramine, e.g. cheese.

Chemotherapy for Solid Tumours

In this section the current management of solid tumours with chemotherapy is reviewed in order to give the reader some indication as to what degree of success can be achieved. With one or two exceptions this is a review only, since current regimes are continually changing and many combinations become outdated almost as rapidly as they are introduced.

Solid tumours may be classified according to their response to chemotherapy (Table 3.6).

Table 3.6. Response according to primary site.

	Primary site
Favourable response	Breast Bronchus (oat cell) Testis Gestational neoplasms Ovary
Possible benefit	Head and neck Bladder Gastrointestinal tract Prostate Cervix
Unresponsive	Brain Kidney Pancreas/gall bladder Bronchus (except oat cell) Mesothelioma

"Favourable response" implies substantial regression of measurable disease in at least 50% of patients and where a statistically significant improvement in survival can be demonstrated compared with untreated patients or those who failed to respond. "Possible benefit" implies useful palliation in some patients, but the numbers achieving complete remission are small and in no instance has a normal life span been attained following "successful" therapy. "Unresponsive" implies inability to control tumour growth and although a favourable response may occasionally be achieved this is generally of short duration and never complete.

Favourable Response

Breast

For patients with metastatic breast cancer it is preferable initially to rely upon hormone therapy, since useful remissions may be achieved with this class of drug with little in the way of toxicity (see Chap. 10). If the decision is made to offer cytotoxic therapy, the clinician must then decide whether to elect to treat the patient with a single drug or a particular drug combination. It is *probable* but not yet proven that drug combinations are more effective than drugs used singly or sequentially for both the quality and duration of remission obtained. There is, however, considerable controversy over the optimal and most effective drug combination and this is particularly important also with respect to toxicity. Though at the time of writing combinations of different drugs produce very similar response rates, it is possible that in the next decade a particular combination will become established therapy in the management of patients with metastatic disease. For the present it is not possible to recommend an optimal schedule other than to say that useful remissions can be achieved with combinations employing the drugs doxorubicin, cyclophosphamide, methotrexate, fluorouracil, and vincristine used with or without prednisolone in various combinations.

Two regimes that have been prospectively evaluated in 216 patients at this Institute were recently compared by means of a clinical trial. The drug regimes were as follows:

Group A Doxorubicin 40 mg/m^2 i.v. day 1, followed by cyclophosphamide 200 mg/m^2 by mouth days 3–6 (from Salmon and Jones 1975)

Group B Methotrexate 60 mg/m^2 i.v. days 1 and 8
5-Fluorouracil 600 mg/m^2 i.v. days 1 and 8
Cyclophosphamide 50 mg/m^2 by mouth daily for 14 days
Prednisolone 25 mg/m^2 by mouth daily for 14 days
(Modified from Canellos et al. 1974)

The response from the two regimes was identical: remission of disease was obtained in 55% in both groups and a complete response was observed in 10% in group A and 13% in group B. The median duration of response was 9 months and 10%–15% of patients in both groups were long-term survivors at 3 years.

The proportion of patients who responded varied according to the site involved, being highest for those with soft tissue or lymph node deposits. Response was more variable and unpredictable in those patients with spread to lung parenchyma and pleura. In the presence of liver metastases the response was more favourable for those patients who received treatment A.

TOXICITY

The doxorubicin combination produced universal nausea, vomiting, and epilation but life-threatening myelosuppression did not occur, except in those patients with liver involvement and jaundice. The other combination, although more acceptable to the patients, occasionally gave rise to severe neutropenia, septicaemia and death.

The response rates obtained with the two regimes are similar to that obtained with other cytotoxic combinations and it must be left to the clinician to select the combination most suitable to manage the individual patient. Particular problems can arise in those patients who have evidence of marrow infiltration, liver deposits or pleural or ascitic fluid. Severe myelosuppression is more likely to occur when the marrow is infiltrated, and reduced doses of any combination must be given. Liver metastases, particularly if the patient is jaundiced, are more likely to result in drug toxicity because of impairment of drug metabolism. A "third space", by producing an extra reservoir for drug, again potentiates toxicity. This can be particularly severe with methotrexate.

It was interesting to note in this particular trial that some patients developed bone metastases whilst actually receiving drug therapy. The inference from this is that even when undetectable microscopic disease is present prior to treatment, chemotherapy is not successfully eradicating spread to bone. This observation must place in question the role of adjuvant chemotherapy. Patients who develop bone metastases only are preferably treated by hormone therapy; chemotherapy is not really effective in producing bone healing except in 10%–15% of patients. Local painful metastases are best treated by irradiation.

If complete remission of disease is achieved the patient is still at risk from cerebral metastases. This is because the majority of drugs currently used to treat metastatic breast cancer do not cross the blood-brain barrier and the patient is therefore continually at risk if metastatic spread has occurred prior to drug therapy.

Bronchus

Bronchial carcinoma remains a major therapeutic challenge in the western world. It is now the experience of most oncological centres that systematic chemotherapy is effective for those patients with pathologically proven small cell carcinoma, and all patients should be considered for treatment. Response is likely to be more favourable in those patients with disease of limited extent, defined as those patients with disease confined to the hemithorax with or without the development of ipsilateral neck node involvement. Again the optimal regime is yet to be determined, but in patients with disease of limited extent a complete remission rate of 60% has been achieved at this Institute using the combined approach of drug therapy and irradiation. Details of treatment are given in Table 3.7. Approximately 20% of

Table 3.7. Treatment of small cell carcinoma of the bronchus of limited extent (from Thatcher et al. 1982).

Methotrexate 100 mg/m^2 days 1 and 14
Day 15—radiotherapy (4 MV) to encompass the thoracic disease, delivered in 8 fractions over 10 days to 3250 cGy through anteroposterior and posteroanterior portals
Cyclophosphamide given 10 days after the final fraction of radiotherapy in three doses, 1.5, 2.5, and 3.5 g/m^2 at 21-day intervals as i.v. bolus injections with hydration

these patients are long-term survivors at 2 and 3 years, but it remains to be seen whether this will be maintained. Prophylactic cranial irradiation was not used in this series, although it does form part of some protocols at other centres. There is no doubt that the incidence of cerebral metastases is increased and several of the patients in this series succumbed from that particular development.

Recently the drug etoposide has been shown to be particularly successful when used as a single agent in patients with metastatic small cell carcinoma. The combination of cyclophosphamide and etoposide has produced a similar complete remission rate to the above and it may be that the duration and proportion of patients remaining in remission is increased by this approach. However, for the present these approaches are experimental and the next 5 years should see a more unified approach to the management of this particular subtype of bronchial cancer.

For the remaining histological types, systemic chemotherapy is never curative and can only produce palliative remission of symptoms (see Chap. 9).

Testicle

Although rare, testicular tumours attract attention because they affect young adult males in the prime of life. The prognosis for patients with metastatic teratoma not amenable to radical radiotherapy was once considered hopeless with the exception of a small number of patients who responded to actinomycin D. However, the introduction of the combination of vinblastine, bleomycin, and cis-platinum by Einhorn and co-workers has produced a substantial improvement in management. This particular combination will produce complete remission in all patients with disease of limited extent and is probably curative.

Since its introduction there have been several modifications, principally for those patients who present with bulk disease, since complete remission can only be achieved in approximately 50% of these patients.

Thus at this Institute two regimes are recommended:

1) For patients with small volume disease the following combination will be effective:
   Vinblastine 6 mg/m^2 i.v. days 1 and 2
   Cis-platinum 20 mg/m^2 i.v. days 1–5 with hydration
   Bleomycin 30 mg i.m. weekly × 12.
   Courses are repeated at intervals of 21 days to a total of four and in some instances six courses. The recommended number of courses is determined by hormone markers and two complete courses should be given once hormone markers have returned to normal. For those patients who do not have marker elevation prior to chemotherapy, reliance must be placed on clinical and radiological assessment of tumour, but it must be recognised that in some instances patients are left with persisting evidence of disease and these patients should then be submitted to appropriate resective surgery or to irradiation.
2) For patients with bulk disease, more intensive chemotherapy is required and the following regime is recommended:
   Vinblastine 6 mg/m^2 days 1 and 2
   Cis-platinum 30 mg/m^2 i.v. days 1–5
   Etoposide 100 mg/m^2 i.v. days 1–3.
   Again treatments are repeated at intervals of 3 weeks to a total of six courses. This latter regime is more myelosuppressive and should

only be administered in specialised centres with appropriate facilities for supportive care.

Metastatic seminoma has until recently been managed radiotherapeutically, but it is now becoming recognised that for patients with bulk disease chemotherapy before radiation is more successful. It is recommended that all patients with demonstrable metastatic disease should first receive the combination of cis-platinum, vinblastine, and etoposide and then appropriate radiotherapy to sites of bulk disease. Current experience suggests that seminoma is equally responsive and this combined approach is again probably curative.

So far there have been no second malignancies reported in patients treated with this approach but 10-year survivors have not yet accrued and it is going to be some years before potential late side effects become evident, particularly second malignancy and the possibility of renal impairment. At the Christie Hospital several patients have recovered fertility after receiving combination chemotherapy unlike that employed for the management of Hodgkin's disease and non-Hodgkin's lymphoma. Patients can therefore be reassured that fertility and sexual function will return to normal after chemotherapy has been completed. Lymphoma of the testicle is rare and should be managed as for generalised non-Hodgkin's lymphoma of poor prognostic type, which is discussed in Chap. 14.

Gestational Trophoblastic Neoplasms

Although rare, this particular group of tumours is important in that it was the first to be effectively controlled by chemotherapy alone. It also provided the first instance where a hormone marker could be identified which provided a reliable quantitative indicator to assess the patient's clinical progress and also predict a relapse. Primary tumours associated with pregnancy must be distinguished from those that arise from the ovary, testis, or other tissues. Most patients will present to an obstetrician, who will therefore be the one who conducts the initial assessment. Further advice may well be sought, however, when the disease is confined locally or metastases have already developed. The ability to measure human chorionic gonadatrophin levels in both serum and urine has provided the oncologist with a unique opportunity to monitor the results of treatment. This particular tumour is very characteristic and whilst several therapeutic regimes are available, the most successful results have been achieved with methotrexate. Once complete remission has been achieved the patient must remain under long-term surveillance and serial human chorionic gonadotrophin levels must be determined in both serum and urine for some years.

Ovary

Carcinoma of the ovary is the most common gynaecological neoplasm and only one third of patients present with disease amenable either to resective surgery or to irradiation. The remainder are doomed to die from progressive disease, although in a number of patients useful response can be achieved with oral alkylating therapy. Until recently the main therapeutic approach has been with alkylating agents used singly, typically melphalan, cyclophosphamide, or chlorambucil. These drugs will produce a partial regression of disease in 40%–60% of patients and in approximately 15% this can be complete. Complete responses are, however, only seen in those patients with minimal residual disease following surgery.

Again, over the last 5 years drug combinations have evolved and these have produced an increase in the number of patients who respond to therapy, but the complete remission rates vary according to the regime evaluated. Cis-platinum, a drug effective in testicular tumours, may also have a useful long-term role to play. Current combinations employ cis-platinum in combination with cyclophosphamide and doxorubicin, and various centres have reported complete remission rates of up to 50% or 60% with various combinations. In some cases these remissions are long-lasting and patients are surviving 3 and 5 years following therapy. It must be emphasised again, however, that current treatments are still under evaluation and it will be some time before an optimum policy of management will be developed.

At present it remains to be decided whether a second-look laparotomy with resection of residual disease is of benefit, while the place of irradiation to sites of residual disease and the need for maintenance treatment have also to be elucidated.

Possible Benefit

For this particular group of tumours chemotherapy may be of value for palliation or may even result in temporary complete remissions in patients with metastatic disease. To date, no schedule has evolved which is curative and each case merits careful consideration before a particular course of treatment is embarked upon.

Head and Neck

Although comprising only 15% of solid tumours in the United Kingdom, tumours of the head and neck attract attention because of the very profound morbidity experienced by those patients who develop recurrent disease or those who present with disease beyond radical surgery or radiotherapy. Cytotoxic therapy is required when the patient presents either with disease no longer amenable to surgery or radiotherapy or with a relapse following previous treatment.

Three drugs find a useful place: methotrexate, bleomycin, and cis-platinum. Several drug combinations have been evaluated, but to date no drug combination is more effective that any of the above drugs used singly. Of the three, methotrexate is probably the drug of choice. Bleomycin will produce remissions but unexpected pulmonary toxicity is not uncommon, particularly in elderly patients. Although cis-platinum is as effective as methotrexate, it is very toxic and has to be administered with great caution in elderly patients.

Methotrexate will produce objective regression of disease in approximately 50% of patients and in a proportion the regression will be complete. The problem with methotrexate is the confusion over the optimum dose required to produce regression. Several studies have consistently failed to show a dose response with this drug, and there is very little to gain from administering high-dose methotrexate with calcium leucovorin (citrovorum factor).

To administer methotrexate safely depends on whether facilities are available to monitor the serum concentration 24 h after treatment. Provided these are available then a dose of 100 mg/m^2 i.v. at 2–3 weekly intervals will produce satisfactory regression of disease and patients who have potentially toxic concentrations can be rescued in the appropriate manner. If facilities are not available it is recommended that a dose of 50 mg/m^2 is not exceeded, since unexplained and potentially fatal toxicity may occur. An alternative drug then is bleomycin, 30 mg i.m. every 2 weeks, as this is indeed safe and non-myelosuppressive.

Several centres have attempted intra-arterial drug delivery but there is nothing to recommend this as primary treatment. Although regressions of tumour can be achieved, local complications are always greater and fatal toxicity can occur even though the drug is administered intra-arterially.

For patients with advanced disease one option to improve the response is to combine irradiation with an effective chemotherapeutic agent as primary treatment. Over the last 15–20 years there has been sporadic interest in the synchronous use of chemotherapy and radiotherapy, particularly with methotrexate. A combination of methotrexate and irradiation will produce complete remission of disease in 45% of patients with stage 3 and 4 carcinoma of the head and neck and all these remissions have been maintained for 2 years. Clinical trials, however, have not conclusively proved that this approach is more successful than conventional irradiation and further trials are currently in progress to determine whether this particular modality should be used as primary treatment.

Gastrointestinal Tract Neoplasms

With the exception of the oesophagus, which is totally resistant to chemotherapy, favourable regression of tumour may be achieved and this is directly related to the primary site, tumours of the stomach being more sensitive than tumours of the colon and rectum. 5-FU is accepted as standard treatment and can be beneficial particularly for those patients with symptoms from metastatic liver disease arising from a colorectal primary. However, bone deposits or large pelvic or nodal masses will not respond. Several variations in drug delivery have been attempted over the years and there is no optimum schedule that can be recommended. Daily administration of 500 mg/m^2 i.v. $\times$5 days is easy to manage on an out-patient basis and is preferable to oral administration as the absorption via the latter route is unpredictable. Toxicity is moderate although severe myelosuppression may occur.

Administration of large doses of 5-FU have been attempted and although improved response rates have been obtained this approach is too toxic for general use. Gastrointestinal neoplasms are more responsive and here drug combinations can be justified. The most common combination is 5-FU, doxorubicin and mitomycin C, which can produce useful palliation in some patients.

Bladder

Advanced metastatic carcinoma of the bladder presents a difficult challenge. Many patients are elderly, their general condition is poor, and their renal function compromised—all factors which potentiate the toxicity of potentially useful cytotoxic drugs. Until 1975 there had been no useful systemic evaluation of cytotoxic drugs in patients with advanced disease. More careful patient selection and the ability to prevent or moderate potentially toxic situations have led to the re-evaluation of two drugs, cis-platinum and methotrexate, that are reasonably active when used as single agents.

Cis-platinum is the most active agent for the treatment of transitional cell carcinoma, where useful regressions of tumour may be seen in 30%–50% of patients. It must be stressed, however, that this particular drug is nephrotoxic, especially if renal function is compromised. There are several different methods of administration, ranging from a single intravenous bolus to fractionated infusions given over a 5-day period. Adequate attention must be paid to rehydration and prevention of vomiting, which is nearly always universal.

A similar situation applies to methotrexate. There is, as yet, no substantial series that has properly evaluated the true response rate of methotrexate in bladder cancer, but it is possible that similar results to those with head and neck cancer may be achieved.

Prostate

Prostatic cancer is a hormone-dependent tumour and useful remissions can be achieved with stilboestrol and its related compounds. Although chemotherapy has been evaluated in this disease as yet no combination has been shown to be capable of prolonging survival in patients with metastatic disease. Although partial remissions can be achieved patients who respond to therapy live no longer than those who do not and when palliation is essentially for the relief of pain it is preferable that appropriate analgesics are prescribed rather than submit the patient to potentially toxic chemotherapy.

Cervix

Until recent times carcinoma of the cervix has generally been unresponsive to chemotherapy. More recently however various groups have reported responses with drugs such as bleomycin, cis-platinum, and methotrexate. Partial and sometimes complete remission of disease can be achieved with these drugs used singly or in combination. The combination of cyclophosphamide, methotrexate, and 5-FU used for breast cancer is capable of achieving partial remissions in up to 50%–60% of patients with cervical cancer. Renal function is, however, often compromised and this can potentiate drug toxicity.

Endometrium

The overall prognosis of this particular tumour is good, approximately 70% of all patients being alive at 5 years after initial treatment. Patients with metastatic disease are therefore not seen in large numbers. For this reason carefully controlled evaluation of cytotoxic drugs is lacking. The mainstay of treatment has been a synthetic progesterone, where responses can be achieved in a third of patients, although survival is not increased. The success of hormone therapy is directly related to the histological type, patients with well-differentiated tumours exhibiting the most favourable response. At the time of going to press there is no current cytotoxic combination that can be of benefit.

Unresponsive Tumours

Brain

The chemotherapy of adult tumours affecting the central nervous system differs between primary tumours of the central nervous system and metastatic involvement.

Primary tumours are treated initially by either surgery or irradiation. Chemotherapy has generally been reserved as an adjunct to controlling local disease, usually with CCNU. The precise place of this and related drugs in the management remains to be fully evaluated, but several groups have reported an increased survival of up to 6–12 weeks when they are given following irradiation. The dose-limiting toxicity is thrombocytopenia, which in some instances requires therapy to be discontinued.

For metastatic disease, the main difficulty is that the majority of cytotoxic drugs do not achieve an adequate cytocidal concentration in the central nervous system. This is because of the particular physiological properties of the blood-brain barrier, but this barrier does become more permeable when cerebral metastases develop. The most effective drug is high-dose methotrexate given with citrovorum factor rescue. This can be effective in carcinomatous meningitis and in lymphomatous infiltration.

Other Tumours

This is a heterogeneous group that so far has proved completely refractory to chemotherapy. It includes primary tumours of the kidney, thyroid, pancreas, gall bladder and biliary tract, liver, and also mesotheliomas. Hopefully, the next decade will see some progress for this rather depressing group of diseases.

References

Benjamin RS, Wiernik PH, Bachur NR (1974) Adriamycin chemotherapy—efficacy, safety and pharmacologic basis of an intermittent single high-dose schedule. Cancer 33: 19–27

Cannellos GP, DeVita VT, Gold LG, Chabner BA, Schein PS, Young RC (1974) Cyclical combination chemotherapy for advanced breast carcinoma. Br Med J I: 218–220

Einhorn LH, Donohue J (1977) Cis-diamminodichloroplatinum vinblastine and bleomycin chemotherapy in disseminated testicular cancer. Ann Intern Med 87: 293–298

Frei E III (1972) Combination cancer chemotherapy. Presidential address. Cancer Res 32: 2595

Henderson ES, Adamson RH, Oliverio VT (1965) The metabolic fate of tritiated methotrexate. Absorption and excretion in man. Cancer Res 25: 1018–1024

Jones SE, Durie BGM, Salmon SE (1975) Combination chemotherapy with adriamycin and cyclophosphamide for advanced breast cancer. Cancer 36: 90–97

Pacciarini MA, Barbieri B, Colombo T, Broggini M, Garattini S, Donelli MG (1978) Distribution and anti-tumour activity of adriamycin given in a high dose and a repeated low-dose schedule in mice. Cancer Treat Rep 62: 791

Skipper HE (1965) The effects of chemotherapy on the kinetics of leukaemia cell behaviour. Cancer Res 25: 1544

Thatcher N, Parker PV, Hunter RD, Carroll KB, Jegarajah S, Wilkinson PM, Crowther D (1982) 11-week course of sequential methotrexate, thoracic irradiation and moderate-dose cyclophosphamide for 'limited-stage' small-cell bronchiogenic carcinoma. Lancet II: 1040–1042

Further Reading

Chabner B (ed) (1982) Pharmacologic principles of cancer treatment. Saunders, Philadelphia

Pinedo HM (ed) (1983) Cancer chemotherapy. Excerpta Medica, Amsterdam

4 Mould Room Practice

R. C. S. Pointon and D. Studd

Treatment Planning Suite

A treatment planning suite in a radiotherapy department should be composed of three parts: (1) a simulator, (2) a mould room, and (3) computer planning facilities with access to a CT scanner. These three units should be sited close together and in close physical relationship to the radiotherapy department itself, so that the most efficient use is made of these facilities. The responsibility for treatment planning is a medical one, with close support from the department of medical physics. Radiotherapists, both qualified and in training, should work and plan their treatments (when appropriate) in collaboration with the technicians involved in making moulds and beam-direction shells. Each completed plan should be reproduced using the computer planning facility and this, along with the treatment prescription, should be checked by a physicist. Before the treatment begins, the final approval rests with the treating radiotherapist.

Functions of a Mould Room

The principal functions of a mould room, with which we are concerned in this chapter, are as follows:

1) The construction of surface applicators (usually described as moulds) designed to carry radioactive sources
2) The construction of plastic shells for small-field beam-directed X-ray treatments
3) The preparation of lead shielding moulds for use with orthovoltage and electron beams—the "lead cut-out"
4) The manufacture of individually prepared lung shields, used for mantle X-ray treatments, and prepared from a low-melting-point alloy
5) The forming and fitting of cervical supports and other splints for those patients who, because of their disease, require some form of immobilisation
6) The provision of prostheses for those patients who suffer cosmetic disability as a result of their disease and/or treatment

Preparation of a Mould or Shell

The following are the stages in the preparation of any mould or shell:

1) An *impression* is taken in a suitable material.
2) A *model* is cast in dental or stone plaster.
3) A *foundation* is formed in an appropriate material to make the basis of the mould or shell.
4) The *mould* or *shell* is fitted to the patient and retained in position by suitable strapping.

These stages result in the construction of a mould or shell which immobilises the relevant parts of the patient and ensures that the chosen position for the treatment is reliably reproduced at each treatment session. The mould is employed to carry radioactive sources at a given distance from the skin for the treatment of superficial lesions, whereas the shell is employed as an essential aid to accurate beam direction.

Preparation of Surface Moulds

Introduction

A surface mould, as the name signifies, is an applicator moulded to the appropriate anatomical site on the patient. The materials to be used depend on the site treated and whether the mould is a continuous or a discontinuous mould. The former type of mould, e.g. an adhesive mould, is designed to remain in place throughout the entire treatment. The discontinuous mould is designed to be worn for a calculated period each day for an overall time of 8 days.

Discontinuous Single-Plane Cobalt-60 Mould

This applicator carries radioactive sources (cobalt-60) in a given position overlying a superficial lesion. As a discontinuous mould it is worn for approximately 8 h per day, fractionated over 8 days. Cellulose acetate butyrate (CAB) is used to construct the mould, as it is non-hygroscopic and therefore unlikely to warp. The mould is prepared as follows: an impression is taken, a model cast, and a foundation is made and fitted to the patient.

When the treatment distance has been decided, the area to be treated is defined on the patient. Since the mould is transparent, the treatment area can be transferred to its surface in ink. An aperture corresponding to the size of the lesion is cut in the mould but the treatment area itself is left intact. Cellophane paper is laid flat over the skin surface of the mould and the treatment area is drawn on it. The surface area on the cellophane is measured in square centimetres, the treatment prescription is calculated and the required number of cobalt sources and their distribution are determined. The cobalt sources are carried at a fixed treatment height, uniformly arranged, directly above the area and parallel to the skin surface below (Fig. 4.1). The applicator is built using the mould as a foundation. It has cylindrical cork pillars, a platform on which the cobalt lies and a cover plate which safely and accurately retains the cobalt sources in their predetermined positions (Fig. 4.2). Corks are used as distance-pieces because they are light, non-compressible, and easily pared down with a knife or filed to the exact height, which is checked with calipers. A line is drawn across the centre of the lower surface of the cork and is projected up the sides and across the top, so that the top and bottom lines are directly above each other. One cork is prepared to support each one of the cobalt sources to be used on the platform. The corks are evenly spaced around the treatment area, cemented to the mould and precisely placed so that the line across the lower surface of each cork lies along the treatment area line on the mould. Sufficient CAB is cut to cover the uppermost surfaces of the corks and intervening space. It is heated and moulded on the top surfaces of the cork pillars forming a platform which will carry the cobalt sources. The height from the skin-surface side of the mould to the top surface of the platform is measured with calipers over many representative points on the mould and any necessary adjustments made. The projected area line on the uppermost surface of the corks is transferred and drawn on the surface of the platform. Non-radioactive dummy rods are temporarily cemented to the platform so that they lie along the line of the projected area as closely as possible (Fig. 4.3). If the tissue surface is convex the projected area will be larger (Fig. 4.4). The platform with the dummies still in position is removed from the supporting corks and a plaster model is cast onto its underside as a support, to avoid distortion while the cover plate is formed. When formed, the edges of the cover plate and platform are trimmed and polished. Nylon nuts and bolts are used to hold the platform and the cover plate together. Clearance holes are drilled, the bolts are introduced from the underside of the platform, and the nuts applied. Thick CAB cement packed around the nuts permanently secures them to the cover plate (Fig. 4.5). The bolts are withdrawn, the two parts prised apart, the dummies are removed and the platform is then precisely cemented in position on the corks ready for radioactive loading. The dummy rods are minutely larger than the active sources. When the cover plate is formed and the rods removed from the moulded cover plate, the little clearance allows

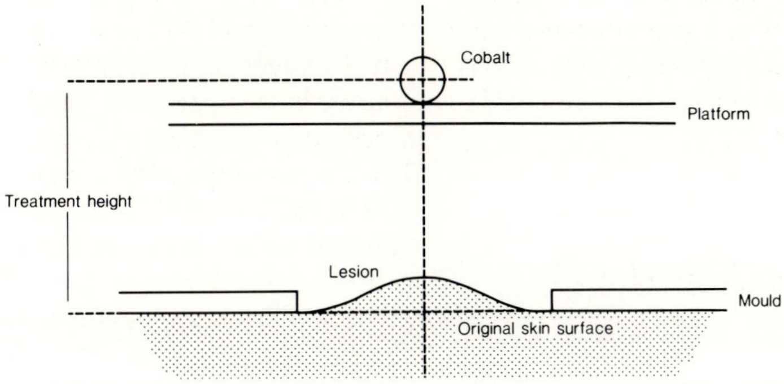

Fig. 4.1.

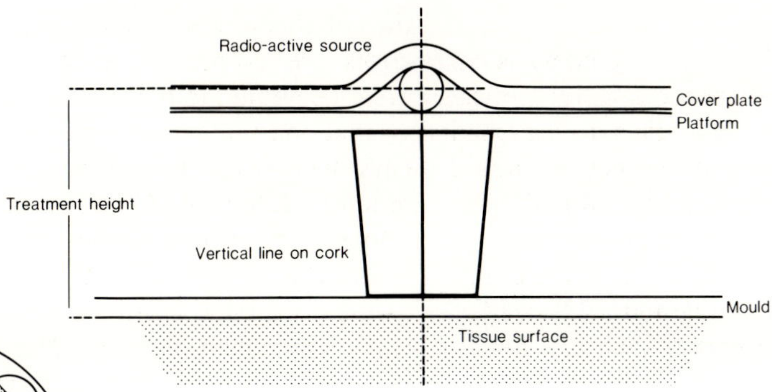

Fig. 4.2.

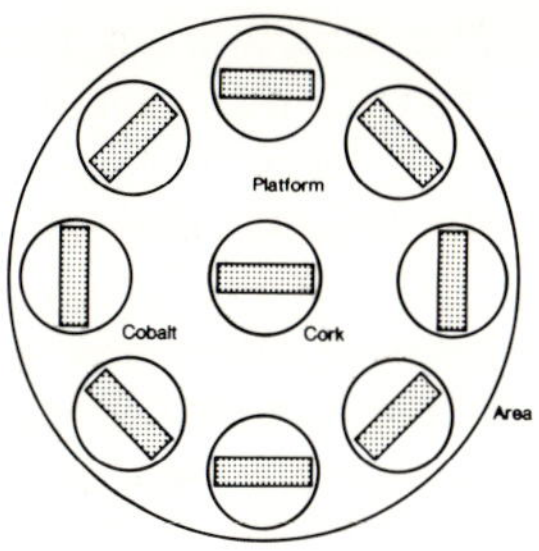

Fig. 4.3.

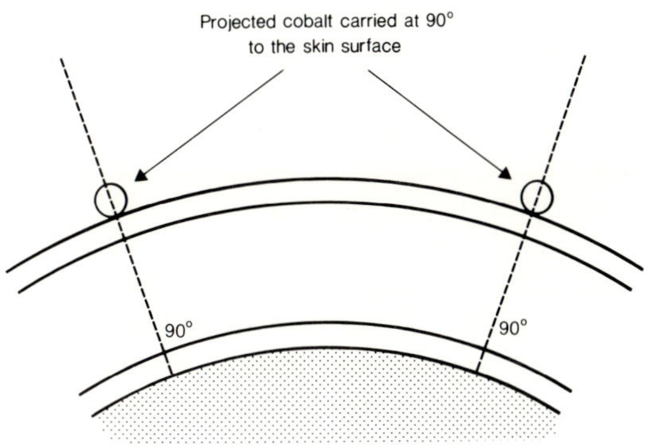

Fig. 4.4.

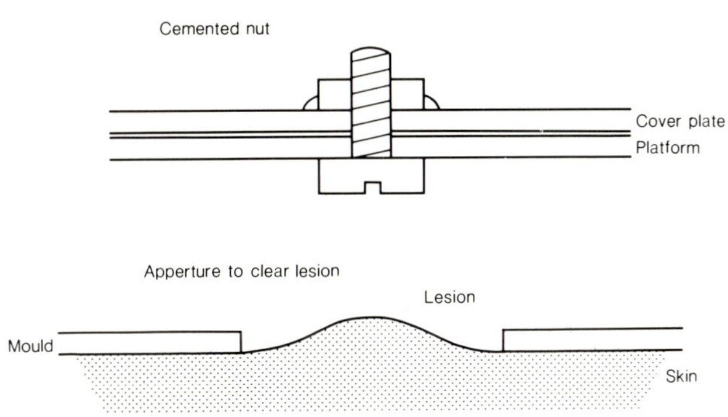

Fig. 4.5.

Figs. 4.1–4.5. Stages in construction of a discontinuous cobalt mould.

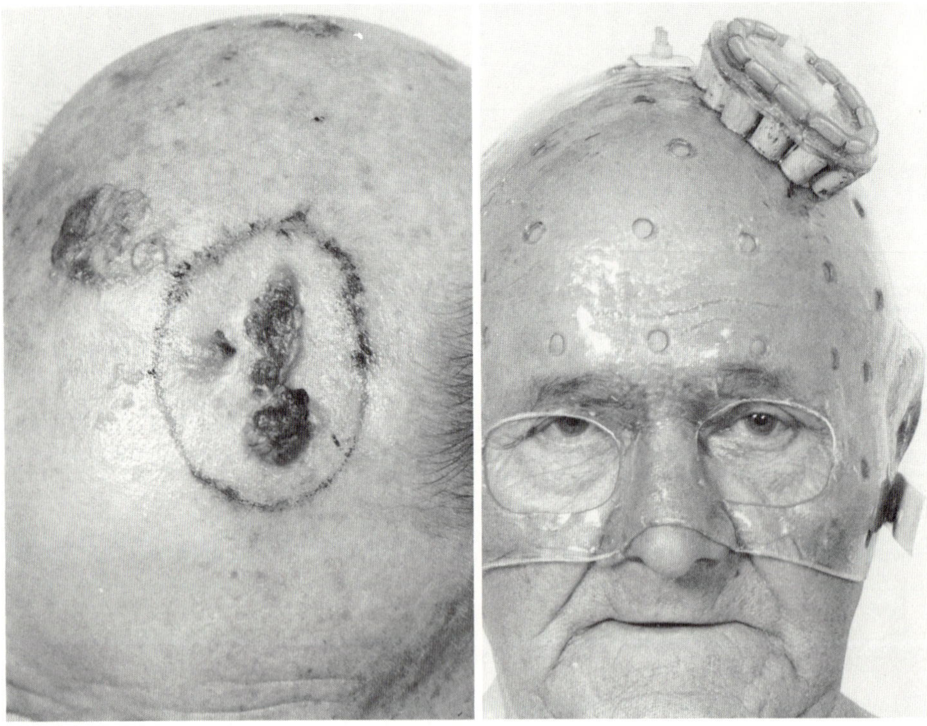

a

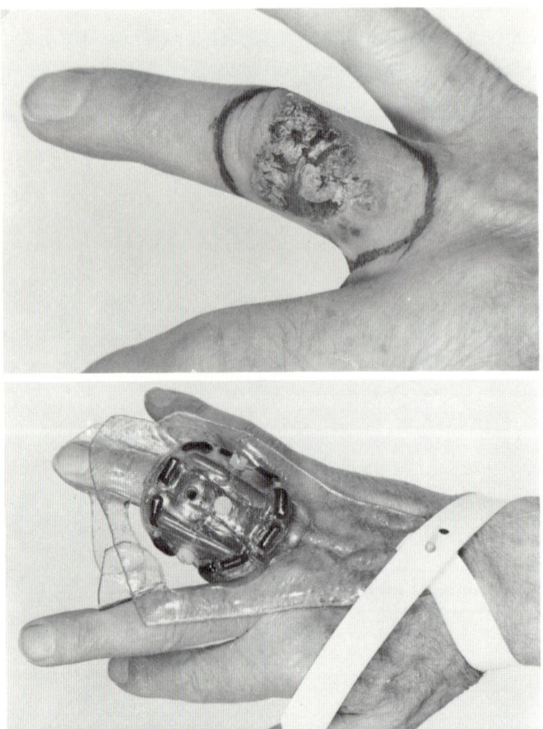

b

Fig. 4.6. **a** Squamous cell carcinoma of scalp—treatment by discontinuous cobalt mould. **b** Squamous cell carcinoma of finger—treatment by discontinuous cobalt mould.

the grooves to accommodate the live sources easily.

The cover plate is turned upside down and a radioactive source is loaded into each of its prepared grooves. The applicator is upturned and placed in perfect apposition with the cover plate, the bolts being re-introduced through the platform and cover plate and tightened into the nuts. If the aperture which is cut to clear the lesion is not sufficiently large to accommodate the screwdriver, for tightening the nuts, it should be enlarged *before* loading begins. Figure 4.6 shows patients wearing typical single-plane cobalt-60 moulds prepared as described above.

Continuous Cobalt-60 Mould

This type of mould is made of a flexible material and carries radioactive cobalt sources in a precise distribution overlying a lesion which is usually situated on a flat surface, i.e. on a leg or arm where there is no necessity to splint the limb in a fixed position. It is worn continuously for 8 days. In general, the treatment height should not exceed 1.5 cm. The mould was originally made from elastoplast-backed orthopaedic felt, but nowadays it is constructed from rubber-reinforced cork sheet

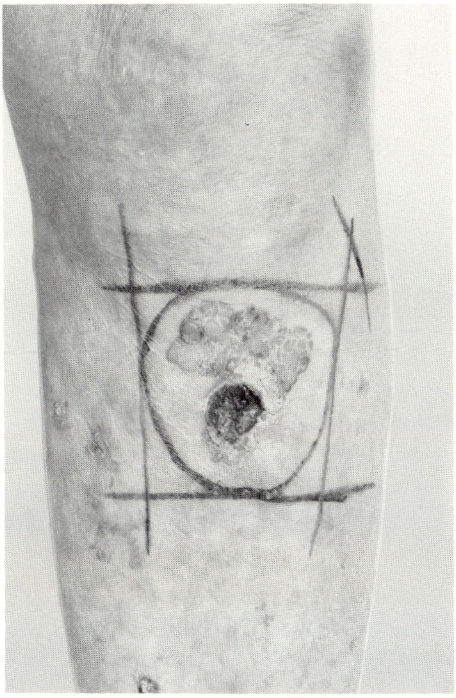

Fig. 4.7.

Figs. 4.7–4.12. Continuous cobalt mould for squamous cell carcinoma of skin of leg (*continued on next page*).

which is flexible but, unlike felt, will not compress.

To prepare the mould the following stages are undertaken. The area to be treated is first defined on the skin. The area may take the shape of a quadrilateral. If so, the four sides are produced a further 2 or 3 cm (Fig. 4.7). These projected lines will be used to mark the exact positioning of the completed mould on the patient. If the area approximates to a circle or an ellipse, four straight lines are drawn around the shape so that it lies within quadrilateral skin marks, again to ensure exact positioning of the completed mould (Fig. 4.8). Following the same procedure described below in the preparation of the larynx shell, a plaster of Paris bandage impression of the patient is taken and a plaster model is cast. Before casting, it is wise to redefine with copying pencil the lines on the impression, to ensure that the area-indicating lines are transferred onto the model from the impression. The proposed size of the mould is then drawn on the model. It must be sufficiently large to support the radioactive sources safely in their precise positions, but, within this limitation, the mould is kept as small as possible. A margin of 1 cm greater than the quadrilateral described on the model is the ideal size (Fig. 4.9).

Layers of cork sheet are built up on the model until the appropriate uniform thickness of the mould is reached. The thickness of the mould is governed by the treatment height. If the contour of the skin is curved, deep slices cut into the surface of the cork allow it to bend and conform to the surface of the model. Further layers of sliced cork are added and bound together with a contact adhesive. The mould is trimmed to the delineated size and temporarily held in position on the model with an elastic band. To project the area onto the upper surface of the mould, each pair of sides of the quadrilateral is projected perpendicularly upwards from the base at each corner and these joined with a connecting line on the upper surface of the mould (Fig. 4.10).

The area to be treated is traced from the model onto cellophane for calculation purposes. If the area resembles a circle the quadrilateral and its produced sides are recorded on the cellophane. Thereafter the area can be transferred from the cellophane to the base of the mould simply by placing the mould in position over the cellophane, lifting the model away from the mould with the undisturbed cellophane, and the area is defined through the cellophane onto the underside of the

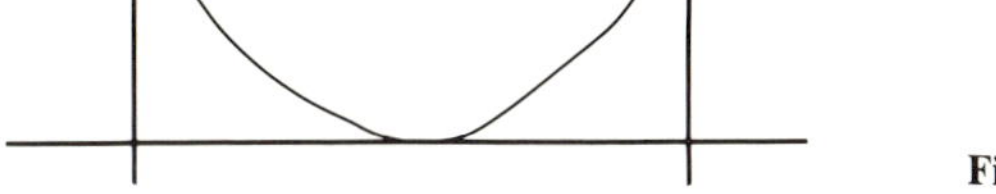

Fig. 4.8.

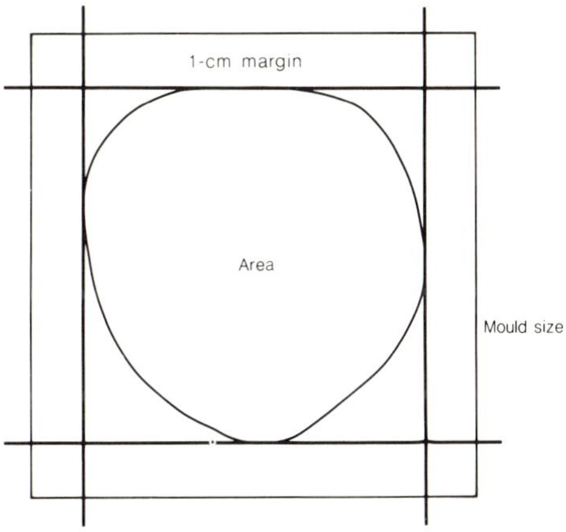

Fig. 4.9.

Figs. **4.7–4.12.** Continuous cobalt mould for squamous cell carcinoma of skin of leg.

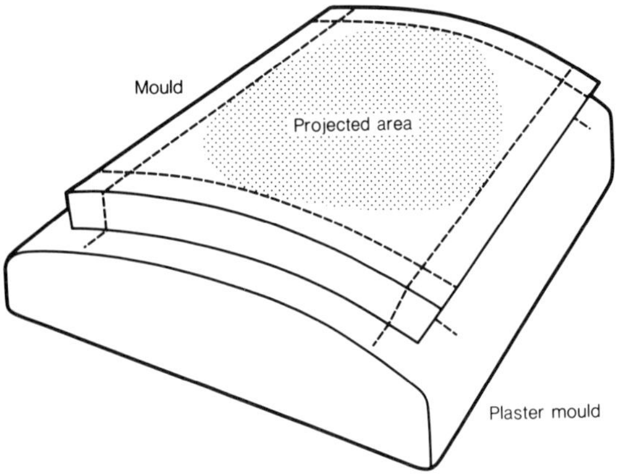

Fig. 4.10.

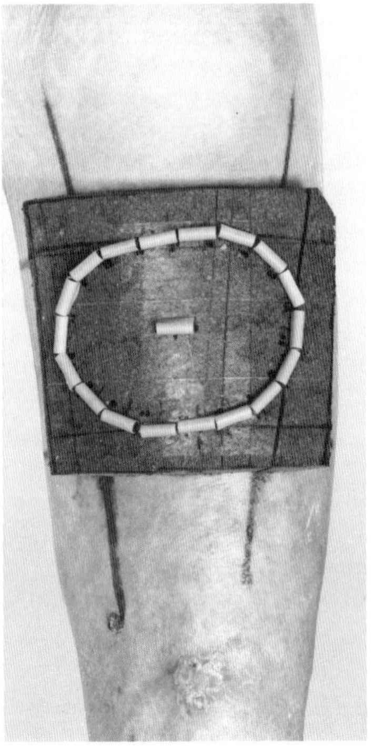

Fig. 4.11.

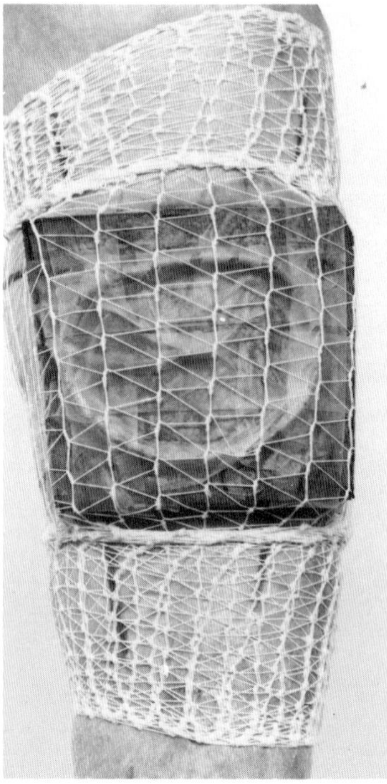

Fig. 4.12.

mould. At each corner the lines of the quadrilateral on the cellophane must meet the lines recorded on the sides of the mould. A hat-pin type of needle, eased through the mould at various points on the circle's circumference, in a direction perpendicular to the contour of the mould's base, will project the shape of the area onto the upper surface of the mould, where it is recorded. The quadrilateral is also projected onto the upper surface for checking purposes. If all is correct, four points on the circumference of the circle will touch the sides of the quadrilateral.

Slow-setting spirit adhesive is applied to the surface of the mould and the prescribed number of cobalt sources are loaded onto the area line. They are secured by transparent plastic adhesive tape, so that it is immediately apparent if a source is displaced during treatment.

The mould is applied to the patient and held in contact by both medical adhesive and plastic adhesive tape. Accurate positioning is achieved by the perfect alignment of the indicating lines on the side of the mould with the produced lines of the quadrilateral on the patient (Fig. 4.11). Tubular elasticated netting is used as an additional aid to holding the mould in position, especially during sleep. Regular checks are made of the mould's position and, of course, any disturbance is easily recognised because neither the tape nor the netting obscures the view of the locating lines on the patient and the mould (Fig. 4.12).

Cellulose Acetate Gold Seed Mould

Moulds carrying radioactive gold seeds have long been used for the treatment of certain lesions arising in the pinna close to the meatus. This device is moulded in clear CAB sheet. The area of the pinna to be treated is drawn on the patient allowing a margin of 1 cm clear of the apparent extent of the lesion (Fig. 4.13). An impression is taken of the area to be treated, allowing for sufficient margin to cover the size of the mould and having due regard to its location and retention. Black tray compound, because of its pliancy and impressibility, is the best available material.

Before the impression is taken the treatment area is defined on the patient and the proposed mould site is painted with liquid paraffin to facilitate separation. The black tray compound is heated in water to a temperature of 56–57 °C until it becomes soft and malleable. Just sufficient compound is moulded into a smooth ball by wet fingers, as excess material is a hindrance. A naked flame played over the surface gives the compound a high polish required to get a good impression. To avoid burning the patient, the compound is repeatedly heated with the flame and cooled to 56 °C in water until it has assumed the appropriate shape. Thereafter, the perfectly shaped compound is packed in the ear, pushed firmly against the tissue surface and held there until the material is cold and hard. It is customary to take two impressions, the better of which is selected for use. A model of the impression is cast in hard plaster (Kaffir Dee). When the plaster is set, it and the attached compound are immersed in hot water. This causes the compound to soften and it is then easily removed from the model. The treatment area previously defined on the patient is exactly transferred onto the model. The treatment height, which is the distance from the central plane of the seeds to the skin, is 0.5 cm. Clear CAB sheets are moulded onto the model using a small thermoplastic forming machine. The sheets are built up in layers to a thickness of 4.5 mm, since the thickness of a seed is 1 mm and the treatment distance of 0.5 cm is measured from the centre of the seeds. The CAB is trimmed to size, the edges are smoothed and polished, and then it is fitted to the patient.

Since the mould is transparent, the treatment area can be transferred from the patient directly onto the surface of the mould. The thickness of the mould is checked with calipers and any deviation from 4.5 mm is corrected. The treatment area is taken from the skin surface of the mould and measured in square centimetres.

When a lesion is protuberant the treatment height is taken from the level of the surrounding normal tissues, so that the upper surface of the mould must be thinned down to the correct height. For the patient's comfort it is desirable to burr a little of the plastic away from the underside of the

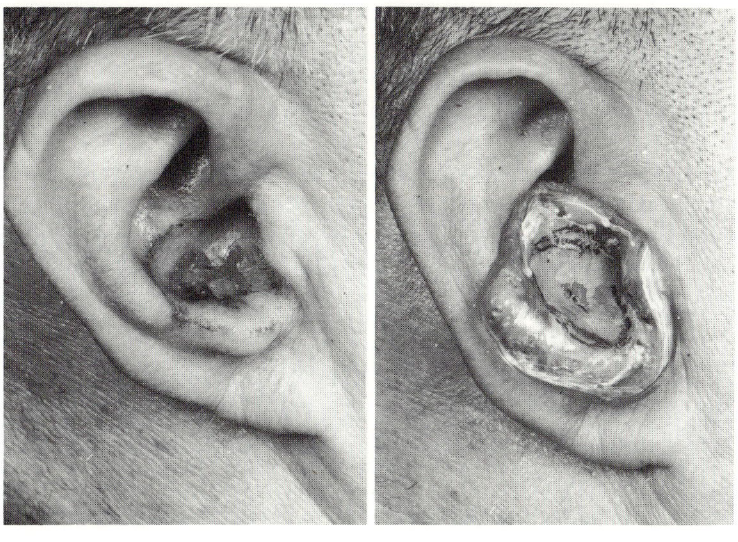

Fig. 4.13. Cellulose acetate gold seed mould.

mould such that it clears the lesion. (If a thermo-forming machine is not available, the mould is first made in wax and then reproduced in acrylic, using the "lost wax" method, as practised by dental technicians.) The mould surface is painted with spirit adhesive and the prescribed number of gold-198 seeds loaded onto the perimeter line. The seeds are secured in position by small pieces of transparent plastic adhesive tape. The mould is applied to the patient (Fig. 4.13) and held in contact with spirit gum; as an additional precaution, adhesive tape is used to hold it in position. The mould is worn continuously over 7 days.

Adhesive Gold Seed Mould

This simple and effective method of treatment for small skin cancers on flat surfaces can be used for out-patients, providing the amount of radioactive sources employed does not exceed the statutory limitations. If these limitations are exceeded it is necessary to admit the patient for one night to allow the sources to decay to an acceptable level.

This type of mould (Fig. 4.14) is of particular value for small superficial skin cancers arising on flat surfaces, e.g. the dorsum of the hand and the lower leg. One other site where it is of great value is for cancer arising from the pinna of the ear, where it may be used either as a single-plane mould or as a double (or sandwich) mould for lesions arising from the free margin of the pinna (Fig. 4.15).

The construction is as follows: Surgical adhesive felt, with adhesive on both sides, in thicknesses of 0.5 and 1 cm, is used to carry the seeds at the necessary treatment distance. The felt is cut to the required shape with a margin of 0.5 cm wider then the area to be treated. Gold seeds are then arranged on one adhesive surface according to the mould distribution rules and covered with a layer of Elastoplast or equivalent to keep them in position. The other adhesive surface is then applied to the skin area involved and the mould secured by additional strips of adhesive material. The loading of the mould is facilitated by the use of a loading former which serves the dual purpose of obtaining uniform accuracy of distribution of sources with consequent reduction of exposure time to staff (Fig. 4.14). Following the prescription and calculation of distribution the gold-198 seeds are loaded in the grooves of the appropriate former. They are then easily transferred by gentle pressure onto one surface of a piece of double adhesive felt of the required thickness. The seeds are then covered by a piece of Elastoplast and the completed mould applied to the skin involved (Fig. 4.14).

The mould is worn continuously for 7 days. The patient is instructed when to remove the mould, and to return it at the next visit to the appropriate clinic.

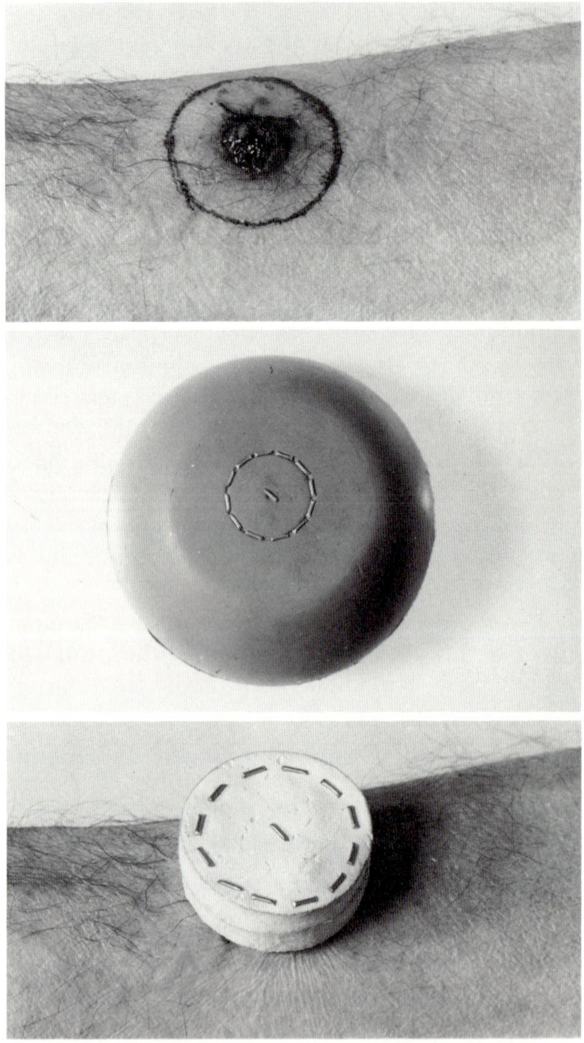

a b c

Fig. 4.14a–c. Adhesive gold seed mould.

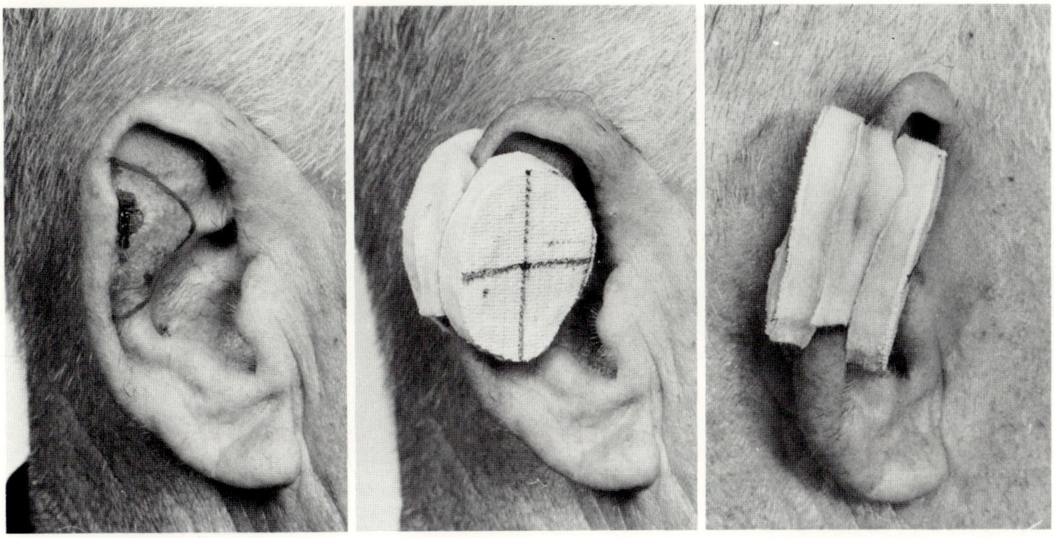

Fig. 4.15. Double adhesive gold seed mould.

Preparation of a Beam Direction Shell

The following detailed example describes the preparation of the shell used in the treatment of the larynx by X-rays from a linear accelerator. The same principles apply to other sites.

Impression

The taking of an impression is a critical stage in the preparation of any variety of mould or shell. It must be accurate and be taken when the patient is as relaxed as possible. The posture of the patient when the impression is taken must be that to be adopted during treatment. For preference, this position is supine, but if the patient cannot lie flat because of respiratory or unusual skeletal disabilities, an inclined board can be used to support the body from the waist up.

The patient with laryngeal cancer is treated lying supine, with the cervical spine extended over a neck support. At the same time, the shoulders are kept well down (Fig. 4.16). The shell must be sufficiently large to immobilise the neck and head of the patient in a reproducible treatment position. To achieve this the shell must be extended upwards onto the chin and jaw and downwards to the clavicles. Plaster of Paris bandage is used as the impression material. It is necessary to use a releasing agent between the patient's skin and the plaster bandage. A barrier cream spread sparingly over the skin surface is suitable for this purpose.

Plaster of Paris bandage is first cut into manageable pieces, approximately 15 cm × 7 cm and double in thickness. It is immersed in warm, not hot, water and the excess moisture is removed by running the pieces of bandage, without creasing, between two straight fingers. The bandage is laid, without wrinkling, on the patient's skin. The bandage is smoothed over the surface of the skin, using the flat of the fingers to chase away any air trapped between the patient and the bandage (Fig. 4.17). Two double layers of bandage are sufficient, but a reinforcing rib wrapped around the curvature of the impression avoids distortion when the impression is removed. It is advisable to use small pieces of bandage which readily follow the surface where the contours are complex. Care must be taken not to carry the impression too far round the cylinder of the neck because, once set, the impression would have to be sprung open and this would distort it when it is withdrawn from the neck. The impression is set within minutes. Before the impression is removed from the patient, the skin is eased away from the bandage around the edges, since this helps to release the vacuum which builds up beneath the impression. The impression is delicate, and to avoid damage it is laid on a sand bag ready for casting the model. Before casting the

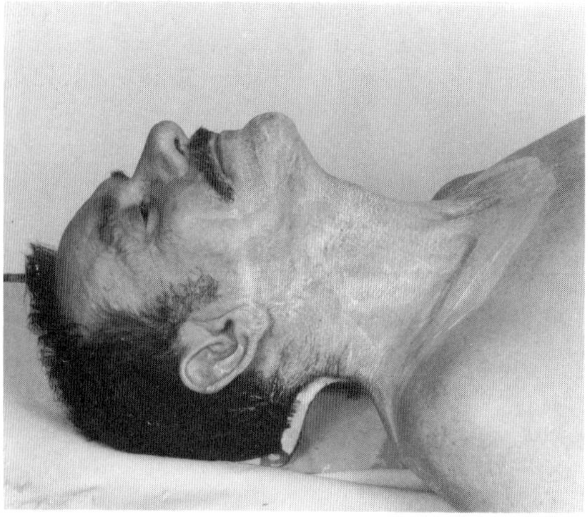

Fig. 4.16.

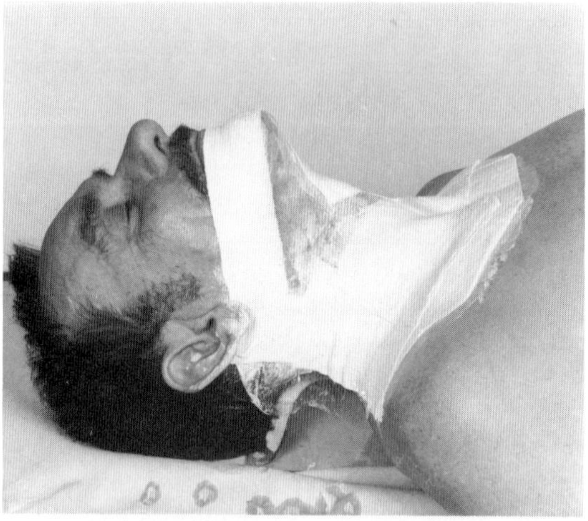

Fig. 4.17.

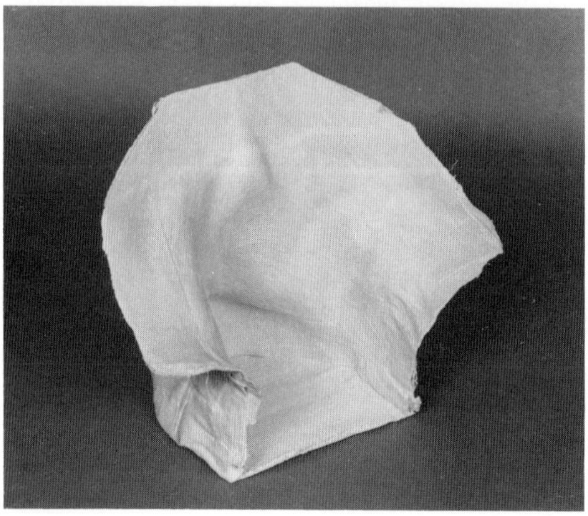

Fig. 4.18.

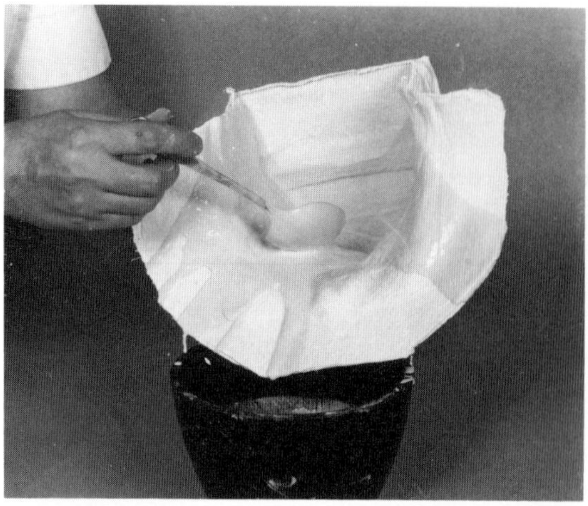

Fig. 4.19.

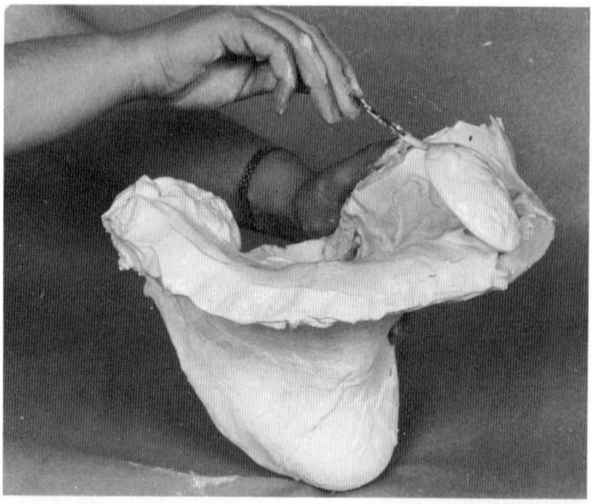

Fig. 4.20.

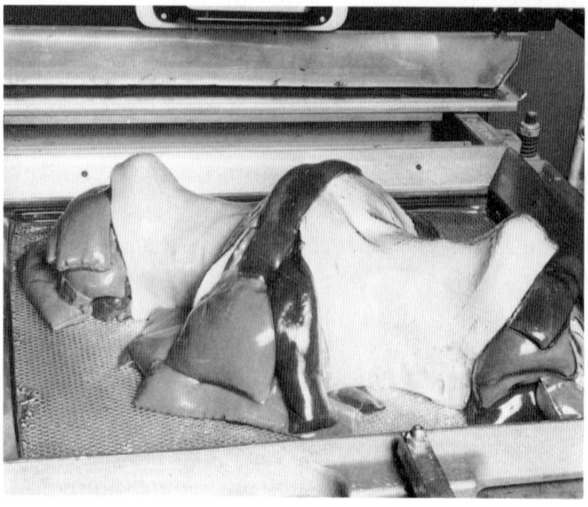

Fig. 4.21.

Figs. 4.16–4.21. Preparation of model for beam direction shell.

model, it is helpful to suspend an additional bandage across the top of the impression. This makes a container for easy casting (Fig. 4.18).

Model

The model is cast in dental plaster of Paris. The plaster powder is sprinkled into a rubber bowl containing cold water until all the liquid has disappeared. The proportions are approximately 50% water to 50% powder by volume. A rubber bowl is used to contain the mixture as it is easily cleaned if the plaster sets too quickly. Cold rather than hot water is used to slow down the setting time of the plaster. The mix is poured into the impression and washed over the surface, thus chasing away trapped air which would form a hole in the positive model (Fig. 4.19). Further mixes of plaster are added, layer by layer, building up to an overall thickness of approximately 2 cm. It is not necessary to fill the impression with plaster. Particular attention is paid to the edge because this is the weakest part of the model; it must be thick and smoothed round with wet fingers when the plaster is firm but not quite set. A thick smooth edge is less likely to be damaged (Fig. 4.20). Within 10 min the plaster is sufficiently hard for the plaster bandage of the impression to be stripped off the model, layer by layer.

The model is a reproduction of the appropriate part of the patient. If the initial impression was a good one there should be no necessity to smooth or alter the surface of the model.

Foundation

The shell is made from 3-mm-thick transparent CAB. This material is an ideal foundation because it is light, is easily worked and machined, and retains its shape. A vacuum forming-machine is used to mould the plastic. For economic reasons the foundations are formed on two models at a time (Fig. 4.21). An experienced technician can speedily form a shell manually with virtually no waste; this is done when only one shell is to be formed. To hand-form, a tissue-paper template is taken from the model and the estimated area of CAB is cut out. Using two pairs of pliers to hold the plastic, both sides are slowly heated over a gas flame using a circular movement to avoid the formation of bubbles in the plastic if it is burnt. At 120 °C the material becomes soft and pliable and in this state it is placed on the model and moulded into shape by hand. Cotton gloves are worn for protection against burns. Small areas which are not in apposition with the model can be locally reheated and persuaded down into position. Surplus CAB is trimmed away from the edges with tin-snips or shears after vacuum or hand forming. The edges are filed until smooth and polished with a solvent. Chloroform dissolves CAB and is suitable for this purpose. If the shell needs to be extended beyond the area originally estimated, a piece of plastic is heated and formed onto the model overlapping the existing shell. This piece can be trimmed when cool, leaving the overlap approximately 0.25 cm wide along the joint. If the edge is bevelled and polished a smart finish can be achieved. Solvent introduced into the joint space causes the two pieces to fuse together.

Fit and Retention

The shell is fitted to the patient and its close apposition with the skin over the whole area is checked (Fig. 4.22). PVC straps passed round the patient hold the shell firmly in position. The straps must be secured in such a manner that the tension does not displace the shell on the patient but holds it snugly in position. Where the straps are fastened, nylon screws are bolted to the shell and holes are punched in the straps to fit over the screw-ends. As "tumour localisations" are carried out on the empty shell, it is important that the shell retains the same shape on and off the patient. The tension of the strap, therefore, must not cause distortion of the shell.

Tumour Localisation

For this procedure the shell is fitted with radio-opaque markers and a lateral radiograph is taken with the patient wearing the shell (Figs. 4.22 and 4.23). A "ladder marker" is made from lead shot which is spaced at approximately 1 cm intervals. The lead shot is held on an adhesive plastic tape and attached to the shell along the midline of the patient. If there is a back portion to the shell, a similar ladder marker is placed along the posterior midline, otherwise a plastic bridge is added to the

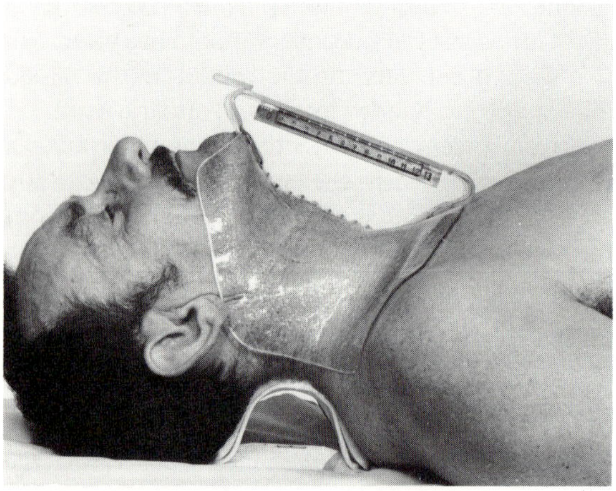

Fig. 4.22. Fit and retention of beam direction shell.

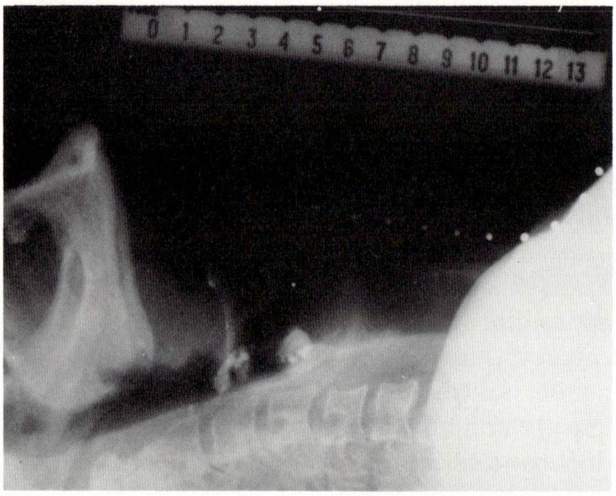

Fig. 4.23. Lateral radiograph for carcinoma of larynx.

shell. The span of the bridge is fixed some 5–6 cm in front of the shell to carry a second marker along the projected midplane of the patient (Figs. 4.24 and 4.25). The bridge is made from a flat strip of CAB 2 cm in width, which is shaped by local heating, modelled to fit on the shell, and the joint is fused with chloroform. To project the midline plane precisely onto the bridge, two thin heated metal rods are pushed through the shell at the inferior and superior ends of the marked mid-line and aligned in an anteroposterior direction along the midplane. The points where the two pin-ends touch the bridge are marked and a straight line drawn between them on the bridge. If the two projected points are correct, the midline on the shell and the line on the bridge are coplanar in the patient's sagittal plane. The second marker is a metal scale (Fig. 4.25). It is fixed by its calibrated edge to the posterior surface of the bridge. It is parallel to the midline and offset from it by 4 mm. Fine metal wire is placed down the outer surface of the bridge for identification on the radiograph (see Fig. 4.24). A lateral radiograph of the patient wearing the shell is taken at a focus-skin distance of 100 cm. Based on the clinical findings, the tumour centre, the vertical and horizontal planes of the treatment volume, and also the treatment plane are drawn on the radiograph. The treatment plane is transferred from the radiograph to the shell (Fig. 4.26) by noting where the plane crosses the

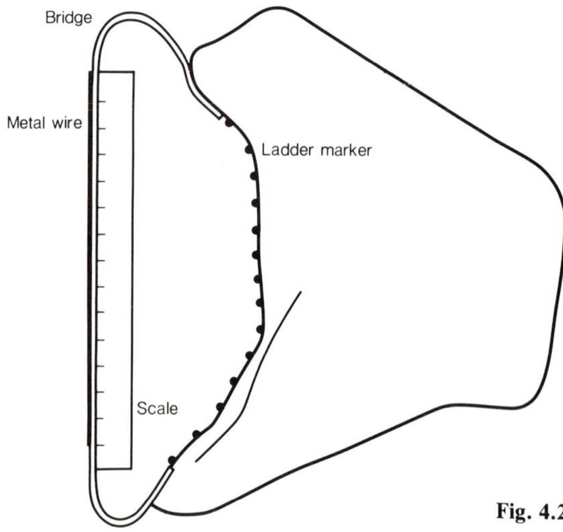

Fig. 4.24.

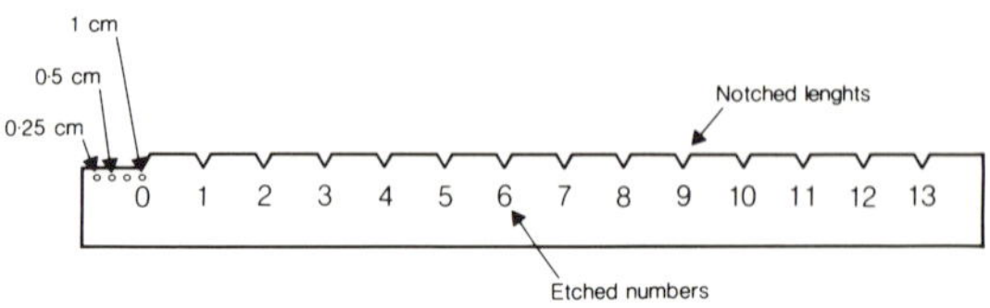

Fig. 4.25.

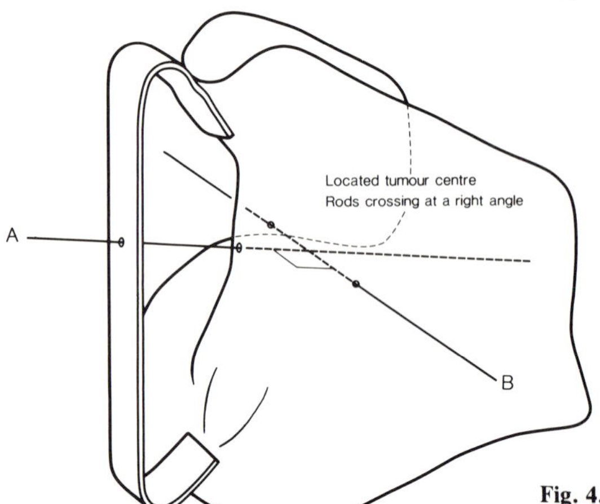

Fig. 4.26.

Figs. 4.24–4.27. Tumour localisation.

Fig. 4.27.

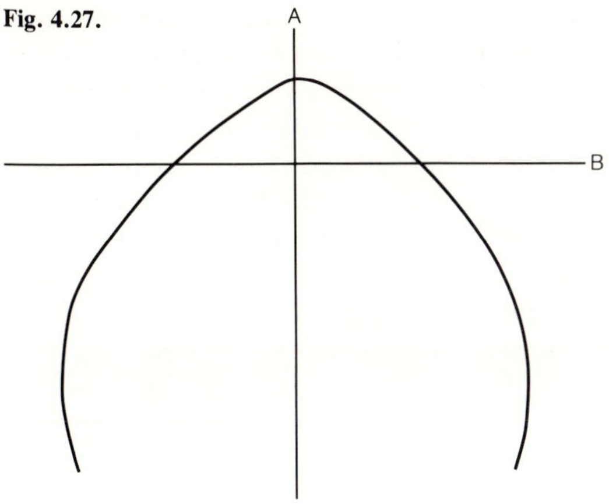

markers and then inserting a heated rod *A* through the lines on the midplane at the appropriate points. This provides an anteroposterior axis of reference. The distance between the tumour centre and the outer surface of the bridge is measured on the radiograph. Because of magnification, the distance when transferred to the shell will need to be reduced. By referring directly to the calibrated scale on the radiograph, the reduced measurement is readily determined. At the predicted tumour centre, a rod *B* is pushed through the shell in a lateral direction, intersecting the anteroposterior rod *A* at a right angle and on the same plane. This provides a lateral locating axis of reference. A *locating table* (described in the section entitled "Mould Room Apparatus" below) is used as an aid in this stage of the preparation.

Verification

Without crossing, rods *A* and *B* support the shell in a *contour table* (also described under "Mould Room Apparatus"). A heated rod, similar in diameter to those used to support the shell, is rested on the table top so that, by sliding the hot end of the rod around the shell, the central treatment plane is permanently etched on the outside of the shell. With the shell in the table, the etched plane and the entrance and exit points of both rods are projected down from the shell onto paper. The points are connected on the paper and the tumour centre is indicated by the intersection of the two axes of reference, anteroposterior and lateral (Fig. 4.27). The position of the tumour centre in the shell and the proposed treatment volume are then verified by a lateral radiograph. To do this precisely, rod *B* is passed through the shell along the lateral axis. A thin metal tube, with a bore minutely larger than the rod, is heated, slid along the rod, welded by its heat into the shell, and allowed to cool. A perfectly flat, highly polished black or mirror-surface Perspex plaque is cut to the size of the treatment volume, and a fine wire fixed around the plaque's perimeter. A hole, of the same diameter as the tube, is precisely drilled perpendicular to the plaque's face and at its centre. The plaque is slid along the rod and eased over the tube (Fig. 4.28). It is held at right angles to the axis and lined up with the treatment plane (Fig. 4.29). The rod *B* is removed, leaving the plaque on the shell at the entrance of the axis; a ball bearing is placed in the exit hole and a short rod is re-introduced through the bridge and into the shell surface. A little adhesive tape on the inside of the shell prevents the rod sticking into the patient.

Because of the complex shape of the shell, the plaque usually stands proud when it is attached to the shell at the correct angle. If the tumour is on the left or right of the patient's midline, the plaque is fixed to the shell on the relevant side, but it must be remembered that the plaque's magnification on the radiograph will be greater than the degree to which the tumour area is magnified.

The shell is fitted to the patient in the treatment position and the pointer of the X-ray machine is lined up to the centre of the plaque. The machine is angled in such a way that the pointer's reflection in the plaque's surface is in a state of "no parallax" and centred on the tube in the middle of the plaque (Fig. 4.30). The film is placed at right angles to the lateral axis, parallel to the plaque. The pointer is removed before exposure. On the radiograph, the treatment plane identified by the anteroposterior rod *A*, the outline of the treatment volume, and the axis *B* passing through the tumour centre are verified. As the tube in the centre of the plaque is observed from the end elevation, it will show on the radiograph as a circle. With precisely accurate alignment the ball bearing placed in the exit hole will be seen as a ball superimposed in the centre of the circle (Fig. 4.31). Reference to the anteroposterior axis on the radiograph confirms the correct angling of the plaque in relation to the plane.

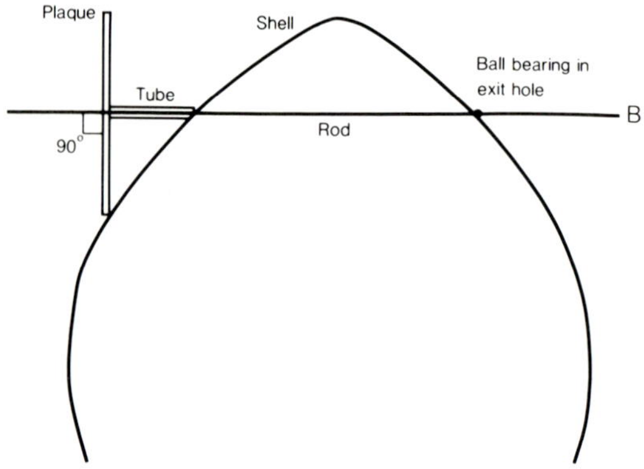

Fig. 4.28.

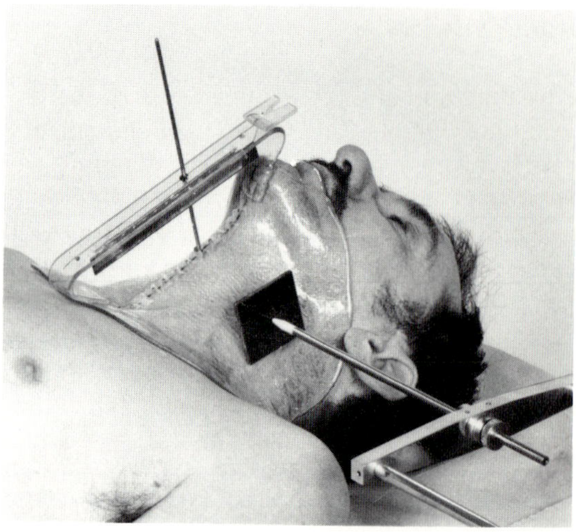

Fig. 4.30.

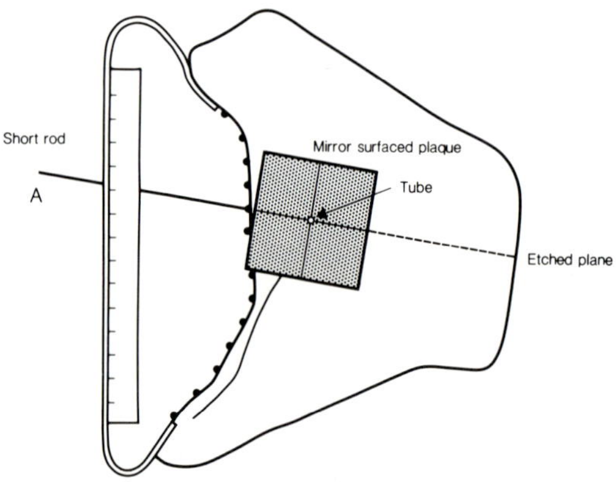

Fig. 4.29.

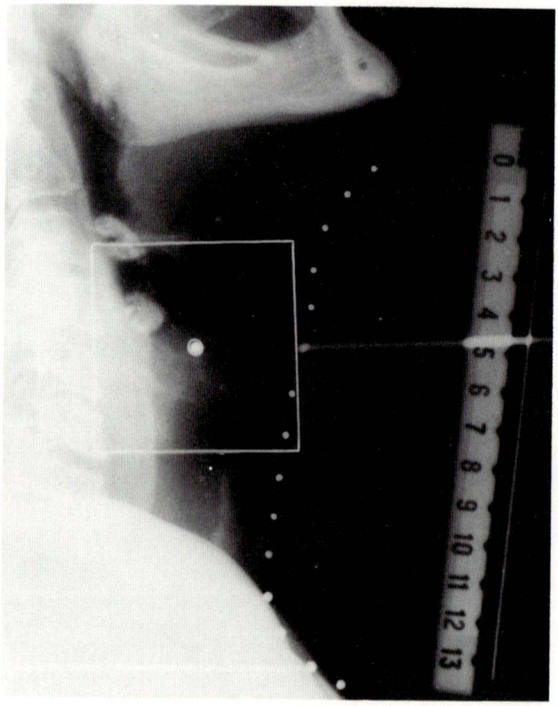

Fig. 4.31.

Figs. 4.28–4.31. Tumour verification.

Plotting of Beams

The treatment beams are arranged and drawn on the contour (Fig. 4.32). The physical and clinical factors involved in field selection and planning are discussed in Chap 1. The entrance and exit points of the central axis of each beam are transferred onto the shell. If the contour was taken from the inside of the shell, these points must be recorded on the same surface. The distance from the verification axis *B* to the entrance and exit points of the axis of each treatment beam are measured with dividers and marked at the appropriate spot on the etched plane on the shell. Rods are pushed through the shell, permanently recording these entry and exit points (Fig. 4.33). The angles at the point of intersection of each beam axis in the shell are checked against those on the plan. If the rods are exactly on the plane (as they should be), it is not possible to introduce more than one at a time into the shell without bending the rods.

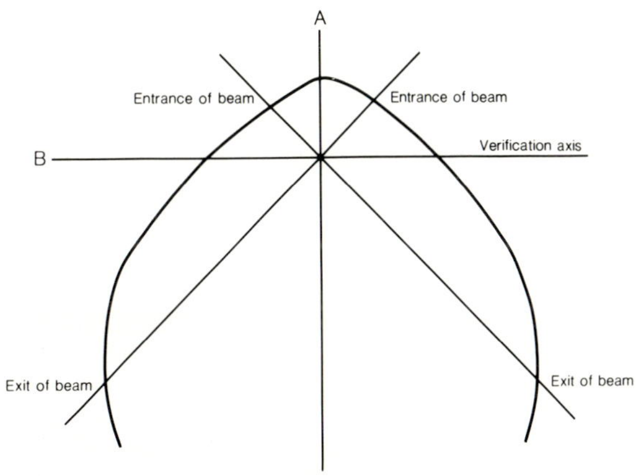

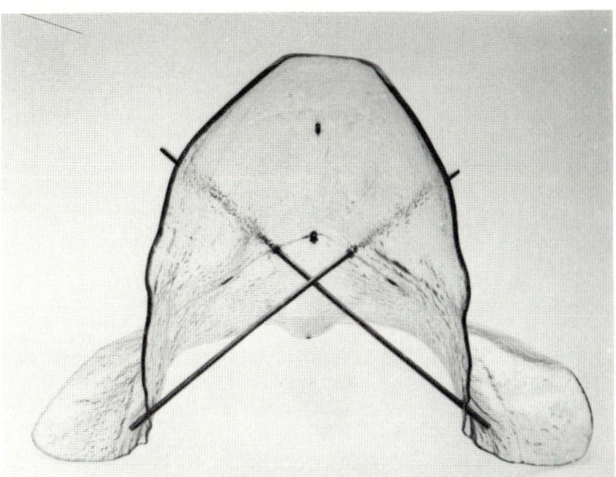

Figs. **4.32–4.33.** Beam plotting.

"Porting" of Field Sizes

The shell is rested in the contour table, supported by a rod which is passed through the entrance and exit points of the central axis of one of the treatment beams. Two rods, supported on the table and held there with lead blocks, are pushed into entrance or exit holes to stabilise the shell in the correct plane. A range of porting guides, simulating the treatment beams' divergence and representing the field sizes from 4 cm×4 cm up to 12 cm×12 cm, are used to define the extent of each field on the shell. The guide is made of brass and has a grooved base which fits over the rod to determine its direction along the treatment axis (Fig. 4.34). Following the edges of the porting guide with a heated flat blade, the upper half of the field outline is etched on the outside of the shell. The shell is then turned upside down, replaced in

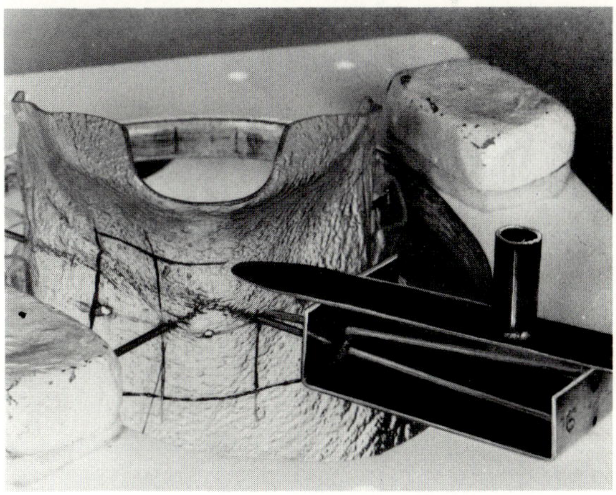

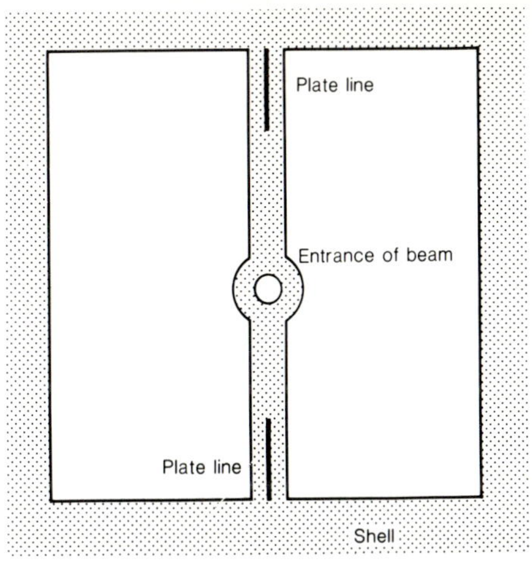

Figs. 4.34–4.35. Porting of fields.

the table, and the lower half of the field outline is defined. To etch the outlines of the other fields on the shell the same procedure is followed. If the field size is rectangular, e.g. 6 cm wide × 8 cm high, two porting guides of appropriate size are used. The vertical midplane of the beam is often used to line up the treatment machine to the correct plane. Therefore, it is necessary to draw the vertical midplane of the beam accurately on the shell. To do this a machine-edged, right-angled block is laid on the contour table in apposition to the beam-axis rod. An identical rod is heated and run up the vertical side of the block, thus projecting the line on the shell. The field size and an additional 0.5 cm around its margin is then cut out with an oscillating saw forming a window in the shell. A central strip, on which the "plate line" (indicating the alignment of the beam) and the entrance point of the beam are marked, remains in the window (Fig. 4.35). The edges are filed and polished to avoid abrasion of the skin. A margin of white plastic emulsion is painted around the field, over the central strip in the window, and over the exit points. The set-up instructions for the treatment, i.e. the "plate lines", centres, field sizes, and the alignment showing the direction and thickness of the wedges, are clearly drawn on the white surface (Fig. 4.36). A colour code identifies the angle and thickness of the wedges.

The characteristics of the shell and the calculations of the prescription are all checked before treatment is allowed to commence. The machine is lined up to the shell on the patient for each treatment, the front and back pointers being accurately aligned. During each exposure the front pointer is, of course, removed, while the back pointer remains in position (Fig. 4.37).

The same procedure, with slight modifications, is followed for the preparation of shells used in the treatments of other sites. In all instances the size of the shell must be sufficiently large to immobilise the patient in a reproducible treatment position and cover the upper and lower limits of the estimated beam margins. If, at the impression stage, it is necessary to cover the eyes or eyebrows, cellophane is the ideal separation material. When the shell is to fit part or all of the hair of the head, tubular nylon hose tied at one end and pulled tightly down over the head is used as the separator. To avoid the patient becoming claustrophobic, a large hole is cut in the nylon exposing the eyes, nose, and mouth. Barrier cream is smoothed over the hose as an extra precaution against the hair protruding through the hose and sticking to the impression material.

To take the impression more than half way round a cylindrical shape, e.g. when preparing a helmet-type shell, it should be done in stages, one half overlapping the other. To do this the first half of the impression is completed and the edges are greased with barrier cream covering a margin of

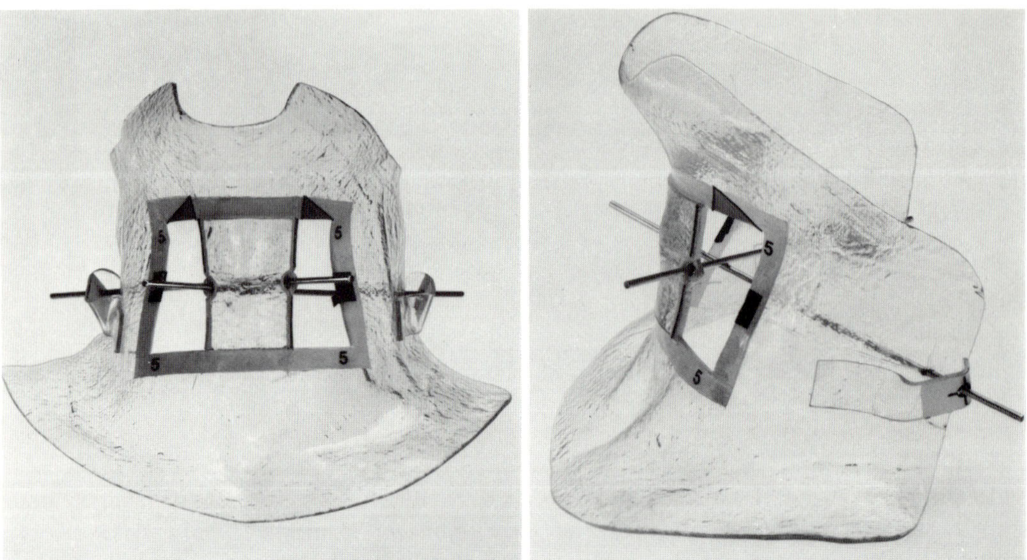

Fig. 4.36. Completed shell for carcinoma of larynx.

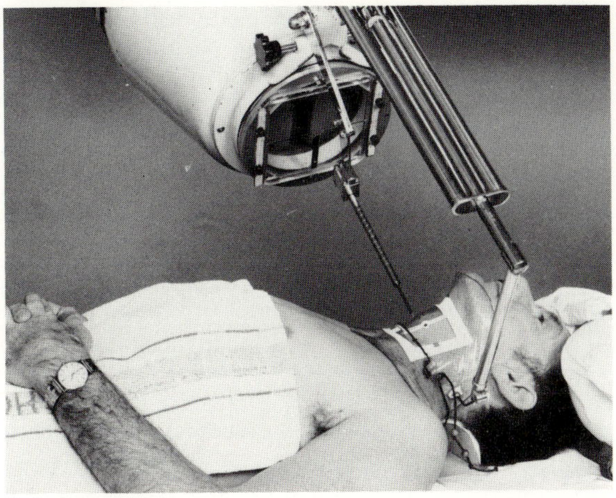

Fig. 4.37. Patient in treatment position.

approximately 2 cm; the second half overlaps this margin. It is advisable to reinforce this seam along the joint with extra pieces of plaster bandage. Locating pencil lines are drawn across the joint for re-alignment of the two sections later. When the impression is set, a flat-edged tool is used to open the joint so that each section can be removed independently. The two parts are slotted together and the alignment of the locating pencil lines checked; bandage applied over the joints holds them together. This additional bandage must lie on the outside of the cast so as not to interfere with the negative impression of the patient when the model is cast.

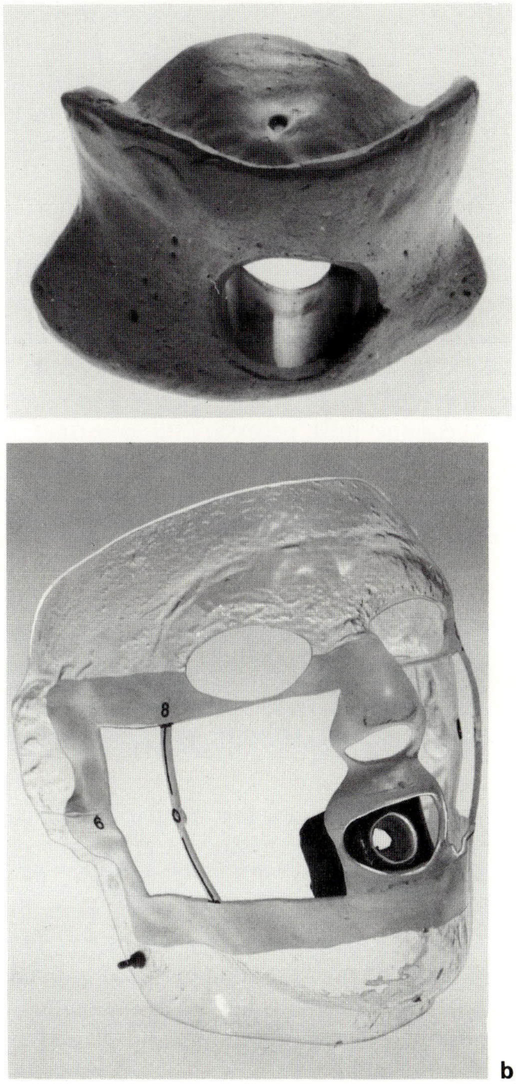

a

b

Fig. 4.38. a Bite-block. **b** Wax-porting.

Bite-Blocks

Used in conjunction with beam direction shells the purpose of a bite block is threefold: (1) to stabilise the jaw of the patient so that the same position of the mouth is reproduced at each treatment, (2) to deflect or depress the tongue away from the high-dose treatment volume, and (3) to fill the natural airspace in the mouth. The decision to employ a bite-block must be taken during the initial clinical assessment of the patient, and the preparation and fitting of the bite-block must, of course, be completed *before* embarking on the preparation of the appropriate beam direction shell.

The bite-block (Fig. 4.38) is easily prepared from dental black tray compound. The compound is softened in water at a temperature of 56–57 °C. Both ends of the barrel of a hypodermic syringe approximately 2 cm in diameter are cut off and smoothed, after which the compound is wrapped around the cylinder, polished, and then a squash bite is taken. The diameter of the syringe is the approximate height of a normal bite, and being hollow it provides an airway for the patient.

The portion of the block which lies on the floor of the mouth is cut away with a sharp, thin-bladed knife, retaining only the groove in which the alveolar ridge fits. To reduce discomfort the compound is also scraped away where it touches the lesion. Where it is desirable to depress the tongue, sufficient additional compound is added to the block on the base of the syringe barrel, spreading posteriorly as far as the patient can tolerate without gagging. If the configuration of the depression is favourable, the soft palate is visible when viewed through the tube. To deflect the tongue towards the midline a similar method is employed and a mass of compound added where the tongue would normally intrude.

It might appear that the wearing of artificial dentures by edentulous patients would be a satisfactory way of stabilising the mouth, but this is seldom practicable because patients with mouth lesions either cannot wear their dentures, or find their tight fit unpleasant as the mouth becomes tender from the radiation reaction.

On occasions it is necessary to construct a tongue depressor for a patient with natural teeth. This type of bite-block can be readily constructed from sheet Perspex and a quick-setting acrylic which cures in air and does not require flasking and heating. However, the curing of quick-setting acrylic is an exothermic reaction and it must, therefore, be used with caution to avoid burning the patient. To prepare the block a flat piece of 3-mm-thick Perspex is fashioned to cover the area of the tongue and the front upper and lower teeth. The edges are filed, smoothed, and polished with a chloroform swab. A doughy mound of quick-setting acrylic is then perched on the upper surface of the prepared Perspex, to which it adheres, and the upper surface of the acrylic dough is liberally coated with a separator of liquid paraffin. The device is placed in the patient's mouth and a squash bite is taken. This impression is taken the moment the acrylic becomes doughy, to avoid a thermal burn. Almost immediately the block is removed from the mouth and allowed to polymerise. When the acrylic has cured, on the underside of the Perspex a small amount of newly mixed dough is laid along the estimated line of the front lower teeth. The block is replaced in the mouth, located on the upper teeth, and the lower impression is taken as the patient closes the mouth. The completed block is removed from the patient, allowed to cure, and any areas causing discomfort are burred or filed away.

Wax Porting on Shells

Wax bolus is used as tissue-equivalent material in three situations:

1) The *wax port* is used if all the surface of the field requires bolus to compensate for excessively oblique incidence in both the vertical and horizontal planes.
2) The *wax curtain* is used if half or part of the field requires bolus to compensate for missing tissues, usually in the vertical plane.
3) The *wax build-up* is used if a uniform thickness of bolus is necessary to bring the dose up to the skin surface, e.g. over nodes or scars and when the tumour is near the skin surface.

Wax Port

The port is faced with a 3-mm-thick Perspex plaque. The plaque is prepared with a 0.5-cm margin greater than the field size. A 3-mm hole is drilled through the centre of the plaque and the field size is drawn on its face along with the central, vertical, and horizontal lines (Fig. 4.39d). Anchorage points, which hold the wax in position on the shell, are necessary because frequent fittings, on and off the patient, loosen the port. Thin strips of 2-mm CAB moulded to the shape of low bridges are cemented to the shell to make the anchors. A thermostatically controlled bath is used to heat the wax, to ensure even malleability. A 3-mm-diameter rod is pushed through the shell along the axis of the treatment beam. A small mass of wax is kneaded well to remove any trapped air. The wax surface which is to come in contact with the shell is heated to a near-melting condition and then packed onto the shell, around the anchors and the rod. The melted wax adheres to the shell surface.

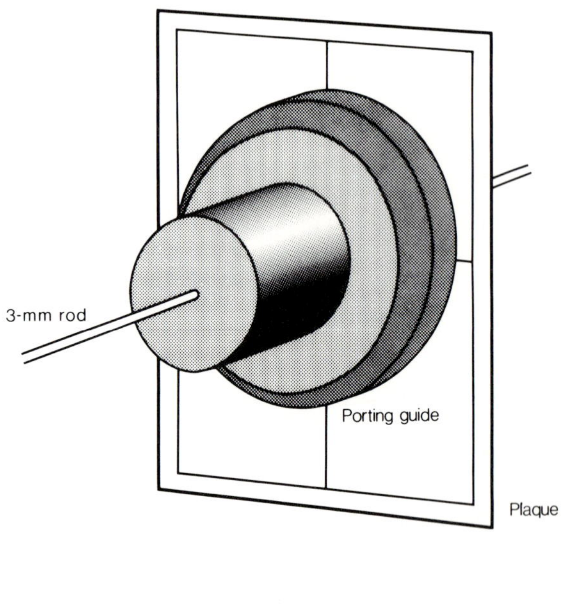

a

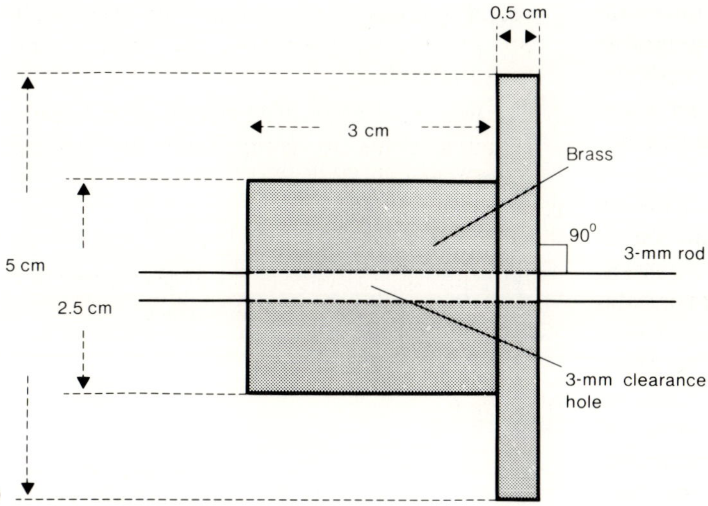

b

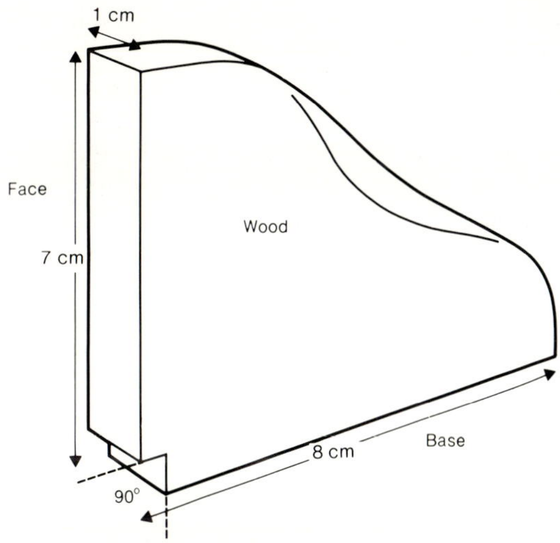

c

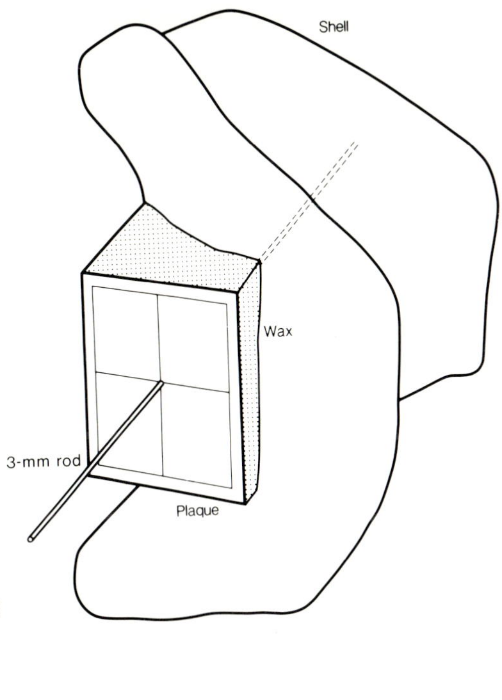

d

Fig. 4.39. Wax porting. **a** Porting guide and plaque, **b** Porting guide, **c** Curtain former, **d** Wax port.

The plaque and the porting guide (Fig. 4.39a) are centred on the rod and held together so that both faces are in close apposition. The pair are slid along the axis until a part of the plaque just touches the shell, at the same time compressing the wax into shape. The distance from the plaque to the tumour centre is kept as short as is practicable, to minimise scattering at the edge of the beam in the wax. If the areas where the plaque and the shell meet are trimmed away, part of the treatment field surface is on the skin and therefore the port is at least 6 mm closer to the plane of the tumour. Since the plaque must lie perpendicular to the treatment axis, excessive pressure may alter this angle and must be avoided. The centre line defined on the plaque must be parallel to the etched plane on the shell. Excess wax is trimmed away and the surface smoothed. The porting guide is not removed until the wax is cool and hard. The angles of the plaque in relation to the rod and the plane on the shell must be checked, since contraction of the wax may cause distortion. The port surface is painted with plastic emulsion on which are drawn the field beam size and the central, vertical, and horizontal lines.

Wax Curtain

Before a wax curtain is applied to a shell, the field sizes are marked out. That part of the field where there is to be no build-up is cut out of the shell. The edge of the shell adjacent to the area requiring build-up is bevelled, so that the curtain begins at the skin surface level, rather than the outside of the shell. Anchors are cemented to the shell to hold the wax. The shell is supported in the contour table in such a way that the area which requires the bolus is uppermost. Soft wax is packed onto the shell and pressed into shape with the aid of a curtain-former (Fig. 4.39c). This former slides over the surface of the contour table until the vertical face butts up against the bevelled edge of the shell. Simultaneously, the former compresses the wax into the required shape of the curtain. If the wax has been kneaded well and the former is moistened with Xylene, the wax does not stick to the former. Wax fragments between the base of the former and the table surface alter the vertical angle and are therefore removed. An additional 0.5-cm margin is left on the wax as a precaution to cover the beam area; the excess is trimmed away and the edges are smoothed. The surface of the wax is painted and the exact field size and plate lines for alignment of the treatment machine are defined on the surface.

Wax Build-up

Where a thickness of up to 6 mm is required, it is usually simpler to use CAB. Layers of CAB are heated and moulded over the shell's surface until the required thickness is attained. The original plaster model must be used to support the shell whilst the heated plastic is added, otherwise distortion is inevitable. However, plastic is not suitable for a build-up greater than 6 mm, because it causes warping of the basic shell. In these circumstances wax is kneaded and packed onto the shell in a layer approximately as thick as is required. A former, similar to the curtain-former, is adapted by introducing a panel pin into its face. The pin is allowed to project the required distance from the former so that it acts as a simple depth gauge. Whilst the wax is still malleable it is pressed down to the desired thickness with the former. Providing the wax is heated to an almost liquid consistency, it will adhere to the shell and anchors are not necessary. Outside calipers are used to check the thickness of the bolus and any necessary adjustment is made. Excess wax around the field is trimmed away and the surface is painted. The fields and their centres are drawn on the surface.

Lead Cut-out

This type of mould is used in fractionated orthovoltage and electron beam treatments of skin lesions, where the contours of the site to be treated do not permit suitable shielding by standard pieces of sheet lead in the treatment room. A tailor-made lead cut-out has the additional important advantage of being able to be repeatedly placed in a stable and reproducible position on the patient.

Impression

Before the preparation of the mould commences, the area to be treated is defined on the skin. The lead cut-out is most frequently made for lesions on the face or ears. Because of the complex shape of these sites an alginate paste is a more suitable impression material than plaster of Paris bandage. Alginate gives a detailed impression, but because of its jelly-like consistency it must be stabilised with plaster of Paris bandage. After application of the alginate a layer of cotton gauze is placed over the setting paste, then a further two layers of plaster bandage are added and allowed to harden. The gauze binds the two materials so that the impression can be removed from the patient without distortion. No separating cream is necessary on the skin when using alginate, but a little grease applied to hairy areas and Vaseline gauze over tender lesions prevent discomfort on removal. Separators should not be used over the defined area since they cause smudging, so that when the treatment area line is transferred to the impression, and later to the model, it may be indistinct. A 4-cm margin around the treatment area is usually adequate for the size of the mould, but for location purposes it may be advisable to extend this further. For instance, the nose is a good anchorage point but it may be necessary to make the mould larger to protect the eyes.

Model

The model is cast in a mixture of 50% Kaffir-Dee (artificial stone) and 50% dental plaster. Though this mix has a longer setting time, a much harder model is produced which will withstand the pressure required to form the lead.

Foundation

The foundation is made from chemically pure lead which is malleable. It is hand-moulded when 1-mm thickness is used, but when shaping a thickness of 2 mm a wooden mallet has to be used. This tool is used to persuade the lead into shape, but swaging actions that might thin the material must be avoided. The lead is cut into sections and soldered together, so that very little hammering is necessary. Paper templates are first made on the model and the most suitable shapes for moulding the lead are then assessed. All the sections are held together with 60Pb/40Sn solder containing flux. This will flow freely providing (1) the adjoining oxidised edges of the lead are scraped clean with a knife or file and (2) the two surfaces of the joint are in close apposition. The lead is cut away precisely, forming an aperture the edge of which follows the delineated area on the plaster model. The perimeter of the mould is trimmed and any sharp projections burnished smooth.

The mould is fitted on the patient and any necessary adjustment made to the aperture. The upper and lower surfaces of the mould are painted with plastic emulsion paint, which protects the patient from lead toxicity and secondary radiation. In general, no strapping is required to retain the mould's position, its own weight usually being sufficient (Fig. 4.40).

If a thickness of 3 mm is required it is best to make the mould first to a thickness of 1 mm. After fitting to the patient it is replaced on the model and a second layer 2 mm in thickness is formed, in a similar manner to the first layer, on top of the mould. These two layers are then held together with solder and are ready for painting. The necessary thickness of the lead varies in relation to the kilovoltage of the machine; 1 mm gives sufficient shielding up to 100 kV, but for 300 kV a 3 mm thickness is required.

The use of electron beam therapy for skin cancer may require appropriate lead protection for surrounding structures. The technical details for preparing a suitable lead cut-out for 10-MV electrons are similar in every respect to those for the 3-mm lead mould for orthovoltage therapy (Fig. 4.41).

Lead Shielding for the Eye

Occasionally a standard eye shield of a suitable size is not available or is inappropriate, in which case an individual eye shield needs to be prepared (Fig. 4.42). This is made from a low-melting-point alloy (MPC70).

To make the shield, an impression is taken of the anaesthetised open eye. Ophthalmic alginate paste is used as the impression material and a model is

a 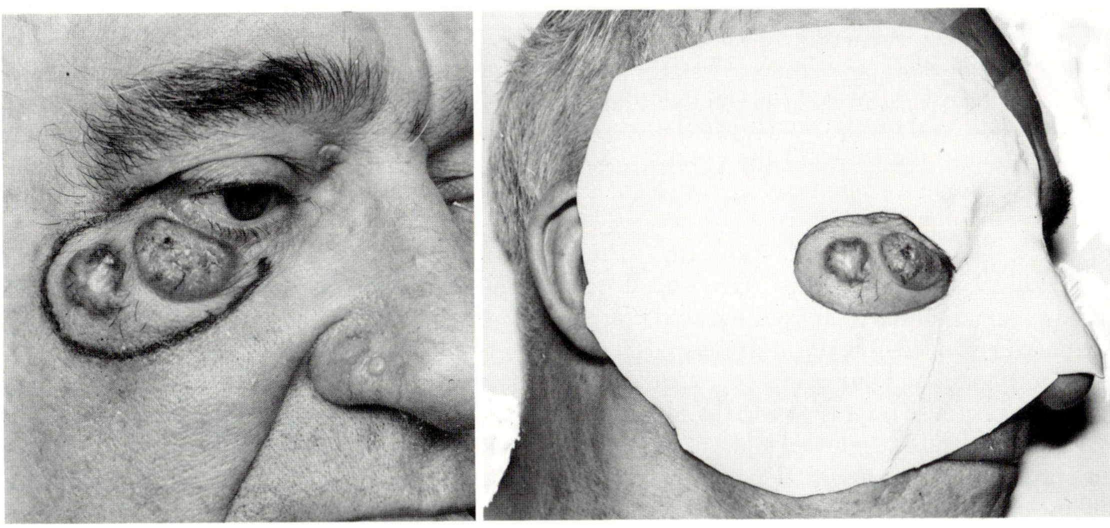 b

Fig. 4.40a,b. Lead cut-out.

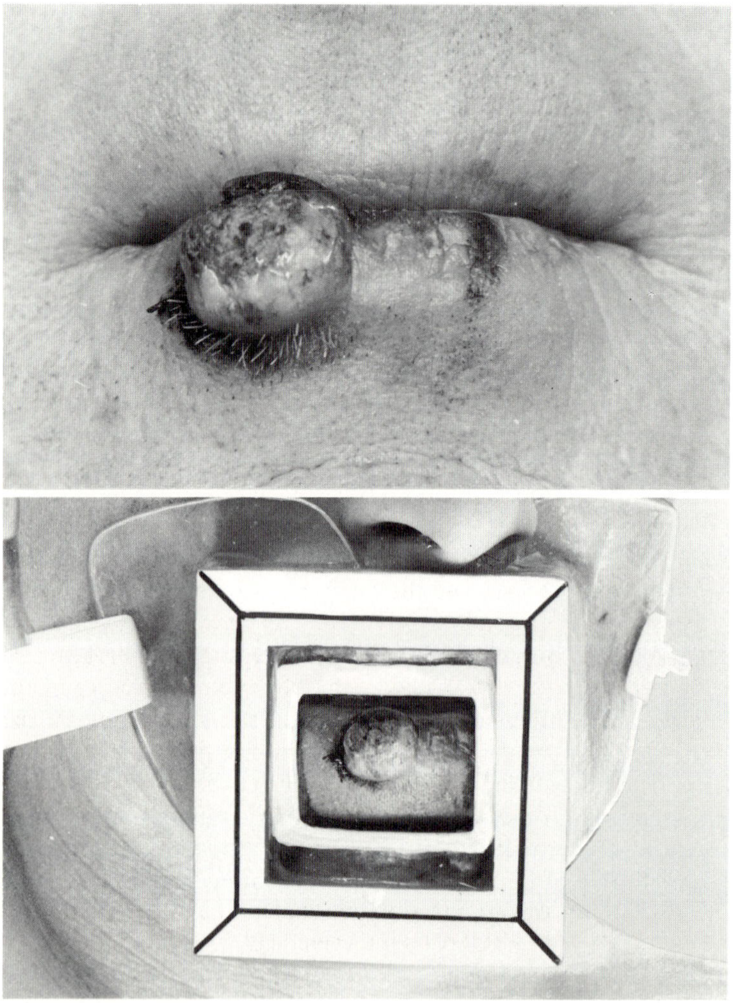

a

b

Fig. 4.41a,b. Lead cut-out for electron beam therapy for carcinoma of the lip.

cast in Kaffir-Dee plaster. A separator of cold mould seal is painted smoothly over the surface of the model. The alloy is heated, and when it becomes fluid it is poured over the eye portion of the model. Particular care is taken to avoid spillage of the alloy on to the model of the eyelids. The alloy is less dense than lead, therefore the shield is built up to a minimum thickness of 4 mm when the patient is to be treated with 300-kV X-rays. The thickness of the shield is built up in layers of alloy, each layer being allowed to cool and harden before the next layer is added. The shield is removed from the plaster model and any sharp edges are filed away. A vinyl varnish is sprayed over the complete surface of the metal and allowed to dry. A further three layers of varnish are added to ensure complete protection for the eye from any possible toxic properties of the alloy. The final application of varnish must be perfectly dry before the shield is used on the patient. When an outer lead cut-out is also required, the shield must be worn by the patient when the impression is taken, otherwise when the outer mould is complete it will not fit or locate in the precise position required to give an accurate treatment. Before each application, the shield is sterilised in a cold antiseptic solution.

Infrequently, because of the site of the disease, it is necessary to treat a portion of the eye itself. It may be possible to avoid cataract induction by directing the gaze of the patient to a marked spot under the lead shield, the position of the spot being chosen such that the pupil is directed out of the X-ray beam. The spot itself is a tiny aperture drilled through the appropriate part of the lead shield. A hood of lead, with sufficient clearance to allow light through, covers the hole.

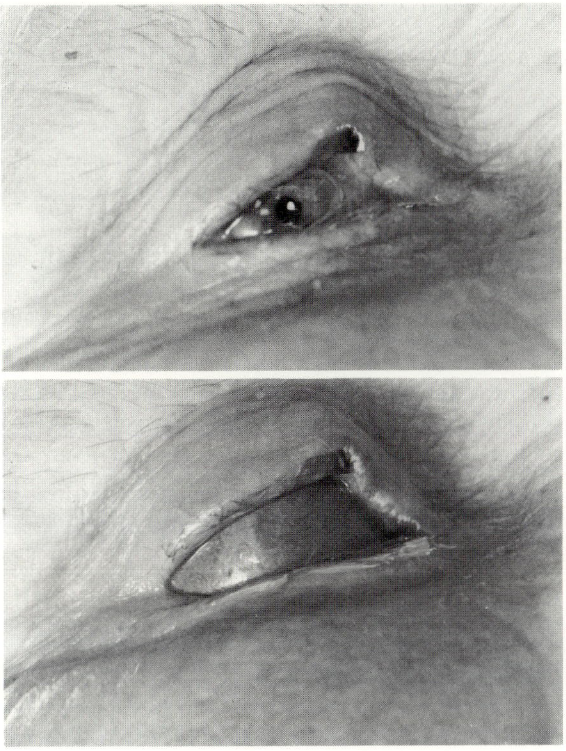

Fig. 4.42. Lead eye shield.

Mould Room Apparatus

The main feature of mould room work, whether for beam-direction shells or for brachytherapy, is the need for precision. Beams of X-rays must be aligned with considerable care and accuracy if a tumour is to be properly irradiated and contiguous normal structures adequately protected. Similarly, the design and fitting of surface moulds, the precise disposition of the radioactive sources, and the reliable maintenance of the exact source-to-surface distance all demand high technical skill. To this end a variety of technical aids have evolved within the mould room and these will be described and discussed below. They are the engineering tools essential to the levels of precision required in mould room work.

Locating Table

The function of this table is to provide a lateral axis through the located tumour centre, at a right angle to the anteroposterior axis. The axes intersect at the predicted tumour centre.

The design of the locating table (Fig. 4.43) is similar to that of the contour table. It has a base and a table top *D*, which are parallel to each other, with an additional calibrated sliding plate *C* which rests on the upper surface of *D*. Four guides support and direct the anteroposterior and lateral rods *A* and *B* along the chosen axes, so that they cross at right angles to one another. The in-facing edge of the anterior guide *E* corresponds to the zero point of the scale on the table. For example, if a long rod were to be placed across the lateral guides and the sliding plate was in its foremost position, the central axis of the rod would intersect the anteroposterior axis at the in-facing point of the guide *E*.

The distance between the outside surface of the bridge and the tumour centre is measured on the radiograph (section on tumour localisation above). By referring directly to the calibrated scale on the radiograph, the actual (unmagnified) distance is found. Using this measurement, the lateral axis guides, which are fixed to the sliding plate *C* on the table, are set at the same reading on the appropriate point of the scale. The position of the plate is fixed with locking nuts. Rod *A* suspends the shell in the mid-treatment plane on the anteroposterior axis guides. It is rotated until it is in a vertical position and held there by the survival arm *F* which locates in a notch in the bridge which is on the central plane of the shell. Heated rods are introduced into the lateral guides piercing the shell in the localised lateral axis *B*.

Forming

It is commonly assumed that a mould room must have a vacuum forming machine. Although this apparatus can be a great asset, it must be used intelligently. A skilled technician can mould plastic by hand onto an uncomplicated model (e.g. a larynx collar) as quickly as it can be done by a machine, and if single moulds are vacuum-formed costly wastage of material is inevitable. It is essential that the apparatus is adequate for the current and anticipated demands placed on it.

At the Christie Hospital three types of machine are used; one is a commercially produced EDL Parnavac (Fig. 4.44), the other two are smaller purpose-built machines. In the Parnavac, no less

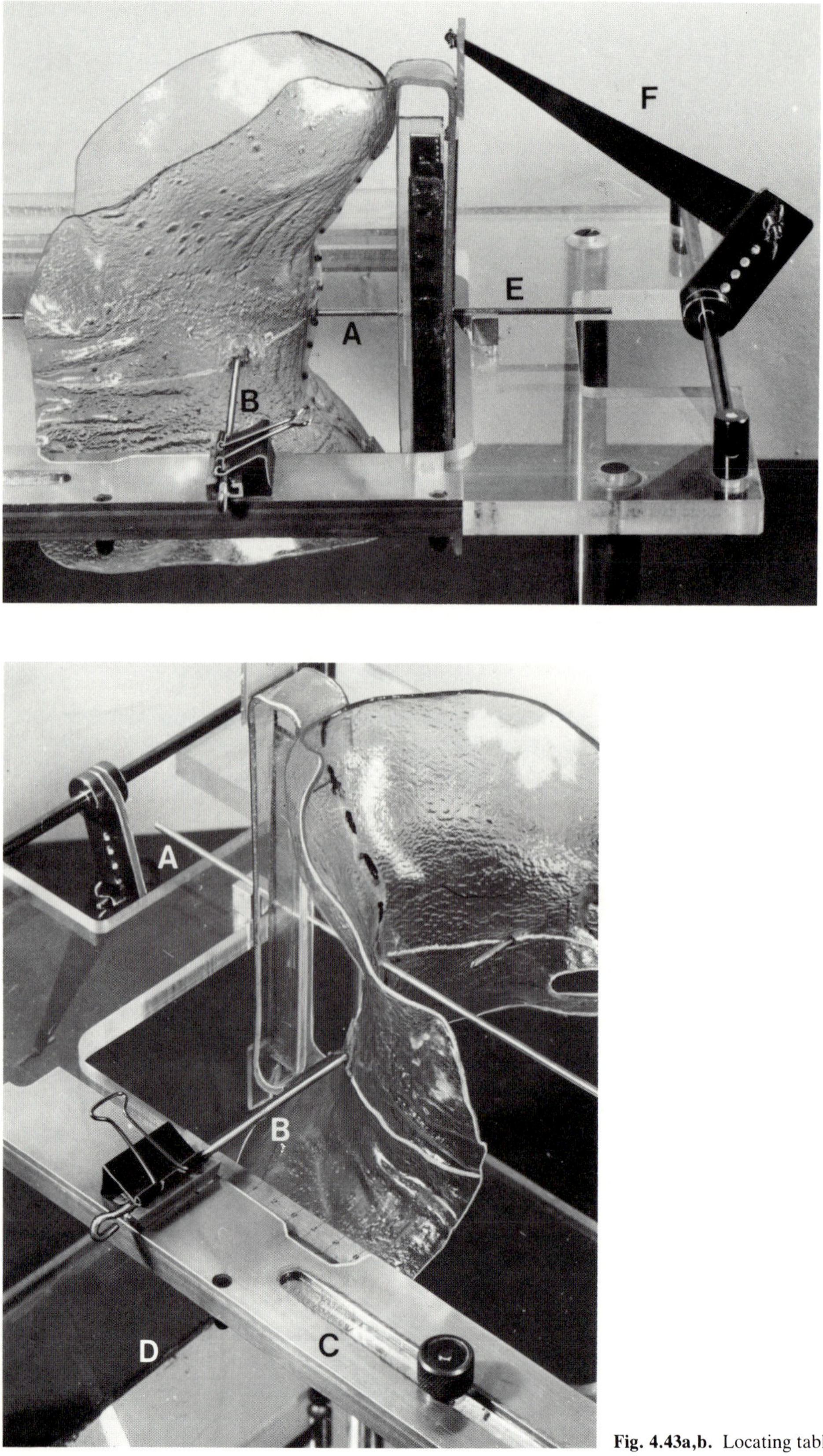

a

b

Fig. 4.43a,b. Locating table.

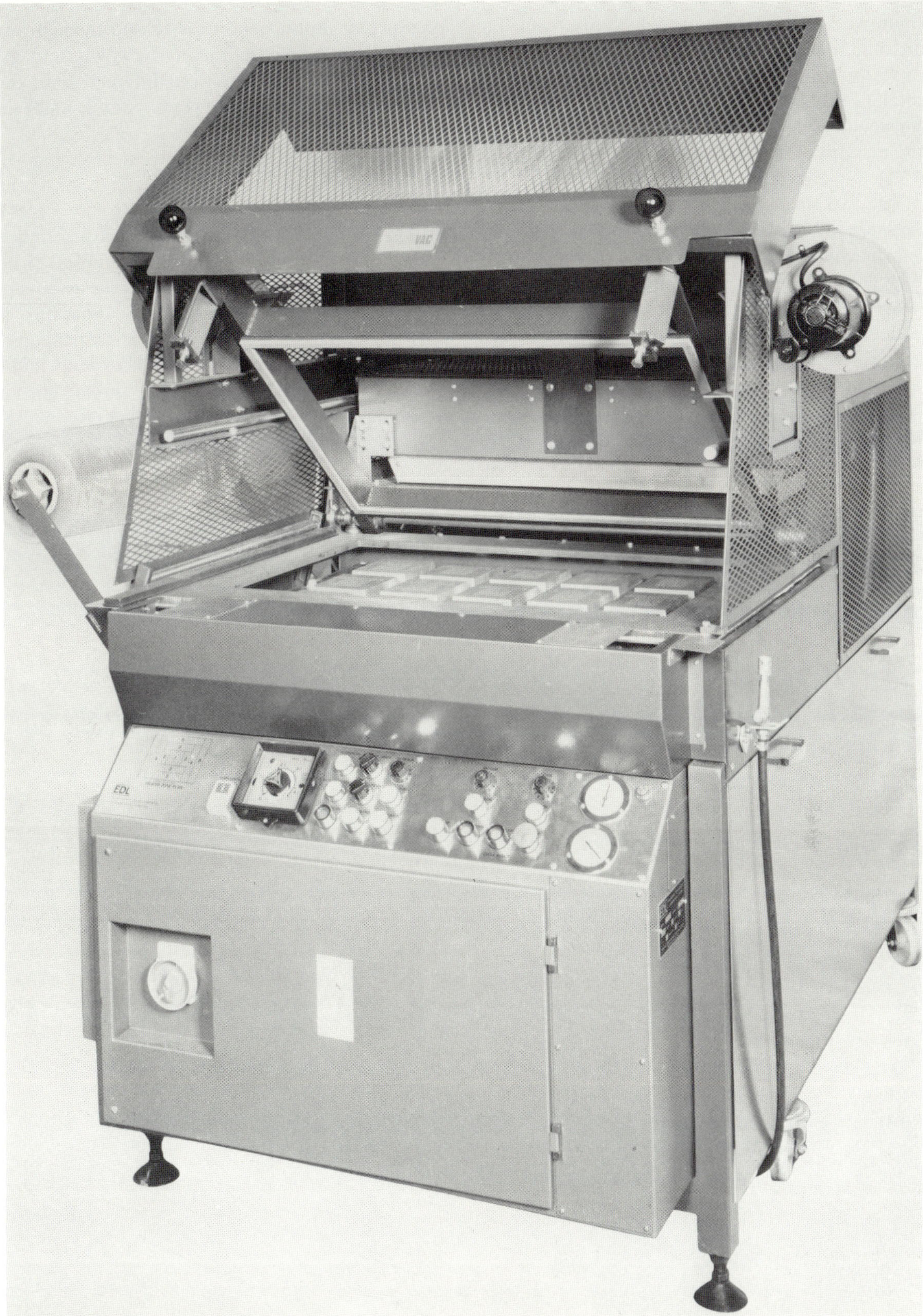

Fig. 4.44. Parnavac vacuum forming machine.

than two head and neck type shells are formed at any one time. To prevent the plastic from tearing or wrapping too far round and locking itself on the model, suitably tailored sand-bags are packed between the models and into the undercuts where the margins of the shells are not required (see Fig. 4.21).

The two smaller machines function by positive pressure rather than by vacuum. The smaller of the two machines is simply constructed from a commercially available dental press. A gasket of rubber sheet 2 mm thick is cemented to the flat undersurface of the press. A hole drilled through the full thickness of the press top, including the adherent rubber sheet, permits a car tyre valve to be introduced into the hole. Any small spaces between the valve and the press are packed with silicone paste, providing an air-tight seal. The sand container is made from aluminium tubing, cut and smoothed so that the top and bottom are parallel. Notches cut in the lower edge of the tube allow air displaced from around the model to escape. A tin lid of suitable diameter forms an ideal base. To operate the apparatus the model is held firmly in damp sand, exposing only the part upon which the mould is to be formed. A piece of 3-mm-thick plastic is heated until it becomes pliable when it is placed over the whole surface of the container. The press is closed, sealing the joint, and air at a pressure of 3 atmospheres is passed through the valve, directly pressing the plastic down onto the model. The air pressure is maintained until the plastic is cool. The result is exact, and is ideal for small mouldings.

The larger of the purpose-built machines (shown in Fig. 4.45) operates in a similar manner to the smaller device, except that the air pressure forces a rubber sheet down onto previously softened material. This method is more economical since only sufficient plastic is used to cover the estimated mould size on the model. The apparatus is constructed from an office press, a stainless steel box 30 cm long, 22 cm wide, and 15 cm deep, and a rubber sheet approximately 34 cm×26 cm. The air

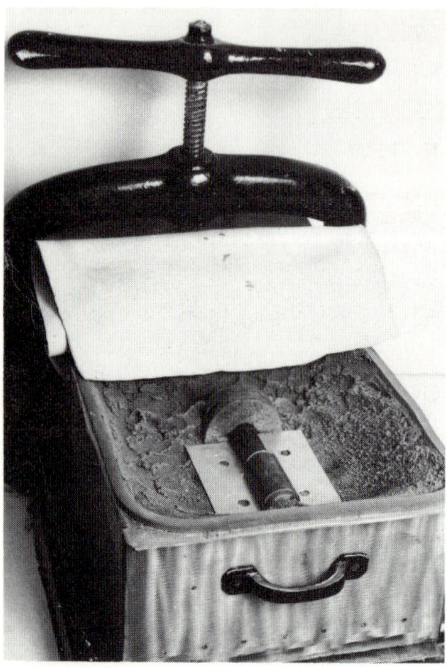

Fig. 4.45. Positive pressure forming machine.

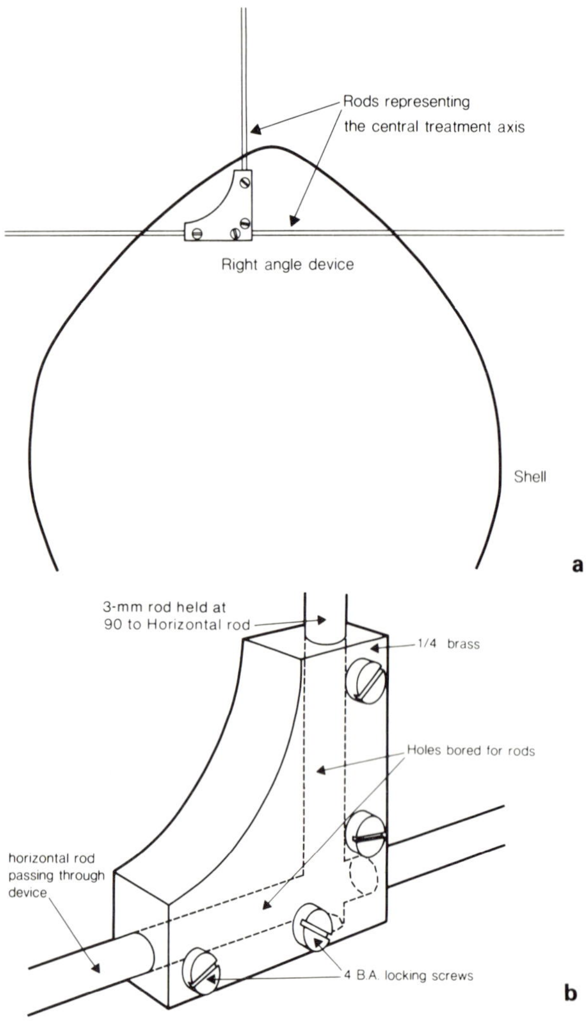

Fig. 4.46a,b. Right angle device.

supply passes through a tyre valve in the top plate. Small holes are drilled through the box to relieve the air pressure below the rubber sheet.

Right Angle Device

This device is used during the preparation of a half shell, at the porting stage. As the name suggests, this simple piece of apparatus fixes, at right angles to one another, two metal rods representing the central axes of the treatment beams (Fig. 4.46). It is an essential aid to precision when there is no exit point within the shell for one of the axes and when the beams are to cross at 90°.

Two-Part Shells

When a shell is made in two parts, it is important that the same relationship of the two parts is maintained on and off the patient. This requirement most commonly arises when a shell is used for the treatment of an intracranial tumour. To ensure the continued close fit of the two parts of the shell, and to fulfil the detailed planning requirements of the treatment, a number of rigid plastic clips are attached in appropriate sites. A rigid strip of plastic is cemented securely to one part of the shell (Fig. 4.47), and this strip extends over the other part, where it slips over a screw in such a position as to ensure the proper degree of tension and a close and comfortable fit.

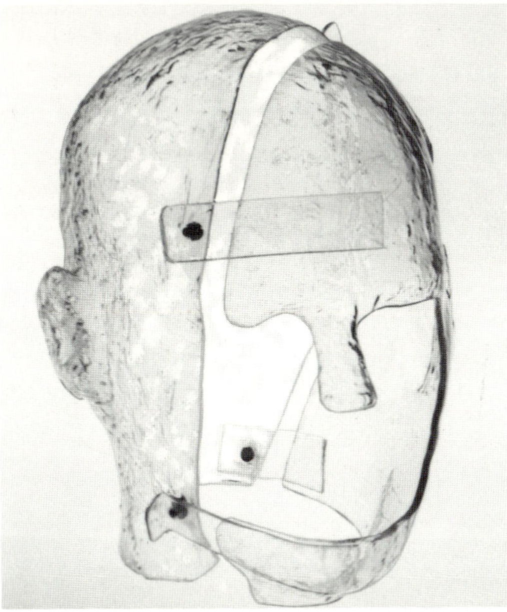

Fig. 4.47. Two-part shell.

Contour Table

The main purpose of the contour table is to transfer onto paper an outline of the chosen treatment plane and tumour-localising axes (Fig. 4.48). The table has a top which is supported on pillars 30 cm above the base and has an elliptical hole in its centre. The size of the ellipse varies

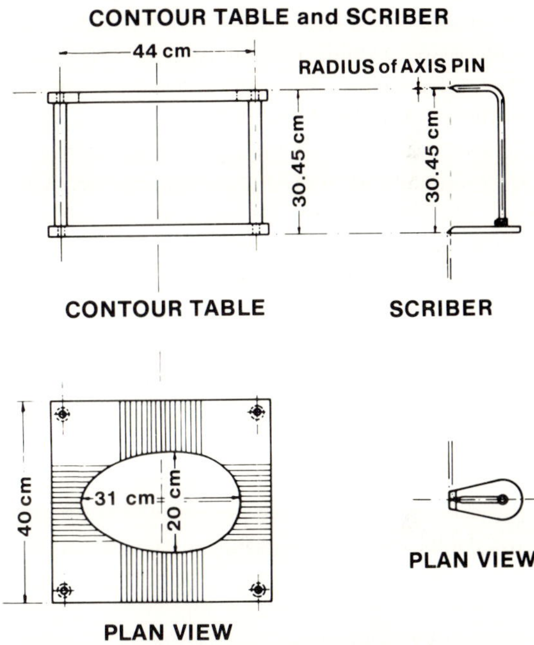

a

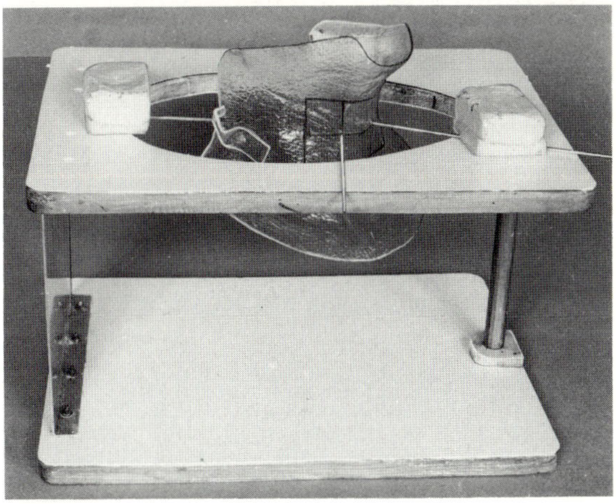

b

Fig. 4.48a,b. Contour table.

according to the size of the shell under preparation. For example, a practical size which accommodates most shells made for the head and neck is 30 cm × 36 cm, whereas an appreciably larger ellipse is required for the jacket-type shell used in the treatment of the lung. The upper surface of the table is marked with a 1-cm graduated grid. Rods supporting the shell are placed over the corresponding lines of the localising axes on each side of the table. These rods must not cross, otherwise the shell will not lie on the correct plane. They are immobilised by lead blocks on the table top. The scriber consists of a wide heavy base carrying a vertical rod. The pointed end of the vertical rod is bent towards the horizontal in such a way as to bring the point vertically above a notch which is cut into the rim of the base. Thus, on a piece of paper pinned on the surface of the base of the contour table, a pencil point inserted into the notch makes a dot vertically below the point of the scriber. In this way a life-size dotted outline of the treatment plane of the shell is transferred to the paper. The crossing axes represented by the rods are likewise projected onto the paper.

The contour table is used:

1) To etch the treatment plane on the shell (using the tip of a heated metal rod).
2) To etch the vertical midplane of each X-ray beam on the shell to ensure the proper alignment of beams during treatment.
3) To provide an outline of the vertical midplane for planning and porting purposes. The shell is suspended between the ends of a rod which has been pushed through the shell, and lies along the central axis of the beam. The shell is rotated about this axis until the vertical plane is horizontal to the table surface. A second rod is heated into the shell, precisely on the plane, and is immobilised on the table top with a lead block. The other outline is transferred in pencil onto paper.
4) To alter the chosen plane, if it proves necessary to raise or lower the plane a given distance, the shell is placed the appropriate way up in the table. A piece of flat Perspex, the same thickness as the specified changed height, is placed on the table, under a heated rod which slides along with the Perspex over the surface of the table as it etches the new plane on the shell.
5) To define the treatment field sizes on the shell.
6) To apply wax build-up as required.

Front Cranked Pointer and Bridge Former

This pointer is used as an alternative to the front-back pointer method of aligning the treatment machine to the shell. It is used when a shell has no beam exit point. This occurs when a half or occasionally a three-quarter type of shell is used, when the back pointer is obstructed by the bed or the pillow or support upon which the patient lies.

The pointer is designed in such a way that, when it is fitted to the treatment head of the therapy machine, its two pointers, which are 9 cm apart, lie precisely on the central axis of the beam (Fig. 4.49). The two points of the pointer locate (1) in a hole on a bridge which is fixed to the shell, and (2) in the entrance hole on the shell (Fig. 4.50).

A simple "distance piece" bridge-forming device, made from tubular plastic, is used to govern the height and position of the bridge. It consists of a hollow shaft 8.5 cm in length with a 3-mm-thick flat cross-piece approximately 8 cm long and 1.5 cm wide. A hole through the centre of the cross-piece accommodates a 3-mm rod, which holds it at right angles to the cross-piece. As there is no beam exit point on the shell, a temporary CAB false back approximately 3 cm wide is fitted to the shell, covering the central axis of the treatment plane. To fix the back, both ends of the

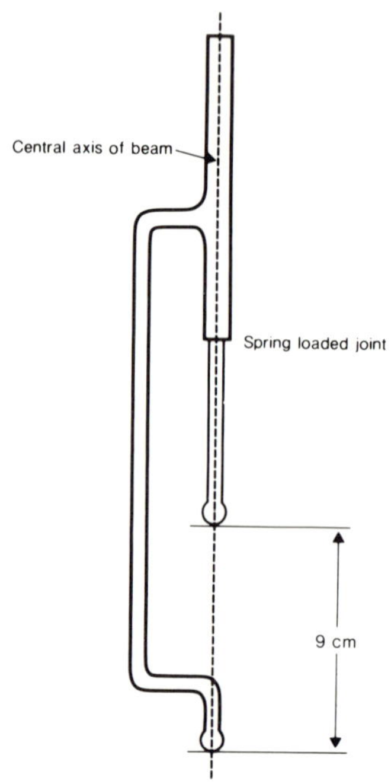

Fig. 4.49. Cranked pin.

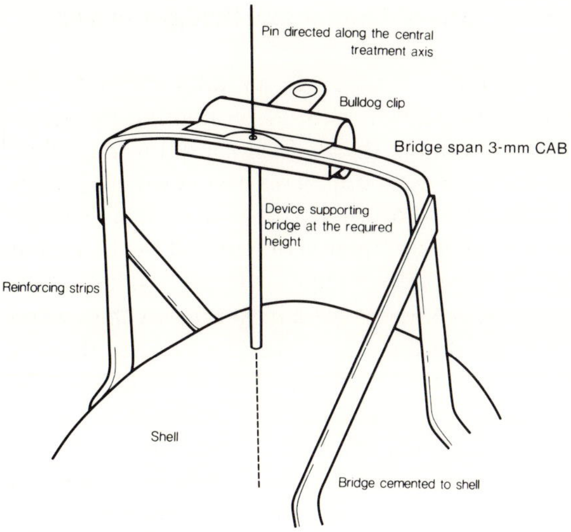

Fig. 4.50. Bridge former.

strip are heated and formed onto the sides of the shell, to which it is temporarily cemented. The plane of the beam is scribed on the back with the aid of the contour table. A hole, punched in the back in the precise position on the plane, fixes the direction of the rod in the correct beam axis. The distance piece is used as an aid to position the bridge on the shell. The device is slid over the rod and allowed to rest on the shell at the entrance point of the beam. A 3-mm clearance aperture is punched in the centre of a long 1-cm-wide strip of 2-mm CAB. The rod is passed through this hole so that the strip is allowed to rest on the cross-piece of the device and held there with a bulldog paper clip. Both sides of the span are then heated with a small flame so that when the sides are soft they fall down to form the uprights of the bridge. The span of the bridge must be greater than the port size to prevent the uprights from impinging on the field of treatment. Where the ends of the uprights meet the shell, they are heated and moulded to conform to the shape of the shell. At these points the bridge is cemented to the shell and then the rod and the former are removed.

The precise position of the hole on the bridge can be checked simply by introducing a rod along another beam axis and sighting through the bridge hole and the beam entrance hole in the shell. If correct, the image will be at the point of intersection of the axes on the rod.

5 General Principles of Radiotherapy

E. C. Easson

The Radiotherapist as Clinical Oncologist

The daily practice of any established branch of medicine should be based on some acceptable principles. This chapter is concerned with the general principles on which the radiotherapy of the Manchester school is based. Though many radiotherapists in other centres would doubtless accept these principles, there are sufficiently wide differences in practice throughout the world to suggest that some therapists adhere to a fundamentally different philosophy. We believe it is important, especially for those beginning their formal training in radiotherapy, to subscribe to an internally consistent school of thought, employing methods of treatment for each type of lesion in each anatomical site that are based on accepted principles and subjected to continuous rigorous scrutiny to test their effectiveness. Not only must each therapeutic technique be evaluated, but the underlying principles too must be questioned if and when this seems indicated. It is a feature of this hospital that similar lesions are all treated by the same technique, so long as statistical evidence justifies such a policy. All members of the staff adhere to the accepted policy until or unless reliable reasons are adduced to change this policy. These views are embodied in the detailed technical descriptions in Chaps. 6–17 and this agreed approach to patient management permits and ensures effective evaluation. Needless to say, these principles are not purely clinical, but also involve physicists, radiobiologists, pathologists, and others jointly concerned with the total care of patients. The radiotherapist is a clinician who should have and should accept full clinical responsibility for his patients from the time the decision is taken that irradiation is the treatment of choice. Who takes this initial decision? Medical men have long been open to the general criticism that when a patient finds himself, virtually by chance, in the hands of a surgeon he is likely to be treated surgically even if an alternative therapeutic approach would have been more appropriate. No doubt patients have been treated by irradiation when surgery would have been preferable. Fortunately, in most established cancer hospitals, it is now appreciated that when dealing with malignant disease the correct choice of treatment is crucial for the patient. The aphorism that the first chance to cure cancer is often the last chance rests on the fact that a wrong first choice of treatment can so readily prove fatal. There is, therefore, a need for consultation between all concerned. The patient with a cancer of the larynx needs expert examination and investigation by a surgical otolaryngologist. But he needs the equally expert advice of a radiotherapist on the prospect of curative irradiation as an alternative to ablative surgery. If a patient is suffering from a tumour of the ovary, the brain, or the bladder, the surgeon concerned would be a gynaecologist, neurosurgeon, or urological surgeon. A chemotherapist or medical oncologist would also take part in these joint consultations and, of course, important contributions to the discussion will be made by the pathologist, diagnostic radiologist, clinical pharmacologist, physicist—indeed anyone whose expertise can be applied to the needs of patient in question.

This team approach to clinical problems is time-consuming, but of the greatest value to the patient. It also has inestimable value for all those taking part by widening their intellectual field of vision and ensuring a proper sense of therapeutic perspective. But when a decision is taken that, for example, a patient's first treatment should be by irradiation, the radiotherapist must then have and accept full clinical responsibility. To this end we feel it essential that a radiotherapy department should have an adequate complement of beds under the sole control of the radiotherapists, in addition of course to all the necessary ancillary staff and equipment. This is equally true for the surgeon or medical oncologist if and when surgery or chemotherapy is indicated. In some cases the agreed programme of management may require initial surgery, then irradiation, and thereafter a course or sequence of courses of chemotherapy. During each of the therapeutic phases the surgeon, the radiotherapist, and the medical oncologist must be clinically responsible for the patient's care. During the long period of surveillance, when no further active treatment is being given, an acceptable follow-up system is required, to ensure that all concerned can again contribute to the patient's after-care and well-being. Joint follow-up clinics also permit evaluation of specific therapeutic regimes and indeed of their component parts.

Having accepted the patient for treatment by irradiation, the radiotherapist has to decide where, when, and how to carry out that treatment. The question of *where* to treat a patient concerns the choice of in-patient or out-patient care. This choice will be influenced by the clinical needs of the patient. Operative treatment clearly necessitates in-patient care, though any aged or infirm patient may likewise require admission. Out-patient treatment, normally acceptable for those who are fit to travel from home to the treatment centre (and who are not too upset by the treatment itself) will naturally depend on geographic features, available transport, and the distribution of treatment centres. In Manchester we have long held the view that it is unwise to fragment our therapeutic resources by creating partially equipped sub-centres to deal with a geographically scattered population. We prefer to maintain a highly equipped centre with sufficient beds for all in-patient needs, but also a dormitory wing providing accommodation for those patients who could have been out-patients had they not lived too far from easy travelling. The dormitory wing aims to provide only hostel accommodation with minimal nursing staff in attendance. The question of *when* to treat a patient involves both clinical and administrative considerations. Clearly it would be unwise to irradiate, for example, a post-mastectomy chest wall too soon after the surgery. Similarly, it would be dangerous to irradiate a large volume of the trunk of a patient whose white cell count was already depressed by recent chemotherapy. Many obvious clinical considerations, such as distressing intercurrent disease, will often compel either cautious initial treatment or a judicious postponement of treatment. But one of the major principles of cancer therapy is that delay is dangerous. However much tumour growth rates may differ from patient to patient, it is logical to suppose that even a slowly growing tumour will spread and metastasise if given sufficient time to do so. Unnecessary delay in starting treatment is therefore to be deplored. This underlines the importance of rapidly establishing a diagnosis, agreeing on the choice of treatment, and instituting appropriate treatment as soon as possible. There is a need, therefore, to examine also the administrative causes of unnecessary delay—slow communication at many points in the chain. The creation of a waiting list is obviously undesirable and dangerous in the context of malignant disease. In general, a patient with cancer should be regarded as a medical emergency requiring urgent attention. The question of *how* to treat a patient by irradiation will be discussed in detail in the body of this textbook. However, it is worth repeating that the planning of a radiation treatment is in our view the responsibility of the radiotherapist. Radiation treatment is to the radiotherapist what a surgical operation is to the surgeon, and the details of a radiation treatment are likewise the homologue of a surgeon's operative technique. There has been an increasing tendency amongst radiotherapists to leave treatment planning to their physicist colleagues, but we would regard this, certainly in its more extreme forms, as the abandonment of the radiotherapist's clinical responsibility. This is seen especially in those patients requiring beam-directed irradiation of very high precision. In our view it is essential for the radiotherapist to carry out an exhaustive examination of the patient in order to determine the precise location and configuration of the tumour to be treated. Moreover, the radiotherapist alone is clinically responsible for deciding on the precise "target volume" to be treated and the contiguous structures that must be protected from too much irradiation—not to mention the variety of dosimetric considerations affecting tumour and normal tissues. The technique of radiation treatment is as clinical a procedure as a surgical operation and the radiotherapist must always accept this fundamental professional responsibility.

Staging of Malignant Tumours

Every patient with malignant disease must of course, like any other patient, be examined systematically and meticulously. It is important not only to examine the patient so far as his or her cancer is concerned, but to ensure that the patient is, for example, not anaemic or suffering from diabetes mellitus, both of which could significantly and adversely affect the response to irradiation. It is also important to know of any other abnormalities even if they are less relevant to the specific care of the malignant disease.

The primary object of staging any malignant tumour is to determine and record in detail the precise site, size, and extent of the lesion. This kind of disciplined description is essential for evaluation of treatment and to permit statistically valid comparisons of like with like (see also Chap. 18). It would clearly be meaningless to compare the success rate, measured in terms of survival, of the surgical extirpation of a large squamous cancer of the tongue which had already metastasised to lymph nodes in the neck, with radium therapy for a small localised cancer confined to the anterior third of the tongue. On the other hand, it would be valid to compare surgery with radium therapy for identical lesions of the tongue, provided both methods of treatment were considered therapeutically appropriate in the first place. The oldest and most pragmatic approach to staging was where a surgeon described a tumour simply as operable or inoperable. A primary tumour may be inoperable because it invades too many contiguous vital structures; but a surgical approach may also be deemed undesirable because of widespread metastases, even when the primary tumour is technically resectable. This simple method of staging was essentially practical and had an immediate bearing on whether or how to treat the patient. A somewhat different problem arises, however, where a primary tumour is technically operable but the patient's general health is so poor that the surgeon's clinical judgement is against any attempt at resection. In such circumstances radiation and/or chemotherapy may be an acceptable alternative to surgery, but such a choice of treatment involves many considerations which will be discussed later. Staging, in the sense of establishing the precise extent of the malignant disease, has obvious prognostic connotations. A patient with a small localised skin cancer has a much better prognosis than a patient whose primary skin cancer is large and invasive and has already metastasised to lymph nodes. But whatever system of staging is employed, the decision that a patient's tumour conforms to an agreed "stage" must not be confused with that patient's prognosis. As we have seen, a patient's tumour may be in a prognostically favourable "stage" while the total clinical assessment of the patient indicates that his prognosis—as a whole—is bad. This commonly arises where unrelated intercurrent disease is a more immediate threat to a patient than his localised tumour. A system of staging must therefore be seen as an important device for statistical evaluation and any associated prognostic significance as incidental and unreliable.

Many different systems have been used and proposed for staging malignant disease. The most important requirement is to decide what is best in each situation and then to adhere to that system with obsessive determination. Since 5- and 10-year survival periods (or longer) are involved in the statistical analysis of different treatments for various types of cancer, stage by stage, it is obvious that apart from the need for the meticulous application of a staging system, any change in that system during the period of study must destroy the validity of analyses. (Equally true is the damaging effect on statistical analyses of any change in the nomenclature of specific diseases, malignant or otherwise, and, of course, the need for consistent as well as reliable histological criteria and diagnoses cannot be overemphasised.) Consistent staging is what is important and this is more readily achieved within any one centre, assuming agreement by all the staff members and uniformly meticulous care by all of them. Even then, it must be accepted that subjective error is inevitable, though hopefully this too is likely to vary within narrow and reasonably constant limits. Efforts to achieve international agreement on a system of staging have been made from time to time, notably by the International Union Against Cancer (the UICC—*Union Internationale Contre le Cancer*). The UICC approach to a "descriptive classification" is known as the TNM system, where details are recorded concerning the tumour (T), the presence or absence of lymph node involvement (N), and the presence or absence of metastases (M). Unfortunately, there has been only a limited agreement on how best to apply this system, though in principle it remains inherently sound. Not all cancers lend themselves to this kind of examination and so far as the Christie Hospital is concerned we have adopted an eclectic approach to the problem, adapting the TNM system to our own well-tried and established system where this seemed wise. The details of our staging system are shown in Appendix 2.

Tumour staging can be considered in three ways—clinical, surgical, and pathological. For *clinical* staging we rely on an examination of the tumour by observation and palpation, supplemented by any of the routine tests of a clinic, such as chest and skeletal X-rays. A malignant ulcer of the skin lends itself readily to direct measurement—for example, "2.5 cm in diameter on the dorsum of the left hand". Palpation of the lesion will determine that it is circumscribed and, of great importance, whether or not it is freely mobile. If mobility is impaired we can assume malignant infiltration into subdermal tissue planes, in this example implying a threat to the extensor tendons. A uterine tumour can be "clinically" inspected only via the vagina, rectum (proctoscopy), and bladder (cystoscopy). Palpation is less easy and therefore less reliable than with a superficial skin tumour, but the mobility of the uterus can be estimated and, by palpation of the parametrial tissues, some estimate can be made of the presence or absence of extra-uterine invasion. With experience, palpation of the pelvis can yield valuable information and permit quite accurate staging—though never free from potential error. The same is true for cancer of the bladder. Abdominal tumours are more difficult to assess by palpation, even when assisted by high-quality radiology. Clinical staging, therefore, has advantages and disadvantages, depending on the nature and anatomical site of the tumour, but where appropriate a high degree of consistency can be maintained.

Surgical staging implies the application to staging of information about a tumour obtained by the surgeon at operation. For example, at laparotomy a gynaecologist may observe tumour which has extended to the outer surface of the corpus uteri; or a urologist may observe tumour extending into perivesical tissues or into para-aortic lymph nodes.

Pathological staging usually implies histological evidence of active tumour. One of the commonest applications of pathological staging is with cancer of the breast. Clinical staging may indicate the presence of a small mobile primary tumour in the upper out quadrant of the right breast and with no lymph nodes palpable in either the related axilla or supraclavicular fossa. At mastectomy the surgeon may or may not find evidence of lymphadenopathy, but the pathologist may find histological proof of axillary nodal metastases. Thus, what was clinically a Stage 1 breast cancer becomes a pathological Stage 2 cancer. Experience has shown that with breast cancers about 30% of patients with no palpable axillary nodes do have histological evidence of nodal involvement; on the other hand, about 30% also of those with clinically palpable nodes before operation prove to have no histological evidence of tumour in these nodes. It is therefore important to make valid decisions concerning how far to pursue staging information. Should all patients with malignant lymphomas be subjected to an exploratory laparotomy to permit more accurate staging? The truth is that laparotomy in a lymphoma patient must be seen not as a "staging" procedure but as part of the total clinical assessment of the patient, and as a prerequisite for adopting the optimal mode of treatment. If a patient with Hodgkin's lymphoma has obvious features of advanced systemic disease (pyrexia, weight loss, anaemia) there is clearly no point in proving the presence or absence of abdominal lymph node involvement. The situation, however, is not always so clear-cut, and careful clinical judgement is necessary. The underlying emphasis is on careful clinical assessment and the choice of optimal therapy. The UICC's "descriptive classification" has interesting epidemiological possibilities that are worth mentioning. Statistical analysis of any one type of tumour aims, amongst other things, at the isolation of important characteristics—for example, a truly curable subgroup of tumours whose special features can be enumerated, provided these data have been recorded. As will be discussed below, certain types of tumour can, under favourable circumstances and by suitable treatment, be permanently cured. Nevertheless, analyses have shown that in this context females are more readily cured than males, though we do not know why femaleness should confer such an advantage. There may well be other recordable data which subsequent analysis might disclose as vital to successful treatment. New knowledge of tumour markers, various receptors, immunological features and the like could well prove of considerable importance in the management of patients with cancer, even though none of these at present play any part in our rather simplified staging systems. The problem is how far to pursue investigative details and how much to record these data. It is always frustrating to embark on a retrospective analysis and be impeded by a lack of recorded data. However, finite resources always demand some compromise, which we can at least try to implement judiciously.

Staging must not be confused with "grading". For many years interest has been shown in tumour grading, which is an attempt to distinguish quantitatively the various degrees of differentiation in the tumour cells. It was long apparent that disease behaviour, prognosis, and the approach to management in the case of a patient with chronic lymphocytic leukaemia were strikingly different from those for a patient with acute lymphoblastic leukaemia. However, the histology of solid tumours is less easily quantified into percentages of well-differentiated, moderately differentiated, and anaplastic tumour cells. Polymorphic tumours of the breast create even greater difficulties, though some workers have devised grading techniques which seem to be acceptably consistent. The grading of a malignant tumour does, at least at the extremes of the differentiation spectrum, have some prognostic significance. Anaplastic bronchogenic cancers do behave more "aggressively" than their well-differentiated counterparts, but the grading of a tumour does not necessarily influence the radiotherapeutic technique required for its treatment. This subject arises again in subsequent chapters, notably those dealing with cancers of the lung and brain and with the lymphomas.

Objectives of Treatment

Having decided that radiation therapy does have something to offer a patient, the therapist must be clear as to his intent. It is sad to discover radiotherapists in some centres around the world who still see their role as providing only palliative treatment. This may be partly related to the fact that many of their patients are referred to them only when their tumours are so advanced both locally and metastatically that even palliative therapy is of very dubious value. But this is not the whole story. Some patients must be encountered whose tumours can be so usefully treated that it should encourage both the radiotherapist himself and also his clinical colleagues in other disciplines to make greater efforts towards earlier referral and more effective treatment.

Curative Treatment

The primary object of radiation therapy should be to cure the patient's cancer. There can be no doubt in anyone's mind that, for example, small squamous cell carcinomas of the skin can be easily cured by an adequate dose of radiation. Such lesions can often be equally easily cured by surgical excision and the choice of method involves many considerations (discussed in Chap. 6). Squamous cell cancer does respond well to irradiation and not only when it occurs in the skin. This type of cancer arises commonly in the buccal cavity and, if localised and technically amenable to adequate radiation therapy, it is just as curable as when it affects the skin. The same is indeed true wherever squamous cancer occurs—skin, buccal cavity, accessory nasal sinuses, larynx, pharynx, bronchus, cervix uteri, vagina, and anus. The only problems presented by squamous cancers in these different sites are that they frequently declare themselves at an advanced stage (as with bronchial cancer) and also create technical difficulties in delivering lethal dosage of radiation to the tumour. How these different technical problems can be overcome, with rewarding results, is the object of this textbook, the object of the radiotherapist's special training, and the basis of his professional expertise.

The time-honoured method of expressing the success of treatment is in terms of the percentage of treated patients who survive 5 years after treatment. This is described as the 5-year survival rate. Sometimes data are presented in terms of the 10-year or 15-year survival rate. The interest in survival rates beyond the 5-year level was prompted by the fact that a proportion of patients die between the fifth and tenth years after treatment, and still more after 10 or even 15 years. The important question which affects any measurement of the true efficacy of treatment is not just survival, but when and from what causes—cancer or otherwise—these patients are dying. Figure 5.1 shows the survival curve, plotted semilogarithmically, for a hypothetical cohort of patients all treated and followed up for 15 years. The continuing mortality is obvious. Figure 5.2, however, shows two survival curves, the lower one being that shown in Fig. 5.1. The upper curve (prepared from life tables) shows the survival rates, year by year, for a normal population matched exactly by age and sex with the cohort of treated cancer patients. Clearly, a proportion of this population of "normal" people is also dying throughout this 15-year period from a variety of causes. Moreover, in this hypothetical case, the two curves are seen to run parallel to one another from the fourth year onwards to the fifteenth year. The parallelism of the two curves implies that the survival rates, or rates of dying, are identical for both populations, the surviving patients and a normal population of the same age and sex. This provides a useful actuarial definition of cure, namely that at some time after treatment (varying in duration according to the type and stage of the treated cancer) there remains a group of survivors who are dying at the same rate and of the same general causes as a normal population of the same age and sex. This subject is further discussed in Chap. 18.

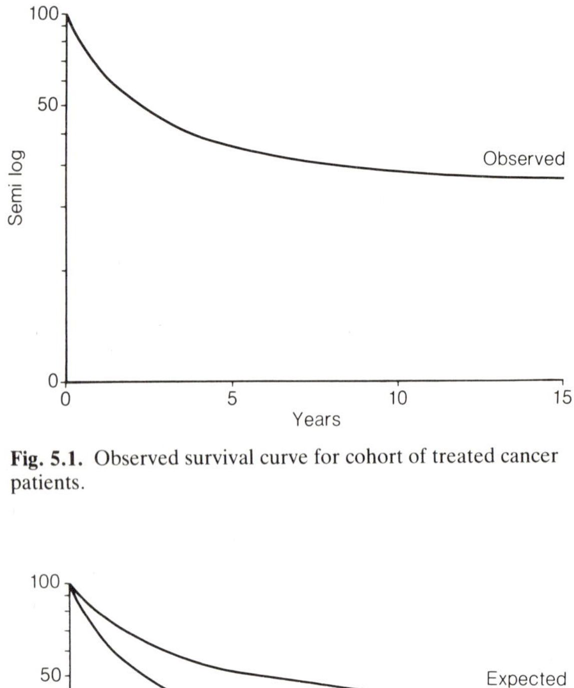

Fig. 5.1. Observed survival curve for cohort of treated cancer patients.

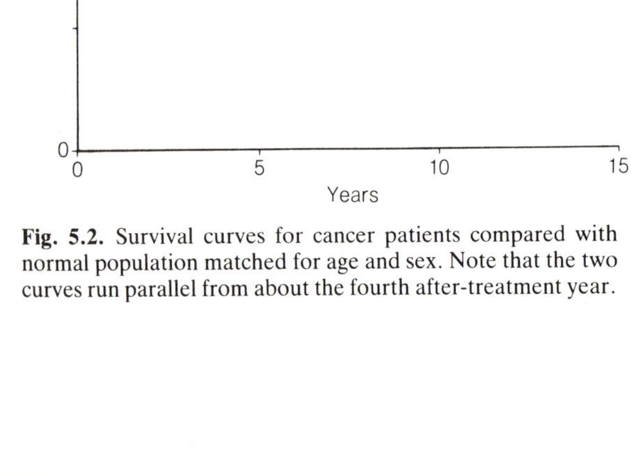

Fig. 5.2. Survival curves for cancer patients compared with normal population matched for age and sex. Note that the two curves run parallel from about the fourth after-treatment year.

Further consideration of this concept of cure confirms that for many patients with, for example, cancer of the cervix, larynx, skin, or testis, high levels of cure can be achieved when the tumour is treated at an early stage of the disease. If the tumour is more extensive at the time of treatment, cure is still possible, but for a measurably smaller percentage of patients. When still more extensive disease is treated the two curves for observed and expected survival (Fig. 5.2) continue to diverge with no evidence of parallelism, and though some patients may survive for many years, definitive cure cannot be anticipated for this cohort of patients. These findings confirm the importance of early diagnosis and treatment, in the context of cure, and they surely invalidate the pessimistic view that earlier diagnosis only extends the survival period between treatment and inevitable death.

Definitive cure of certain types of cancer can, therefore, be achieved and, since this is the object of treatment, it is important to consider the various factors that influence the prospect of cure. These relevant factors concern the tumour itself, the specific method of treatment, and the dosage of radiation given. The *tumour* may arise in an anatomical site, such as the larynx, where a malignant tumour will almost certainly be of squamous cell type (though unusual tumours do occur in that site). As such, the tumour is likely to respond to radiation therapy provided it is not too extensive. A lesion of the vocal cord will fortunately alert the patient by creating persistent symptoms, even when the tumour is small and easily cured. Even quite extensive cancer in the pyriform fossa, however, may remain symptomless for too long, and curative treatment may prove either unlikely or impossible. Each anatomical site gives rise to its own type or types of cancer, each with different prospects of cure. The radiotherapist is therefore guided in his endeavours by the site, histology, and clinical stage of the disease in each patient. As previously mentioned, however, even a favourable lesion may occur in a patient who, for other reasons, could not tolerate the radical treatment essential to his cure.

The *method of treatment* is largely determined by the site, type and stage of the tumour. The factors which influence this choice of treatment and also the various choices available to the radiotherapist will be discussed shortly. If the wrong choice is made, however, a potentially curable tumour may extend and kill the patient just as surely as if a surgeon performed the wrong type of operation. The *dosage* of radiation delivered to the tumour by whatever chosen technique is also vital to success. Though the inhibition of tumour growth is directly related to the dose of radiation reaching the tumour, there is clearly a need to consider the damage done to the host as well as to the tumour itself. This question is discussed in detail in the section entitled "Optimum Dose" below.

Palliative Treatment

Some types of cancer are therefore curable provided a number of preconditions are satisfied. In our experience, however, some types of cancer do not respond well, or at all, to maximum tolerable dosage levels. Even those cancers that are amenable to curative treatment may present at a stage when this objective is no longer feasible. Under these conditions the radiotherapist must consider the possibility of helping the patient by relieving distressing symptoms, i.e. by palliative treatment. It is important always to keep in mind that the object of palliative treatment is the palliation of a symptom or symptoms. For example, pain arising from a metastasis in bone from a primary cancer of the breast can be readily relieved by irradiation. Equally important is the fact that this pain relief can be achieved by a simple and often a single treatment with X-rays. This usually means that there are no unpleasant side-effects from the treatment, and no new symptoms are created by the treatment itself. The distress of superior vena caval compression, associated with an anaplastic bronchogenic cancer in the anterior mediastinum, can also be relieved by a simple X-ray treatment of short duration, and without inducing new problems attributable to the irradiation. Sometimes a short treatment with X-rays will lead to healing of an ulcerated lesion with relief of local discomfort and discharge, even though known metastases may ultimately prove fatal. Some symptoms are difficult or impossible to palliate, such as vomiting arising from gross intra-abdominal disease, or dysphagia created by a large oesophageal or bronchial tumour. Though alternative approaches to palliation may be worth considering (such as one of the variety of oesophageal tubes) it is sometimes in a patient's best interests to avoid the possibility of making matters worse by striving injudiciously to help. It is a truism that more clinical judgement is required to know when and how best to attempt palliative care, than to treat a small cancer radically.

The criteria of good palliation can therefore be summarised as follows: The symptom must first be judged sufficiently disturbing and persistent to justify an effort to relieve it; the radiation therapy necessary to relieve the symptom in question should be preferably of short duration and should thus make no significant demands on the patient; the radiation dosage should be sufficient to achieve the desired object without creating distressing side-effects of any kind. Ideally, a patient would have his symptoms controlled for a prolonged period, his life qualitatively improved, and his terminal illness would be short. Simply to prolong life, especially a life distressed by uncontrolled pain, vomiting and/or dyspnoea, would be bad palliation and even worse clinical judgement. These comments also have obvious relevance to surgery and chemotherapy.

Before leaving the subject of palliation, brief mention must be made of another important consequence of the choice between a radical (curative) and a palliative approach to management. Palliation is ideally a technically simple treatment of short duration. This implies selection of those patients who can gain most, in the sense of potential cure, from radical treatment, which is time-consuming and demanding not only for the patient but also for the radiotherapist and his entire department. A common view, with which we would disagree, is that when radical treatment fails it nevertheless gives the best palliative results for the patient. This notion ignores the fact that the sometimes serious side-effects of radical radiotherapy are acceptable only if the prospects of cure are substantial. It would, therefore, be bad palliative treatment which created more symptoms than it relieved. But to subject all patients to radical treatment is both clinically injudicious and administratively unwise. Radical treatment absorbs all the resources of the radiotherapy department and to direct this time-consuming effort to patients who have nothing to gain must delay the urgent treatment of those who are—or were—potentially curable. Though there are many reasons for hospital waiting lists, and some beyond the control of the clinicians concerned, this initial choice, between attempting radical treatment or accepting the more limited objective of palliation, remains vital to the best interests of our patients. This choice demands good clinical judgement—a subtle combination of wide experience and commonsense.

Optimum Dose

The variations in the reactions of different tissues to different doses of ionising radiation were discussed in Chap. 2. At the risk of being repetitious it is proposed here to discuss the concept of optimum dosage in the context of clinical radiotherapy. A small squamous carcinoma of the skin, measuring say 2.0 cm in diameter, can be cured in nearly, but not all, cases by an adequate single treatment with X-rays. If a very small dose of X-rays is given—what might be described as a futile dose—no response would be seen or expected. If a larger but still inadequate dose is given, the tumour might show some temporary resolution, but would sooner or later display its former growth rate. Such a treatment is usually described as providing only growth retardation, and though this is sometimes of value in terms of temporary palliation, it would have no place in the context of curative treatment for a small and potentially curable skin cancer. If a still larger dose of X-rays is administered to such a tumour, permanent inhibition of tumour growth—cure of the cancer—may be expected in a small but definite percentage of cases. There would still, however, be a majority of such tumours that would display only temporary growth retardation. Such a level of dosage could therefore be regarded as adequate for only the more "sensitive" variants of squamous cell cancers affecting the skin of a mixed population of patients. A still larger dose of X-rays would prove lethal to a larger percentage of tumours, but if we continue to increase the administered dose a point is reached where these further increases result in a falling level of lethal effect. This dose-response curve is shown graphically in Fig. 5.3. This sigmoid curve, characteristic of many biological systems, demonstrates clearly the more sensitive response at one extreme, the more resistant minority at the other (upper) extreme, and the intermediate group showing a rapid increase in percentage response following small increases in dose.

To understand the concept of optimum dosage it is essential to examine the relationship of the sigmoid curve of tumour response to the equally sigmoid curve of the normal tissues in and around the tumour, shown in Fig. 5.4. The sigmoid curve of the normal tissues lies, under favourable circumstances, at a higher dosage level than that for the tumour lethal effect. For squamous cancer of the skin, as shown here in general terms, it is clear that if the dosage of X-rays is increased, with the object of achieving 100% cure, the price paid would be a very high and clinically quite unacceptable level of morbidity. Moreover, if a decision were made to avoid all risk of morbidity the dosage would have to be reduced to the level where, in view of the shape of the sigmoid curve, the cure level would fall rapidly to equally unacceptable levels. The optimum dose can therefore be defined as that level of dosage which will result in the highest percentage of cures consistent with an *acceptable level of morbidity*. In the hypothetical (though clinically realistic) situation shown in Fig. 5.4 it can be seen that the optimum dose will cure more than 90% of the tumours at the acceptable price of some 5% morbidity. In this case the morbidity would take the form of persisting high-dose effects on the skin with atrophic changes affecting the skin appendages (hair follicles, sweat

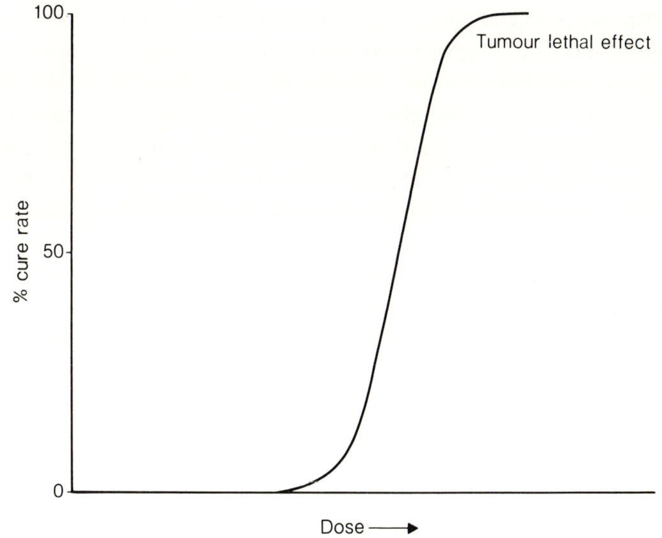

Fig. 5.3. Sigmoid dose-response curve showing sensitive response (*bottom left*) and resistant response (*top right*).

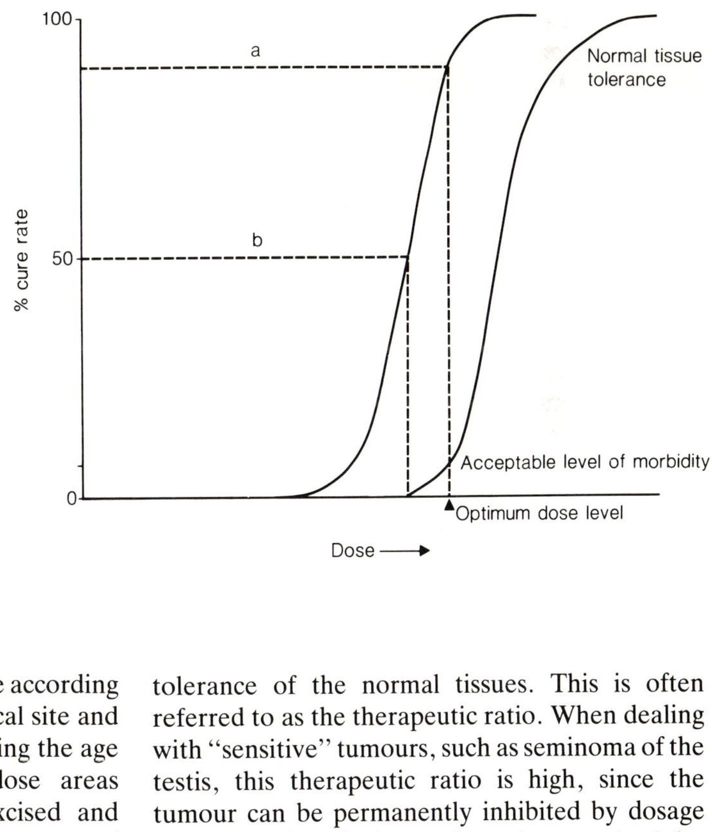

Fig. 5.4. Relationship between dose-response curve of tumour and dose-response curve of related normal tissues. Note that optimum dose level (*a*) accepts some morbidity in return for high cure rate. Relatedness of these two curves demonstrates that demand for no morbidity (*b*) involves dramatic fall in tumour cure rate.

and sebaceous glands) varying in degree according to dose and influenced by the anatomical site and local as well as systemic factors, including the age of the patient. Troublesome high-dose areas affecting the skin can usually be excised and grafted if necessary, so that a modest percentage of morbidity is acceptable, especially since the treated cancer previously within the damaged area has doubtless been cured in the overall damaging procedure. For small squamous cancers of the skin, therefore, there is a favourable balance between the responsiveness of the tumour and the tolerance of the normal tissues. This is often referred to as the therapeutic ratio. When dealing with "sensitive" tumours, such as seminoma of the testis, this therapeutic ratio is high, since the tumour can be permanently inhibited by dosage levels significantly lower than that required for squamous cell cancers. (The need to irradiate large volumes of tissue when treating seminoma, and other equally sensitive tumours, creates different problems in terms of "normal tissue tolerance"; see Chap. 13.) With radioresistant tumours, such as chondrosarcoma, the therapeutic ratio is low, in that the dosage necessary to be effectively lethal to the tumour is at tolerance levels for normal tissues in too high a percentage of patients. The "morbidity level" is, of course, a strictly quantitative expression. Though skin atrophy may be clinically acceptable, even in 5% of patients, some forms of morbidity raise serious questions of acceptability. Bone necrosis, though it can be a tiresome and debilitating problem, is often acceptable finally, in that the spontaneous extrusion of a sequestrum or its removal by radical surgery (for a now non-malignant lesion) can lead to complete healing. But how far should one risk transverse myelitis of the cervical spinal cord and consequent para- or quadriplegia? Even if the treated cancer were cured, to create such morbidity would be a Pyrrhic victory indeed. Thus, radiation morbidity must be considered qualitatively as well as quantitatively, site by site. Nevertheless, we would hold to the view that any centre which never had any patients at any time requiring appropriate care for high-dose problems was habitually operating at too low a level of general dosage.

For a squamous skin cancer of diameter 2.0 cm, using superficial X-rays of 60–100 kV through a 3.0-cm-diameter applicator, the optimum dose, for a single-exposure treatment, is 2250 cGy. If a fractionated course of treatment is preferred (though scarcely necessary for such a small skin lesion) the optimum dose has been established, in our experience, as 4000 cGy for 4 daily treatments, 4500 cGy for 8 treatments, and 5000 cGy for 15 treatments. For squamous cancer in other sites, such as the larynx or cervix uteri, the optimum dose levels have been established by experience over many years. This is equally true for tumours of different histological types and complex techniques of treatment. The dose/time and other technical details are described in the appropriate chapters later. Before leaving the subject of optimum dose, some comment must be made concerning comparisons between different techniques of treatment. New methods of treatment for different cancers are constantly being proposed and some of these are rightly subjected to critical study. When comparing two regimes of treatment it is first necessary to select lesions that are identical in every way, so that the only variables to be compared are the two different methods of treatment—the old established method and the new one. But with each method of treatment it is essential to compare the optimal treating conditions—hence the need to compare (so far as radiation therapy is concerned) the optimum dose for each treatment. If, for example, treatment *A* was a well-established method resulting predictably in 85% cures and 5% morbidity, it would be wrong to claim that treatment *B* was better because 95% cure rates resulted, if this 95% tumour effect cost a 15% morbidity level. In short, when comparing two methods of radiation therapy it is essential first to establish the optimum dose levels for both, *equating the morbidity levels*, and only then compare the tumour cure rates.

From what has been said about optimum dosage in radiotherapy, it will be clear that this concept is accepted as a feature of the Manchester School. While it would be quite inaccurate to describe this as just giving the maximum tolerable dosage, the notion of an optimum dose for each tumour type and treatment regime does accept the *need* for an acceptable level of morbidity. Accepting this as a need is quite distinct from accepting only a risk, a possible chance of morbidity. Trial and error leads to establishing the acceptable morbidity level, while the cure rates that follow such an established regime can be regarded as optimal. How then does such an approach to treatment compare with the common practice of prescribing 200 cGy daily with the intention of continuing this daily fraction for "4–6 weeks"? Many centres, in our view unwisely, adopt this latter approach to prescribing dosage of X-rays. It is commonly expressed as an intention to give "from 4000 to 6000 cGy in from 4 to 6 weeks". This could raise the question as to how many patients might receive 4000 cGy in 6 weeks, or 6000 cGy in 4 weeks. These two extremes are logically implicit in the initial statement and many other permutations are possible—5000 cGy in 5 weeks, for example, or even 5000 cGy in 4 weeks. From what has been said about optimum dose levels, and the dose-response curves in Fig. 5.4, it is obvious that 4000 cGy in 6 weeks could prove therapeutically inadequate, while 6000 cGy in 4 weeks could create unacceptably high levels of morbidity. In short, a prescription of X-ray dosage based on a regular daily fraction of 200 cGy but with no "standard" end point is, in our view, an unsatisfactory approach to treatment. It must be added that where we prescribe, for example, the optimum dose for a laryngeal cancer with a planned 16 exposures in an overall time of 3 weeks, this does not mean that the prescribed dose will always be given regardless of the individual patient's local and/or general reaction. Constant clinical observation is essential and though the established optimum dose will not be exceeded, any unusually severe reaction occurring before the normal end of the course of treatment would lead us to stop the planned procedure short of the accepted optimum level. This need rarely arises in practice, but continuous clinical observation and care must take priority over a desire to reach an accepted optimum level of dosage, however carefully this may have been established. One further point must be made before leaving this critical comparison between the concept of optimum dose and the "constant daily input" practice of many other centres. It must be conceded that with experience and care the "end point" with both schools of thought is remarkably constant. The statement "4000–6000 cGy in 4–6 weeks" works out, within fairly narrow limits, at something close to the Manchester optimum dose for any similar lesion. It remains our view, however, that our concept is scientifically sound in principle as well as in practice and permits much more precise evaluation of different treatment regimes. Indeed, it is the absence of this kind of dosimetric precision which makes comparisons between different centres so difficult and so often invalid. These difficulties have, in fact, given rise to various attempts to validate comparisons, the nominal standard dose (NSD) approach being one. However, they all suffer from a variety of inbuilt errors and uncertainties and in Manchester we prefer to continue to build on the solid foundations of five decades of experience.

It is clear, therefore, that the anatomical site, the histology of the tumour, and its extent and configuration will together determine if radical radiotherapy is feasible. The volume to be irradiated will be determined and the entire prescription for the course of treatment will be planned, usually along well-tried lines. The optimum dose levels being known, the course of treatment will begin and end along a predictable pathway. Nevertheless, if an out-patient fails to appear for a few days (for whatever reason), or if the machine on which his treatment has been planned and is being executed should break down, how does this affect his "optimum dose"? Radiobiological studies over a number of years (Chap. 2) have only confirmed the extensive clinical experience that, other things being equal, an unplanned extension of the overall time in which a fixed dosage is delivered will reduce the biological effectiveness of that dosage. Thus, the defaulting patient will receive a less effective treatment and the problem then is how to correct this defect. With the best will in the world any dosage correction must be a guess, but at least it can be an informed guess. For example, in a 21-day treatment an unplanned gap of 1 day might be ignored on the grounds that the consequent slight loss of effect would be unlikely to put this patient into the dose level associated with no morbidity and reduced cure rate. However, a gap of a week in a 3-week course of treatment could be catastrophic and only an inspired guess can be made to adjust the dosage upwards, perhaps erring on the high rather than the low side. From what has been said about optimum dosage, and from an understanding of the radiobiology underlying this problem, it will be appreciated why we regard a *course* of treatment, with all of its connotations, as sacrosanct.

Radiosensitivity of Tumours

In Chap. 2 there was some discussion of the various factors involved in the resolution or otherwise of a tumour following irradiation. It is sometimes difficult, however, to disentangle radiobiological experimental fact from biological hypothesis. It is nevertheless important to appreciate the biological and histological differences between tumours, the different ratios of tumour cells to stromal cells, different proportions of growing to resting cells, varying repopulation and absorption rates, areas of hypoxia, necrosis and the like. These factors must be kept in mind, especially when observing the response of a tumour in a particular patient, since an awareness of the many subtle influences on tumour resolution can and should govern clinical judgement.

In spite of the experimental and theoretical factors which might affect the rate of resolution of a tumour, clinical experience has long demonstrated wide differences in response. A tumour such as a seminoma testis, which rapidly resolves in response to a modest dose of radiation, is described clinically as a radiosensitive tumour and this description remains true whatever the radiobiological explanations may be for this kind of response. Some tumours, for example chondrosarcoma, habitually show little if any discernible response in volume even after large doses of radiation that come close to the maximum tolerance of the contiguous normal tissues. These tumours are described in clinical practice as radioresistant. A large number of tumours, essentially epidermal cancers, fall into an intermediate category, described as moderately sensitive, where slow resolution follows optimum dosage. As will be made clear in subsequent chapters, high radiosensitivity can be associated with high levels of definitive cure (e.g. seminoma) or with lower but still rewarding levels of cure (e.g. medulloblastoma of the cerebellum, Hodgkin's lymphoma, and others). Unfortunately, similar degrees of high radiosensitivity may result in rapid resolution only to be followed by equally rapid local recurrence and metastasis (e.g. anaplastic tumours of the lung and thyroid). On the other hand, epidermal carcinomas of the skin, the head and neck, and the genito-urinary tract can, when appropriately irradiated in their early stages, yield high cure rates even though they resolve relatively slowly in response to high localised dosage. These moderately sensitive tumours represent the radiotherapist's main field of success, his "bread and butter" work. Tumours which, with few exceptions, display little discernible resolution even after high-dose irradiation—the radioresistant tumours—include the various types of connective tissue sarcoma. This apparent lack of response is probably because most of the bulk of these tumours consists of differentiated and nonproliferating cells, the malignant tumour cells being a small though potentially lethal minority. It is difficult to establish the true radiosensitivity of these tumour cells, but for the radiotherapist they still represent a rather disappointing therapeutic challenge. Recent attempts to combine radiotherapy with surgery and chemotherapy have yet to demonstrate any substantial gain in overall curability. Another kind of problem arises with adenocarcinoma of the gastrointestinal tract—stomach, colon, and rectum. Here again it is difficult to estimate the intrinsic radiosensitivity of the adenocarcinoma cells but they would certainly not seem to be highly sensitive. If they are, as we suspect, of the same general sensitivity as epidermal carcinoma, high localised dosage might lead to local tumour control. Unfortunately, such high localised irradiation is not only technically difficult in the anatomical sites involved, but the normal tissue damage induced can create clinically unacceptable problems. Apart from early perforation through an ulcerated tumour, the late effects of ischaemic fibrosis can lead to progressive obstruction of the affected segment of gut.

Experience in the clinical field has demonstrated therefore that tumours do fall roughly into one of the three general categories of sensitivity: highly sensitive, moderately sensitive, or resistant. For each single tumour type, however, the clinician can expect a range of sensitivity, as shown in the dose-response curve in Fig. 5.3, and the optimum dose should be given in each case. A special problem sometimes arises where a patient with, for example, a tumour of the tonsillar fossa is diagnosed as having a localised squamous cell carcinoma and treatment by beam-directed megavoltage X-rays is instituted. After a few daily treatment fractions the tumour displays high radiosensitivity and virtually disappears. Under these circumstances it is prudent to review the histological sections on which the initial diagnosis was made, since review might then suggest that the tumour is not epidermal but lymphomatous in nature. It may then be wise to change the treatment plan to include the lymph nodes of the neck—a regional technique rather than localised beam-direction. This problem is not common, but when it arises it underlines the importance of reliable histopathology (which begins incidentally with an adequate and representative biopsy!) and alert clinical observation throughout a course of treatment.

Choice of Treatment

The choice of treatment appropriate to an individual patient's needs is a product of three components discussed above: the tumour type, the stage of the disease, and the therapeutic objective. The resulting decision to employ a specific radiotherapeutic technique presupposes that it is technically feasible and that the necessary facilities are available. The radiation sources required will include beams of X-rays or gamma rays and radioactive isotopes (solid or in solution).

Beam Therapy

That tumour response is dose-dependent is a fundamental clinical and radiobiological fact. However, effective radiotherapy demands much more than simply "a dose" of ionising radiation. Of the many connotations of "dose"—quantity, quality, volume, time, fractionation, etc.—one vital requirement which underlies the correct choice of treatment technique is that *all parts of a tumour must be adequately irradiated*.

Single Beams

It is obvious, though often forgotten, that to irradiate a substantial tumour with a single beam of X-rays must place that tumour in a falling gradient of dosage. The tumour nearest the surface (and the radiation source) must receive a higher dose than that part of the tumour farthest from the surface. This is equally true for the normal tissues lying in the same X-ray beam. Thus, the only way to ensure an adequate dose to the most distal part of such a tumour would be to give a very high and damaging dose to the proximal part—and to the contiguous normal tissues. This is unacceptable and is also unnecessary provided appropriate steps are taken to correct such dosimetric imbalance. When a tumour is not a substantial one, for example when treating a slender plaque of basal cell carcinoma in the skin, the deepest surface of the tumour lies so close to the skin surface that a single beam of X-rays can adequately irradiate the entire tumour without exceeding the tolerance dose level at the surface. As the thickness of a skin tumour increases, as with an invasive squamous carcinoma of the skin, further thought must be given to the adequacy of dosage in depth from a single beam of X-rays. Failure to take this requirement into consideration is a potent source of failure to cure a curable cancer.

Details of the various techniques suitable for treating tumours of the skin are discussed in Chap. 6.

Parallel Opposed Beams

In spite of the obvious dose gradient in a single beam of X-rays, it is curious how often a

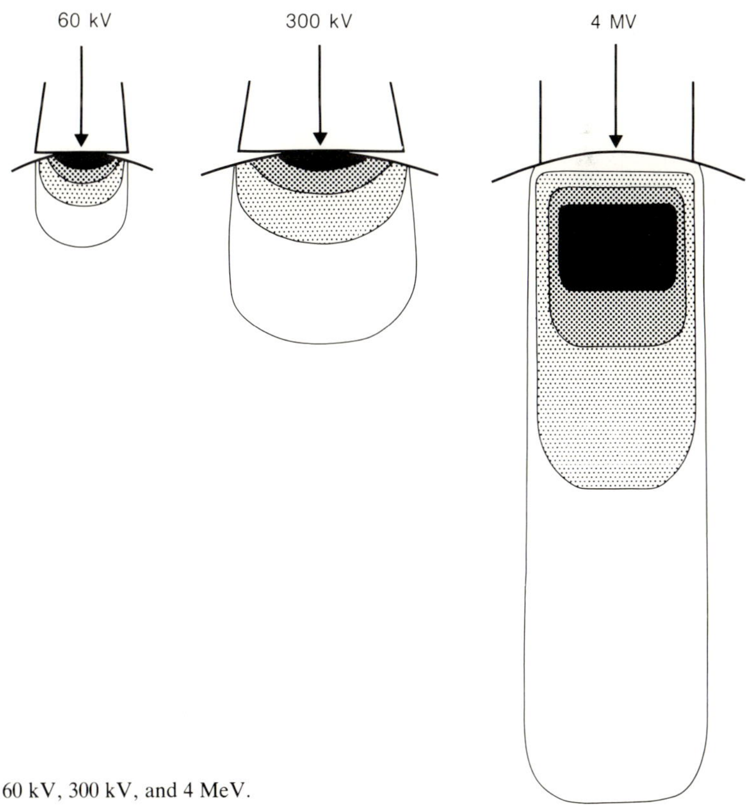

Fig. 5.5. Single-beam dose distributions for 60 kV, 300 kV, and 4 MeV.

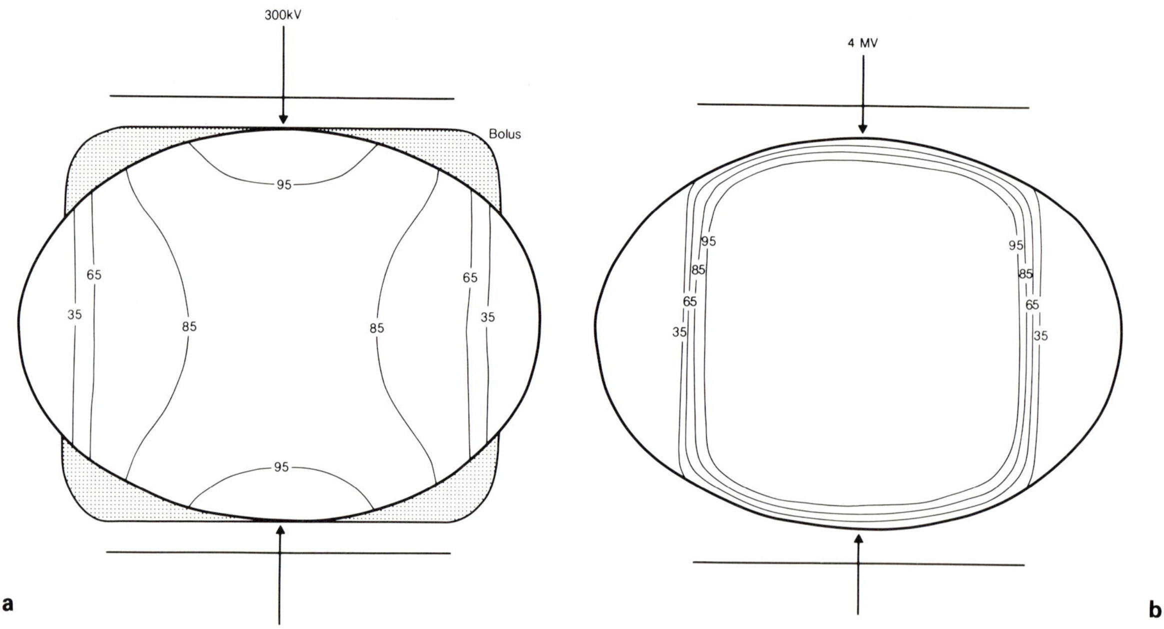

Fig. 5.6a,b. Parallel pair dose distributions. **a** 300 kV, **b** 4 MeV.

substantial deeply situated tumour is treated, apparently with radical intent, by a single beam of X-rays. By employing two parallel opposed beams it is easy to negate the falling gradient of a single beam and to ensure that the entire tumour lies within a suitably homogeneous zone of irradiated tissue. This technique is seen typically in the regional type of therapy required for testicular tumours (Chap. 13) and lymphomas (Chap. 14).

The dose distribution created by large parallel opposed beams of megavoltage X-rays is remarkably homogeneous and clearly superior, where radical treatment is intended, to a single beam.

Beam Direction

Tumours of moderate sensitivity—most commonly epidermal carcinoma—require high-dose treatment when cure is the therapeutic objective. This approach to treatment is feasible only when the target volume is of limited dimensions, since only then could the essential high levels of dosage be tolerated. Various arrangements of two or more X-ray beams, either wedged or unwedged, can be directed at the tumour in such a way as to ensure the necessary high and homogeneous dosage in and immediately around the tumour and also to ensure a rapid fall-off of dosage within the normal tissues outside the target volume. This small-field, high-dose, beam-directed technique is described in Chap. 7. It is the treatment of choice for tumours in the head and neck, for certain intracranial tumours, for the bladder, and for various other sites requiring accurately circumscribed irradiation.

Another important feature of beam-directed radiotherapy is that the judicious use of wedged and unwedged beams permits the creation of a three-dimensional volume of high dose, in any anatomical site, and appropriate to virtually any shape imposed by the configuration of the tumour. The precise choice of technique for any patient is critical and, as always with malignant disease, considerable care and skill are essential to success, and failure is lethal.

Radioactive Isotopes

Solid radioisotopes include the time-honoured naturally occurring radium as well as a variety of solid artificial isotopes, sometimes described as radium substitutes, of which cobalt-60, caesium-137, and gold-198 are most commonly used. These solid radioactive sources each have unique physical features on which their special clinical usefulness depends. They may be used as intersti-

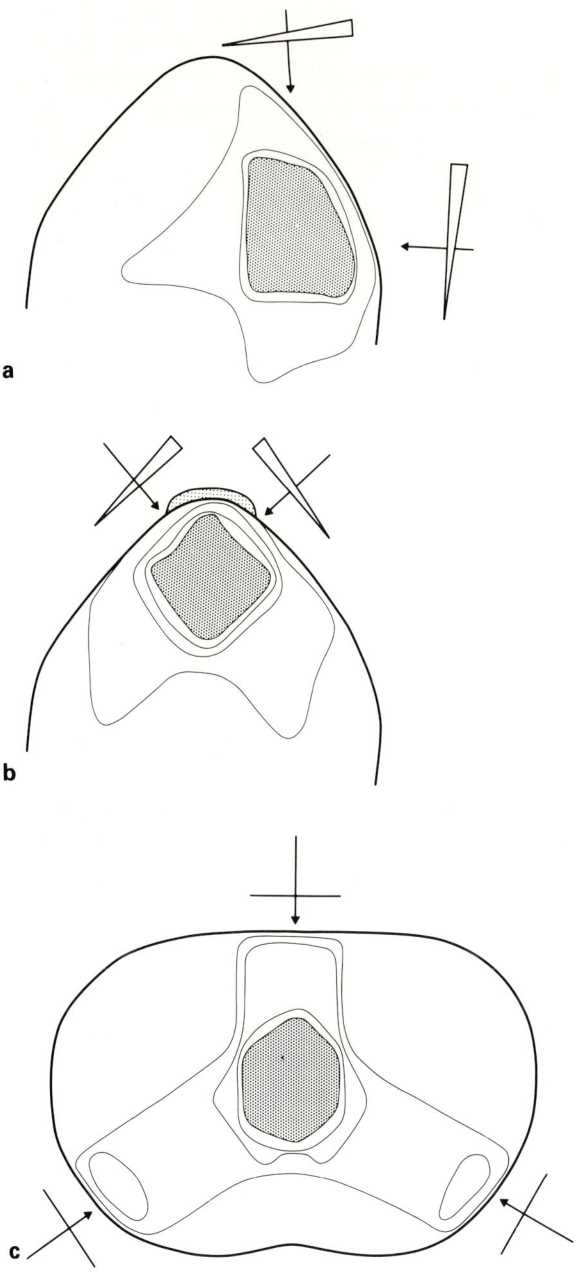

Fig. 5.7a–c. Beam direction. **a** Floor of mouth, **b** larynx, **c** bladder.

tial implants, as intracavitary sources of radiation, or on surface applicators (moulds). In this Centre we still prefer radium needles for interstitial therapy, though iridium-192 and tantalum-182 have been used (and are preferred in some centres). Radium needle implants are mainly used for squamous cancers of the buccal cavity and anus, and for selected cases of vulval and vaginal cancers. Occasionally an awkward cancer of the skin may be treated by a radium implant. Permanent implants of gold-198 seeds are ideally suited to treat relatively small areas of plaque-like squamous cancer in the mouth, bladder, vagina, and skin (see Chaps. 6, 7, 11, 12, and 17).

The important dosimetric feature to note concerning interstitial implants is that the dose around each source is exceedingly high but falls off rapidly in all directions. In the context of making a correct choice of treatment, the essential requirement is to ensure that the *entire* tumour, e.g. a squamous carcinoma of the tongue, lies within a zone of radiation which at no point falls below a lethal dose level, however high the dosage may be in close proximity to each needle or seed in the implant as a whole. The dose-distribution that can be achieved in and around a single-plane, two-plane, or volume implant must, therefore, be clearly appreciated before choosing to treat a patient's cancer. If in doubt it may be wise to examine the feasibility of a beam-directed X-ray treatment as a better alternative to interstitial radium (Chap. 7).

Radium, cobalt, and caesium lend themselves well to intracavitary use, for cancers of the corpus and cervix uteri. The once common use of intracavitary radium for treating cancers of the maxillary sinus has now been superseded by beam-directed megavoltage therapy. Radium for uterine cancer, invaluable and highly effective for more than half a century, is also being progressively replaced by caesium and cobalt. This is partly because of the easier handling characteristics of caesium and cobalt and partly the result of an increasing trend towards remote afterloading, a technique for which radium is unsuitable. As with interstitial sources, intracavitary therapy is characterised by a very high dose level close to the radiation sources and a steep gradient outwards from the centre. So long as all of the tumour lies within an adequate level of dosage, the very high dose centrally can be ignored. Where the tumour extends beyond the minimum acceptable dose level, steps must be taken to balance this falling dose gradient by appropriately planned X-ray beams. This technique is described in detail in Chap. 11 and the importance of choosing the appropriate treatment method in relation to the stage of the disease is discussed.

Cobalt-60 has now replaced radium for treatment involving surface applicators or moulds. Small sources of cobalt-60 can be obtained in a range of sizes suitable for mould treatment.

Moreover, the relatively rapid radioactive decay of cobalt-60, about 1% per month, can be exploited to create a wide range of source strengths. The clinical usefulness of short-distance gamma-radiation therapy (brachytherapy) rests on the rapid fall-off in dosage. As with a single beam of X-rays, a cobalt mould can deal effectively with a superficial lesion. The choice of this treatment as an alternative to X-ray therapy (or even to surgery) is governed primarily by the anatomical site of the tumour—as well, of course, as its stage and histology. For example, a circumscribed squamous carcinoma of the skin on the dorsum of the hand can be ideally treated by a short-distance (0.5-cm) cobalt-60 mould. The high dosage to the tumour does not penetrate far enough to damage the underlying extensor tendons and their sheaths. Superficial X-ray therapy can also be used for such a lesion, though when possible we prefer a cobalt mould and gamma radiation. Surgery as an alternative carries the risk of leaving malignant cells behind because of the surgeon's natural urge to avoid damage to tendon sheaths. In some sites and with smaller tumours, cobalt-60 may be replaced by gold-198 seeds. Certain sites lend themselves to small adhesive moulds, while others require more elaborate preparation and fixation. In every case the precise technique used is dictated by the individual clinical picture (see Chaps. 6 and 7).

Soluble radioisotopes used for malignant disease include iodine-131 and phosphorus-32. The place of iodine-131 in the management of certain thyroid cancers is discussed in Chap. 7. The object is to exploit the selective absorption of iodine-131 in relation to the various histological types of thyroid tumour. Phosphorus-32 has its place in the overall management of the chronic leukaemias, polycythaemia vera, and thrombocythaemia. Other methods of treatment are also available and the judicious choice and timing of each type of treatment is of paramount importance. This subject is discussed in Chap. 14.

Re-treatment

Sometimes after an apparently successful course of radiation therapy a malignant tumour shows signs of local recurrence within the irradiated volume. The radiotherapist is then faced with the problem of further management. It may be possible to resort to radical surgical resection, and if this can be curative it may be advisable. Chemotherapy may be considered as a possible alternative to surgery. Inevitably the question will arise as to the value and wisdom of giving further radiation treatment. Bearing in mind what was said above concerning optimum dosage, it will be appreciated that if a patient has already received a level of dosage which carries a significant incidence of high-dose morbidity, then further irradiation to the same tissue must increase the irreversible tissue changes leading to overt morbidity. The nature of this morbidity will depend on the anatomical site involved. For example, to re-treat recurrent cancer of the bladder, after a previous course of X-ray therapy to optimal dose levels, would greatly increase the probability of considerable and permanent contraction of the organ. Another important consideration is the response of the recurrent cancer to further irradiation. If the initial treatment was properly executed and to the maximum safe level of dosage there seems no reason to expect another similar treatment to be any more effective. To give a larger dose on the second occasion could be to court disaster. To give a smaller dose is likely to fail as before. Even to attempt palliation, by growth retardation, would in such circumstances run a risk of undesirable morbidity, sooner rather than later. We have argued that the best chance to cure is the first chance to cure. Where the first course of treatment has been suboptimal, it could be claimed that a second treatment might prove helpful. On the other hand, had the first course been at optimum dose levels, there might well have been no recurrence requiring treatment.

Radium, whether by interstitial, surface, or intracavitary treatment, is always used at optimum dosage levels. Any local recurrence following radium therapy must therefore be dealt with surgically, if feasible, or alternatively by some appropriate chemotherapy. Small-field beam-directed X-ray therapy, as mentioned above, relies on high localised dosage at optimum levels. Any local recurrence following this kind of irradiation would, as with radium therapy, require surgical resection if feasible, or chemotherapy if appropriate. A somewhat different problem arises, however, with local recurrence of a radiosensitive tumour treated initially by regional, large-field X-ray therapy. Having irradiated the whole abdomen (as for seminoma testis) any attempt to repeat this treatment to the same dosage level and to the same volume of tissue would carry grave risks of (1) bone marrow failure, (2) renal failure, and (3) malabsorption problems arising from damage to the small bowel. Nevertheless, it is sometimes possible and clinically justified to attempt to control a *localised* recurrence by irradiating a substantially smaller volume of the abdomen; this would be to a modest level of dosage, which may yet prove effective, even if only with palliative intent. In short, though regional X-ray therapy creates its own regional problems of tissue tolerance (lung, kidney, bone marrow) the total dose given to these large volumes is low enough to permit some additional irradiation *confined to a smaller volume*. In this carefully restricted sense we would and do accept the possibility of re-treatment (see also Chap. 13). In short, the temptation to re-treat a recurrent tumour should be tempered with caution and with a careful assessment of alternative management.

Causes of Failure

It is salutary to give some attention to why we fail, especially if we confidently anticipated success. We may fail to cure a patient's cancer, on the one hand, or we may fail to provide effective palliation, on the other. It seems clear that our failures arise (1) from errors of judgement, (2) from errors of omission, and (3) from errors of commission.

Failure to Cure

Errors of judgement can arise at many points in the whole process of management. For example, it would not be surprising if we failed to cure a malignant melanoma because it had been wrongly diagnosed as a pigmented basal cell carcinoma, and treated as such. Many other examples could be quoted to underline the importance of reliable histological diagnosis. It would also be no surprise to fail to cure a tumour which a more experienced radiotherapist would have recognised as simply too large for curative irradiation. (The experimental radiobiological explanation for this kind of failure was discussed in Chap. 2.) When we speak of failure to cure we tend to think of "curing the tumour" when in fact we should be thinking always of curing the patient. Sometimes a tedious course of radiotherapy is completed and the tumour successfully "cured" but metastases are then discovered which soon kill the patient. The error of judgement in this case rests on the failure to detect the metastases before exposing the patient to an unnecessarily upsetting radical treatment for the primary tumour. In such circumstances a more modest palliative approach to the primary lesion might have been adequate, depending of course on the anticipated rate of general deterioration from widespread disease.

Errors of omission arise, for example, from failing to give an adequate level of dosage, i.e. from a less than optimum dose. It has already been said that too many radiotherapists seem to regard morbidity of any kind as too high a price to pay for potential cure. In fact radiation morbidity, in the sense of persisting high-dose effects requiring special intervention, must be accepted in a small percentage of patients, just as postoperative problems such as colostomy or tracheostomy are acceptable to the surgeon. The brisk reactions following radical radiotherapy are, of course, unpleasant but they are transient and are as unavoidable and as clinically acceptable as postoperative discomfort or pain. Inadequate dosage, therefore, is a major error of omission and is often the sole cause of failure and death. This sub-optimal dosage is not of course, to be confused with the previous example of failure where a tumour is so large that even the maximum tolerable level of dosage is bound to fail.

Errors of commission can simply be described as carelessness. This kind of error in radiotherapy may not always be dramatically obvious but, for example, the habitual use of a poor technique will in time be reflected in a lower cure rate than might have been expected. A badly planned X-ray treatment may result from carelessness or bad training—both equally undesirable. Errors in dose calculation are much more common than we realise, and for this reason some systematic double-checking procedure is essential in a radiotherapy department. Badly positioned X-ray applicators can lead to a part of a tumour lying outside the treated volume, the so-called "geographic miss", with the inevitable result of failure to control the growth. Another variation of this type of error is to fail to ensure that an adequate margin of "normal" tissue around a tumour is included in the target volume of high dosage. Badly positioned or slipped radium applicators, when treating cervical cancer for example, represent another common cause of failure. Here again, appropriate checks should be standard procedure in the radiotherapy department. The wrong use of dosage tables is another error of commission—for example, reading a radium dosage table for a treating distance of 1.0 cm when the treatment intended, and given, is at 0.5 cm. This leads to a substantially larger quantity of radium being implanted into the tissues than was intended, with disastrous results. Many errors result from a lack of alert observation, as when a dose-monitor in an X-ray console is ignored at some crucial period.

There are, therefore, many controllable causes of failure to cure a potentially curable cancer. To attribute these failures simply to human error is too complacent. The radiotherapist, when planning and executing any treatment, however "simple", must be obsessively precise. Moreover, the entire department needs to have inbuilt checks to reduce these human risks to a minimum. In spite of all our efforts, however, it must be admitted that we sometimes fail for no discoverable reason, even with some patients whom we confidently expected to cure. Patients in this category deserve very special study, by all available means, in the hope of learning how we may fail less often.

Failure to Palliate

Most of the causes of failure to cure are equally relevant to the failure to palliate. Errors of omission and commission are ever-present problems, but perhaps the greatest obstacle to successful palliation arises from errors of judgement. When to attempt palliative treatment by irradiation requires experience and sound clinical judgement. As noted above, the object of palliative treatment is the relief of a distressing and persistent symptom, provided that irradiation can in fact influence that symptom. To irradiate an impossibly large and painful cancer of the buccal cavity, using two large parallel opposing X-ray beams, will fail to relieve the pain from invaded bone and nerve, will fail to achieve any worthwhile tumour control, and worse, will make the patient even more miserable by inhibiting secretion from the parotid glands. In short, not only is failure to palliate bad clinical judgement, especially if the clinical situation is made worse rather than better, but the patient and his relatives will attribute his predictable deterioration directly to the radiotherapy: "He wasn't so bad until he had X-ray treatment". This attitude is unfortunately sometimes shared even by our medical colleagues who themselves had urged the unwise attempt at palliation. We must learn to recognise when not to treat and when to resist firmly the many pleas for help. No patient is immortal and, apart from opiates, it is often wise and kind to withhold all medication and allow our patient to die with dignity.

Control of Factors that Influence Prognosis

It is important to consider how, if at all, we can influence the prognosis of a patient with cancer. There is a great deal of epidemiological information showing striking geographical, racial, and cultural differences in the incidence of specific types of malignant disease. This is not the place to discuss this interesting subject in detail, but though we clearly cannot influence where we are born, it is important to appreciate that being born in Japan carries a high risk of gastric cancer, with a poor prognosis. Being born in Latin America carries a high risk of cervical cancer, with a good prognosis of proper action is taken, while someone born in the Caspian littoral has a high risk of oesophageal cancer, with a very poor prognosis. The importance of the site of a tumour has already been emphasised, since this influences the histological nature of the disease and the possibility of detecting the tumour when it is still small enough to be potentially curable. But again we cannot influence in what site a patient will develop his cancer and to that extent we cannot influence his prognosis. The same is true for the age of the patient, though one reason for a worsening prognosis as age increases is related to apathy, and this at least is open to some effort at persuasive education. Some cancers have also been shown to respond better in females than in males, all relevant factors being otherwise identical. Why this should be so is unknown, as indeed is the actuarial fact that women have an overall longer life expectancy than men. But again, we cannot choose our own sex.

What then remains within our control so far as prognosis is concerned? Since we cannot control the site and therefore the histology of a tumour we can at least try to diagnose the disease as soon as possible. To this end the radiotherapist can combine with other involved colleagues to pursue any and all potentially useful avenues towards prevention and earlier detection of various cancers. Different countries, as mentioned above, present different risks and require different strategies. Education and information about cancer for the public is no less important than for the medical and paramedical professions. Research and development into effective screening procedures, including cervical cytology, mammography, immunodiagnosis, and other subtle tumour markers at present unknown need to be supported and encouraged. Apart from these methods of influencing prognosis, once the diagnosis has been established, the most crucial factors on which success or failure depends are to make the correct choice of treatment and to execute it with skill. The remaining chapters of this textbook are concerned with the practical details of how to apply radiation therapy with skill, albeit according to the Manchester school of thought.

6 Skin

R. D. Hunter

Introduction

Malignant disease involving the skin represents a significant work load to the general radiotherapist and can involve interesting diagnostic and therapeutic decisions. Primary skin cancer is also relatively common and there is a need to provide an efficient service in which the first treatment is successful in the majority of patients. The reward for careful attention to technique is very considerable both in terms of clinical cancer control and functional results. Squamous cell carcinoma, basal cell carcinoma, and intra-epidermal carcinoma constitute the majority of the lesions dealt with clinically, but metastatic disease, lymphomas, and malignant melanomas are also referred regularly for opinions and may require radiotherapy. Lymphomatous involvement of the skin is dealt with in Chap. 14.

The general principles of the techniques of assessment and radiotherapeutic management to be described are equally applicable to any malignant skin tumour once the decision has been made to accept it for radiotherapy. Dosage and fractionation may have to be adjusted to allow for the nature of the disease process and the intent of the treatment.

All the primary skin carcinomas carry a good prognosis. In the United Kingdom they tend to be smaller than cancers in other sites, are diagnosed accurately at an earlier stage, and they are referred for specialist opinion without delay. Both surgery and radiotherapy offer very similar overall results in experienced hands and often the availability of a satisfactory service dictates the treatment method.

Surgical management is often straightforward on the trunk, neck, and proximal limbs. The more common sites for skin cancer on the face, around the eyes, the ears, the dorsum of the hand, and the anterior tibial region are less suitable for surgical excision and primary closure with good cosmetic results. Radical radiotherapy has very definite advantages at these sites and can spare the patient grafting or difficult reconstructive surgery. Some of the radiotherapy techniques which will be described to treat these lesions appear complicated, but the practical results, in experienced hands, justify the efforts.

Chemotherapy

Chemotherapy has a very limited place in the management of skin cancer. The majority of lesions encountered can be cured by radical radiotherapy or surgery. The rare aggressive, invasive, and metastatic varieties of these tumours do not respond to the systemic chemotherapeutic agents available at the present time. The only effective place for chemotherapy is in the management of very superficial or intra-epidermal basal and squamous cell carcinomas and benign hyperkeratoses. These lesions can be cured or controlled by topical application of cytotoxic drugs. The bulk of clinical experience is with 5-fluorouracil ointment. Twice-daily application to lesions produces a skin reaction very similar to an acute radiation reaction at 2–3 weeks, which then settles spontaneously over the next month, if the ointment is discontinued. Tumour resolution often accompanies the resolving reaction. Treatment can be repeated as required, long-term control can be achieved, and necrosis with late effects is not seen. Excessive application of the ointment produces severe skin reactions and similar reactions are seen on uninvolved sites if the ointment is not confined to the lesion.

Clinical experience of intra-epidermal skin neoplasia is required when initiating treatment, since lesions which are physically too thick for topical chemotherapy will sometimes heal superficially under the influence of the ointment while continuing to progress more deeply.

The use of topical chemotherapy in primary skin carcinomata should be confined to cooperative patients whose general health or extent of disease precludes radical treatment and whose lesions are truly intra-epidermal. Locally recurrent superficial disease beyond further radical treatment may also respond to a trial of treatment.

Assessment

The radiotherapist must take certain factors into account before accepting a patient with skin cancer for treatment.

Anatomical Consideration

All the primary skin cancers arise in the dividing cell population of the basal layers of the epidermis. Skin varies slightly in thickness and texture between individuals and between different sites on the same individual. It can be of help when attempting to assess dosage for infiltrating tumours to remember that the epidermis is approximately 0.2 cm thick and is supported by a dermis 0.3 cm thick. What is more important is to remember that the skin at some special sites has a minimum of supporting subcutaneous tissue separating it from bone or cartilage. The bone of the skull and anterior tibia and the cartilage of the ear and the nose are so close to the skin that superficial X-ray therapy at 100–150 kV can result in the delivery of large absorbed doses to these subjacent tissues. This increases the risk of necrosis and a poor functional result. Some of the high-energy electron and special mould techniques in use at the Christie Hospital, to be described later, are used at these sites because the better quality of radiation avoids the risk associated with a high absorbed dose.

Pathological Considerations

Squamous cell carcinoma, basal cell carcinoma, and intra-epidermal carcinoma all respond satisfactorily to radical radiotherapy and are correctly regarded as radiocurable tumours. Malignant melanomas are very unpredictable in their response to radiation, and this fact, when viewed in the light of the excellent results of primary radical surgery for early-stage lesions, should influence the radiotherapist against accepting melanomas for primary treatment.

Metastatic melanoma and metastatic carcinoma can be accepted for therapy so long as the palliative nature of the treatment is understood.

Many varieties of the common skin cancers are seen in practice but they are readily recognisable with clinical experience. Basal cell carcinoma and intra-epidermal carcinoma rarely need biopsy. Squamous cell carcinoma must be confirmed histologically because that diagnosis demands a careful follow-up policy for the first 2 years. This must be directed towards the early recognition of regional lymph node metastases. These are very rare with small head and neck tumours but more common with large ear or limb lesions. Keratoacanthomas should be treated as squamous cell carcinomas unless they have been radically excised and the whole base of the lesion examined histologically.

Malignant melanomas should not be casually biopsied. If clinical opinion is in favour of melanoma, primary radical surgery should be anticipated. In elderly people the tendency for basal cell carcinomas to become pigmented should not be forgotten.

It cannot be stressed too strongly that larger than necessary biopsies are potentially harmful. They make subsequent accurate clinical assessment impossible because of distortion of the tumour and may result in patients receiving a treatment using an unnecessarily large field or a more penetrating type of radiation.

Another common practical problem arises with the referral of patients whose skin cancers have been histologically incompletely excised. The long and non-metastatic natural history of basal cell carcinomas allows a policy of observation to be pursued, reserving active treatment only for clinical recurrence. Histologically residual squamous carcinomas should be irradiated as if the primary disease were still present.

Size

Clinical radiotherapists accept that the larger the carcinoma, the more difficult it will be to control.

The visible tumour is a mixture of normal and malignant cells and the true tumour volume is a function of the area of skin involved and the thickness of the lesion both above and below the skin. This is a difficult concept to apply in daily practice when assessing the patient. In practice the area of skin involved has acquired considerable importance when attempting to assess the probability of control. Christie Hospital experience suggests that infiltrating tumours greater in mean diameter than 6 cm are rarely controlled by radical radiotherapy. Extensive non-infiltrating intraepidermal carcinomas, especially of the trunk, are controllable, even if very significantly larger than 6 cm, but only after allowing a considerable time for healing and accepting a protracted, more severe skin reaction than normal.

Age

Skin cancer is commoner in elderly patients, but both squamous cell and basal cell carcinoma are seen in adults below 40, particularly when they have been exposed in their youth to excessive amounts of ultraviolet light, or when there is a family history of the rare basal cell naevus syndrome. These tumours are no less radiosensitive than those seen in older patients, but younger adults, with their longer life expectancy, will be exposed to long-term risks associated with radical skin radiotherapy. The principal problems are thinning of the skin, telangiectasia, and radiation necrosis, particularly on exposed or chronically traumatised skin. Carcinogenesis is only a theoretical risk.

It is not our routine practice to irradiate primary skin cancers under the age of 40. It is also worth considering primary surgery in patients under 50 with tumours on conspicuous or exposed sites.

Age becomes an important factor again particularly over 70. Skin tolerance is reduced especially for small fields on the head and neck, and in these patients a dosage reduction should be made (dosage is discussed in a later section).

With very elderly or infirm patients who have relatively large skin tumours there is also a need to consider giving the simplest treatment possible. This may involve giving a single exposure of relatively low dose to a large field. The treatment may not be strictly curative, in terms of dosage, but in a patient whose limited life is complicated by a discharging or bleeding skin cancer, very gratifying healing of lesions is commonly observed.

Site

Site is also an important factor during the clinical assessment. The majority of cancers arise in the skin of the head and neck and this skin, along with that on the dorsum of the hand, tolerates radiation best. If, on the basis of all other factors, a small range of dosage seems possible then the highest dose should be used at these sites. The trunk and proximal limbs are much less tolerant and the lowest radical dose should be used. Unfortunately, lesions in these latter two areas also tend to be larger than those of the head and neck. The problems of poorer tolerance and size may incline the therapist to advise primary surgery, especially if the skin is relatively redundant. The radiotherapeutic alternative is a more severe reaction progressing to moist desquamation and slower healing.

The groins, perineum, and scrotum are very difficult sites for radiation reactions. External beam therapy is so poorly tolerated that it must only be used in the absence of any alternative. Acute reactions at these sites are invariably more severe and protracted and often call for specialist nursing. The best radiotherapeutic techniques for these areas employ interstitial implantation, which if appropriate often offers a good alternative to difficult perineal surgery.

The management of the acute reactions is not the only important factor when the site is under consideration. Radically irradiated skin tolerates chronic trauma poorly and necrosis can be precipitated. Lesions on sites like the lateral forearm and under ladies' clothing straps and belts should be considered for primary surgery.

Surface Irregularities

Primary skin cancers, arising potentially at any site on the skin, are inevitably found on irregular surfaces and present some problems because of convexity or, more rarely, concavity. Most irregularities can be dealt with radiotherapeutically (see treatment section below), but circumferential skin lesions, e.g. on the fingers, or when convexity and concavity are present in the same treatment area, e.g. lesions *over* the bridge of the nose and lesions extending into finger webs, may call for primary surgical management.

Steps in Treatment

Defining the Area

The area of normal skin supporting the tumour to be irradiated must be clearly defined by the radiotherapist. Skin cancers must be examined in a good light and the clinical margins noted. Intra-epidermal carcinomas and superficial cicatrising basal cell carcinomas can produce very significant involvement of surrounding apparently healthy skin and this may be more apparent if the lesion is viewed obliquely. Careful palpation of the skin to define the margin and depth of infiltration is an essential aspect of the assessment. Lesions confined to the epidermis have no substance, dermal involvement allows for thickening with free mobility over subcutaneous tissue, while deeper involvement can be felt as varying degrees of fixation of the tumour on underlying tissues.

Treatment Planning

1) The area to be treated should include a margin of normal skin not less than 0.5 cm and not more than 1 cm all round the tumour.
2) It is good practice to mark out the whole circumference of this area with gentian violet or other suitable skin-marker (see Fig. 6.1).
3) The majority of small skin tumours can be treated with circular or elliptical fields of modest size (2–4 cm) and with these there is nothing to be gained by creating irregular areas.
4) A set of dummy Perspex applicators which allow direct observation of the tumour and margin is helpful for checking the intended set-up before completing the prescription.

As fields become larger, irregular margins must be accepted otherwise unnecessarily large volumes of healthy skin will be treated. Standard-sized applicators on X-ray machines can be individually adapted by the use of lead cut-outs shaped to allow only the tumour and margin to be irradiated. For energies up to 100 kV, 1-mm lead is all that is required physically to reduce the exposure to less than 5% of the given dose. This thickness of lead is soft and malleable. Cut-outs can be made in the X-ray department by tracing the required field on to cellophane, transferring the outline to 1-mm lead, and cutting it out with scissors. This cut-out is then matched to the smallest standard applicator that will allow treatment of the whole area. The use of a lead cut-out calls for an exposure adjustment factor which must be applied by the treating radiographer. This varies with the area to be treated (Fig. 6.2).

When energies higher than 100 kV are in use and surfaces become very irregular, formal impressions of the treatment area and surrounding normal tissues must be taken and lead cut-outs of appropriate thickness can then be moulded to the model before treatment starts. For energies up to 300 kV, 3-mm lead is appropriate and gives a robust cut-out (Fig. 6.3; see Chap. 4).

Square and rectangular fields are rarely necessary in practice and do leave more conspicuous stigmata. They have a place only when multiple, small, individual treatments can be envisaged over an area of skin. This is a problem when patients have very dysplastic skin, coincidental multiple tumours, or a familial tendency to multiple basal cell carcinomas (basal cell naevus syndrome).

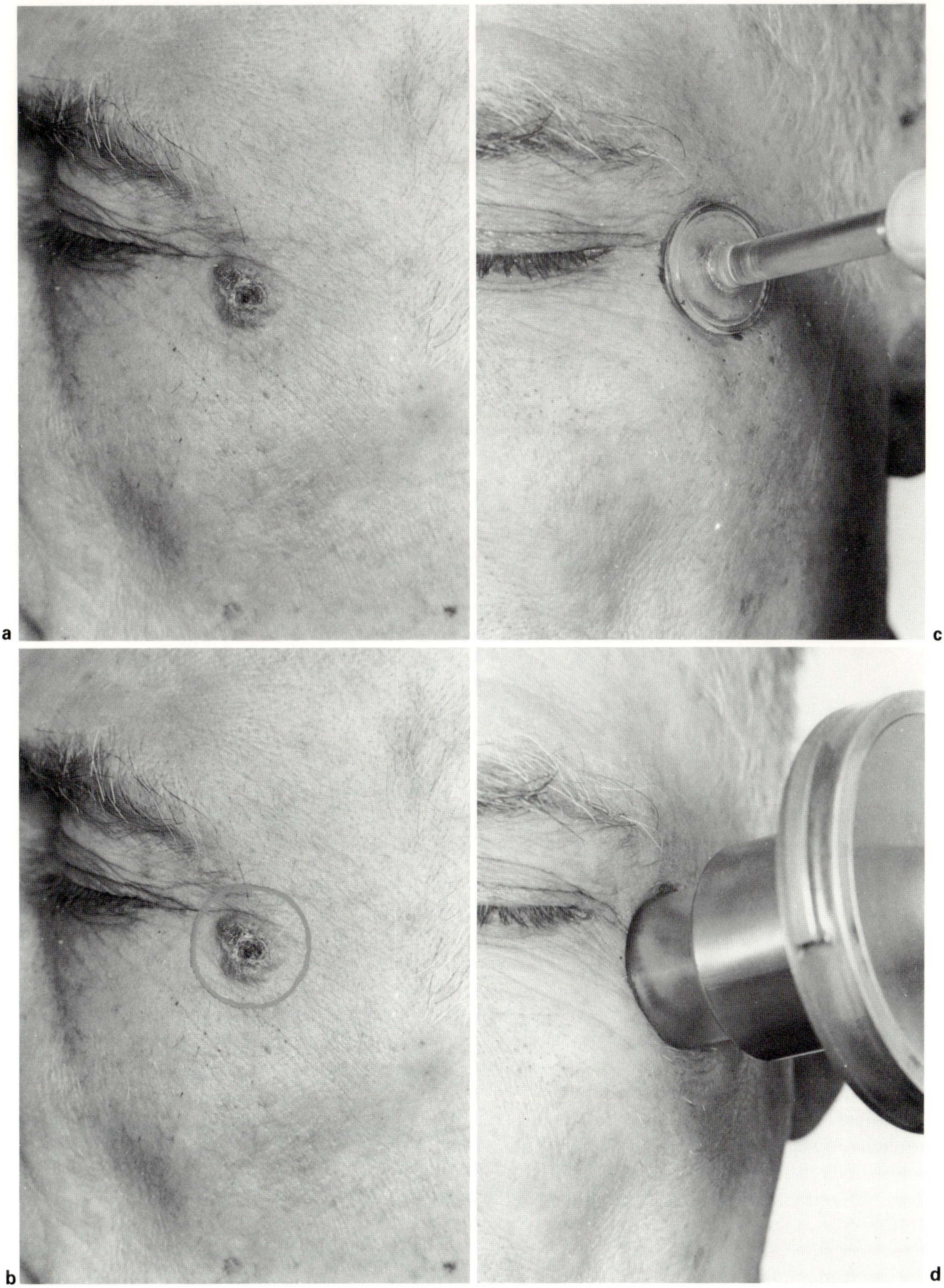

Fig. 6.1a–d. Stages in treatment planning for a small basal cell carcinoma overlying the left zygoma. **a** The lesion; **b** the treatment area defined; **c** checking the area with dummy applicators; **d** treatment set-up with circular applicator applied to defined area.

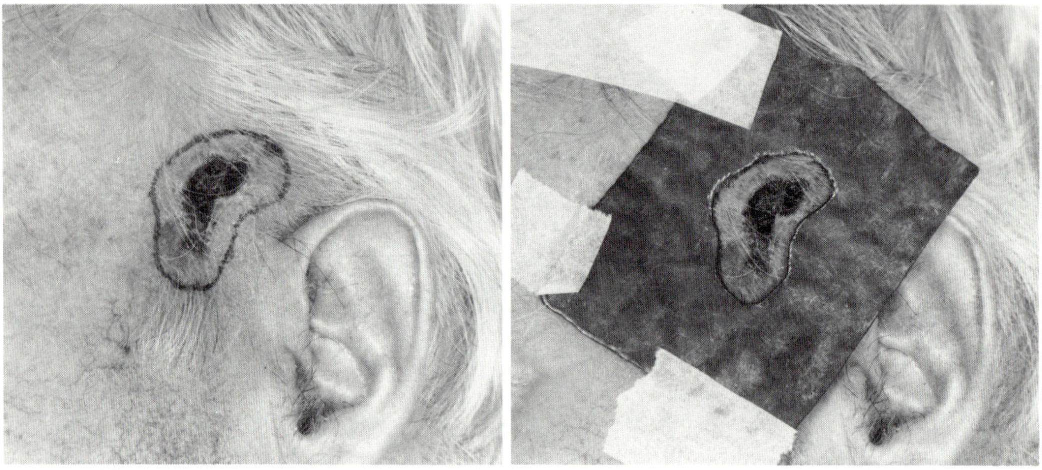

a b

Fig. 6.2a,b. Individual lead cut-out made in therapy department from 1 mm thick lead. **a** Irregular basal cell carcinoma in left pre-auricular region; **b** irregular 1-mm-thick lead cut-out in position.

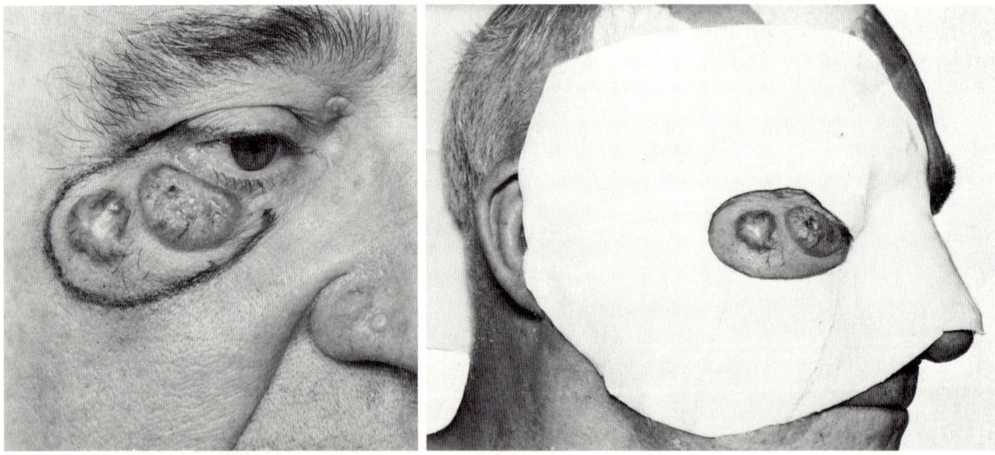

a b

Fig. 6.3a,b. Robust lead cut-out in 3-mm lead for fractionated treatment. **a** Treatment area defined on patient; **b** patient in treatment position wearing cut-out.

Selecting the Energy

Treating skin cancers radically with kilovoltage X-ray therapy or surface applicators is very different from radical radiotherapy for tumours in other tissues. No attempt is made to achieve homogeneity. Dosage is expressed only as the given dose and refers to the dose on the surface of the skin, not to the "tumour dose". To eradicate the tumours, a cancerocidal dose must be delivered to the malignant cells. The level of penetration of the tumours can only be assessed and expressed very crudely. The dose that can be delivered to the surface of the skin, i.e. the classical "skin tolerance", is dictated by the field size, site, and age of the skin, as discussed previously. The only methods of increasing the depth dose in a penetrating tumour are by increasing the energy of the radiation or increasing the treating distance. The majority of skin tumours can be successfully treated with radical given doses at 100 kV and 45 kV at a focus-skin distance (FSD) of 10 cm.

Clinical experience is the only sure way of achieving an understanding of this difficult problem, but it is our experience that epidermal lesions respond to energies of 45–65 kV, tumours involving the dermis require 100 kV, and subcutaneous extension requires energies of at least 200–300 kV. It is a potential source of error to operate equipment at too many different voltages. Successful practice and safety are best met by having available in any department only *one* energy level for each degree of tumour extension.

Avoiding Unnecessary Inhomogeneity

Since homogeneity is never achieved in depth with single field treatment, an attempt must always be made to deliver a homogeneous dose to the tumour-bearing area of skin. Because of the natural contours of the human body, treatment often has to be given to slightly concave or convex surfaces bearing a central tumour. In the majority of situations this presents little difficulty, since open-ended applicators of the required size, brought firmly down on the previously defined treatment area, in a position of skin apposition, will flatten the skin and allow the tumour to lie inside the applicator (Fig. 6.4), where its surface

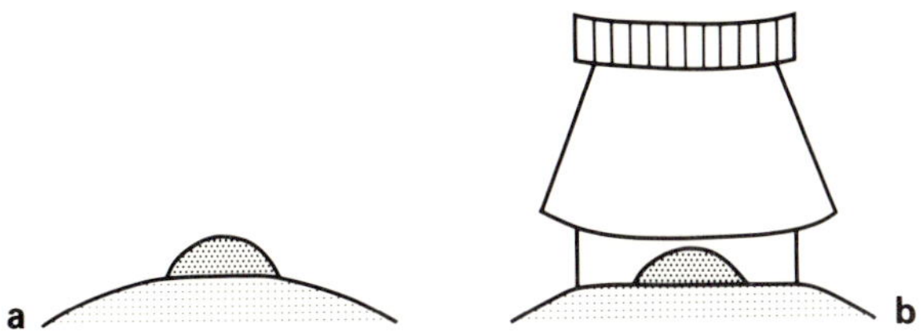

Fig. 6.4a,b. **a** Diagrammatic skin tumour on a slightly convex surface; **b** applicator in skin apposition flattening skin treatment surface and allowing lesion to lie inside open-ended applicator.

dose will be even higher than that intended for the skin. If there is any anxiety about a concave surface, e.g. in the inner canthus, where the tissues cannot be flattened by the applicator, a treating energy higher than seems necessary for the lesion itself may be chosen to ensure an adequate depth dose. When convexity becomes a serious problem, e.g. on the fingers themselves or around their webs, on the anterior tibia, and on the back of the skull, an alternative form of treatment should be considered. Christie Hospital practice is to use high-energy electrons or surface moulds in these situations.

Another problem occasionally encountered with lesions immediately anterior to the ear, or of the skin invading the vermilion surface of the lip, is the presence of an air gap in part of the margin of the treatment area. Because of the importance of lateral scatter in kilovoltage X-ray therapy this gap must be filled with a bolus material up to the level of the skin surface. Moist cotton wool or gauze is satisfactory for this purpose and can easily be adjusted to produce the required flat treatment surface (Fig. 6.5).

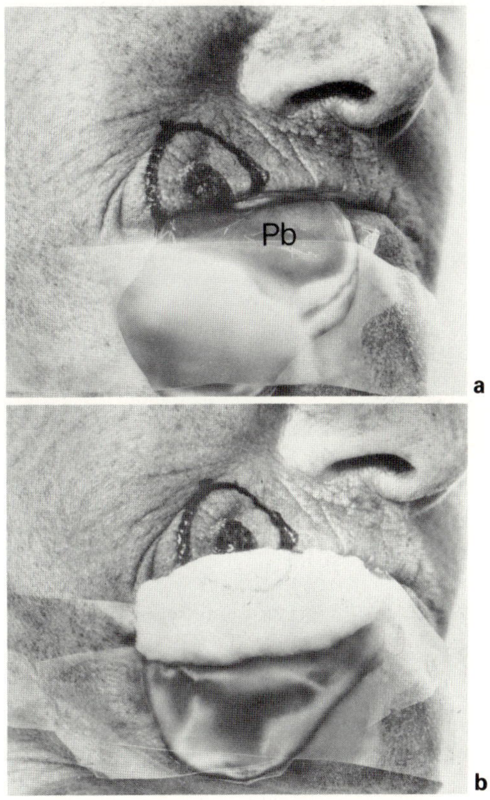

Fig. 6.5a,b. Primary basal cell carcinoma on right upper lip extending to vermilion border. **a** The treatment area is defined and a moulded 1-mm lead sheet covers the right lower lip; **b** moist cotton wool is used to fill the air gap on the lower margin of the field, flattening off the treatment surface.

Bolus is also required over megavoltage electron fields to avoid the build-up zone, and formal shells, with wax bolus, are wise if fractionated electron treatments are envisaged (see later section).

Lead Shielding

Normal uninvolved tissues can be spared unnecessary radiation reactions in some situations by the careful use of lead. The easiest example is a lesion low on the lateral surface of the nose, where a thin

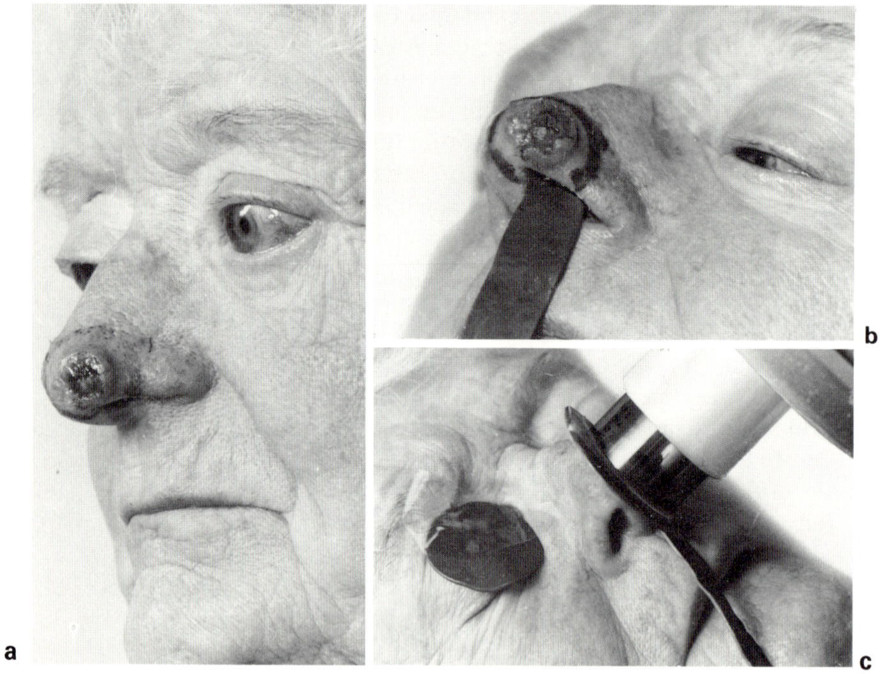

Fig. 6.6a–c. Lead shielding. **a** Lesion defined on tip of left nose; **b** tongue of 1-mm lead in left nostril to protect medial wall of nose; **c** final set-up with lead in nostril and additional 1 mm lead shielding of right eye.

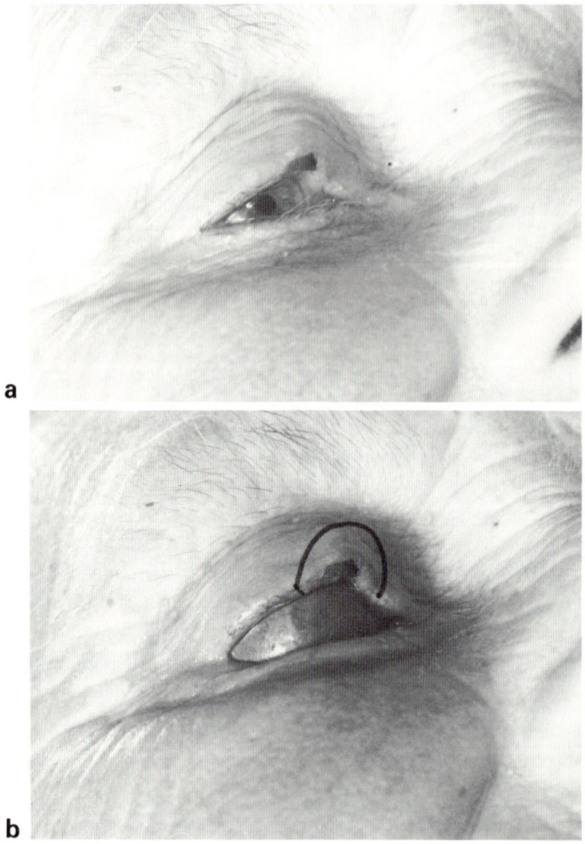

Fig. 6.7. a Awkward lesion on margin of right upper eyelid; **b** full 1-mm lead eye shield in conjunctival sac with treatment area defined.

sheet of lead inserted in the nostril will shield the medial wall of the nose from radiation passing right through the lateral nostril (Fig. 6.6). A similar technique can be used when lip or skin lesions overlie the anterior buccal mucosa. Lead shielding appropriate to the energy of radiation being used, if placed carefully inside the lips or buccal mucosa, will spare the alveolus and tongue from the reaction.

Lead shielding is particularly important when treating skin lesions around the eye, where transmitted radiation could result in a significant unnecessary dose being given to the retina, lens, or bulbar conjunctiva. Instillation of a sterile mixture of local anaesthetic in glycerine will allow carefully moulded lead eye-shields to be placed behind the lids. The eyelids must be mobile and great care taken when inserting these shields.

A lead shield entering only the lower conjunctival sac is quite adequate when skin lesions are present in the middle of that lid (half eye-shields). When lesions involve the upper lid, or both lids and angles, or when half eye-shielding is not satisfactory, the potentially more damaging full eye-shields must be inserted. These are only appropriate when skin lesions have not involved the bulbar conjunctiva but where there is a danger of unnecessary radiation reaching the globe. With eye-shields in position the overlying skin lesion is then treated as described above (Fig. 6.7).

It is our practice to use the minimal fractionation compatible with tolerance and tumour control when eye-shields are in use. The majority of these lesions are successfully treated by single exposures at 100 kV.

Dosage and Fractionation

As outlined in the discussion on energy selection, the principles of radical radiotherapy for skin cancer are different from those of radical radiotherapy at other sites. The radical dose is the given dose on the surface of the normal skin supporting the tumour. Tolerance doses must be used for all skin carcinomas. When one is treating a general population, some stigmata and a proportion of necroses must be accepted. Stigmata are a nuisance if large conspicuous areas are treated, but it must not be forgotten that a major contribution to those stigmata is often the irreversible destruction of normal tissue by the invading tumour present before treatment.

There is a school of thought that fractionation helps to prevent stigmata in skin treatment. In our view, however, radiation stigmata are a consequence of giving tolerance doses of radiation and they can be avoided only by reducing dosage below tolerance limits. Since reduction of the given dose implies a reduced dose to the tumour, the consequence is likely to be an increased failure rate. Because of the steepness of the dose-response curve for squamous cell carcinoma, especially larger tumours (see Chap. 2), there is a danger that substantial reduction of dose to avoid high-dose effects will very significantly increase primary failure rate and therefore negate the purpose of the treatment. The best control rates for skin cancer come from tolerance doses, and Christie Hospital practice is to deliver these on every occasion when the decision has been made to treat such a lesion by radiotherapy. In clinical practice with superficial X-ray therapy, these results can be achieved by single exposures for all head and neck lesions where the mean diameter of the field is not more than 4 cm. This group of lesions constitutes the majority referred to the radiotherapist. For the patients, this policy avoids unnecessary hospital visits. It also allows efficient use of resources in departments with a large work load.

Skin tolerance falls as field size increases and demands either a reduction in the given dose or fractionation of the treatment. Since reduction of dose means a poorer primary control rate, this approach with single-exposure treatments over 4 cm in diameter is reserved for senile patients with unpleasant, bleeding, or infected lesions. In all other situations fractionation must be used to achieve good results, and in Christie Hospital practice the majority of these bigger tumours can be dealt with by tolerance doses delivered in eight fractions over 10 days. Many of these larger lesions are irregular and call for individual lead cut-outs.

Table 6.1 shows standard tolerance doses and represents cumulative experience over many years, treating in excess of 2000 such patients a year.

Tolerance limits are very well established for single-exposure and eight-fraction treatments. In all situations where a range of dose seems possible the upper dose is applicable to head and neck lesions in younger patients and the lower doses to trunk or limb lesions or those in whom the skin is in poor general condition.

Table 6.1. Tolerance doses (in cGy) 45–100 kV.

	Up to 2.0 cm	2 cm–4 cm	4 cm upward
Single exposure	2250[a]	1800–2000	1500–1800[b]
Four days daily	—	(4000)	—
Eight days daily	—	4500	4000–4500
Sixteen days daily	—	(5000)	4500–5000

[a] Only in patients under seventy
[b] May represent palliative dose but be indicated by patient's general condition

Reactions

Acute Reactions

A slight erythema of normal treated skin is sometimes obvious in the first few hours after radiotherapy, but the true reaction appears as an erythema with heavy central crusting of any ulcerated lesion in about 10 days. The dose and fractionation outlined above will produce dry desquamation in the majority of the patients. They should be encouraged not to interfere with the crusting and to allow it to take its normal course. Some patients find the reaction itchy and they often report that topical lanolin ointments relieve that symptom. Large treatment areas, particularly those for superficial lesions on the trunk, will often progress to moist desquamation. Without proper care these can become infected. A topical antiseptic ointment is all that is required for mild moist desquamation on an exposed area, but similar reactions, particularly of large intra-epidermal carcinomas on the trunk, will require regular dressing. A paraffin-impregnated gauze dressing, changed daily for 1–2 months, is not an unusual requirement in large trunk lesions and is compatible with very satisfactory healing of the skin. All acute reactions with this regime will have healed by 8 weeks. Crusting is often heavy for the first weeks and then gradually settles. The surrounding erythema of the normal treated skin may not fade for a number of months.

The most difficult problems are presented by the rarer perineal skin reactions. Moist desquamation is usually present and this is aggravated by rubbing of the surfaces during normal movement. These reactions are best managed by rest, often in hospital, regular antiseptic or salt baths, and local antiseptic creams.

Tumour Response

Tumour response rates can be very variable and results must not be prejudged at a standard time. Squamous cell carcinomas have normally resolved at 2 months, but cystic basal cell and intra-epidermal carcinomas can take more than a year to disappear. Occasionally the epidermis will heal but the distortion (or defect) produced by the tumour may remain. This "ghost" lesion is not a cause for concern and should be left alone. It appears more commonly when patients do not wash the treated area satisfactorily while the reaction is settling. Patients should only be advised not to wash irradiated areas when there is a danger of introducing local infection, for example when moist desquamation is present. It is more important to dry treatment areas satisfactorily after washing than to avoid water altogether.

Late Reactions

Some degree of thinning of the skin, often accompanied by telangiectasia, is regularly seen after successful treatment. It is rare for this to require treatment. The more serious complication of skin necrosis can appear anything from 1 to 20 years after successful treatment of skin cancer. The history of local pain and rapid ulceration, often following trauma or a sudden change of external temperature, is very characteristic. Although there may be doubt about the clinical picture, the history is often so clear that biopsy can and should be avoided. Many necroses will heal with scarring under the influence of time and topical antiseptic ointments.

Persistent, painful ulceration should be dealt with by local radical surgery carried out by a surgeon experienced in operating on irradiated tissues. Radiotherapists who see no necrosis after irradiating skin malignancy are not treating to tolerance levels, and in the interests of maximum cure rates we believe that a necrosis rate of 5% is acceptable. In the early months after treating large squamous cell carcinomas, recurrent painful ulceration can present a difficult diagnostic and management problem since there is a danger of missing recurrent carcinoma. These patients should have the benefit of radical surgery if it is technically possible. Squamous cell carcinoma so rarely recurs after 2 years that new ulceration at this time can more readily be accepted as necrosis. Basal cell carcinomas may recur some years after therapy, but lesions of this type are slow-growing and they should be assessed over some months before submitting to surgical excision, especially in the elderly.

Radical treatment of a hair-bearing surface inevitably produces permanent alopecia. Inner canthus treatments can result in permanent lacrimal duct damage. In most situations this is a mild nuisance, but if it remains troublesome, plastic surgical reconstruction of the duct may be considered in a younger patient.

High-Energy Electron Therapy

This type of beam therapy has become more widely available over the last decade. The linear accelerators producing the electrons are relatively expensive. In view of the excellence of the results of treating most skin cancer with the simpler kilovoltage X-ray therapy, the clinical advantages of using electron therapy are strictly limited.

There are two advantages of electron beams. The first is the pattern of distribution of energy in tissue. This is evident only in beams generated at 2–15 MV. These beams have a short build-up zone, a relatively homogeneous plateau, and a rapid fall-off. This contrasts with the exponentially falling kilovoltage dose distribution (Fig. 6.8). Provided a skin tumour can be treated within the plateau zone, homogeneous irradiation can be delivered to cancers up to 3 cm thick.

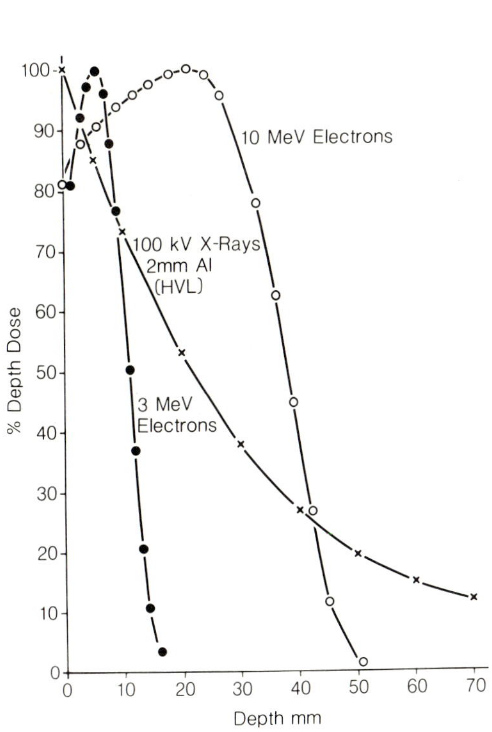

Fig. 6.8. Isodose distributions in soft tissue for 10-MeV electrons, 3-MeV electrons, and 100-kV photons showing the different patterns of energy distribution. The electrons show a "plateau" zone followed by a rapid fall in dose at depth, and contrast with the exponential fall of the photons.

The other advantage comes from the better quality of the electron radiation. These megavoltage beams are absorbed by pair-production and not by the photoelectric effect which operates at low kilovoltage. Electron treatment thus avoids the high absorbed doses seen in cartilage and bone with kilovoltage X-ray therapy. This can be of advantage especially in treating skin lesions on the pinna, scalp, dorsum of the hand, and anterior tibial region.

The finite range of electron beams and the presence of a build-up zone means that careful planning must be done. Field size is defined in a similar manner to kilovoltage X-ray therapy. Lead cut-outs of appropriate thickness (e.g. 3 mm for 10 MeV) are commonly required to adapt standard electron applicators, while lead shielding (e.g. behind the ear; see Fig. 6.9) can be used very successfully. The problem of finite range and the use of lead cut-outs should encourage the preparation of individual treatment shells for fractionated electron treatments (see Chap. 4).

The energy of the electron beam used to treat an individual lesion must be sufficient to include the tumour and treating margin (in depth) within the plateau region of the beam. The "treatment depth" or "effective range" available for an individual beam includes any build-up zone and plateau region and is, in centimetres, approximately one-quarter of the accelerating voltage when this is expressed in megavolts. For example, the range provided by 10-MeV electrons is 10/4 cm, i.e. 2.5 cm.

It is important to note that this is independent of the field size provided the mean diameter used is greater than twice the *range* as previously defined. For smaller field sizes the dose distribution is less satisfactory and individual isodose information must be available. For example, when using a 10-MeV beam the "range" is 2.5 cm. Individual isodose information will be necessary when field sizes smaller than twice the range (i.e. in this case 5 cm) are being used. These technical complexities result in electron treatments being used at the Christie Hospital only for moderate-sized, fractionated beam therapy of difficult skin cancers.

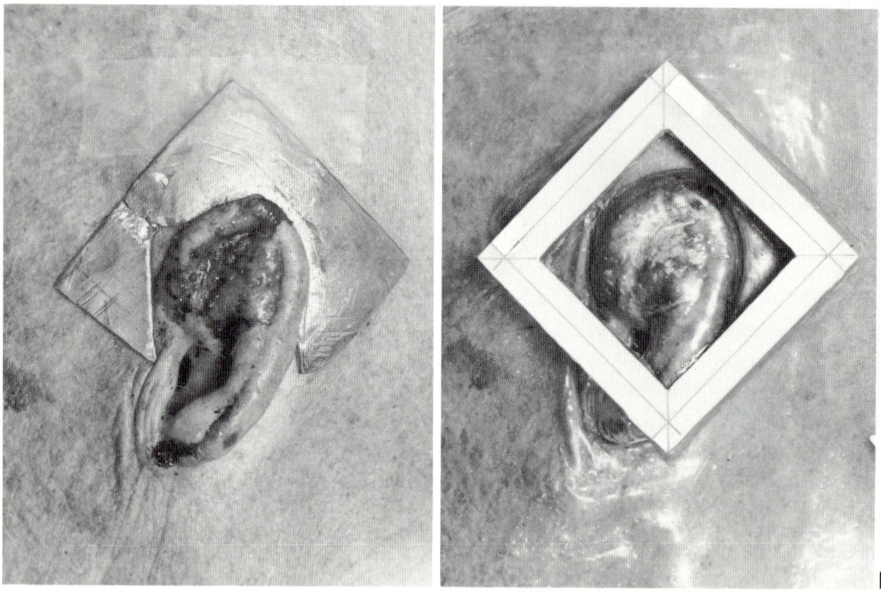

Fig. 6.9a,b. Treatment shell for use with high-energy electrons during fractionated treatments. **a** Squamous cell carcinoma in skin of left upper pinna; 3-mm lead is positioned behind the ear to protect the scalp. **b** Treatment shell in position. This example has bolus incorporated in the shell and an applicator mounting to enable easy accurate daily set-ups.

Dosage

Megavoltage electron beams have an RBE in soft tissue equal to megavoltage photons, and significantly less than that seen with kilovoltage photons. Clinical experience has, however, demonstrated that an RBE correction should not be applied and that doses for megavoltage electrons should be prescribed within the tolerance dose limits shown in Table 6.1. Attempts to increase these doses will result in unacceptable normal tissue reactions. This anomalous situation probably arises from the different pattern of distribution of energy in tissue seen with electron beams when compared with kilovoltage photons.

Moulds

Kilovoltage techniques and electron beam therapy allow the radiotherapist to deal quickly and efficiently with the majority of skin cancer problems. Unfortunately a small number of patients have lesions on their skin which, because of surface irregularity, proximity to bone or cartilage, or poor intrinsic tolerance, cannot be satisfactorily treated by beam therapy. Radiotherapeutic techniques to treat these special lesions were developed many decades ago and have been in continuous use at the Christie Hospital since then. This large experience of control rates and tolerance forms the basis of the following sections.

All the techniques involve mounting sealed radionuclides on surface applicators, colloquially known as "moulds" (see Chap. 4). They can be applied to a wide variety of lesions, but their use results in a small though significant radiation protection problem. This, coupled with the availability in some situations of an equally successful alternative, restricts their use to very special problem lesions. Four different types of mould will be described to illustrate their advantages.

The basic principles of all the different mould treatments are the same. Sealed radionuclides are mounted on an individually constructed carrier surface and placed over the skin cancer. The quantity of the radionuclide is dictated by the treatment area, the treating distance (h), the time the mould is to be worn, and the required dose. The treatment area is decided and defined using identical principles to those described for kilovoltage X-ray techniques. Treating distances may vary from 0.5 to 2.0 cm (at 0.5-cm intervals) and this will dictate the depth-dose pattern given by the mould. For epidermal and superficial dermal lesions 0.5–1.0 cm is sufficient. Thick dermal lesions with or without subcutaneous invasion need moulds at 1.5-2.0 cm. Treating distances beyond 2.0 cm require such large quantities of radionuclide that they present an unacceptable radiation hazard and are therefore not used nowadays.

If splintage of the lesion and its surrounding skin is not a problem the moulds are worn continuously for 7 days (168 h). More commonly, for the patient's comfort and convenience they are worn intermittently for 6–12 h per day for 8 days. This results in a wide variety of surface dose rates but no radiobiological allowance has been found necessary in clinical practice.

Dosage is expressed, as with kilovoltage X-ray therapy, as a surface dose. In practice the tolerance dose for the planar moulds, to be described, is 5250 cGy using the time periods described above.

The distribution of the sources on the surface of the mould is according to the Manchester Radium Dosage System (see Chap. 1) and this results in homogeneous dose rates to the treatment surface, even in the presence of surface convexity or concavity.

The sealed radionuclides used at the Christie Hospital for mould treatments are gold-198 and cobalt-60. The former sources produce gamma radiation of a quality that does not present a protection problem, but the half-life is very short. Gold-198 is used on moulds of small area and at short treating distances. Patients wearing continous gold-198 moulds mounted with less than 30 mCi (1110 MBq) can be treated as out-patients. The moulds can also be transported and applied at peripheral clinics or at patients' homes—a considerable advantage to infirm elderly patients. Larger treatment areas and greater treating distances require greater quantities of a more suitable long-term radionuclide, and cobalt-60 sources are preferred. Mould room skills are required in the construction of comfortable individual planar cobalt-60 moulds (see Chap. 4).

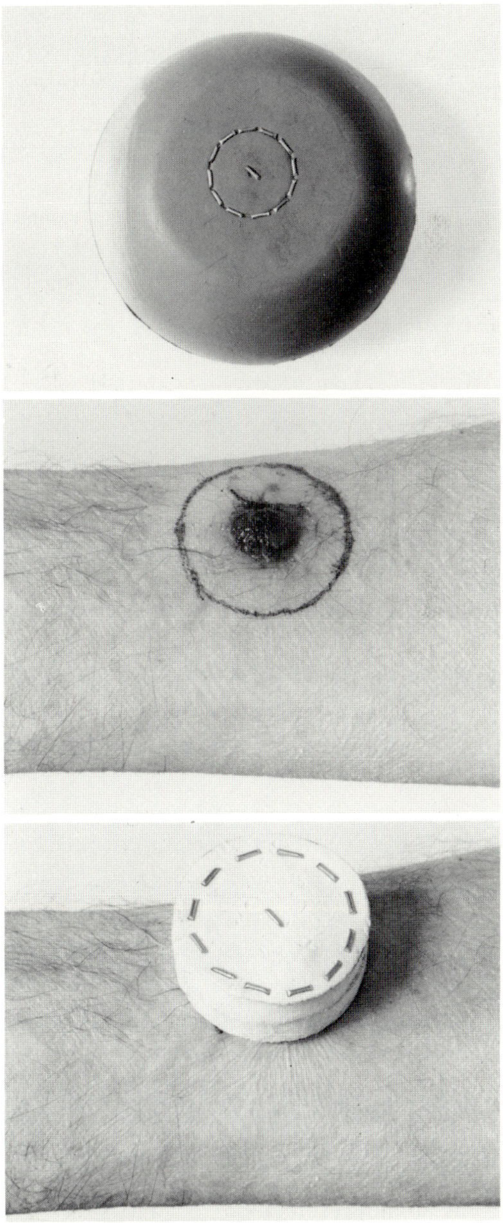
a
b
c

Fig. 6.10. Elastoplast gold seed mould.
Calculation
Intended dose 5250 cGy at 1 cm in 7 days
Treated zone a circle of diameter 2.5 cm
Area=4.9 cm^2
Treating distance=1.0 cm
From mould tables
1000 cGy=328 mg h
∴ 5250 cGy=1722 mg h
Initial MBq gold 198 required=1722×1.66
=2870 MBq
Final distribution: 95% on perimeter, 5% at centre
Use 12 sources 225 MBq on perimeter=2700
1 source 150 MBq on centre = 150
Total MBq 2850
Final time=169 h for dose 5250 cGy at 1.0 cm
Note: 1 mg h (radium) is equivalent to 1.66 MBq of ^{198}Au for 7 days.

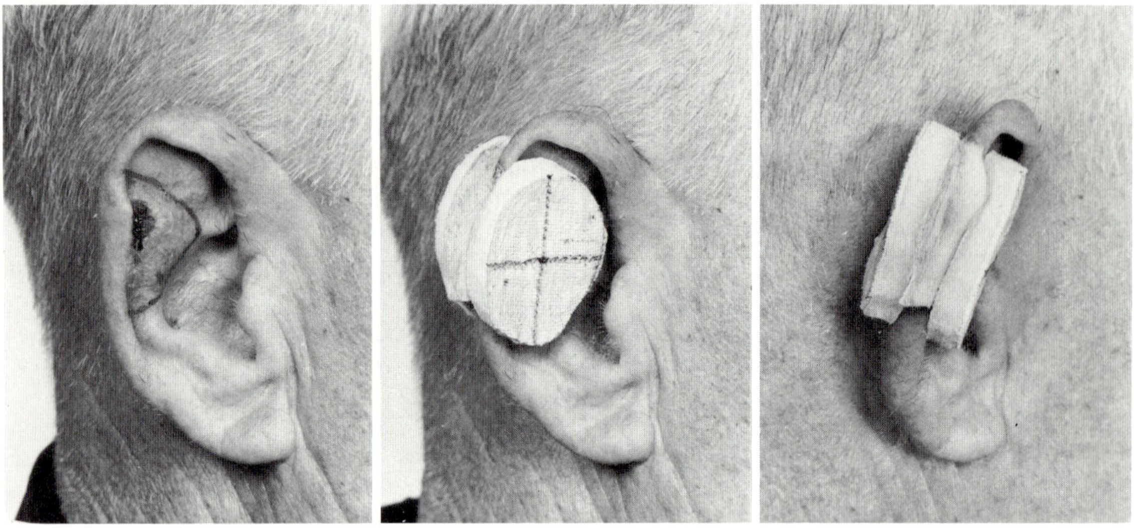

Fig. 6.11. Double Elastoplast gold seed mould.

Calculation

Ear thickness 1 cm
Diameter 2.5 cm

Treating distance 0.5 cm
Skin dose 5500 cGy

Treatment time 7 days
Midplane dose 4350 cGy

	Skin surface (1)	Midplane	Skin surface (2)
Area cm^2	4.9	4.9	4.9
Distance cm	0.5	1.0	1.5
mg h/1000 cGy	172	328	536
Percentage depth dose	100	52	32

$$5+0.325=5500$$
$$5=4170\text{ cGy}$$

Considering each mould separately an applied dose of 4170 cGy must be given from each mould to the adjacent skin surface.
Total mg h per mould=172×4.17=717
1 mg h (radium) is equivalent to 1.66 MBq of ^{198}Au for 7 days.
Initial activity required per mould=1195 MBq
Distribution of activity for each mould

		Required MBq	Number of sources	MBq per source	Total MBq
Centre	5%	60	1	70	70
Circumference	95%	1135	9	125	1125

Total activity used=1195 MBq per mould

Elastoplast Gold Seed Mould

This small mould is ideal for small superficial invasive skin cancers on the forearms, the back of the hand, and around the ears. A lesion on such an area of skin can be easily immobilised without disturbing any joint function.

In practice, for treatment areas up to 4 cm in diameter, regular circles or ellipses are employed. Treating distances of 0.5 and 1.0 cm are used. The mould construction material is double adhesive felt and this is cut a little larger than the previously defined treatment area. Radioactive gold seeds of the required number and strength are distributed,

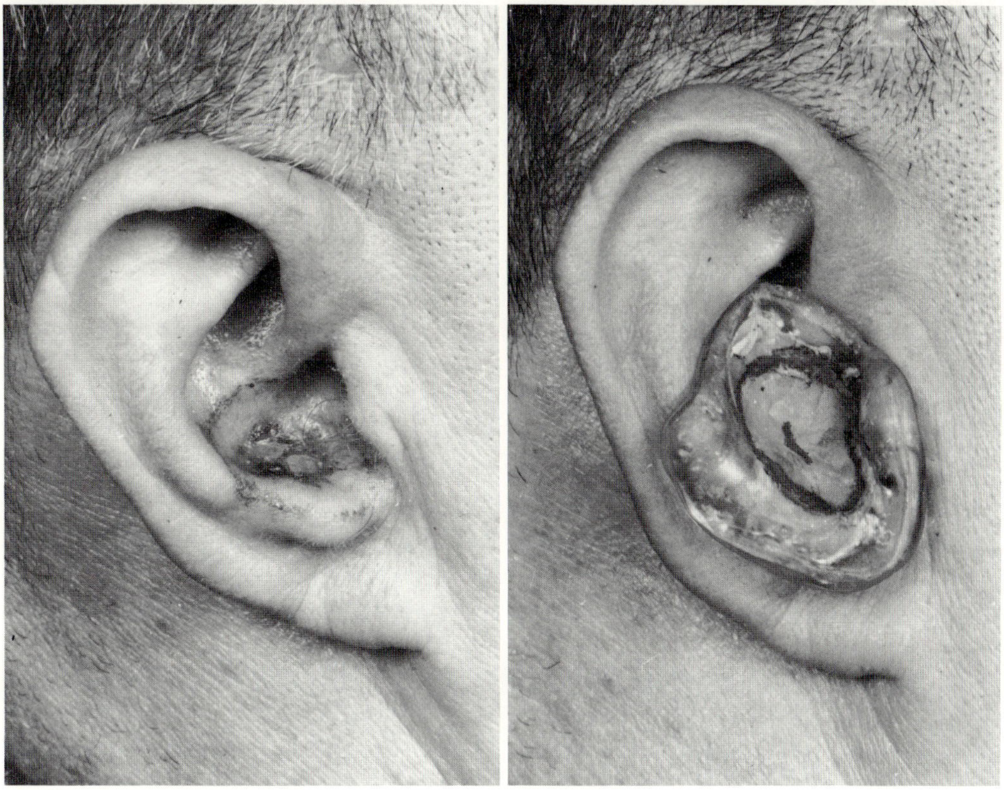

Fig. 6.12. Cellulose acetate gold seed mould.
Calculation
Intended dose 5250 cGy at 0.5 cm in 7 days
Treated zone a circle of diameter 2.5 cm
Area=4.9 cm^2
Mould distance=0.5 cm
From mould tables
1000 cGy=170 mg h
5250 cGy=892.5 mg h
Initial MBq gold-198 required=892.5×1.66=1481 MBq
Final distribution: 95% activity on the perimeter, 5% at centre
Use: 7 sources 700 MBq on perimeter=1400
1 source 100 MBq on centre = 100
1500
Giving final time=166 h to deliver 5250 cGy

according to the above-mentioned rules, on a small flat-topped stone/plaster "table" (Fig. 6.10a). One adhesive surface is applied to the table, transferring the seeds, which are then sealed in position with a second layer of Elastoplast. The mould can then be applied to the treatment area and strapped securely in place (Fig. 6.10b,c). The patient is issued with written instructions giving the date and time of removal. After removal the patient stores the mould and returns it at the follow-up clinic. The decaying gold seeds can be recovered and sent for reactivation.

A particularly useful modification of this mould can be used for small skin cancers on the margin of the pinna. A two-plane "sandwich" mould can be made by placing the lesion between two Elastoplast moulds. This gives an excellent cosmetic result on a difficult site (Fig. 6.11).

Cellulose Acetate Gold Seed Mould

A very special small gold-198 mould can be constructed for superficial skin cancers arising in the concavity of the pinna. The lesion must not extend to the external acoustic meatus and the whole lesion must be comfortably within the concavity of the pinna. Mould construction (see Chap. 4) utilises a firm carrier material and a treating distance of 0.5 cm is employed. The mould can be individually made and fitted in 2 h. This is normally an out-patient procedure and instructions are given to the patient as for an Elastoplast mould (Fig. 6.12).

Continuous Cobalt-60 Mould

This mould is used almost exclusively for larger skin cancers arising on easily immobilised convex surfaces. On the limbs it is particularly useful for moderate-sized squamous cell carcinoma in the anterior tibial region, where skin texture and tolerance to beam therapy are poor. It is a continuous mould, constructed in the mould room, and mounted with cobalt-60 sources. After careful positioning and strapping, the limb should be kept horizontal as much as possible. Results are excellent provided the lesion is not more than 6 cm in diameter. This treatment can spare elderly patients protracted hospitalisation for excision and skin grafting (Fig. 6.13).

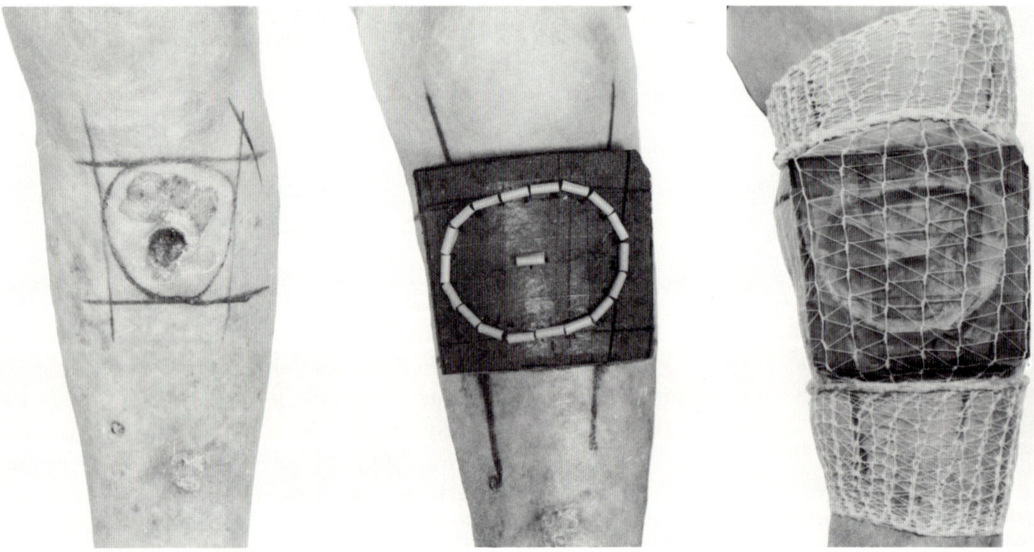

Fig. 6.13. Continuous cobalt mould.
Calculation
Intended dose 5250 cGy in 8 days (192 h)
Treated zone a circle diameter 6.6 cm
Area=32.5 cm^2
Treating distance=1.5 cm
From mould table
1000 cGy=1295 mg h
5250 cGy=6799 mg h
Approximate treating time=192 h
∴ Approximate mg required=35.41 mg
Length of periphery=20 cm
Final distribution: 95% of activity on the periphery, 5% at centre
Linear density of periphery=1.68 mg/cm
Use: 18 sources cobalt-60 1.87 mg Ra Eq on periphery=33.66
1 source cobalt-60 1.87 mg Ra Eq at centre = 1.87
35.53
Giving final time=191 h 30 min for 5250 cGy

Intermittent Cobalt-60 Mould

The most sophisticated moulds are those worn intermittently, constructed of cellulose acetate butyrate, and mounted with cobalt-60 sources. These are used for moderate-sized, bulky lesions overlying or adjacent to joints, often where convexity and/or concavity is also present. They are most commonly used on the scalp, around the wrist joint, the metacarpophalangeal joints, and on the fingers; also when superficial infection or bleeding make an adhesive continuous cobalt-60 mould inappropriate on the anterior or posterior tibial region (Fig. 6.14).

Construction (Chap. 4) aims to produce a comfortable mould which is easily fitted and removed by the patient, supervised by a trained nurse. Clinical instructions are given that the mould should be worn for a specified number of hours and minutes each day for the required 8 days. While not in use the mould is stored in a suitable safe near the ward, and a record is kept by the nursing staff who must supervise each event.

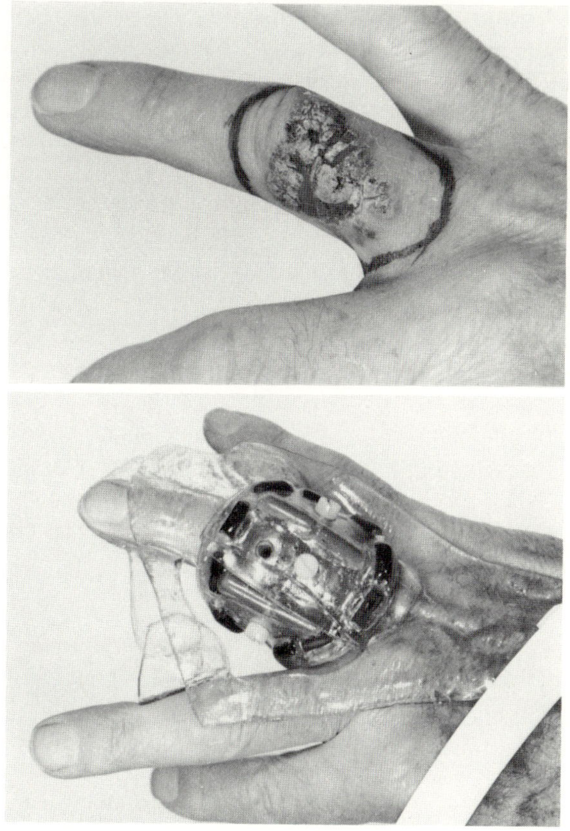

Fig. 6.14. Intermittent cobalt mould.
Calculation
Intended dose=5250 cGy in 8 days treating 10 h/day=80 h
Treated zone an ellipse treated as a rectangle, 4.5×5 cm
Area=16.5 cm^2
Treating distance=1.0 cm
From mould tables
1000 cGy =621.5 mg h
+ Elongation correction (0.5%)=624.5 mg h
5250 cGy=3278 mg h
Approximate treatment time=80 h
Approximate mg required=40.98 mg
Length of periphery=15 cm
Final distribution: periphery of uniform linear density and two bars each of 2/3 linear density of periphery.
Use 11 sources on periphery each 2.89 mg Ra Eq=31.79
2 sources on each bar each 2.89 mg Ra Eq =11.56
43.35 mg
Giving final time of 9.5 h/day for 7 days and 9 h/day for 1 day for 5250 cGy

7 Head and Neck

M. B. Duthie, N. K. Gupta and R. C. S. Pointon

Carcinoma of the Lip

Clinical Features

Cancer of the lip arises from the vermilion border of the lip. Lesions arising from the skin of the lip are not included in this classification. Cancer of the lip occurs most frequently in those geographic areas subject to long hours of sunlight and in workers who have a long outdoor exposure. It occurs most frequently between 50 and 80 years with a mean age of 64 years and occurs predominantly in males, the ratio of male to female being approximately 12:1.

Site

The lips are classified into three anatomical sites:

1) Upper lip
2) Lower lip
3) Commissure

The lower lip is involved in 90%–98% of cases; approximately 1% occur at the commissure and the remainder on the upper lip. The great majority of cancers of the lip are well or moderately differentiated squamous cell carcinoma.

The lesion usually presents in an early stage as an indurated nodule, superficial erosion, or fissure. As the lesion progresses it develops the typical everted raised edges and indurated base. Less commonly, it may present as a papillary form which projects from the surface of the lip. As the lesion progresses it extends into the substance of the lip and as it advances may invade the cheeks, alveolobuccal sulcus, and other neighbouring structures. The principal form of metastasis is to the regional lymph nodes. Other tumours of the lip are rare. Tumours may arise from the mucous glands of the lip and are either mixed adenomas or adenoid-cystic carcinoma: they usually occur on the upper lip.

Lymphatic Drainage of the Lip

The lymphatic drainage of the lips is to the submandibular and submental nodes but occasionally may be directly into the deep cervical node chain. The lymphatics of the upper lip also drain into the submandibular and submental nodes but occasionally may drain into the preauricular or parotid lymph nodes. The submandibular node is by far the commonest node involved. Approximately 7% of cases present with significant nodes and about 10% subsequently develop secondary node involvement.

Diagnosis

As an orificial lesion, lip cancer is usually easily diagnosed and its extent is readily defined. Any persistent ulcer on the lip should be regarded with suspicion and a biopsy is mandatory. Equally, before any treatment is commenced a biopsy should be taken.

Treatment Policy

Cancer of the lips can be cured by any well-conducted method of radiotherapy or surgery and failure to control the primary should be very rare. A high cure rate with an excellent functional and cosmetic result can be achieved by radiotherapy and it is therefore the treatment of choice in the majority of cases.

The selection of the method to be used will be influenced by the site, size, and thickness of the lesion; by the age and general condition of the patient; by the facilities available and the preference of the treating centre.

Methods

1) X-ray therapy
   a) Superficial X-ray therapy (100–140 kV)
   b) Orthovoltage X-ray therapy (300 kV)
2) Electron therapy (8–10 MV)
3) Surface applicator (double mould)
4) Interstitial irradiation, i.e. radium needle implant or equivalent. Permanent gold (^{198}Au) seed or grain implant

X-ray Therapy

Superficial X-ray Therapy (100–140 kV)

As the average lip thickness is 1 cm, X-rays of energy 100–140 kV and HVT 2–3 mm Al provide an adequate depth dose. The mouth is shielded by the use of a black tray compound bite-block to which is attached a moulded lead sheet of 1 mm thickness. The block should fit comfortably behind the lip in the alveolobuccal sulcus, holding the upper lip away and protecting the mouth and tongue. The mouth block may be combined with an external lead shield or "cut out" to reduce the volume of normal tissue irradiated to the required minimum. This form of treatment is suitable only for T_1 and T_2 lesions.

The dose is 4500 cGy in eight treatments over 10 days.

In aged subjects with small lesions a single exposure of 1850–2000 cGy is a simple and effective treatment.

Orthovoltage X-ray Therapy (300 kV)

For substantial and thick lesions, orthovoltage X-ray therapy (300 kV, HVT 2.4 mm Cu) may be used. A single field is used, subtending the lesion together with an adequate margin of normal tissue, not less than 1–1.5 cm clear of known disease. Shielding of the mouth and teeth is carried out as described for superficial X-ray therapy, but the lead employed should be 2.5 mm thick.

The dose is 4500 cGy in eight treatments over 10 days or 5000–5500 cGy in 15 treatments over 21 days.

Double Cobalt-60 Mould

For the majority of carcinomas of the lower lip, a surface applicator using radioactive cobalt-60 is a very satisfactory method of treatment. The method used is that of the double mould. This is a precise and accurately calculated treatment resulting in a high cure rate and excellent cosmetic result. There is an absence of high-dose areas and a reasonably homogeneous dose is delivered to the treated volume. A double mould may be used particularly when there is extension from the commissure to the buccal mucosa, but its use is restricted when there is extension of tumour downwards into the alveolobuccal sulcus. To make a good double mould a high degree of technical skill is necessary. The mould must be easily removable and replaceable with certainty. It must be comfortable to wear yet must be closely applied to the lip so that the amount of movement is negligible. The materials used for the mould must be easy to manipulate, impervious to body fluids, and stable at body temperature and must retain their shape throughout the treatment.

Construction

The applicator consists of two parts (Fig. 7.1), an inner and an outer plane, bearing radioactive cobalt-60 sources which are parallel to each other. The area to be treated must include the lesion with a margin of 1–1.5 cm of normal lip.

Each applicator must be made for the individual patient.

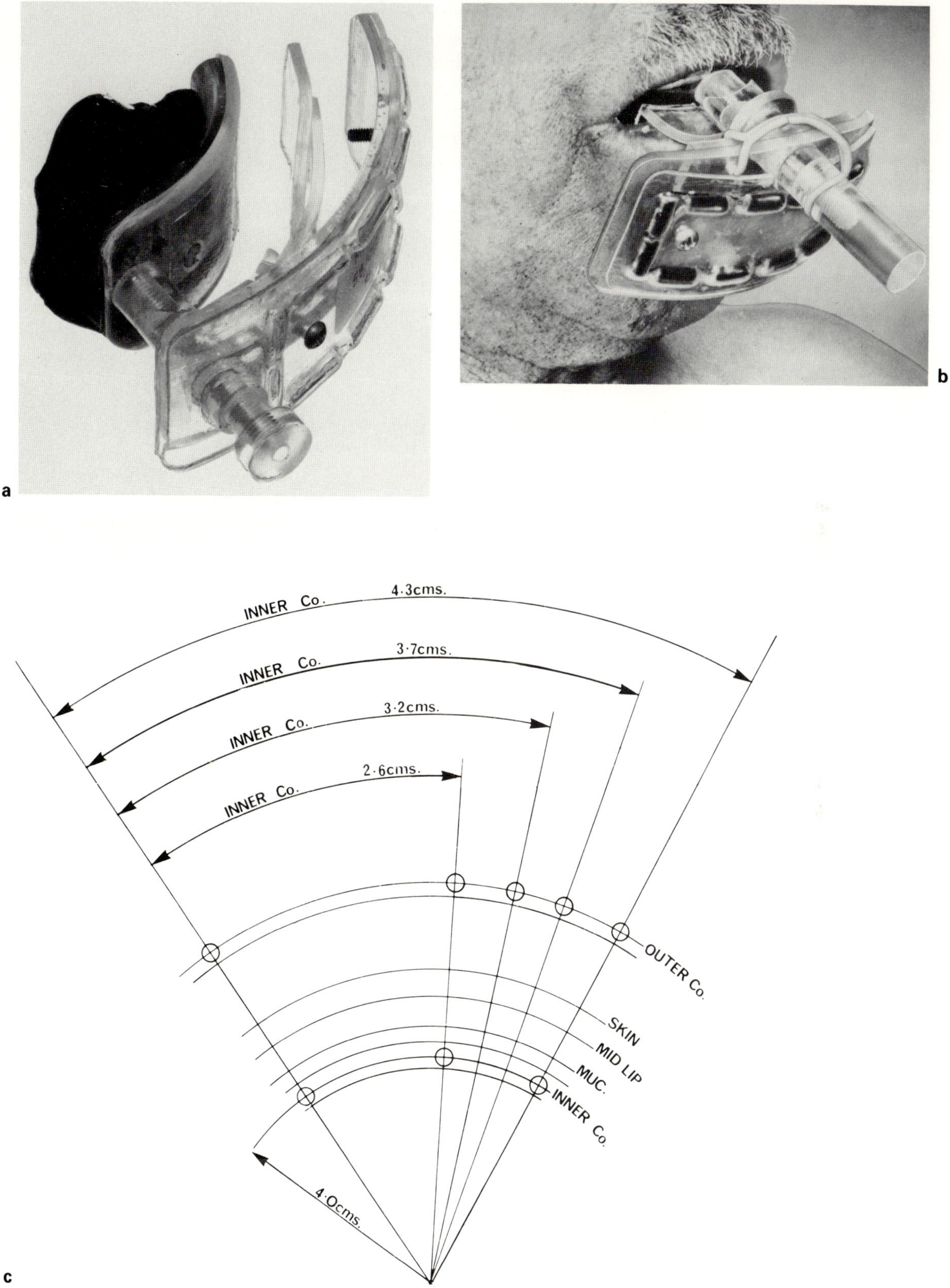

Fig. 7.1a–c. Double mould for carcinoma of lower lip. **a** Construction of mould. **b** Mould as worn. **c** Diagram of dimensions.

Inner Mould

A rectangular plaque of Perspex 0.5 cm thick is curved to form a sector of a cylinder of radius 4.5 cm, of sufficient size to subtend the proposed mucosal area. This plaque is fitted behind the lesion and the area to be treated is accurately marked on its convex surface. The plaque extends 0.5 cm below the treated area and 1.5 cm above it. To the top of the plaque is fixed a Perspex sleeve through which passes the holding screw joining the two planes. This sleeve engages in a similar sleeve fixed to the outer mould and maintains the distance between the two planes. This junction is designed to prevent any rotation of either plane independently of the other.

A second Perspex plaque is made, curved to form a sector of a cylinder of diameter 4 cm. The outer surface of this plaque is "troughed" and the resulting trough will carry the radioactive sources. These two plaques are then joined by means of small screws. To the lingual aspect of the combined plaque is connected a flange of Perspex. Since a bite-block is required to hold the double mould in position, soft black tray compound is inserted into the mouth and a comfortable bite-impression is made. The bite-block is removed, allowed to harden, and then attached to the lingual aspect of the Perspex plaque. The area which will bear the cobalt-60 can now be marked out in the troughed plaque.

Outer Mould

For a lip thickness of 1 cm, the treating distance is 1.5 cm; for a lip thickness of 1.5 cm, the treating distance is 2 cm. The outer plane is made of a rectangular plaque of Perspex, 0.3 cm in thickness, which is curved to be parallel to the inner plane. To the upper part is connected a Perspex sleeve through which the holding screw passes. The radioactive sources on the outer mould are maintained in position by means of a thin Perspex cover fashioned such that it closely fits the individual sources. The two parts of the mould are then joined and held together by means of the Perspex nut which engages on the holding screw. The mould is then checked to ensure that both planes are parallel and the interplane separation is as prescribed. When the treatment prescription has been completed (see example in Table 7.1) and the number and strengths of the radioactive cobalt sources to be used are known, the inner and outer plaques can be prepared to receive the sources.

Treatment

The mould is worn for approximately 6 h a day for 8 days, so that the average total treatment time is 48 h.

For a lip thickness of 1 cm the dose is 6500 cGy on the mucosa of the lip and 5500 cGy on the skin. For a lip thickness of 1.5 cm the respective doses are 7000 cGy on the mucosa and 5500 cGy on the skin. The mid-lip dose will be 5000 cGy or higher.

Electron Therapy

Low energy (8–10 MV) electrons afford a serious alternative method of irradiation (Fig. 7.2). The energy of the electron beam is such as to give an adequate depth dose while permitting simple shielding of the rest of the mouth. The use of a beam scatterer obviates the need for any build-up, except where there is excessive curvature.

The mouth is protected by the use of a black tray compound bite-block which is mounted on a lead shield as described for X-ray therapy.

The dose with 10-MV electrons is 4250–4500 cGy in eight treatments over 10 days.

Interstitial Treatment

Interstitial irradiation by means of a radium needle or iridium-192 implant is perfectly satisfactory treatment for carcinoma of the lip and is the preferred treatment for lesions arising on the upper lip. A single-plane implant is used and is planned to deliver a dose of 6000 cGy in 7 days at 0.5 cm. To avoid splinting of the lip, an interleaving implant is preferred (Fig. 7.3). Great care should be taken in implanting the superior needles so that they lie just 0.5 cm below the surface of the lip. The obvious disadvantage of a radium needle implant is the need for a general anaesthetic and hospitalisation during the course of the treatment.

Table 7.1. Cobalt-60 double mould treatment record.

Name: Hospital No:

Treatment by:	Date: Biopsy:
Intended dose: Mucosa =6500 cGy in 8 days Skin =5500 cGy in 8 days Hours per day=6 approx. Inner "h" =0.5 cm Outer "h" =1.5 cm Lip Thickness=1.0 cm	*Elong.* *Corr.* 1.13 0.5% 1.27 1.5% 1.41 2.0% 1.56 3.0% 1.98 5.0% *Area (cm^2)* Inner Co. 2.3×2.6 = 5.98 Mucosa 2.3×2.92 = 6.72 Mid Lip 2.3×3.25 = 7.48 Skin 2.3×3.57 = 8.22 Outer Co. 2.3×4.55 =10.47

M+0.56S=6500 cGy — —
0.33M+S=5500 cGy — All shorts
0.33M+0.185S=2145 INNER DISTRIBUTION
s=4115 cGy
M=4190 cGy

S L S
S S
S L S
OUTER DISTRIBUTION

	COBALT-60 USED		
Type	Ks	Os	OL
Strength	1.55	5.3	7.95
Number	10	6	2
	Inner		Outer

Treatment started on........at.....

INNER	*MUCOSA*	*MID LIP*	*SKIN*	
Area (cm^2)	←	6.0	→	Co^{60} required= 192×4.19/48=16.76 mg
Distance (cm)	0.5	1.0	1.5	ρ=16.76/13.3=1.26 mg/cm
mg–h/1000 cGy	191	360	579	Long sides (3.28)=2×1.55
E.F.	(0.5%)1	(0.5%)2	(0.5%)3	Vert. sides (2.90)=2×1.55
Corr. mg–h/1000 cGy	192	362	582	Bars (2.19)=2×1.05
% DD	100	53.0	33.0	All Shorts. Total=16.6 mg

OUTER	*MUCOSA*	*MID LIP*	*SKIN*	
Eff. area (cm^2)	6.75	7.5	8.25	Co^{60} required= 675×4.12/48=57.94 mg
Distance (cm	2.5	2.0	1.5	ρ=57.94/11.76=4.93 mg/cm
mg–h/1000 cGy	1188	904	655	Long sides (17.59)
E.F.	(1.5%)18	(2%)18	(3%)20	=5.3×2 (short)+7.95×1 (long)
Corr. mg–h/1000 cGy	1206	922	675	=18.55
% DD	56.0	73.2	100	Short sides (11.34)=5.3×2 (short)=10.6 Total=58.3 mg

DOSE RATE cGy/h				
Inner	86.5	45.9	28.5	
Outer	48.3	63.2	86.4	
Total	134.8	109.1	114.9	
DOSES cGy	6500	5260	5540	

Doses on mucosa 6500 cGy
Final Treatment Time 48.2 h
Approved by:

Skin Dose 5540 cGy
(6 hours per day for 7 days)
(6.2 hours per day for 1 day)

Calculation checked by:
Mould checked by:
Sources supplied by:

Sources loaded by:
Source loading checked by:
Time slip issued by:

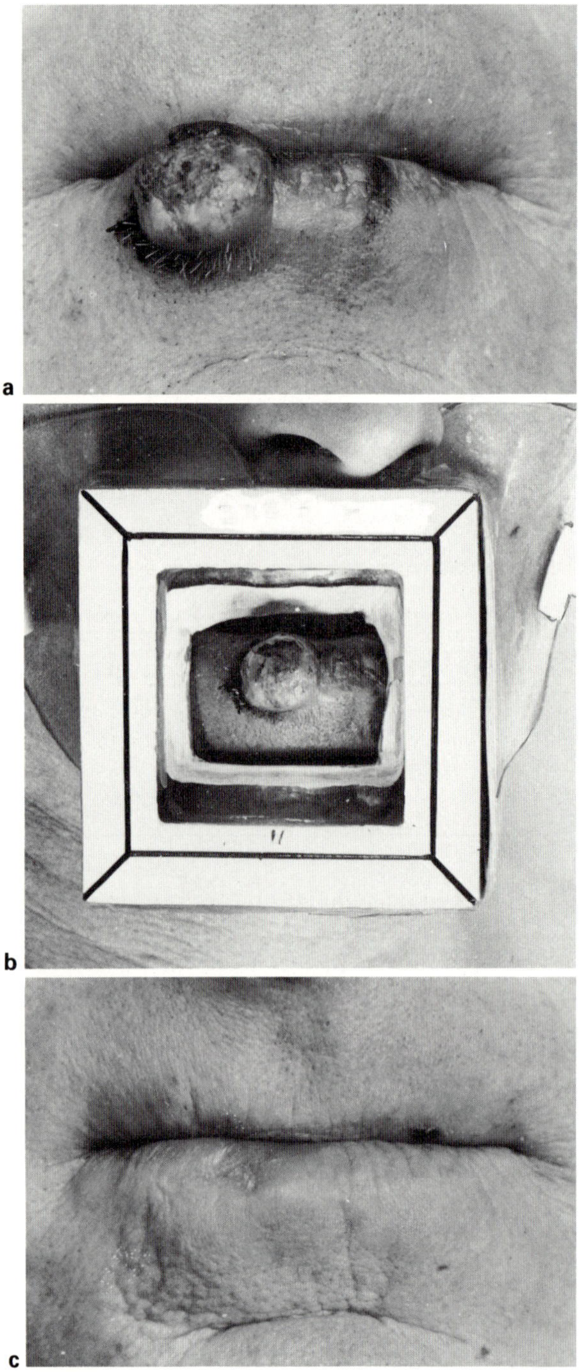

Fig. 7.2a–c. Carcinoma of lower lip—10-MeV electron therapy.

Gold Seed or Grain Implant

Small lesions may be treated by means of a permanent implant using gold (^{198}Au) seeds or grains. Implants of this type in the lip are technically difficult and their use should be reserved for uncooperative aged patients when a suitable X-ray treatment cannot be carried out. The dose aimed at is 6000 cGy at 0.5 cm.

Complications

Recurrence

Following well-planned radiotherapy, failure to control the primary disease in lip cancer should be exceptional. Treatment is by the appropriate surgical excision and repair.

Necrosis

Significant necrosis following radiotherapy for lip cancer is rare. If there is definitive loss of tissue, excision and appropriate plastic surgical repair are indicated.

Second primary

Second primary lip cancer occurs in about 1% of cases. It should be treated on its merits. Further radiotherapy is possible if there is an adequate margin between the new and the previously treated lesion, otherwise surgical intervention is the wisest course.

Results

The results of treatment of lip cancer are excellent and cure is to be expected in over 90% of cases.

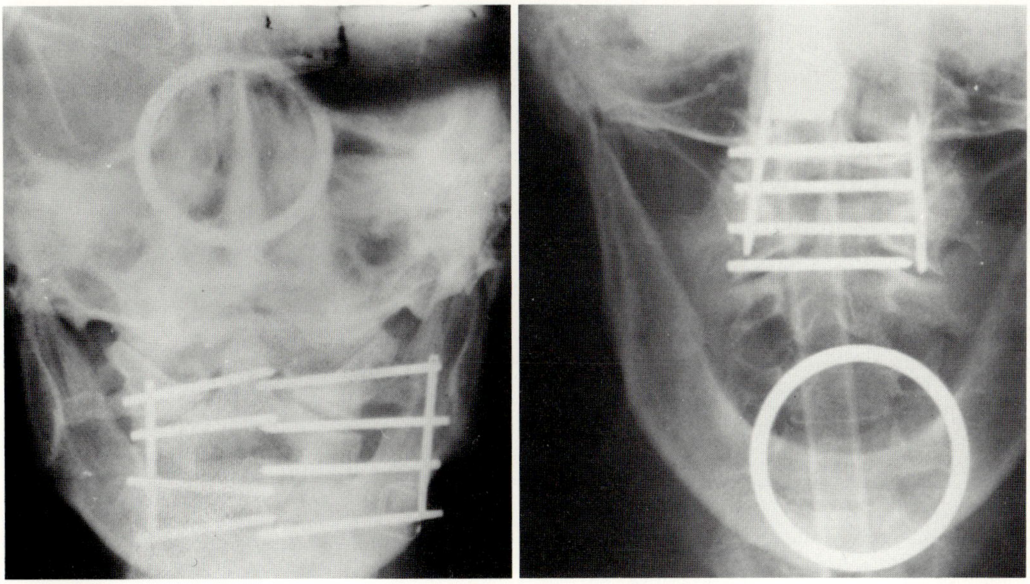

Fig. 7.3a, b. Carcinoma of lip—radium implant.
Calculation for **a**.
Lip. Single-plane implant
Implanted area=18.75 cm^2
Dose required=6000 cGy
Approximate treatment time=68 h
mg h/1000 cGy=380
mg radium required=13.57 mg
Needles used 2×2 mg active length 3.0 cm
2×1 mg active length 3.0 cm
4×1.5 mg active length 2.25 cm
2×0.75 mg active length 2.25 cm
mg radium used=13.1 mg (including filtration correction)
Final treatment time=174 hours

Carcinoma of the Oral Cavity

Clinical Features

Incidence

Oral cancer accounts for 2% of malignant tumours in the United Kingdom. This contrasts with an incidence of 13% in certain parts of India. The incidence of oral cancer in the United Kingdom has continuously declined. This has been due to a decrease of the disease in males, the female incidence remaining largely unchanged.

With the progressive decline of oral malignancy in men, the present male to female sex ratio is about 1.6:1.

In the Manchester region 50% of patients are aged between 65 and 80 years, the mean age for males being 68.5 years and for females 67.3 years.

Aetiology

The commonly recognised aetiological factors are: poor dental hygiene, tobacco, alcohol, syphilis, iron-deficiency anaemia, chronic hyperplastic candidiasis, and betel nut chewing.

With the exception of the last-mentioned, their relevance to the individual patient is frequently obscure. An enhanced risk for oral cancer has been demonstrated in textile workers, particularly in those workers exposed to the dust created by the initial "carding" of raw cotton and wool.

Leucoplakia

Leucoplakia is defined as a raised white patch of oral mucosa measuring 5 mm or more, which cannot be scraped off and which cannot be attributed to any other diagnosable condition.

Three main clinical types are described, namely homogeneous, ulcerated, and speckled. Homogeneous leucoplakia is characterised by raised, white plaques with irregular edges. It may be limited in extent or involve wide areas in a confluent manner. Ulcerated leucoplakia usually results from trauma due to chewing or equivalent injury. Speckled leucoplakia has the characteristic appearance of white patches on an erythematous base. Often superimposed on florid leucoplakia is a candida infection. Other oral precancerous conditions, seen mainly in Asia, include oral submucous fibrosis, leucokeratosis, nicotine palate, and erythroplakia. Of all cases of leucoplakia, probably not more than 3% undergo malignant change. Where a malignant lesion arises from a patch of leucoplakia, then the whole of the leucoplakic area should be included in the treatment volume. On the other hand, where there is widespread leucoplakia involving much of the oral mucosa, then the treatment volume should be confined to the known malignancy and the patient kept under close surveillance.

Histology

The majority of carcinomas of the oral cavity are squamous cell carcinoma, comprising some 96% of all oral malignancy. These tumours are normally well-differentiated squamous carcinoma—undifferentiated lesions are rare. Histological grading has not been found to be of significant value. One variant of squamous cell carcinoma occasionally seen is the so-called verrucous carcinoma, which is characterised by its papilliferous appearance; the response to irradiation of this variant is no different from that of the more commonly seen lesions (Fig. 7.4).

The rare forms of malignancy occurring in the oral cavity are mainly tumours of the minor salivary glands, and soft tissue sarcomas.

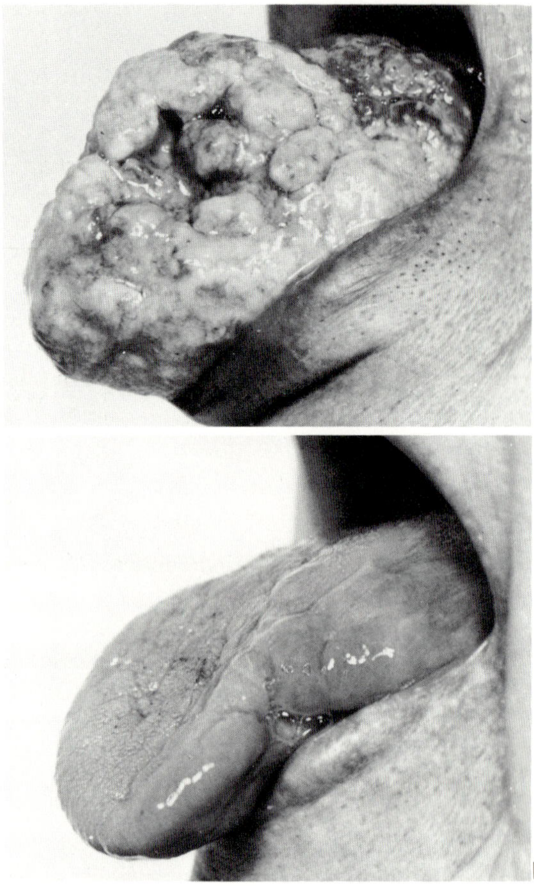

a

b

Fig. 7.4. **a** Verrucous carcinoma of tongue. **b** Post single-plane radium needle implant.

Clinical Presentation

Squamous cell carcinoma of the oral cavity presents as an indurated fissure, ulcer, or nodule. Less commonly there may be a papilliferous element, illustrated in its grossest form by the verrucous carcinoma. There may be an admixture of these variants. Leucoplakia may be present and, rarely, frank evidence of syphilitic glossitis. The lesion extends locally to involve other sites in the oral cavity. In advanced cases there will be fixity of the tongue, involvement of bone and skin. Clinical features of advanced disease are otalgia, slurred speech, excessive salivation. Lesions arising in the retromolar region may extend to the pterygoid fossa, resulting in trismus, which implies a very poor prognosis. Metastasis is to the regional lymph nodes. Distant metastases are rare.

The differential diagnoses include simple traumatic ulcers and epulis from ill-fitting dentures, while oral syphilis and tuberculosis are rare but should not be discounted. It is essential to obtain histological proof and a biopsy should always be taken of any persistent lesion in the oral cavity, even if there be positive serology for syphilis.

Lymphatic Drainage

The lymphatic drainage of the oral cavity is similar to that described for the lips. The predominantly involved nodes are the submandibular and upper deep cervical nodes. Involvement of the submental, mid-cervical, and lower deep cervical nodes is uncommon except in advanced disease. The lymphatics of the oral cavity anastomose freely in the midline, so there may be contralateral node involvement, particularly if the primary lesion is situated in or near to the midline. The most common primary site from which metastases spread to contralateral nodes is the tongue.

The percentage lymph node incidence on presentation is shown below:

N_0 74%
N_1 14%
N_2 2%
N_3 10%

Thus three-quarters of patients with oral cancer present with clinically uninvolved nodes. Of these, one third will subsequently develop node involvement.

The principal factors influencing node involvement are (1) the stage of the primary lesion and (2) the site of the primary lesion within the oral cavity. Thus, related to size of primary, the percentage node incidence on presentation is:

Primary size	*No nodes on presentation*
2 cm	95%
2–4 cm	84%
4 cm	51%

The size of the primary principally determines the degree of local control obtained, and thus also affects the subsequent development of node metastases.

Of the primary sites in the oral cavity, carcinomas of the tongue and the floor of the mouth yield the highest incidence of metastatic lymphadenopathy and carcinoma of the buccal mucosa the least.

The secondary involvement of cervical lymph nodes occurs almost entirely within 2 years of the primary treatment. Secondary involvement arising after 2 years is rare and is complicated by the occurrence of other primary malignancies in the head and neck.

Examination of block dissection specimens indicates that the clinical detection of metastatic lymphadenopathy is correct in 86% of cases.

Distant Metastases

Blood-borne metastases from oral cancer are rare, the principally involved sites being the lung, liver, and bone. It is frequently difficult to be certain whether such metastases originate from a primary in the oral cavity or from a second primary outside the head and neck.

Anatomical Subdivision of the Oral Cavity

Table 7.2 shows the anatomical subdivisions of the oral cavity which are clinically important to the radiotherapist, while Table 7.3 shows the relative frequency with which carcinomas have presented in each of these sites at the Christie Hospital.

Table 7.2. Anatomical subdivisions of the oral cavity.

1) Buccal mucosa	i) inner surface of lips
	ii) lining of cheeks
	iii) retromolar triangle
	iv) buccoalveolar sulci, upper and lower
2) Lower alveolus and gingiva	
3) Upper alveolus and gingiva	
4) Hard palate	
5) Tongue	i) dorsum and lateral borders of anterior two-thirds (i.e. anterior to the valleata)
	ii) ventral surfacee
6) Floor of mouth	

Table 7.3. Carcinoma of oral cavity.

Site	% Incidence
Buccal mucosa	18
Upper alveolus and gingiva	6
Lower alveolus and gingiva	15
Hard Palate	4
Tongue	34
Floor of mouth	23
Total	100

Treatment Policy

The successful management of oral cancer is the product of a multidisciplinary approach involving surgeon, radiotherapist, and chemotherapist. Ideally, the patient should be seen initially by all three together and an agreed treatment policy decided.

Whatever mode of therapy is decided upon, the aim should be to eradicate the primary lesion. The principal curative methods of treatment remain surgery and radiotherapy. Similar results may be obtained with each method in early and moderately advanced lesions. Well-planned radiotherapy is the preferred method of treatment of oral cancer, affording as it does good results, the preservation of function, and minimal morbidity.

While treatment for each patient is individualised, it is essential to maintain a definitive policy to permit analysis of methods.

The basic premise of the radiotherapeutic treatment of cancer of the oral cavity is to irradiate the primary lesion with an adequate margin of normal tissue, while sparing the remainder of the mouth. Interstitial irradiation affords the best method of achieving this by ensuring that a high dose is accurately placed. Modern megavoltage techniques can also achieve this objective, with the advantage of a wider margin in sites where interstitial irradiation is rendered difficult by the extent of the lesion and the anatomy of the part. As a result, 30% of our cases are now treated by interstitial irradiation and the remainder by megavoltage X-ray therapy.

The role of surgery is primarily reserved for salvage in cases of residual or recurrent disease following irradiation. The indications for primary surgical treatment are few and relate to the site of the lesion, unusual histology, and the underlying aetiological process.

Interstitial Treatment

The inherent limitations of this form of therapy are:

1) Accessible tumours only can be treated, which usually means that the extent of the tumour can be more accurately determined.
2) Effective dosage is restricted to a plane of little depth, but because of this restriction the dose permitted is a high one.

A high dose, strictly confined and accurately placed, represents the ideal concept for irradiation of squamous cell carcinoma of the oral cavity.

Interstitial techniques fall into two main groups:

1) Removable implants, the classic example of which requires implanted radium needles. This will be described in detail below. Radium may be substituted by equivalent isotopes, e.g. cobalt-60, caesium-137, and iridium-192.
2) Permanent implants, in which isotopes with a short half-life are used and the sources allowed to decay to inactivity in the tissues implanted. The most common sources employed are gold (^{198}Au) seeds or grains with a half-life of 2.7 days. Although the treatment is given with a falling dose rate, no effects differing from those of a removable implant are detectable clinically.

Radium Needle Implants

The initial assessment of the lesion to be implanted entails:

1) A careful measurement of the tumour in all dimensions, to determine the physical extent of the lesion. In particular, care should be taken to ensure that an adequate margin of normal tissue (1–1.5 cm) is available all round the lesion, to permit implanting the peripheral needles. As the majority of intraoral implants will have an uncrossed lower end, it is essential to be sure of an adequate lower margin of clearance of the tumour.
2) The selection of the appropriate type of implant. This will, of necessity, be decided by the size of the tumour and the anatomical site in the oral cavity from which it arises.
3) A decision on the dose to be delivered.

Once these decisions have been made, it is necessary to have a clear idea of what is intended, and to endeavour to carry out the appropriate implant as closely as is practicable. To this end, the lesion must be measured accurately and a pre-implant calculation made. As a result, the precise geometry of the required implant can be decided.

Single-plane Implant

The single plane is by far the commonest form of implant used in the oral cavity. The most frequent application is for carcinoma of the tongue and buccal mucosa. The normal single-plane implant is designed to treat a slab of tissue not greater than 1 cm thick. This limitation must be recognised in planning the implant. It is therefore essential to adopt a methodical approach.

1) Careful preoperative examination to determine

whether the lesion is suitable for this form of treatment. Determination of the extent of the lesion with measurement of all its dimensions. Using the Paterson-Parker distribution rules, the implant should be planned and a diagram of the distribution of sources should be made. Following this, the necessary sources may be ordered.

2) Intraoral implants are best carried out under general anaesthesia with an endotracheal tube and the pharynx packed off. Opportunity should be taken at this stage to re-check the dimensions of the lesion.
3) Distribution and spacing of sources. The sources will be distributed following the Paterson-Parker rules. Allowance must be made for the difference between the position of the tongue in the anaesthetised state and the normal anatomical position, so that the angle of introduction of the needles is adjusted accordingly. Great care should be taken to ensure that the needles are superficial and follow the anatomy of the part. Normally the spacing between sources will be 0.8–1 cm. Each needle following insertion should be secured with a retaining suture of suitable absorbent material. Before completing the implant, an image intensifier may be used to check the distribution. At completion, the silks from the needles are secured together by a retaining suture and then led out of the mouth through a shaped rubber tube (to avoid chafing at the angle of the mouth).
4) The sources, whose strength is identified by the use of different coloured silks, are checked by the ward nurse.
5) Radiographs of the implant are taken using a pair of perpendicular views, a metal ring being included in the views as a magnification ring. From these films the physicist will calculate the *actual* area of the implant and the final time to deliver the prescribed dose will be determined (Fig. 7.5).

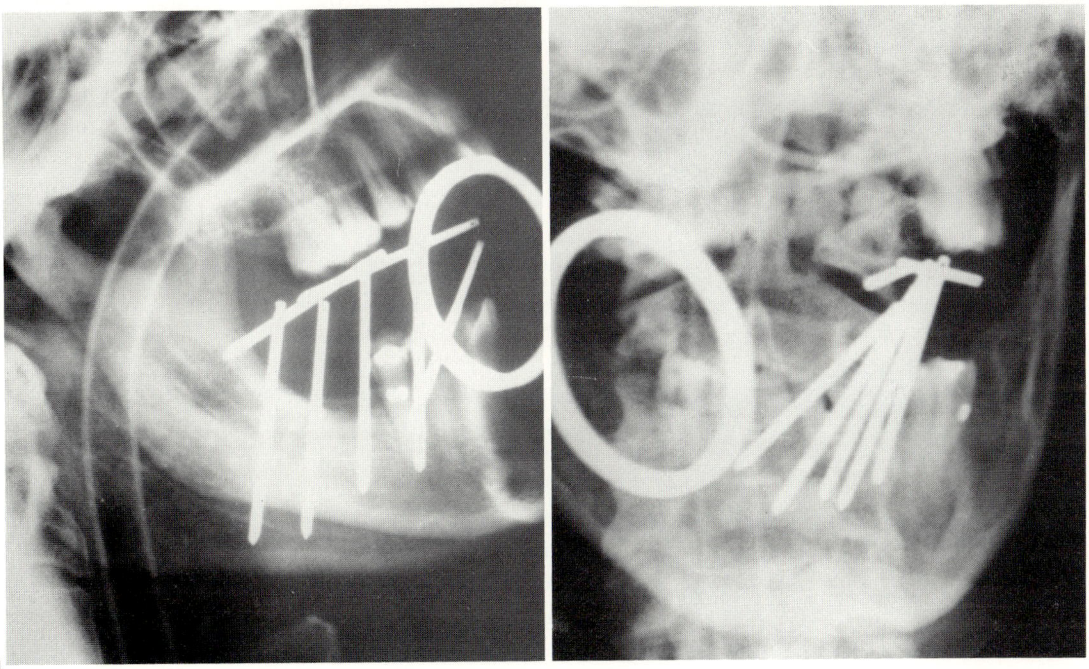
a b

Fig. 7.5a, b. Carcinoma of tongue. Single-plane radium needle implant.

Calculation.

Tongue. Single-plane implant
Implanted area=11.8 cm^2
Dose required=6500 cGy
Approximate treatment time=168 h
mg h/1000 cGy=279
mg radium required=10.79 mg
Needles used 2×2 mg active length 3.0 cm
3×1 mg active length 3.0 cm
2×1.5 mg active length 2.25 cm
mg radium used=9.8 mg (including filtration correction)
Final treatment time= 185 h

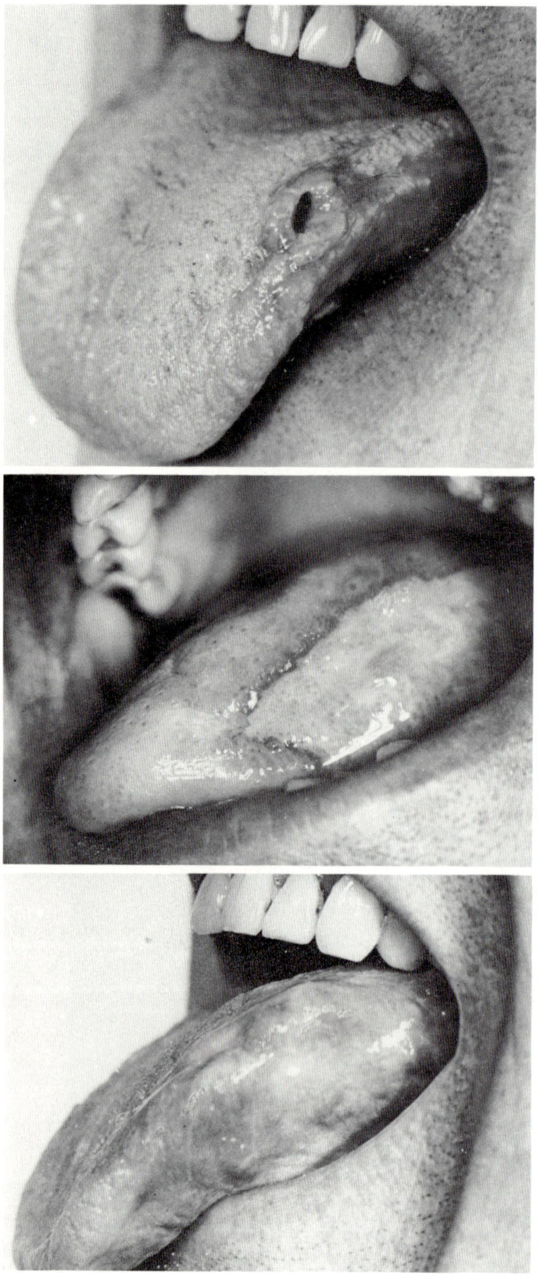

a

b

c

Fig. 7.6. **a** Carcinoma of tongue. **b** Reaction post single-plane radium needle implant. **c** Result.

6) There will be some postoperative oedema but this usually settles within a day. Thereafter simple irrigation of the mouth is normally all that is necessary by way of postoperative care. The patient is given a fluid or semifluid diet while the needles are in situ. Routine use of antibiotics is unnecessary.
7) At the completion of the final time, the sources are removed in the ward without an anaesthetic, although some sedation may be required (Fig. 7.6).
8) The dose aimed at is 6000–6500 cGy in 7 days.

Thick-plane Implant

This form of single-plane implant is used for carcinoma of the lateral border of the tongue where the lesion is greater than 1 cm thick but can be encompassed in a slab of tissue 1.5 cm thick. To do this, it is necessary to express the dose at 0.75 cm and thus accept a higher dose at the customary expressed treating distance of 0.5 cm. The implant is carried out as for a single-plane implant but the sources used are full-strength needles throughout. The dose aimed at is 6500 cGy at 0.75 cm in seven days.

Two-plane Implant

Because of its technical difficulty, this is the least common form of implant used in the oral cavity. Its use is confined to the treatment of carcinoma of the lateral border of the tongue, too thick for treatment by a single-plane implant. A two-plane implant will treat a slab of tissue greater than 1 cm in thickness. The planes should be clear of the limits of the lesion and should include the whole tumour between them. One of the prime difficulties in this implant is that the lateral plane cannot be clear of tumour and thus the needles need to be as superficial as possible. The insertion of this lateral plane can be very difficult if the tumour is friable or considerable destruction of the margin of the tongue has occurred as a result of the lesion. For this reason, preference is usually given to the "thick" single-plane implant or to a volume implant of the tongue (Fig. 7.7).

For both two-plane and volume implants, in order to obey the distribution rules and have a sufficient number of sources, the needles, while of the same active length, are preferably of a lower linear density, i.e. 0.5 mg and 0.75 mg per centimetre. The dose aimed at in a two-plane implant is 6000–6500 cGy in 7 days expressed at 0.5 cm from the planes.

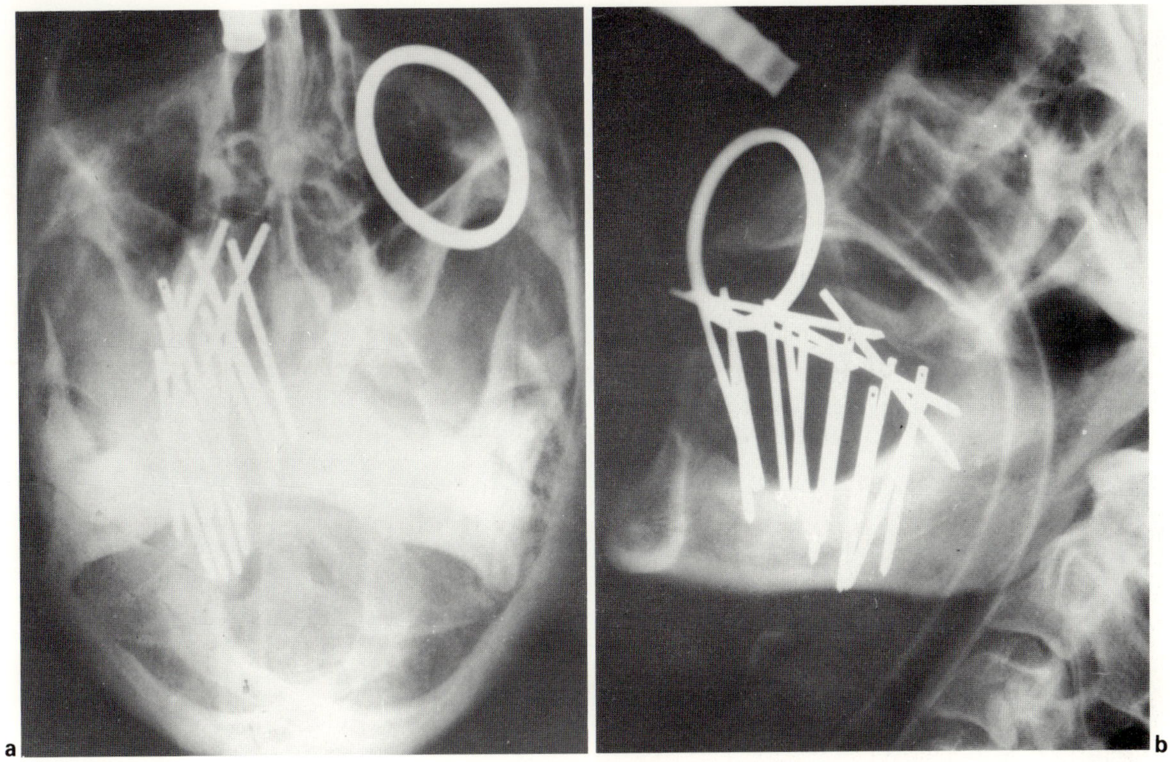

Fig. 7.7a, b. Carcinoma of tongue—two-plane radium needle implant.

Volume Implant

This form of implant is used (1) for carcinoma of the tongue where the tumour is not suitable for a single-plane implant, by virtue of either its thickness or its site and (2) for carcinoma of the floor of the mouth where there is a clear margin between the tumour and the lower alveolus. In use, the volume must be defined by the needles and takes the form of a cylinder, circular or elliptical in shape. Normally it is practicable to cross only the upper end; the lower end may be "crossed" if deemed necessary by the use of Indian club needles.

In the majority of cases the tongue is immobilised by a stitch which is inserted through the skin of the submental region, through the floor of the mouth and the tongue wide of the lesion. The stitch is tied so that the tongue is held down to the floor of the mouth. To prevent any implantation of tumour cells by the stitching needles, two needles are used, one at each end of the suture material. To prevent the suture from cutting the skin and the tongue, a small piece of rubber or plastic tubing is incorporated and the stitch tied over it. The implant is then carried out through the dorsum of the tongue (Fig. 7.8).

The needles are inserted following the Paterson-Parker distribution rules, with a minimum of eight sources in the peripheral "rind". The preferred needles are of 30 mm active length and, to achieve the desired 7-day implant, the strength of the peripheral needles used is 0.75 mg instead of the 1-mg needles preferred for a single-plane implant. In addition to the routine post-implant anteroposterior and lateral radiographs, a submentovertical view is helpful in defining the volume of the implant for the physicist. The dose aimed at is 6000–6500 cGy in 7 days.

Dose/Time Correction

The object of dose/time correction is to permit treatments at different dose rates to produce the same biological effect and to permit control over graduated dosage at whatever rate it is applied. In practice, equivalent doses can only be arrived at by the collected data resulting from the study of many cases treated by similar methods. As a consequ-

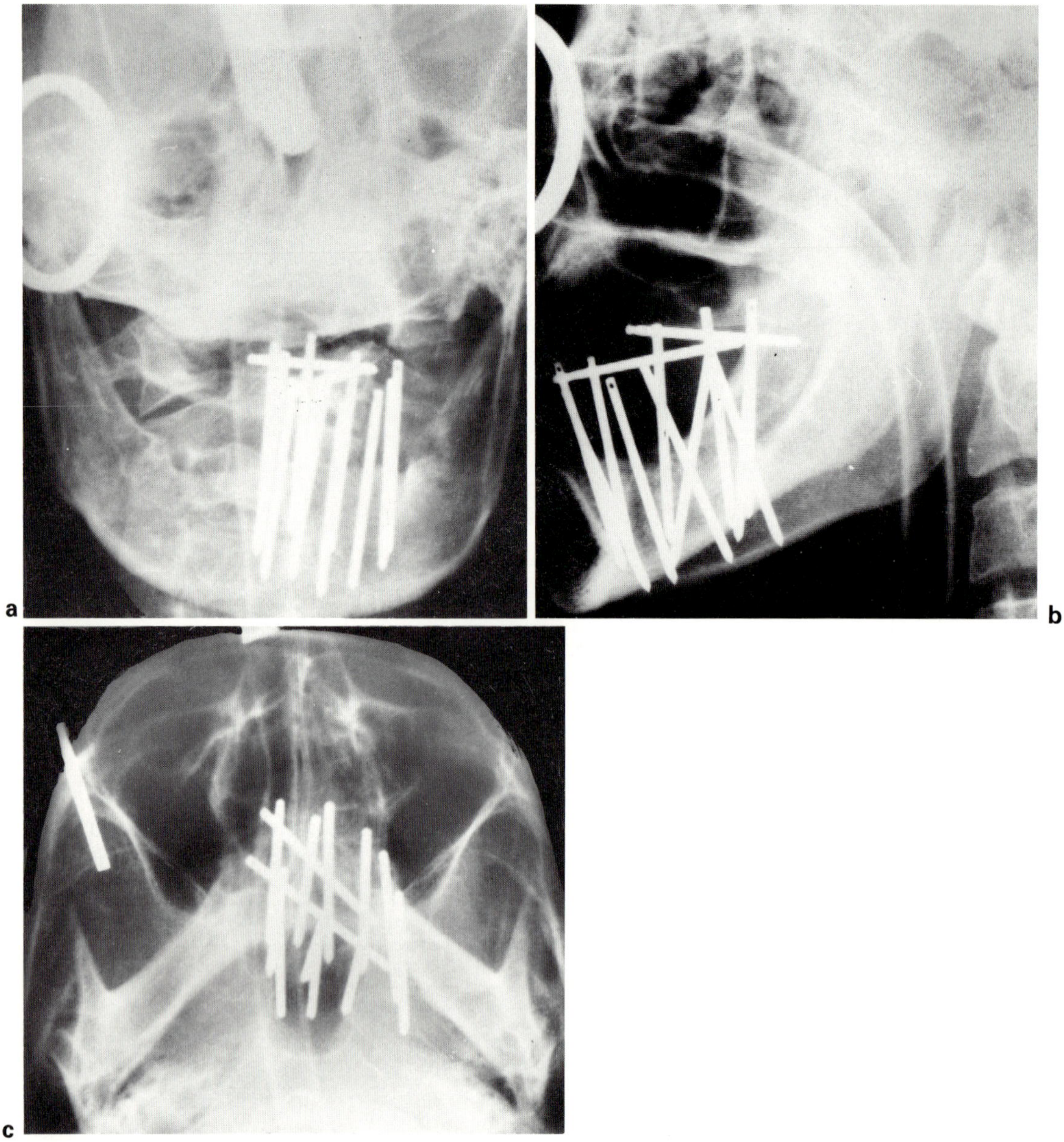

Fig. 7.8a–c. Carcinoma of tongue—volume implant.

Calculation.

Tongue. Volume implant
Implanted volume=18.8 cm^3
Dose required=6500 cGy
Approximate treatment time=168 h
mg h/1000 cGy=260
mg radium required=10 mg
Needles used 9×0.75 mg active length 3.0 cm
4×1.5 mg active length 3.0 cm
mg radium used=12.5 mg (including filtration correction)
Final treatment time=135 h

ence, an empiric curve can be constructed which demonstrates the connection between dose rate and time to produce the effect of 6500 cGy in 7 days. Such a curve has been used with good effect. However, analysis has shown that with good techniques using the radium distribution rules with the appropriate source strengths, the variation between the planned dose and the actual dose delivered is small. Thus, observing the above provisions, time correction is unnecessary in the majority of instances. In certain conditions, i.e. where the dose rate is considerably higher or where the implant is of an unusual type, it may be desirable to apply some time correction. A simple rule for determining this correction is as follows: for every 24 h by which the time calculated for the *actual* dose rate falls short of or exceeds the *intended* 7-day interval, the time prescribed should be reduced or increased respectively by 8 h.

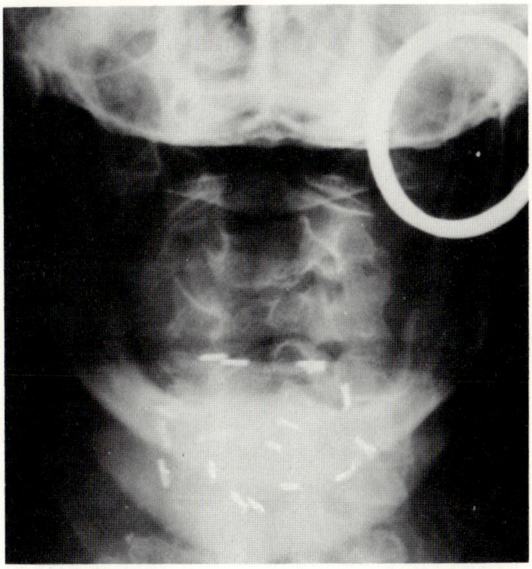

Fig. 7.9. Carcinoma floor of mouth—gold seed implant.

Gold Seed Implants

Permanent implants using gold seeds, or grains, or equivalent isotope afford a simple and effective method of treatment for small carcinomas of the oral cavity. As the sources are small they can be applied to highly curved surfaces or to surfaces inaccessible to needles because of the anatomy of the part, e.g. hard palate and alveolus. With a permanent implant, accuracy must be as precise as possible since the dose given is inevitably that resulting from the total decay of the isotope implanted (Fig. 7.9).

As most permanent implants are small and the tolerance of the oral mucosa is good, some excess of dose is acceptable, but as overdosage is the more common fault, the implanter would be wise to aim at a lower dose than the considered optimum. Underdosage can be rectified by a small supplementary X-ray contribution. The problem which may arise is where the distribution of sources is poor and as a result there is a patchy distribution of dose. This can be partially obviated by the use of an image intensifier during the implantation. While it is not practicable to remove sources already implanted, gaps may be filled by the insertion of extra sources, accepting that as a result there will be some degree of overdosage.

Practical points worthy of consideration are:

1) While permanent implants may be carried out under local anaesthesia, for implants in the oral cavity, general anaesthesia is to be preferred. The procedure should not be time-consuming and anaesthesia of this type is well tolerated even in old and frail subjects.
2) It is advantageous, because of anatomical curvatures, to have a small flexible lead strip available so that the area of the implant may be simply measured.
3) Easily visible in the theatre should be information on the strength of the sources available, together with a table indicating the number of megabecquerels required for a given dose and area (see App. 1).
4) A larger number of weak sources makes for a more uniform dose distribution.
5) When inserting the sources, cognisance should be taken of the elasticity of the tissue implanted so that the track made should be a little longer than that considered necessary, thus preventing the sources springing back.
6) In implanting sources deep to the mucoperiosteum, it is helpful to make a preliminary track with a blunt probe before inserting the gun.
7) As these implants are usually on considerably curved surfaces, it is desirable that the standard postoperative anteroposterior and lateral radiographs be supplemented by stereo views to permit allowance in the calculation of dosage for any "cupping" that may have occurred.

Permanent implants have a very useful place in the treatment of small oral cancers in aged subjects. In spite of the lack of physical control obtainable with a removable implant, local recurrence and necrosis is uncommon following a permanent gold seed implant.

Megavoltage X-ray Techniques

The evolution of wedge filter techniques with megavoltage (4 MV) X-rays has permitted the development of treatment methods allowing homogeneous irradiation of the desired volume with a minimum margin of additional irradiated tissue. Furthermore, there is the considerable advantage of very little differential absorption in bone from radiation of this quality (Fig. 7.10).

To capitalise on these advantages, the use of full beam-directed techniques, as described previously, cannot be overemphasised. Small-field beam-directed X-ray therapy using wedged fields requires a full shell to take advantage of the precision characteristic of this form of treatment. With this approach, the necessary volume can be treated while sparing the remainder of the mouth from high-dose irradiation. Accurate localisation is essential and to facilitate this it is useful to insert gold seed markers to indicate the extent of the lesion on the localising radiograph. Thereafter, the process of verification and treatment planning can be implemented.

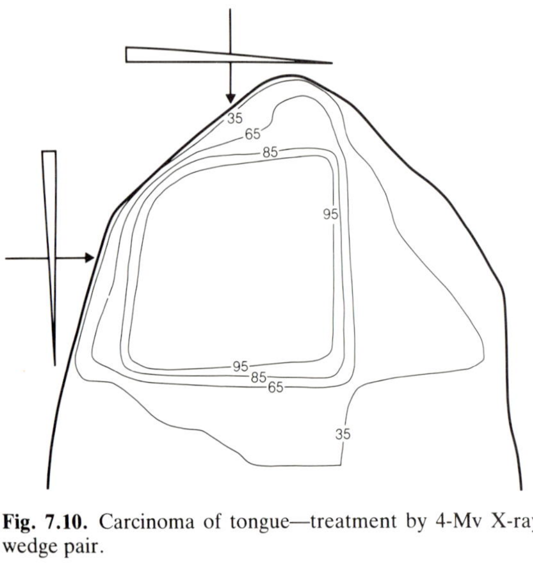

Fig. 7.10. Carcinoma of tongue—treatment by 4-Mv X-rays wedge pair.

As oral cancer is relatively superficial, it lends itself to treatment by means of wedged fields using 4-MV X-rays. There are two basic techniques:

1) For unilateral lesions, e.g. carcinoma of the lower alveolus, a wedge pair approach
2) For lesions crossing the midline, a parallel pair using a wedge to overcome oblique incidence

Using the wedge pair approach, the treatment volume can be accurately shaped to subtend the tumour to be irradiated along with precise normal tissue margins. The technique is facilitated by the availability of a number of wedge filters of different angles, as described in Chap. 1. The technique can be made more versatile by combining the use of wedges with a suitable build-up material, e.g. wax or CAB. Build-up may be necessary in certain sites where the skin is menaced, to extend the high-dose volume to the surface. The standard practice is followed of localisation, followed by verification of the accuracy of the localisation, and confirmation of the adequacy of the field size selected. The treatment plan is prepared either by hand, using isodose curves, or by resort to a treatment planning computer. It cannot be overemphasised that this is a small-field beam-directed technique and the average size of field employed will not exceed 35 cm^2. It is, therefore, possible to create a range of shaped volumes adapted to the shape of the tumour and of the part involved, with a very sharp cut-off. Examples are shown in Figs. 7.10, 7.12, and 7.14.

Normally the dose delivered is given in five fractions per week to a total of 15 or 16 fractions over 21 days. The dose delivered is 5250–5500 cGy. Where the patient is aged or frail, resort may be made to a shorter overall time and delivering e.g. a dose of 4500 cGy in eight fractions over 10 days.

Buccal Mucosa

The buccal mucosa is subdivided into the following sites:

1) Inner surface of lips
2) Lining of cheeks
3) Retromolar triangle
4) Buccoalveolar sulci, upper and lower

Inner Surface of Lips

Squamous cell carcinoma arising primarily in this site is rare; it is usually an extension from an adjacent site, e.g. floor of mouth or alveolus. The rarity of carcinoma at this site means that the treatment method used must be highly individualised, depending on the extent of the lesion. Interstitial irradiation at this site is difficult and our preference would be for external beam irradiation. Electron beam therapy, if available, affords an adequate method of treating the primary lesion while sparing much of the mouth from high-dose irradiation by the use of lead shielding mounted on a bite-block. With a normal lip thickness an electron beam of 10-MV energy should prove adequate. Using a single-field approach, a dose of 4500 cGy is given in eight exposures over 10 days.

Lining of Cheek

The factors influencing the choice of treatment are (1) the site of the lesion, (2) the degree of infiltration into the substance of the cheek, and (3) the relationship of the lesion to the buccoalveolar sulci. In addition, recognition of the increasing thickness of the cheek from front to back and the close application of the mucosa to the ascending ramus of the mandible must be taken into consideration when planning treatment. Lesions close to the commissure of the lips may be treated very satisfactorily by means of a double mould, as described for carcinoma of the lip. When the lesion is arising from the centre of the cheek and is well clear of the buccoalveolar sulci, the treatment options are (1) interstitial irradiation, (2) electron beam therapy, and (3) beam-directed megavoltage X-ray therapy.

Interstitial Irradiation A single-plane implant by definition will only treat a slab of tissue 1 cm thick, so that its use must be confined to relatively superficial lesions. The implant may be carried out intraorally, but is often simpler through the skin of the cheek. If carried out in the latter manner the needles are first introduced vertically until the point can be felt just deep to the mucosal aspect and are then run horizontally submucosally. The anterior end of the plane is crossed with a vertical needle or needles, but crossing the posterior end with needles is usually impracticable. Posterior crossing may be carried out by the use of Indian club needles, which contain a double cell at the tip of the needle. In practice this is not necessary provided long enough needles are used to ensure adequate clearance posteriorly (Fig. 7.11). The dose delivered is 6000 cGy at 0.5 cm in 7 days.

For small superficial lesions, particularly in the aged subject, a permanent gold seed implant is a simple practical alternative. The dose aimed at is 6000 cGy at 0.5 cm.

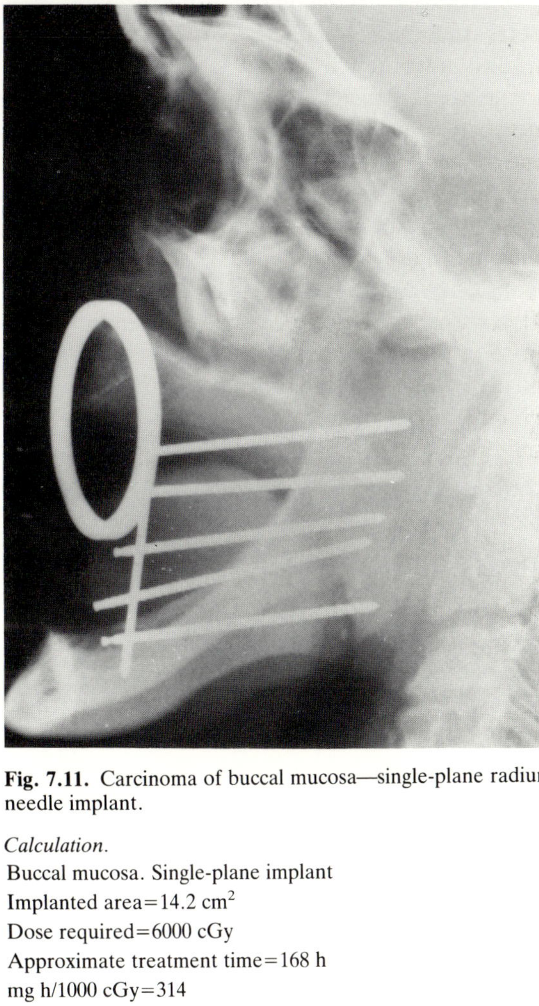

Fig. 7.11. Carcinoma of buccal mucosa—single-plane radium needle implant.

Calculation.
Buccal mucosa. Single-plane implant
Implanted area=14.2 cm^2
Dose required=6000 cGy
Approximate treatment time=168 h
mg h/1000 cGy=314
mg radium required=11.21 mg
Needles used 2×3 mg active length 4.5 cm
3×1.5 mg active length 4.5 cm
1×2 mg active length 3.0 cm
mg radium used=12.15 mg (including filtration correction)
Final treatment time=155 h

Electron Beam Therapy Electron beam therapy of medium energy (10 MV), using a single-field approach, affords a simple method of treatment while sparing much of the mouth from the high-dose volume. As with all electron beam therapy, a substantial margin around the lesion should be subtended. The limited penetration of the beam must be taken into consideration in the selection of cases for this form of therapy. Using a single field, suggested doses are 4500 cGy in eight treatments over 10 days or 5250–5500 cGy in 15 treatments over 21 days.

Beam-directed Megavoltage X-ray Therapy This is the treatment method of choice for deeply infiltrating lesions and when the lesion involves the buccoalveolar sulcus. The standard cellulose acetate shell is made. To facilitate verification, gold seed markers are inserted just beyond the periphery of the lesion. Using 4-MV X-rays a wedge pair approach is used. Normally some build-up on the skin will be necessary, and usually 4 mm of cellulose acetate will be adequate, but when the skin is menaced build-up should be at least 8 mm in thickness. The average field size used will be 5×5 cm–6×6 cm. The dose delivered is 5500 cGy in 16 exposures over 21 days (Fig. 7.12).

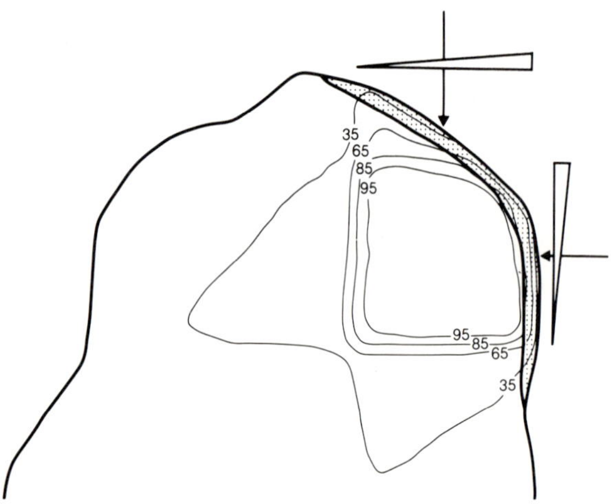

Fig. 7.12. Carcinoma of buccal mucosa—treatment by 4-MV X-rays wedge pair. Note build up.

Retromolar Triangle

This site carries the poorest prognosis of all buccal mucosal lesions. Direct spread to adjacent sites is common, and extension to the pterygoid fossa will produce trismus. Trismus is indicative of an extensive lesion and is associated with an extremely bad prognosis (Fig. 7.13).

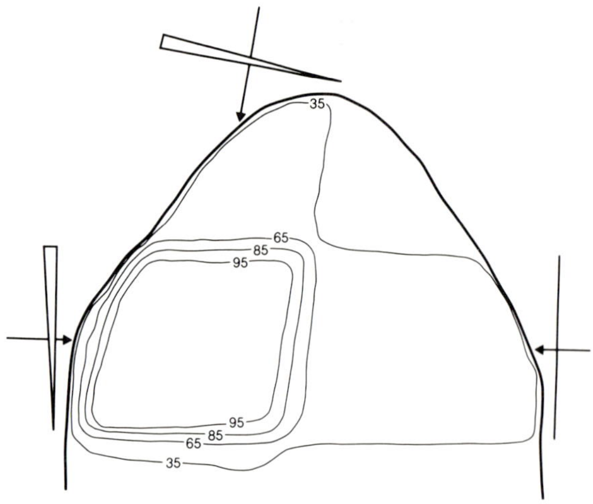

Fig. 7.13. Carcinoma of buccal mucosa (retromolar)—three-field technique.

Treatment is by means of megavoltage X-ray therapy using the wedge pair technique described above.

Buccoalveolar Sulcus

Involvement of the buccoalveolar sulcus is usually the result of direct extension from a lesion arising in the lining of the cheek. When the upper buccoalveolar sulcus is involved it is essential to exclude a primary cancer arising in the maxillary antrum and presenting in the sulcus. Full sinus radiology should be carried out and exploration of the antrum may be necessary if there is any doubt as to the origin of the lesion. Lesions involving the lower alveolar sulcus may arise from the alveolus. Treatment is by means of megavoltage X-ray therapy using a wedge pair approach as previously described.

Lower Alveolus The optimum treatment for carcinoma of the lower alveolus is a wedge pair approach using two fields, one anterior and one lateral. Build-up is only necessary if there is extension to the buccal mucosa. A bite-block is worn during treatment, designed to displace the tongue from the high-dose volume; it also acts to reduce air gaps in the mouth. The very little differential absorption in bone from megavoltage X-ray therapy permits the treatment of lesions even where there is demonstrable bone involvement, without significant morbidity. In practice, the average field size is 5×5 cm and the dose

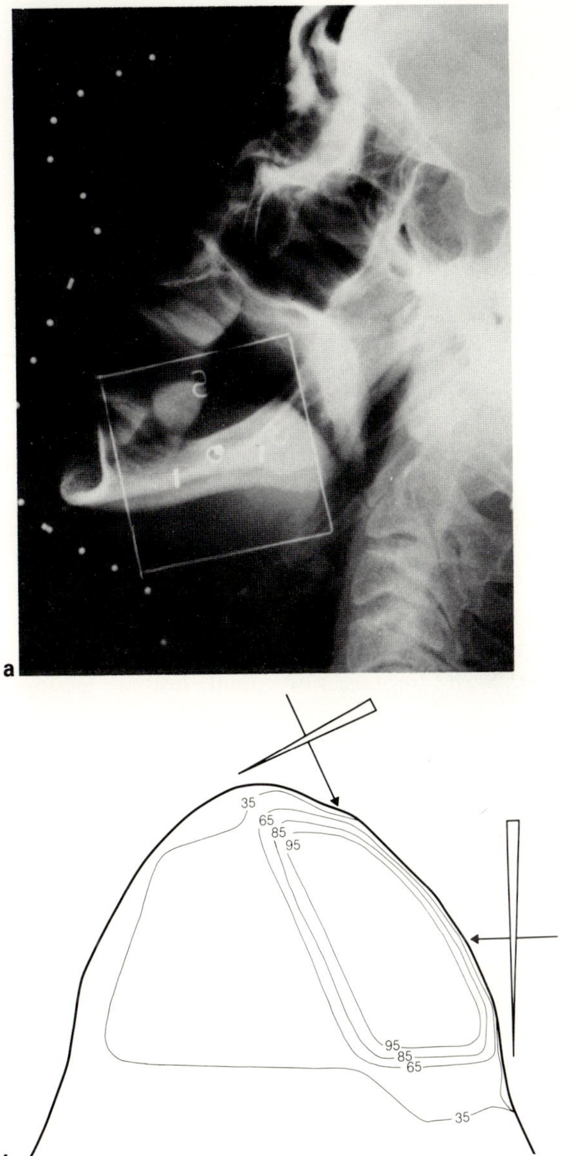

Fig. 7.14a,b. Carcinoma of lower alveolus. **a** Verification film tumour demarcated by gold seeds. **b** 4-MV X-rays wedge pair.

delivered 5500 cGy in 16 exposures over 21 days (Fig. 7.14).

In aged subjects with a small lesion, consideration should be given to the use of a permanent gold seed implant. The anatomy of the region and the close application of the mucoperiosteum make consistently good implants difficult to achieve. The dose aimed at is 6000 cGy at 0.5 cm.

Upper Alveolus and Gingiva Carcinoma of the upper alveolus is an uncommon lesion. It is essential to establish that the lesion is truly primary and not an extension from a primary carcinoma of the maxillary antrum. The situation is usually clarified by radiology of the nasal sinuses. In some extensive cases, involvement of the lower half of the antrum will occur by direct involvement. This lesion is best managed by beam-directed megavoltage X-ray therapy, usually a wedge pair of fields.

Hard Palate

As for carcinoma of the upper alveolus, it is essential to eliminate a primary lesion arising in the maxillary antrum. The demonstration of the integrity of the bone of the hard palate is an important clinical observation. Extension to involve the soft palate is common.

Small lesions may be treated by a permanent gold seed implant (Fig. 7.15). This type of implant is difficult at this site due to the close application of the mucoperiosteum, which tends to strip as the seeds are inserted. It is useful therefore to make a small tunnel with blunt forceps before attempting to insert a seed.

The majority of lesions will be treated by megavoltage X-ray therapy; unilateral lesions by means of a wedged pair of fields, anterior and lateral. Where the lesion is midline or has crossed the midline, a parallel pair of fields is preferred. Where there is evidence of involvement of the floor of the maxillary antrum, the lower half of the antrum should be included in the high-dose volume.

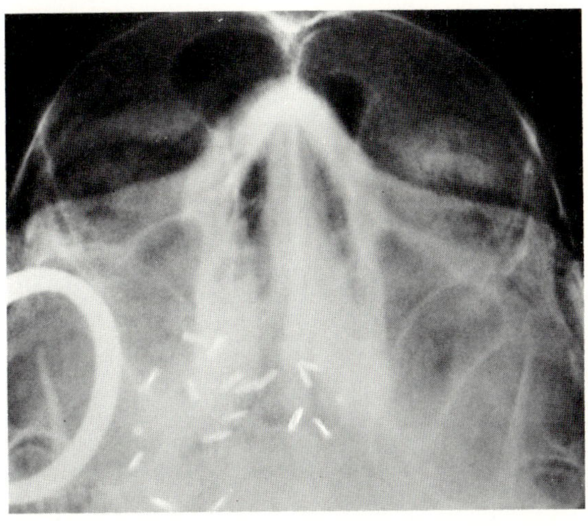

Fig. 7.15. Carcinoma of hard palate—gold seed implant.

Tongue

The treatment of choice for early and moderately advanced carcinoma of the anterior two-thirds of the tongue is by means of interstitial therapy. The selection of the type of implant will depend on the extent of the tumour or upon the form of implant that will best fit around it so as to include an adequate margin of normal surrounding tissue. As the majority of carcinomas of the tongue arise from the lateral border, the commonest form of implant employed is the single plane. For the uncommon tumours arising from the dorsum of the tongue, a transdorsal single-plane implant may be used. The next commonest form of implant is the volume implant. This type of implant is most suitable for tumours that have penetrated the body of the tongue. For lesions more than 1 cm thick arising from the lateral border of the tongue, resort may be made to a two-plane implant. This is difficult to perform and preference may be for a "thick" plane single implant, expressing the dose at 0.75 cm and accepting a higher dose at 0.5 cm. The commonest dose employed is 6000–6500 cGy in 7 days.

Where the lesion is too extensive for interstitial therapy or where there is extension to other sites beyond treatment by an implant, then resort must be made to external beam therapy. When the lesion is clearly unilateral, a wedge pair approach using 4-MV X-rays is used. If, however, there is considerable extension across the midline, a parallel pair approach is used, often using a wedge to compensate for oblique incidence (Fig. 7.16).

The field sizes employed should be kept to the minimum necessary to subtend the tumour with an

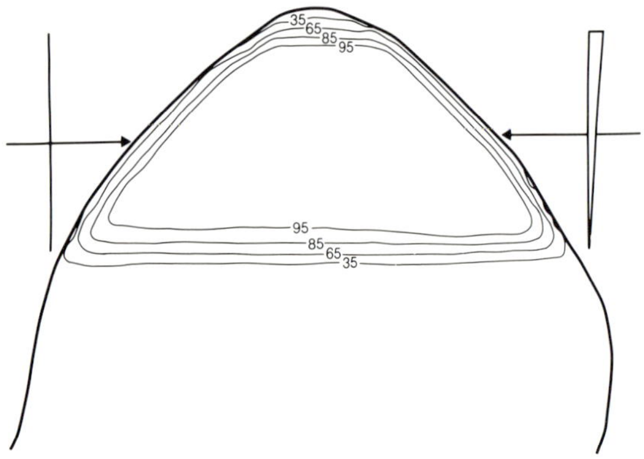

Fig. 7.16. Carcinoma of floor of mouth—4-MV X-rays parallel pair wedge used to compensate for oblique incidence.

adequate margin of normal tissue. The dose given, according to the volume treated, will vary from 5000 to 5500 cGy in 15 fractions over 21 days.

Floor of Mouth

The choice of treatment method will be influenced by the direction of spread of the lesion. There may be extensions to the alveolus, anteriorly or laterally, or posteriorly to the ventral surface of the tongue. In advanced cases the alveolus will be involved and the tumour may rarely present with gross destruction of the lower alveolus with involvement of the soft tissues overlying the symphysis menti. Similarly there may be gross invasion of the substance of the tongue with limitation of movement of that organ.

Interstitial Irradiation

Gold Seed Implant For small lesions arising centrally in the floor of the mouth, clear of the alveolus and not extending into the tongue, implantation of gold (^{198}Au) seeds remains a perfectly satisfactory method of treatment. As with all permanent implants it lacks the advantage of precise physical control. It is of particular value in the management of these lesions in aged subjects.

The dose aimed at is 6000 cGy at 0.5 cm.

Radium Needle Implant This method of treatment is particularly suitable for centrally placed floor of mouth lesions clear of the alveolus. Extension on to the frenum or ventral surface of the tongue does not invalidate this form of treatment provided that the involvement of the tongue is not gross. The type of implant used is the volume implant. The volume will be defined by the needles and takes the form of a cylinder or circular or elliptical section, with one or both ends of the implant closed by crossing needles. The technique for this implant requires that the tongue be sewn down to prevent lifting of the implant by postoperative oedema. The dose aimed at is 6500 cGy in 7 days.

X-ray Therapy

Where the lesion is closely applied to the lower alveolus or when there is considerable involvement of the tongue, it is better to use external beam therapy. Where the lesion is unilateral, a wedge pair approach using 4-MV X-rays is used. When the lesion crosses the midline, a parallel pair approach is preferred using a wedge to compensate for oblique incidence. Excessive irradiation of the lips should be avoided. The average field size is 5×5 cm and the dose delivered 5500 cGy in 16 fractions over 21 days.

Dental Care

In the United Kingdom 85% of patients presenting with oral cancer are edentulous. Where teeth are present and sound, no dental interference apart from hygiene is necessary and radiotherapy may be commenced immediately. Where there is poor dental hygiene and gross caries is present, then dental clearance is indicated. This should be carried out under antibiotic cover and care should be taken to avoid interference with the vascular supply to the jaw. Following clearance, there would normally be an interval of 10–14 days before radiotherapy could be commenced as patients would not tolerate the intraoral manipulations necessary to make a suitable bite-block. Occasionally teeth may impede the preparation of a suitable mould or bite-block. Under those circumstances the offending teeth should be removed.

Following radiotherapy the patients should be instructed in simple oral hygiene and warned that before undergoing dental treatment they should inform their dental surgeon of the nature of the treatment they have received. Subsequent dental treatment should be as conservative as possible and large-scale extractions avoided.

Necrosis

Following a well-planned interstitial or megavoltage treatment for carcinoma of the oral cavity, soft tissue necrosis is rare. When it does occur, it is usually of a minor nature at the site of a localised "hot spot" and normally settles down with simple conservative measures. Failure to respond to such measures should be regarded as suspicious of recurrence and a biopsy should be taken. Necrosis of bone is almost entirely confined to the lower jaw and particularly to the mid third of the mandible. The blood supply to this segment of the mandible diminishes with advancing age and may be further reduced by recent dental extractions. The management of bony necrosis is essentially conservative, with the use of dental hygiene and long-term antibiotic therapy. Serial radiography is essential to determine the extent of bone destruction and to demonstrate sequestration.

Surgical intervention should be delayed until the full extent of the necrosis has been shown. It may be that simple removal of a sequestrum will suffice, but a more formal resection of the jaw may be required.

Necrosis of the jaw following treatment for oral cancer occurs principally within 2 years of the primary treatment—late necrosis is exceptional. The primary site most commonly associated with bone necrosis is the floor of the mouth.

Second Primary

Approximately 6% of patients treated for carcinoma of the mouth will develop another primary in the oral cavity. Some patients with very unstable mucosa will develop multiple malignancies. The management of the second lesion will depend, to a large extent, on its proximity to the original lesion. In the majority of cases further radiotherapy is feasible. If embarked upon it must be planned with great care and should aim to be as precise as possible. Interstitial irradiation is of particular value in this situation. Under certain circumstances it is justifiable to extend the new treatment into the previously irradiated volume, provided that the extension is kept to a minimum and the risk of a limited subsequent necrosis accepted.

Where further irradiation is considered inadvisable then surgery should be resorted to. In selected cases treatment with a laser may be of considerable value.

Recurrence

Recurrence following a radical course of radiotherapy occurs mainly in the first year following treatment. Certainly, recurrence after 2 years is exceptional and most probably represents the development of a second primary in the oral cavity.

The most important feature affecting the development of a recurrence is the initial size of the primary lesion. Using the treatment methods described for the various sites in the oral cavity, the primary control rates are similar.

Once the presence of recurrence has been established, surgical opinion should be sought as to the feasibility of radical excision. Even if excision is not possible, useful control may often be obtained by the use of the laser or cryoprobe. If surgery is considered inadvisable, then consideration should be given to chemotherapy which, while only palliative, can give very satisfying pain relief.

Advanced Disease

As indicated earlier, in the management of carcinoma of the oral cavity, primary control is the aim of all treatment. If the lesion is clearly beyond a radical treatment, careful consideration should be given to the fact that the patient would gain very little from palliative treatment, whether it be by radiotherapy or surgery. It is unkind to submit a patient to a radiation reaction in the mouth when clearly the primary disease will not be controlled. Better palliation will be secured with opiates and supportive measures.

For patients in good general condition with advanced lesions, consideration should be given to measures to supplement conventional X-ray therapy. Clinical trials to evaluate neutron therapy, radiosensitisers, and the combination of chemotherapy and X-ray therapy are currently being undertaken. There is at present no clear indication of a significant advantage from any of these approaches.

Follow-up

Long-term studies in oral cancer show that the great majority of subsequent incidents will occur within 2 years of the primary treatment. It follows that the maximum surveillance should be maintained during this period. In the first year following treatment, the patient should be seen monthly or more frequently if the clinical state demands it. In the second year, the interval between visits may be increased to 2 months. After the second year, the interval between visits may be steadily increased. The possibility of a further primary lesion in the mouth should not be overlooked.

Prognostic Factors

The prime prognostic factor in oral cancer is the size of the primary lesion on presentation. The site of the lesion is less important, but carcinoma of the buccal mucosa has a better prognosis than other sites. The influence of sex is less marked than previously observed, but females with oral malignancy have a better prognosis than males. Age appears to have a definite effect on prognosis, with the younger age groups having a positive advantage. Older patients tend to present with more advanced disease.

Cervical Nodes

Of equal importance to the successful treatment of the primary is the treatment of involved nodes. Radical block dissection of the neck remains the treatment of choice for mobile involved nodes. Elective block dissection of the neck has not been practised at the Christie Hospital. The maximum incidence of lymph node involvement occurs within the first 2 years following treatment of the primary. Approximately 50% of block dissections of the neck will be carried out within 3 months of the primary treatment and most of the remainder within 2 years of the primary treatment.

Where there are involved nodes on presentation, and if they are mobile and discrete in the immediate lymph drainage area, the primary is treated by the appropriate irradiation method and block dissection is carried out after an interval of 4–6 weeks in order to avoid the radiation reaction phase. In those cases where it is felt that delay is undesirable, the following policies may be followed:

1) Block dissection of the neck followed by radiation treatment of the primary.
2) Radiation treatment of the primary followed by immediate block dissection. This is most practical where the primary treatment is by means of interstitial irradiation.
3) Radiation treatment of the primary plus a localised "holding" X-ray treatment to the involved nodes, followed by block dissection of the affected neck after an interval of 4–6 weeks.

In general, completion of the radiation treatment of the primary is preferred before surgical treatment of the involved nodes.

Radiotherapeutic Management of Cervical Lymphadenopathy

Radiation therapy may be directed to the lymph drainage areas of the neck in the following circumstances:

1) Elective radiotherapy to the neck
2) Inclusion of involved nodes in primary treatment volume
3) Use of a "holding" dose of X-ray therapy while the primary treatment is completed, with subsequent block dissection
4) Treatment of subsequent nodes where the primary is well and block dissection is not feasible

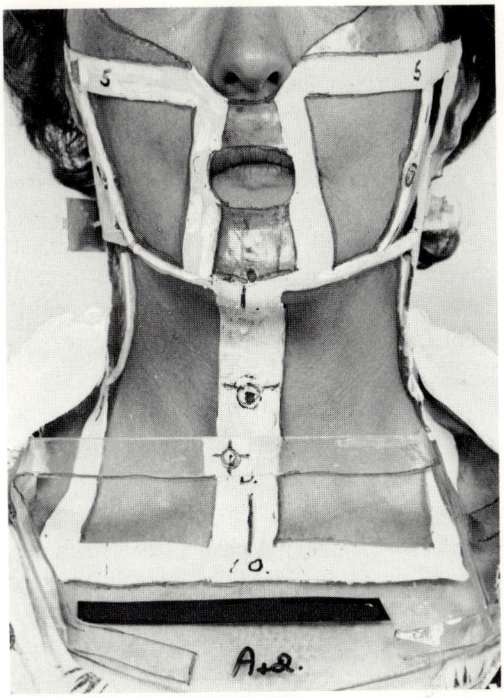

Fig. 7.17. Treatment of cervical nodes by anterior field shielding spinal cord.

Elective Radiotherapy to the Neck

Routine elective radiotherapy to the clinically negative neck has not been found to be a justifiable procedure. It is, however, an effective treatment in reducing the subsequent node incidence. Its use should be reserved for:

1) Cases where adequate surveillance is not feasible
2) Cases where the patient's general condition precludes block dissection

Two treatment methods will be discussed: 4-MV X-ray therapy to the whole neck, and 10-MV electron therapy to the unilateral neck.

4-MV X-ray Therapy to the Whole Neck This therapy is given concurrently with X-ray treatment to the primary lesion. The object is to irradiate both sides of the neck, from the junction with the lowest margin of the primary treatment volume to the clavicles. A single anterior field is used with a 2-cm leaded central strip to protect the pharynx and the spinal cord. To plan this treatment, a single shell is made which will subtend the primary treatment volume and the neck. The primary treatment is planned and radiographs are then taken with an opaque wire at the lowest margin of the primary volume to be irradiated. The field size necessary to subtend the neck is then selected. This is facilitated by the use of a graduated grid and an anteroposterior radiograph will confirm the position of the anterior neck field relative to the fields used to treat the primary. The necessary area for lead shielding is then indicated on this film. Apart from the central strip, the fields are cut out except where there are palpable nodes, when the cellulose acetate sheet is retained to provide build-up (Fig. 7.17). If the homolateral neck only is to be treated, the procedure followed is similar, but with a field size necessary to subtend this volume. Treatment is given in 15 fractions over 21 days, delivering a dose of 5000 cGy.

10-MV Electrons for Unilateral Neck Treatment This technique is of particular value when a unilateral carcinoma of the tongue has been treated by means of interstitial therapy. Treatments is carried out by means of a lateral field whose boundaries are demarcated by means of a lead cut-out. The treatment field can, therefore, be shaped to subtend the regional lymph drainage of the primary organ. The penetration of a 10-MV electron beam is such that the regional nodes are adequately irradiated without provoking any gross reaction in the deeper structures. Treatment can be planned as soon as the sources are removed from the primary site. No build-up is required. The dose delivered is 5000 cGy in 15 fractions over 21 days.

Inclusion of Nodes in Primary Treatment Volume

Involved nodes on presentation may be included in the primary treatment volume provided the whole treatment volume remains small. Substantial enlargement of the treated volume in order to include the involved nodes will mean a reduction of the tumour dose and therefore a greater risk of failure at the primary site. Under such circumstances, consideration should be given to the use of a separate field to treat the involved nodes.

Holding Dose Followed by Block Dissection

As a general rule, treatment of the primary should be undertaken before block dissection of mobile involved nodes. Occasionally, the situation arises where the mobility of the node is becoming limited and delay before block dissection is therefore undesirable. Under such circumstances the use of a holding dose of X-ray therapy to the node is useful. During the course of the primary treatment a single field large enough to subtend the involved node is used and a single exposure of 1500 cGy is given. The block dissection can then be carried out at the optimum time following completion of the primary course of therapy.

Subsequent Nodes with Primary Site Well

As indicated, the treatment of choice for involved cervical nodes from cancer of the oral cavity is block dissection of the neck. Where block dissection of the neck is contraindicated because of the general condition and/or the age of the patient, or where the node is fixed, then treatment is by means of X-ray therapy. If it is to be successful, treatment should be confined to as small a volume as possible. This may be carried out by the use of a single field to the involved volume, using either electron beam therapy or megavoltage X-rays. In the latter case, some build-up over the node(s) is desirable.

Practical dose schedules are 1750 cGy in a single exposure or 4000–4500 cGy in eight exposures over 10 days. Where there is substantial node involvement and palliation only is the aim, then the use of growth restraint X-ray therapy may be of considerable value. This technique consists of giving a dose of 400 cGy to the affected volume once weekly and continuing to a total dose of 7000–8000 cGy, or less if local tolerance has been exhausted.

Results

The degree of primary control that may be obtained by radiotherapy in early and moderately advanced carcinoma of the oral cavity is high. Where the primary lesion is not greater than 2 cm in diameter, over 90% of tumours will be cured by radiotherapy and a substantial proportion of the failures will be salvaged by surgery. Where the primary lesion is not greater than 4 cm in diameter, three-quarters will be controlled by radiotherapy and approximately half of the failures will be salvaged by subsequent surgery. However, where the lesion is greater than 4 cm in diameter, primary control falls to about 50% and only a few of the failures will be amenable to surgical salvage.

Cancer of the Oropharynx

Clinical Features

Anatomy

This part of the pharynx lies between the inferior surface of the soft palate and the level of the floor of the vallecula. The posterior third of the tongue, the vallecula, and the anterior surface of the epiglottis form the anterior boundary. Posteriorly, it lies at the level of the second and third cervical vertebrae. The lateral walls are formed by the tonsils and the faucial pillars.

It is worth noting especially that the lymphatic drainage of this area is complex and abundant. The tissues comprising Waldeyer's ring are richly supplied with lymphatics which drain freely to the upper deep cervical nodes and also directly to the lower neck nodes. It is also a characteristic of this drainage system that many of the lymphatics cross the midline, so that contralateral metastases in nodes are commonly seen.

Incidence

Oropharyngeal cancer accounts for rather less than half of all pharyngeal neoplasms. The highest incidence in the world is said to occur in India, where it is about 6 per 100 000 of the population: in the United Kingdom this figure is less than 1 per 100 000. It is more common in men that women.

Site

The tonsils and their fossae are the commonest sites of origin and represent half of oropharyngeal malignancies. The posterior third of the tongue and the vallecula are the second commonest sites.

Pathology

Squamous cell carcinoma is the most common type and occurs in all degrees of differentiation. Because of the abundance of lymphoid tissue, malignant lymphomata, particularly lymphosarcoma and reticulosarcoma (non-Hodgkin's lymphoma) are relatively common. Adenocarcinoma, cylindroma, and malignant melanoma, though rare, may also occur in the oropharynx.

Spread

Early involvement of the neighbouring region is frequent. A lesion arising in or around the tonsillar fossa may at an early stage extend to the lateral pharyngeal wall, the soft palate, the floor of the mouth and the tongue. A tumour arising from the base of the tongue usually spreads to the middle third of the tongue, the floor of the mouth and the vallecula.

Early lymph node involvement from oropharyngeal cancer is common in patients with tumours arising from the posterior third of the tongue and the tonsillar fossa, usually appearing first in the upper deep group. Involvement of nodes on both sides of the neck is frequent, particularly from a midline lesion.

Investigation and Diagnosis

The commonest presenting symptom is a feeling that a foreign body is lodged in the throat. Pain or discomfort when swallowing is also common. The lesion is sometimes first noticed at a routine dental examination. A visible lump in the neck may lead the patient to seek medical advice, even though the primary lesion is small and asymptomatic. Otalgia may develop from involvement of the glossopharyngeal nerve, and dysphagia may develop, causing malnutrition and weight loss.

Examination of the mouth and the pharynx under good illumination should show the extent of a lesion in the oropharynx, A lesion at the base of the tongue or the vallecula needs especially careful examination, for a small area of ulceration or a minor swelling may easily be overlooked by an inexperienced physician. Indirect laryngoscopy must always be performed for adequate visualisation of the base of the tongue, the vallecula and the posterolateral pharyngeal walls. At the same time the full extent of the spread should be determined for staging and treatment planning. Occasionally, the disease may be multifocal in origin.

Digital examination is essential to ascertain the local infiltration of the tumour. It is not uncommon to be able to palpate a tumour at the base of the tongue when the mirror examination shows no obvious abnormality. Careful and systematic examination of the neck, each side in turn, is mandatory, for it is not possible to concentrate fully on all one's finger tips if both hands palpate each side of the neck at the same time. We prefer to carry out this important examination standing behind the seated patient.

A lateral soft tissue X-ray of the neck and postnasal space is often helpful in defining the extent of the tumour. A chest X-ray should also be done.

The clinical and radiological findings should be confirmed at the time of examination under anaesthetic and at the same time a biopsy must be obtained.

Treatment Policy

The common squamous cell carcinoma of the oropharynx is a tumour which, if not too advanced, is often curable by radiotherapy. Moreover, for advanced tumours the prognosis is poor irrespective of the mode of treatment. The value of adjuvant chemotherapy is under investigation and the initial findings are encouraging. For malignant lymphoma of the tonsillar area or the posterior third of the tongue, radiotherapy is the treatment of choice.

Metastases of carcinoma to the lymph nodes are frequent and the local nodes should preferably be included in the primary treatment volume if this can be done without unduly increasing the field size. If the nodes persist following radiotherapy, a block dissection of the neck should be considered, provided the primary lesion has disappeared, or residual primary tumour is resectable. If, however, the nodes are positioned in the lower neck, the primary lesion should be treated radically and a separate single dose of radiation should be given to the nodes, merely to delay the progress of the disease until the patient is ready for a block dissection of the neck. If there is bilateral cervical lymph node involvement, the prognosis is poor and only palliative treatment should be given. This may relieve distressing symptoms and delay fungation of the neoplasm.

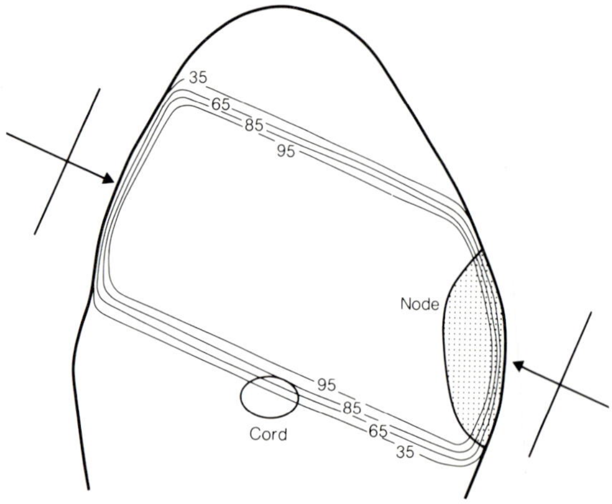

Fig. 7.18. Carcinoma of oropharynx—oblique parallel pair to avoid spinal cord.

Treatment Techniques

The basic principles of small-field beam-direction techniques have already been described. For squamous cell tumours arising in or near the midline of the oropharynx, both sides of the upper neck should be included in the treatment volume, so that all the local lymph drainage areas are included. This is best achieved by an opposed parallel pair of fields, using wedge filters or compensators as necessary. The field sizes required for such lesions range from 6×5 cm to 8×6 cm, depending on the extent of the tumour. When planning the treatment, care must be taken to avoid including the spinal cord in the path of the beams. When palpable nodes are included in the treatment volume, the fields may need to be angled forwards a few degrees to keep the spinal cord out of the beam (Fig. 7.18). Alternatively, if it is impossible to avoid the spinal cord, the dose must be kept below the radiation tolerance of the cord. If nodes are already palpable lower in the neck, or are spreading too posteriorly, it may be desirable to limit the volume of the high-dose region from the opposed parallel pair of fields, and treat the nodes below this volume by an additional single field. Such a treatment, however, is really beyond what is usually considered to be "radical" in the sense of being curative.

The treated volume should be restricted to the affected side for a squamous cell carcinoma localised to the tonsillar fossa or the faucial pillars. This avoids a radiation reaction in the other half of the oral cavity and oropharynx, and reduces discomfort for the patient. A wedge pair technique is appropriate (Fig. 7.19). Using this arrangement, the given dose on the anterior wedge field usually exceeds the acceptable tolerance dose for the lip. For this reason a given dose of 3000 cGy from the anterior field should not be exceeded when given in 16 fractions over 22 days. In practice, 75% of the tumour dose is delivered by the wedge pair technique, and the remaining 25% from an opposed parallel pair. The usual field sizes are from 5×5 cm to 7×6 cm.

Some superficial lesions arising in the soft palate or uvula may be treated effectively by a permanent implant. Radioactive gold seeds may be used, and

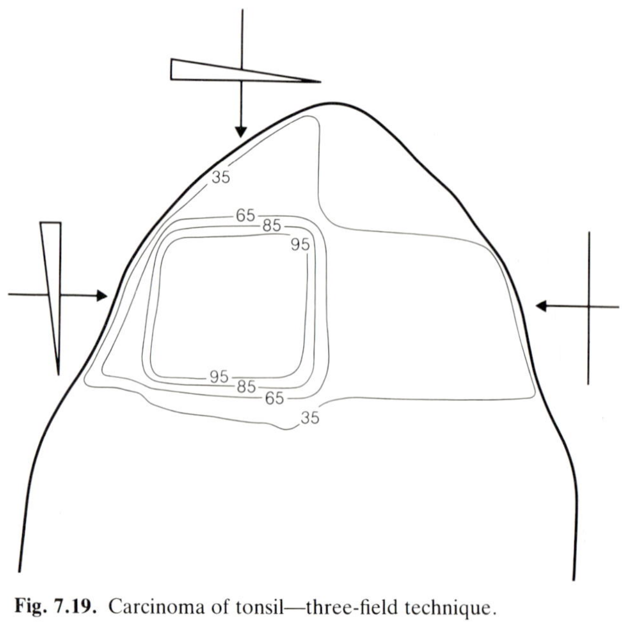

Fig. 7.19. Carcinoma of tonsil—three-field technique.

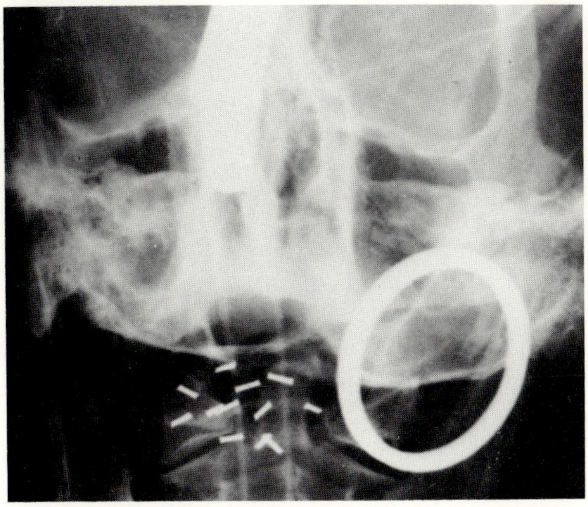

Fig. 7.20. Carcinoma of soft palate—gold seed implant.

Calculation.
Soft palate. Single-plane gold seed implant
Implanted area=4.96 cm^2
Dose required=5500 cGy
mg h/1000 cGy=173
1 MBq Au-198 to decay is equivalent to 0.72 mg h (radium)
Initial activity required=1322 MBq
Seeds used 12×111 MBq
Total initial activity used=1332 MBq
Final dose=5500 cGy

the technique is simple (Fig. 7.20). It is particularly suitable for elderly patients, and there is very little discomfort from the localised radiation reaction, in contrast to that from external radiotherapy. The patient need only stay in hospital for a few days.

Wedge Filters

It can be seen from Fig. 7.19 that in the horizontal plane through the centre of the treated volume, the oblique incidence of the surface contour is minimal, in contrast to that of a contour through the neck. For such a situation two plain (unwedged) fields suffice, placed on either side of the patient to achieve a homogeneous dose. Rarely, it may be necessary to use a low wedge angle of about 20° against a plain field from the opposite side, to correct a small oblique incidence.

For the wedge pair technique, two 50° wedges are usually required with a hinge angle of 90°. The thick ends of the wedges should lie close to each other.

Dose and Fractionation

When the whole of the oropharynx is included in the treatment volume, a dose of 5000 cGy is the optimum for 16 fractions given over 22 days. For advanced tumours requiring the treatment of a large volume, this dose needs to be reduced.

For the wedge pair technique, the high-dose volume is limited to the affected side only, and a dose of 5500 cGy may be given.

A dose of 6500 cGy is appropriate for a small gold seed implant.

Malignant lymphomas are often quite bulky tumours, and need treatment to a greater margin of tissue outside the palpable limits of the tumour than is necessary for squamous cell carcinoma. In addition, nodes often extend posteriorly in the neck so that the fields, if they are to cover the posterior tumour limit with a margin, often necessarily include the spinal cord. For this reason, and because the treated volume is large, the tumour dose has to be reduced considerably, and is in the order of 2500–3000 cGy in 21 days depending on the field sizes (see also Chap. 14).

Cancer of the Nasopharynx

Clinical Features

Anatomy

The nasopharynx (the postnasal space) is bounded posterosuperiorly by the basisphenoid and basiocciput. It lies anterior to the upper two cervical vertebrae. The lateral wall is formed by the superior constrictor muscle and the fossa of Rosenmüller with the opening of the Eustachian tube. Anteriorly it opens into the nose, and inferiorly to the oropharynx.

There is a rich lymphatic plexus in the postnasal space which drains primarily into the retropharyngeal nodes, and lies in close relation to the last four cranial nerves and the sympathetic chain as they emerge from the base of the skull. Upper deep cervical nodes may receive lymphatics from the retropharyngeal nodes or directly from the nasopharynx.

Incidence and Aetiology

Nasopharyngeal cancer occurs in an unusually high frequency in the southern Chinese, and is known to have a close association with the Epstein-Barr virus independent of geography. Males are more frequently affected. The cause is uncertain, although there are suggestions that feeding salted fish to southern Chinese "boat people" in early childhood, in the absence of vitamin C while at sea, may be a contributing factor.

Site

Common sites of origin are the roof of the nasopharynx and the fossa of Rosenmüller, though when the tumour is extensive it is usually not possible to determine its site of origin.

Pathology

Squamous cell carcinoma is the commonest histological type and occurs in all degrees of differentiation. Because of the presence of lymphoid tissue, malignant lymphomas are relatively common. Lymphoepithelioma, which is a poorly differentiated carcinoma diffusely infiltrated by lymphocytes is commonly seen in young patients. Adenocarcinoma and chordoma, though rare, may occur.

Spread

It is characteristic that neoplasms arising from the nasopharynx metastasise early, even before the primary lesion produces symptoms. The tumour soon spreads posterolaterally to the parapharyngeal space and may involve the last four cranial nerves and the sympathetic chain, or the mandibular branch of the trigeminal nerve as it emerges from the foramen ovale. The trigeminal and the facial nerves may be involved intracranially by superior extension of the growth through the foramen lacerum. Displacement of the soft palate downward, a mass in the lateral pharyngeal wall, or spread to the posterior nares may be seen when the tumour extends to the oropharynx. Destruction of the basiocciput, basisphenoid, and the petrous temporal bone is often seen. Involvement of the Eustachian tube is common.

Metastases to the neck nodes are frequent. The retropharyngeal nodes and any of the deep cervical nodes may be affected. Bilateral metastases to the neck nodes is common.

Haematogenous spread to the lung, liver, and bones may occur.

Investigation and Diagnosis

The lack of early symptoms is often responsible for delay in diagnosis and unfortunately many physicians fail to suspect a growth in the nasopharynx until it is too late. By then the vast majority of patients have developed metastases to the nodes, or evidence of obvious cranial nerve palsy.

Nasal obstruction and discharge are common presenting symptoms. Epistaxis is not often seen unless there is extension of the neoplasm to the posterior nares. A conductive type of deafness develops when the Eustachian tube is blocked by the tumour.

The most common neurological symptom is pain in the face from involvement of the mandibular division of the trigeminal nerve. Diplopia is frequent when the abducent nerve or less commonly the oculomotor or trochlear nerves are affected. Palsy of the last four cranial nerves produces dysphonia, dysphagia, and weakness of the shoulder girdle. Involvement of the optic tract from intracranial extension of the neoplasm causes homonymous hemianopia. When the disease is advanced, eye movements and vision may be impaired by direct extension into the orbit.

Delay in diagnosis often occurs because of the relative inaccessibility of the postnasal space. All patients suspected of having a tumour in the nasopharynx must be seen in a joint clinic by a radiotherapist and an ENT surgeon, to determine the site and extent of the growth. The cranial nerves must be systematically examined for possible involvement. The neck should be palpated carefully. It is common to detect no abnormality, even though the clinical presentation arouses suspicion of a nasopharyngeal neoplasm.

A lateral soft tissue X-ray of the postnasal space, a radiograph of the base of the skull including a submentovertical view, and a radiograph of the paranasal sinuses may reveal tumour. CT is a useful tool for detailed radiological study. A chest X-ray must be taken.

Examination of the postnasal space under

general anaesthesia is the most valuable single investigation. There must be a thorough and meticulous inspection of the area and a biopsy must be taken. When there is no obvious growth, several blind punch biopsies (including a biopsy from the basisphenoid by splitting the soft palate) should be obtained and may reveal carcinoma.

Patients with malignant lymphomas require other investigations in addition. Lymphoma at this site may develop as a primary focus without involvement elsewhere.

The lack of early symptoms, the delay in diagnosis and the rapid and early spread of the tumour are responsible for the dismal prognosis.

Treatment Policy

Radiotherapy is the only available treatment for a neoplasm at this site, and there is no place for surgery in primary control.

When a malignant lymphoma occurs in the nasopharynx and the disease is localised, radical radiotherapy should be curative. The treated volume should be generous and must include the postnasal space, Waldeyer's ring, and both sides of the neck. The lower limit of the field should extend to the level of the clavicle.

The treatment policy for the common squamous cell carcinoma and lymphoepithelioma depends on the extent of the growth. For simplicity it is best classified according to the various patterns of presentation:

1) Tumour limited to the nasopharynx
2) Tumour in the nasopharynx with extension to the posterior nares
3) Tumour as above (1 or 2) but with ipsilateral or bilateral neck nodes
4) Tumour as above (1 or 2 or 3) with evidence of bone destruction and/or cranial nerve palsy
5) Cervical adenopathy with no visible tumour in the nasopharynx, but with biopsy proof of carcinoma
6) Advanced disease with distant metastases
7) Malignant lymphoma

The extent of the tumour and the histological type determine the irradiated volume and the treatment technique. The base of the skull is routinely included in the volume whether or not there is radiological evidence of bony erosion.

Treatment Techniques

Groups 1 and 2

It is rare to find patients with such limited tumours, but accurate beam direction is worthwhile because the 5-year disease-free survival may reach 60%. With a three-field arrangement as for a carcinoma of the ethmoid (see Fig. 7.29), a high-dose zone in the desired volume can be obtained. This is achieved by using an opposed parallel pair of fields each wedged horizontally at about 40° and a third plain field (unwedged) placed anteriorly between the eyes. The anterior field is essential when the tumour encroaches on the posterior nares and the nasal cavity. The lateral field sizes usually range between 6×6 cm and 8×6 cm. The anterior field lies between the pupils of the eyes and does not exceed 4.5 cm in width. Care must be taken to avoid inclusion of the spinal cord in the path of the lateral beams. The base of the brain must be shielded on the lateral fields to avoid a high dose to the brain stem. A dose of 5000–5250 cGy can be given in 16 fractions over 3 weeks.

Group 3

The primary tumour should be treated as described earlier either by a three-field technique or, in the absence of anterior extension of the neoplasm to the nose, by an opposed parallel pair. Irrespective of the group of cervical nodes involved, both sides of the neck should be treated. This can be achieved by a megavoltage single anterior field, encompassing the whole neck but shielding the midline by a 2-cm lead strip to protect the larynx and the spinal cord (Fig. 7.21). The upper edge of the field normally lies just above the ramus of the mandible and should preferably be parallel to the lower edge of the nasopharyngeal field without a significant gap between them. This ideal situation may not always be accomplished because of a large mass of nodes high up in the neck. The neck field in such circumstances needs to be adjusted to include the nodes, and as a result there may be an overlap of the fields which cannot be accepted. The area of overlap should be marked on the lateral fields and must be shielded. By careful planning, it is thus possible to leave a wedge-shaped area in the oral cavity untreated

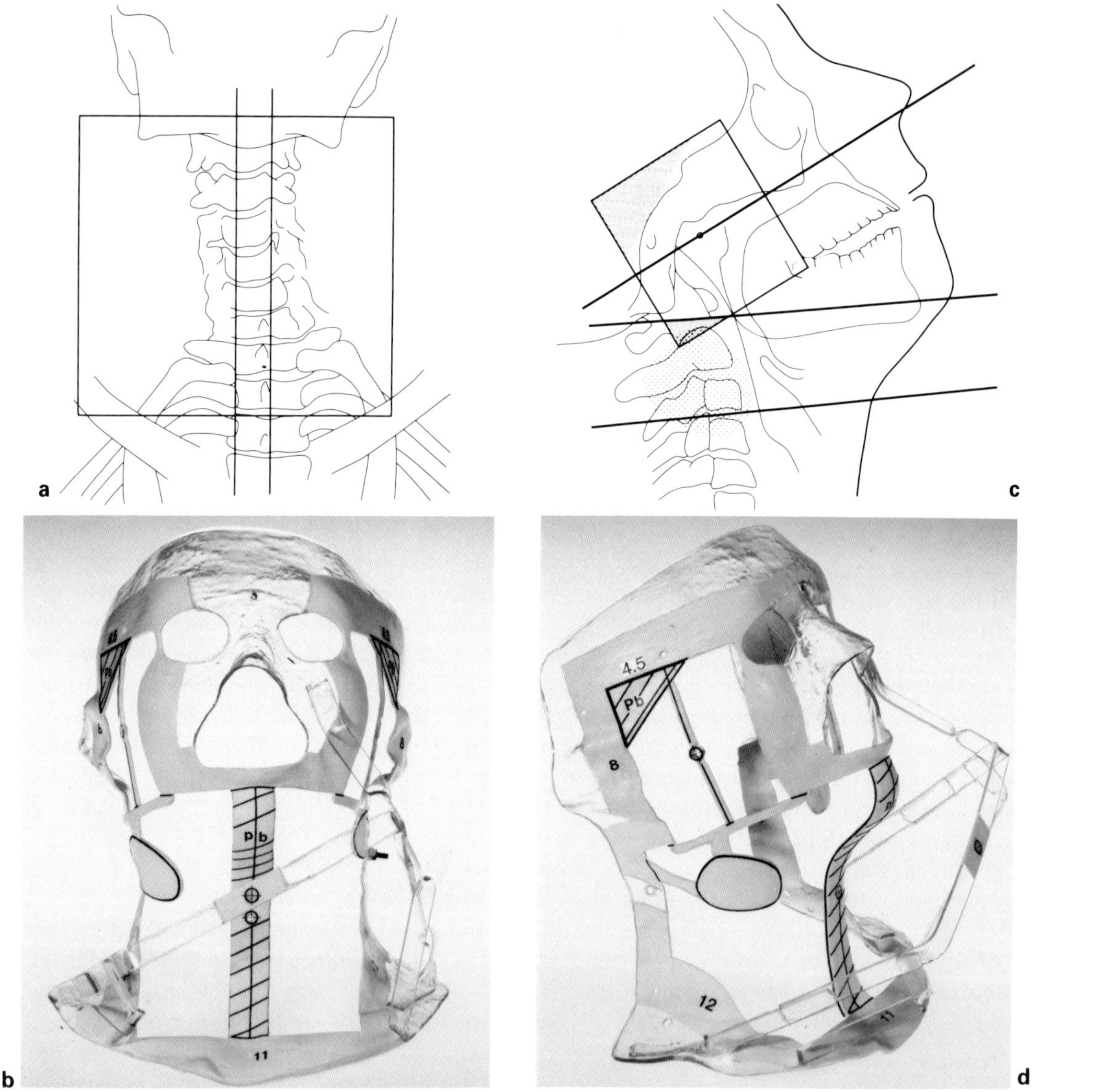

Fig. 7.21a–d. Carcinoma of nasopharynx—Treating primary and cervical nodes.

(Fig. 7.21). The field size ranges from 12×12 cm to 15×15 cm.

When the postnasal space and the neck are treated concurrently, the dose needs to be reduced and a dose of 4500 cGy in 3 weeks to each area would be optimal. If, after a successful treatment to the nasopharynx alone, nodes develop in the neck months later, the neck can be given a dose of 4750–5000 cGy in a similar overall time.

It is often necessary to treat the primary tumour and the nodes in continuity when there is no gap between them. The fields need to be long and a parallel pair of fields suffices. When possible, the spinal cord should be placed outside the path of the

Table 7.4. Spinal cord tolerance.

Fractions/overall time		Dose (cGy)		
16	3 weeks	5000	4250	3500
8	2 weeks	4250	3500	2750
Length of cord (cm)		less than 7	7–15	more than 15

beam and a dose of 4500 cGy can then be given. If, however, the cord has to be included because of the posterior position of the node mass, the dose should be kept within the cord tolerance level (see Table 7.4) and must not exceed 3500 cGy over 3 weeks for a field size more than 15 cm long. Such treatment would of course only be palliative.

Group 4

The treatment for patients in this category is palliative because the prognosis is virtually hopeless. An opposed parallel pair of fields is used. The top end of the fields must cover the base of the skull and the dose should be kept below the level of tolerance of the midbrain. For treatment over 3 weeks, a dose of 4000 cGy is the maximum that can safely be given. More commonly, the general condition of the patient and the advanced state of the disease justify only a short palliative course of X-ray treatment. A dose of 3000 cGy in eight fractions over 2 weeks is appropriate. No attempt should be made to encompass both nodes and primary tumour for such extensive tumours. If, however, the nodes can be included without using unduly long fields this should be done, but the dose needs to be reduced accordingly.

Group 5

The treatment technique is as for group 3.

Group 6

The patients in this category are in a poor physical state and are only suitable for simple palliative X-ray treatment. Treatment should be given according to the need for palliation for symptoms, for example to prevent impending fungation of a nodal mass or to relieve local or bony pain. Alternatively, administration of morphine or heroin in sufficient dosage and at frequent intervals will control pain.

Group 7

Malignant lymphoma, when limited to the head and neck, has a much better prognosis than the more common squamous cell carcinoma and lymphoepithelioma. The fields often necessarily include the spinal cord in order to encompass nodes in the posterior triangle, and the irradiated volume needs to be large to give a generous margin. A dose of 2500–3000 cGy, depending on field size, is given over 3 weeks (see also Chap. 14).

Cancer of the Hypopharynx

Clinical Features

Anatomy

The hypopharynx lies anterior to the fourth and fifth cervical vertebrae, and extends from the level of the floor of the vallecula to the opening of the oesophagus at the level of the inferior border of the cricoid cartilage. Anteriorly is the larynx with the pyriform fossa on either side.

The lymphatics from the hypopharynx may drain into any level of the deep cervical chain of nodes. The lymphatics from the postcricoid area drain directly to the lower deep cervical nodes and to the pre- and paratracheal nodes. Bilateral involvement of neck nodes is frequent when a lesion crosses the midline, particularly from an annular postcricoid growth.

Incidence and Aetiology

The incidence of cancer of the hypopharynx is very similar to that of oropharyngeal cancer. It is common in India and affects about 8 per 100 000 population; in the United Kingdom the incidence is much lower and it is said to occur in less than 1 per 100 000. The disease is commoner in males than females, except for tumours arising from the postcricoid region, which are much more frequent in women and often associated with the Paterson-Brown-Kelly syndrome.

For most patients with hypopharyngeal cancer, the cause is unknown. There is no doubt, however, that a few tumours are radiation-induced after a latent period of about 20 years, the radiation usually having been given for thyrotoxicosis.

Site

Tumours arising from the hypopharynx are listed according to their anatomical sites of origin, for example pyriform fossa, postcricoid, and posterior pharyngeal wall lesions. The pyriform fossae and the postcricoid region are the commonest sites.

Pathology

Unlike tumours of the rest of the pharynx the hypopharyngeal lesions are almost always squamous cell carcinomas and are usually well differentiated. Though solitary plasmacytoma is a rare enough tumour in any site, the hypopharynx appears frequently in published series as a relatively common site, along with the paranasal sinuses (see also Chap. 15).

Spread

Squamous carcinoma of the hypopharynx has a tendency to spread submucosally beyond the visible tumour—a point worth remembering during radiotherapy planning. A lesion arising from the pyriform fossa soon involves the aryepiglottic fold and the ventricular band, and the hemilarynx may become fixed. Involvement of the thyroid gland and the thyroid cartilage is frequent. The postcricoid lesion soon produces narrowing of the lumen by its characteristic circumferential growth, and tends to spread to the larynx superiorly and downwards to the cervical oesophagus.

Early involvement of the lymph nodes is frequent, usually appearing first in the middle deep cervical group. Bilateral involvement is common.

Because of the short survival time of these patients, blood-borne metastases are rarely seen.

Investigation and Diagnosis

A history of a persistent "foreign body" sensation at the back of the throat or discomfort during swallowing, and evidence of obvious weight loss, are strongly suggestive of a tumour in the pharyngo-oesophageal region. Tumours arising from the pyriform fossa or the posterior pharyngeal wall do not usually give marked symptoms until the disease is advanced locally and has spread to nodes, so that the prognosis is bad. The postcricoid tumour produces obstructive symptoms early, but because of the submucosal spread and the early lymphatic involvement the prognosis remains poor. Frequently, a visible lump in the neck is the only reason for a patient to seek a medical opinion, without any symptom attributable to a pharyngeal cancer. In advanced cases there may be gross dysphagia for both solid and liquid foods, sometimes associated with pain and excessive salivation, resulting in malnutrition and weight loss.

Examination of the oral cavity under good illumination may reveal a posterior pharyngeal lesion. Indirect laryngoscopy must be done for a patient having dysphagia, and may reveal a hidden primary tumour in the laryngo-pharyngeal region, particularly in a patient whose only presenting sign is a visible lump in the neck. An exophytic tumour with a pool of mucus in the pyriform fossa can easily be seen. It is often difficult to visualise adequately a tumour in the postcricoid area by indirect examination.

A chest X-ray should be done routinely. A lateral soft tissue view of the neck is often useful to demarcate the extent of the neoplasm. Widening of the prevertebral space in a lateral radiograph of the neck is sinister, and should raise suspicion of a growth in the hypopharyngeal area. Coronal tomography of this area is particularly helpful in defining the extent of the growth, and is also useful in radiotherapy planning. For postcricoid lesions a barium swallow examination is indicated, and may show an irregular filling defect.

Direct laryngo-pharyngoscopic examination under general anaesthesia is mandatory in order to assess the site and extent of the tumour accurately, and confirm the clinical and radiological findings. A biopsy must be obtained at the same time.

Careful and systematic examination of the neck must be carried out. When nodes are involved the disease is advanced and for most patients the prognosis is hopeless.

A routine full blood count should be done and for postcricoid tumours the serum folate and serum iron should be estimated.

Treatment Policy

A carcinoma of the hypopharynx usually produces symptoms only when the tumour is well advanced and has already spread to the regional lymph nodes. Most patients when first seen therefore have advanced disease with gross dysphagia. They may be in pain and show signs of malnutrition.

Unfortunately the vast majority of patients are not suitable for curative treatment, whether by surgery or by radiotherapy. Palliative radiotherapy in such advanced cases is of dubious benefit, and should be withheld. For patients in reasonably good general condition, a simple regime of chemotherapy such as one or two injections of methotrexate (100 mg/m^2) at an interval of 3–4 weeks gives the best palliation without adding much discomfort.

Radiotherapy remains the primary treatment of choice for lesions which are not too advanced and which can be encompassed by modest field sizes up to 10×5 cm. Surgery is mutilating and requires laryngo-pharyngectomy with restoration of continuity of the alimentary tract. The 5-year survival figure of between 20% and 30% following radiotherapy is very similar to that of most surgical series. The value of chemotherapy in conjunction with radiotherapy is under investigation and the preliminary findings are encouraging. Unlike cancer of the larynx or of the oropharynx, it is often difficult to assess the state of the hypopharynx at follow-up, so that salvage surgery is not often possible.

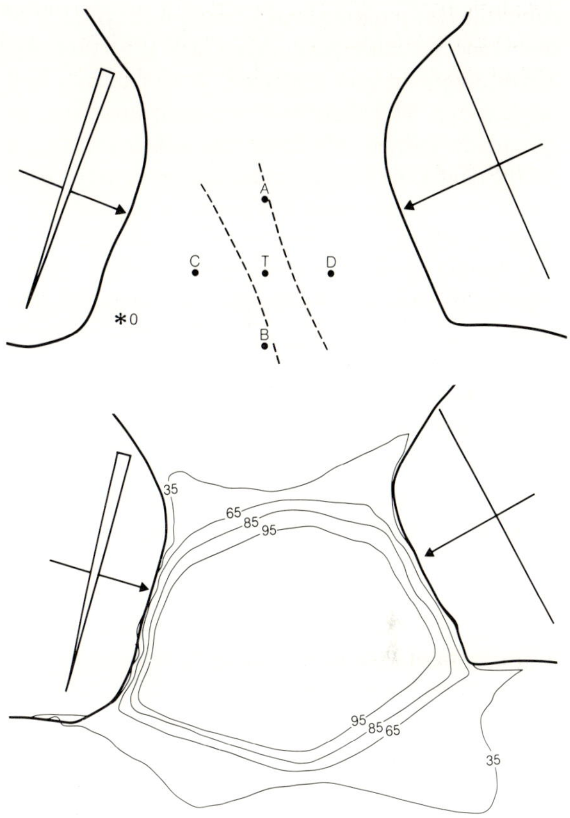

Fig. 7.22. Carcinoma of hypopharynx—tipped parallel pair technique.

Treatment Techniques

Because bilateral involvement of cervical lymph nodes is so frequent from hypopharyngeal neoplasms, both sides of the neck should be included in the treatment volume. This is achieved by an opposed parallel pair of fields, using wedge filters or compensators as required (see Fig. 7.24). The field sizes range from 7×5 cm to 10×6 cm. These sizes are necessary in order to give at least 2 cm clearance from the visible edge of the growth and to cover the lymph drainage system. For a postcricoid tumour, however, an opposed parallel pair of fields would not be feasible because the lower margin of the fields would impinge on the shoulders. For this site the fields need to be tilted so that their upper ends are closer together, and a vertical wedge filter is required to compensate for the vertical obliquity of the surface contour of the neck (Fig. 7.22).

Any palpable nodes must be included in the treatment volume and this may mean angling the fields forwards a few degrees to exclude the spinal cord from the beams. Care must be taken not to miss the primary tumour in the treated volume by angling the fields to much. If the spinal cord has to be included in the treated volume because of the posterior position of the nodes, the dose must be kept below the radiation tolerance of the cord.

The treatment technique is very similar to that for laryngeal carcinoma and is described in the next section. For an area up to 40 cm^2, a dose of 5250 cGy is the optimum, given in 16 fractions over 3 weeks.

Cancer of the Larynx

Introduction

Cancer of the larynx is relatively common, and when the lesion is limited to the vocal cord, the 5-year cure rate following radiotherapy is of the order of 90%. Laryngectomy does indeed produce a comparably high cure rate for early tumours but cannot justifiably compete with the much superior functional result following radiotherapy, and the sophisticated electronic larynx is in no way a substitute for a natural voice, even if the quality of the voice remains poor after radiation therapy. Early diagnosis and treatment are of paramount importance. The chances of a patient surviving for 5 years drop drastically from about 90% for stage I glottic cancer to 60% for stage III and a mere 10% for stage IV tumours. It should be stressed that accurate beam direction to a minimum volume and a radiation dose to the maximum normal tissue tolerance are necessary to achieve the best results. Inadequate treatment technique and inadequate dosage fail to achieve the maximum possible cure rate and this leads to a high laryngectomy rate for radiation failure. By contrast, the supraglottic and subglottic cancers produce symptoms relatively late and have a high incidence of metastases to the neck nodes, so that the overall 5-year cure rate in these sites is only about 40%.

Clinical Features

Anatomy

The larynx is bounded superiorly by the posterior surface of the tip of the epiglottis, the aryepiglottic folds, and the inter-arytenoid region; and inferiorly by the lower border of the cricoid cartilage. The region superior to the lower border of the false cords is referred to as supraglottic, and that below the true cords as subglottic, the true cords themselves, with the anterior and posterior commissures, forming the glottic region.

Lymphatics

The true vocal cords are devoid of any lymphatic vessels. The supraglottic region has a rich lymphatic plexus which drains primarily to the upper deep cervical nodes. The lymphatics from the subglottic region drain into the prelaryngeal, lower and middle deep cervical, and paratracheal nodes. The supraglottic and subglottic regions have a lymphatic "watershed" in the midline, across which lymphatic communication is free, so that metastases from these regions commonly occur to either or both sides of the neck. The incidence of metastases to nodes clearly varies according to the primary site, occurring more often from supraglottic (33%) and subglottic (20%) tumours and rarely from the glottic region except when the tumour involves the anterior or posterior commissure.

Anatomic Subdivisions

The divisions of the larynx have been classified by the UICC as follows:

Supraglottis Epilarynx including marginal zone.

1) Posterior surface of suprahyoid epiglottis including the tip
2) Aryepiglottic fold
3) Arytenoid

Supraglottis excluding epilarynx

4) Infrahyoid epiglottis
5) Ventricular bands (false cords)
6) Ventricular cavities

Glottis

1) Vocal cords
2) Anterior commissure
3) Posterior commissure

Subglottis

Incidence and Aetiology

Cancer of the larynx accounts for about 2% of all malignant conditions. It is commoner in men than women in a ratio of 7:1. The incidence in great Britain is about 4 per 100 000 population, and the highest incidence reported is 14 per 100 000 of the population in both Brazil and the Indian subcontinent. The aetiology is uncertain, but heavy smoking and chewing of tobacco may be contributory factors.

Histology

Squamous cell carcinoma is by far the commonest histological type. The tumours of the vocal cords are generally well-differentiated, whereas those arising from the supraglottic and subglottic regions are often poorly differentiated. Other malignant tumours are rare and include adenocarcinoma, transitional cell carcinoma, malignant melanoma, plasmacytoma, fibrosarcoma, and chondrosarcoma.

TNM Classification (Summary)

Glottis	T_{IS}	Carcinoma in situ
	T_1	Limited/mobile a. one cord b. both cords
	T_2	Extension to supra- or sub-glottis/mobile
	T_3	Fixation of cord(s)
	T_4	Extension beyond larynx
Supra- and subglottis	T_{IS}	Carcinoma in situ
	T_1	Limited/mobile
	T_2	Extension to glottis/mobile
	T_3	Fixation of cord(s)
	T_4	Extension beyond larynx
All regions	N_0	No node involvement
	N_1	Homolateral movable
	N_2	Contra- or bilateral movable
	N_3	Fixed
	M_0	No evidence of metastases
	M_1	Evidence of distant metastases
	M_X	Minimum requirements to assess the presence of distant metastases cannot be met

Spread

The glottis is the commonest site of origin of laryngeal carcinoma. The tumour usually arises from the anterior two-thirds of a vocal cord and spreads forwards to the anterior commissure. Posterior spread to the arytenoid is less common. The glottic tumour may be unilateral or bilateral, and may extend to the supraglottic or subglottic region (T_2) with normal or impaired mobility of the vocal cords. In more advanced cases one or both cords may be fixed (T_3) and the tumour may progress by direct extension beyond the larynx (T_4). Thyroid cartilage acts as a barrier against anterior spread of the true vocal cord tumour for a long time, but because of the lack of an effective barrier posteriorly, the tumour can easily gain access to the pyriform fossa and to the postcricoid region.

A supraglottic cancer may arise anywhere from the posterior surface of the tip of the epiglottis superiorly to the ventricular cavities inferiorly. Until a supraglottic tumour is moderately advanced there are few symptoms. For tumours involving the infrahyoid epiglottis the mode of spread is primarily towards the pre-epiglottic space. Tumours arising from the false cords or the ventricular cavities, however, spread more easily to the pyriform fossa. Extension of tumour to the posterior third of the tongue or the vallecula commonly occurs from a primary epilaryngeal cancer (that is, the posterior surface of the suprahyoid epiglottis including the tip, the aryepiglottic fold, and the arytenoid). It may be difficult, on occasions, to ascertain the precise site of origin of the tumour, but careful laryngoscopic examination during and after treatment may indicate the site of origin if the path of tumour regression is followed. Metastases to both ipsilateral and contralateral nodes occur frequently.

Primary subglottic tumours are rare. Extension of disease to the cricothyroid membrane, thyroid gland, or deep fascia and strap muscles is more frequent than from the remainder of the larynx. Lymphatic spread is early. Because of the lack of early symptoms, and easy access of the tumour to adjacent structures, the prognosis for a subglottic tumour is disappointing.

Investigation and Diagnosis

Hoarseness of voice is the first and most persistent symptom of a glottic tumour. Hoarseness may also occur when the vocal cords become involved secondarily by the extension of a primary tumour arising in the supraglottic or subglottic region, but late in the course of the disease. When the tumour obstructs the airway, stridor develops. If the pharynx is involved, the patient complains of a sore throat and may eventually develop dysphagia. In a few advanced cases pain may be referred to the ear on the affected side.

The clinical history of intermittent or persistent hoarseness, possibly in association with a sore throat, recent stridor, or earache, should suggest the diagnosis. The neck should be observed from the front for any visible mass of nodes, which may be the presenting feature in a few cases. In addition, the neck should also be observed for any asymmetry or abnormality which may be caused by the expansion of the larynx, or involvement of the thyroid cartilage or the surrounding skin by the primary tumour. Stridor, if present, is obvious.

Palpation of the neck may reveal expansion of

the larynx and normal laryngeal crepitation may be lost because of fixation of the larynx posteriorly by tumour infiltration. The cartilages should also be palpated for any abnormality. Because involvement of the cervical nodes is common, careful palpation of the neck should be carried out in an orderly manner. The tip of the styloid process, the transverse process of the second cervical vertebra, the anterior cornu of the hyoid, and the carotid bulb are normal structures which must not be mistaken for lymph nodes. A palpable mass in the neck may be an extension of the primary tumour.

Indirect laryngoscopy is essential to assess the extent of spread of the disease. At the same time, the oropharynx and hypopharynx should be inspected for any abnormality. A local anaesthetic spray to the orpharynx may be necessary in difficult cases, if the patient gags uncontrollably. Rarely, an overlying "infantile" epiglottis may make visualisation of the larynx difficult or impossible.

All patients should have a chest X-ray to exclude metastatic deposits, or even a second primary bronchial carcinoma. The latter is not common but has been estimated to occur in about 5%–10% of cases. A lateral radiograph of the neck is useful, and may reveal a defect in a calcified thyroid cartilage. Sometimes a careful examination of the radiograph will show a soft tissue mass in the larynx, the limits of which can easily be defined. The normal prevertebral space may be widened, if the tumour involves the hypopharynx. The opportunity should be taken to look for any abnormality in the bones. Tomography of the larynx is an important radiological investigation to study the extent of the disease and is particularly useful in defining the subglottic spread and the extension of a laryngeal lesion to the hypopharynx. The knowledge gained from the tomogram is also helpful in treatment planning.

A full blood count should be done routinely.

Direct laryngoscopic examination under a general anaesthetic is mandatory in order to assess the extent of the disease accurately and confirm the previous findings. A biopsy must be taken to confirm the diagnosis.

Treatment Policy

The management of laryngeal carcinoma is best carried out by a specialist team. Patients should be seen in a joint consultative clinic by a surgeon and a radiotherapist to assess the extent of the tumour and to decide treatment and subsequent management. The object of treatment in most cases should be curative irrespective of the methods chosen, whether by radiotherapy alone or by a combination of surgery and radiotherapy. There is no indication for palliative radiotherapy for laryngeal cancer, for though radiation in such cases may help to reduce pain and possibly prevent fungation, the dose of radiation which needs to be given to a moderately large volume necessarily produces a brisk reaction with increasing oedema of the larynx, making swallowing more difficult for the patient. The mucus becomes viscid and difficult to expel, adding much discomfort.

Surgery and radiotherapy are the only methods of curative treatment for cancer of the larynx. For early lesions limited to one vocal cord in its middle third, laryngofissure is an excellent treatment, although at the price of a permanent voice impairment. In more advanced cases with involvement of both vocal cords, extension to the supraglottic or subglottic region, or fixation of a cord, total laryngectomy is the only safe surgical approach. Supraglottic laryngectomy has been advised for some carcinomas arising from the epiglottis, but there is always a danger of leaving malignant disease behind. Radiotherapy as an initial treatment spares about half of these patients from having a primary laryngectomy, will often achieve a cure, and is therefore the treatment of choice. If radiation treatment fails, subsequent laryngectomy is still possible.

Indications for Primary Surgery

1) An advanced tumour with impaired airway where tracheostomy will be required
2) A glottic cancer with supraglottic or subglottic spread associated with mobile neck nodes
3) An advanced tumour with clinical involvement of the cartilage

Indications for Surgery After Radical Radiotherapy

1) Recurrent or residual malignancy following initial treatment by radiotherapy
2) Chondronecrosis following radiotherapy

Indications for Radical Radiotherapy

1) Glottic cancer T_{1-3} without neck node involvement
2) Supraglottic cancer T_{1-3} with or without neck node involvement
3) Subglottic cancer
4) Primary surgery is indicated, but the patient is unfit for surgery for medical reasons or refuses surgery

Carcinoma in situ

The choice of treatment for carcinoma in situ is primarily determined by the site and extent of the lesion. If it is limited to the vocal cords, stripping the mucosa of the affected area may be sufficient. Such cases, however, need close follow-up, and if laryngoscopy shows recurrence, a biopsy should be taken to exclude the presence of an invasive carcinoma for which radical radiotherapy would be necessary.

If the in situ lesion is extensive when first seen, especially if it extends beyond the true cords, radiotherapy is the treatment of choice. There are a few patients who have a small area of in situ disease, otherwise suitable for stripping, who cannot for one reason or other guarantee to attend regularly for their follow-up examinations, and such patients are also best treated initially by radiotherapy.

Treatment is given using a wedge pair, as described for an early carcinoma (T_1 glottic carcinoma) of the larynx. Cordectomy is still occasionally done for these cases, but the functional result is of course much inferior.

Glottic Tumours

T_1 Surgery or radiotherapy give identical cure rates for this group of tumours, but radiotherapy is universally preferred because the patient retains his larynx, and usually a good voice also. Before the introduction of megavoltage radiation, the Finzi Harmer operation using radium needles achieved an excellent functional result and a high percentage of cures. In the last 25 years megavoltage radiation has been accepted as a better alternative because it does not involve operation, and avoids the trauma of radium needles. The dose distribution, unlike that of an implant, can be arranged to be virtually perfect.

T_2 When there is extension of tumour off the cord to the supraglottic or subglottic areas, treatment by megavoltage X-ray therapy gives results almost identical to those obtained in T_1 glottic lesions.

T_3 For more advanced tumours with fixation of the cord, but without involvement of the neck nodes, radical radiotherapy alone achieves more than 60% 5-year survival and avoids many unnecessary laryngectomies. When radiation fails, subsequent laryngectomy is still possible, and is no more difficult than a primary laryngectomy.

T_{1-3} N_{1-3} Metastases to the cervical nodes may occur when the vocal cord lesion extends to the anterior or posterior commissure or spreads beyond the true cord to the supraglottic or subglottic areas. In such cases, if the nodes are mobile, laryngectomy with block dissection of the neck gives the best chance of cure. If, however, the nodes are fixed, radiotherapy should be given to the primary tumour and the node-bearing area in one volume. If the primary regresses completely, leaving residual palpable but mobile nodes, block dissection can be considered.

Supraglottic Tumours

T_{1-3} N_{1-3} The incidence of metastases to nodes from cancer at this site may reach 40%. Because surgery for supraglottic cancer necessitates laryngo-pharyngectomy with bilateral block dissection of the neck, radical radiotherapy should be tried as the primary treatment, and should be expected to cure 40% of cases. If tumour regression is unsatisfactory, or the nodes persist, salvage surgery should then be considered.

Subglottic Tumours

Primary tumours in the subglottic area are rare. Treatment may be by surgery or by radical X-ray treatment, both of which give 5-year cure rates of the order of 40%, but radiotherapy is the preferred treatment because it avoids the functional defects of surgery. Visualisation of the subglottic space is often difficult by indirect laryngoscopy, and endoscopy under anaesthetic is usually necessary.

Treatment Techniques

Energy of Radiation

The use of megavoltage radiation has produced a marginal improvement in survival figures compared with kilovoltage radiation, but the real benefit has been derived from the skin sparing effect, lack of penumbra, superior collimation, and the lack of preferential absorption in cartilage. These factors help by minimising the radiation reaction of the surrounding normal tissues and by achieving more effective shielding of the spinal cord. Homogeneity of dose distribution in the treated volume is easily obtained. An energy between 2 and 6 MV is more than adequate for treating any tumour of the head and neck region, when photons are used.

Immobilisation

The patient lies supine with the neck extended and held in position on a neck rest. Immobilisation of the neck during treatment is achieved by a well-fitted cellulose acetate or Perspex shell reaching from the level of the angle of the jaw down to just below the level of the clavicle, thus fixing the head in relation to the thoracic inlet.

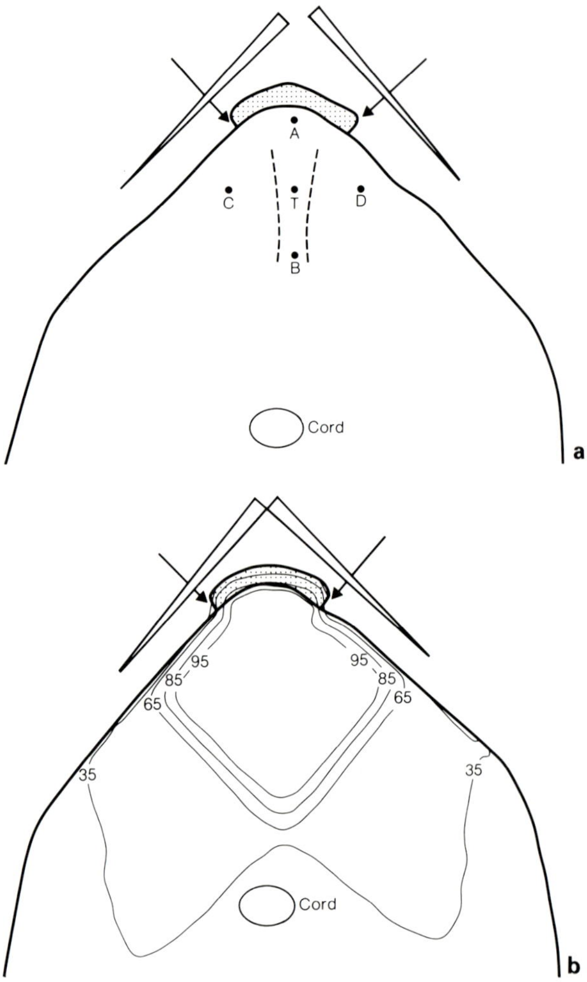

Fig. 7.23 Carcinoma of glottis—wedge pair technique.

Field Arrangement

For a T_1 glottic tumour two anterior oblique wedged beams are used. The beams are angled at about 90° to give a homogeneous dose to the treatment volume (Fig. 7.23). A 4–6 mm thickness of unit-density material (normally one or two layers of the Perspex), depending on the energy of radiation, is required to be placed anteriorly on the shell as a "build-up", between the entrance points of the central axes of the beams. This extends the high-dose zone anteriorly so as to include the anterior commissure. This technique minimises the tissue reaction at the sides of the neck but is only suitable for early cord lesions. For T_{2-3} glottic tumours and all supraglottic and subglottic tumours, both sides of the neck should be included in the treatment volume so that the lymph drainage areas are included. This is achieved (Fig. 7.24) by an opposed parallel pair of fields, using appropriate wedge filters or compensators to correct for the oblique incidence of the surface of the neck. Treatment by plain (unwedged) fields would create an inhomogeneity of up to 20% (Fig. 7.24a), and must not be used.

Field Size

It is important that the tumour should be localised accurately. This is done by taking a true lateral radiograph of the tumour region whilst the patient wears the shell, on which are fitted two sets of radio-opaque markers. By relating these to the anatomical landmarks, localisation and final verification should be accurate. Care must be taken to avoid placing the spinal cord in the path of the beams. The field sizes usually range from 5×4

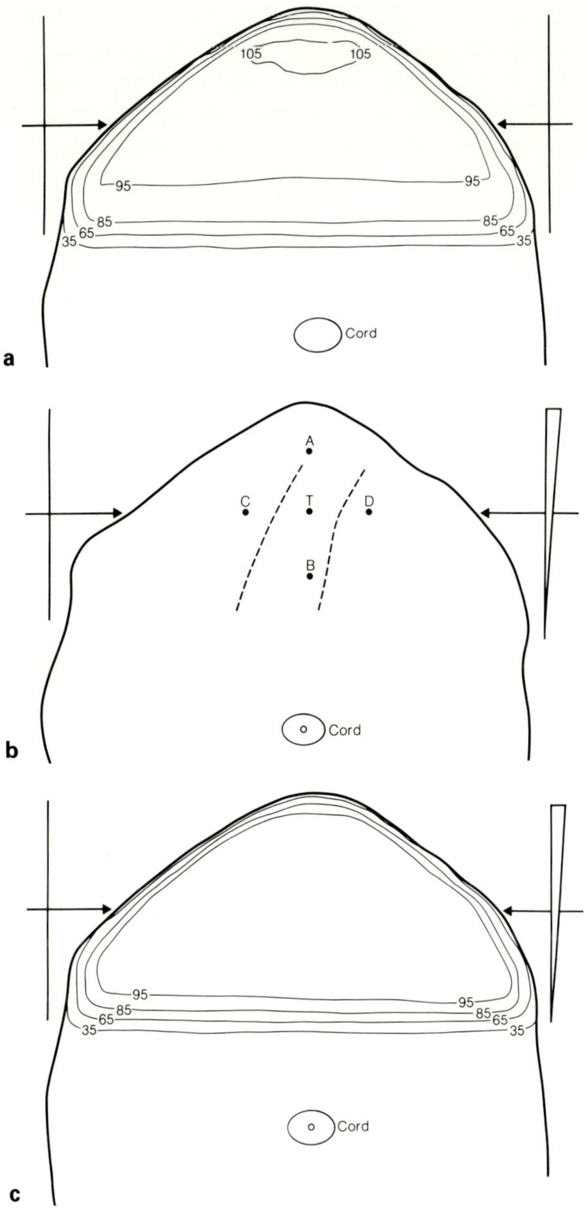

Fig. 7.24. a Carcinoma of supraglottic larynx—parallel pair without wedge. **b** Carcinoma of supraglottic !arynx—parallel pair with wedge.

cm to 5×5 cm for early lesions. For more advanced tumours field sizes up to 7×5 cm may be necessary for radical treatment. If the neck is short, or if there is considerable subglottic extension, two parallel opposed fields may not be feasible because the lower margins of the fields would impinge on the shoulders. In such cases the fields need to be tilted so that their upper ends are closer together, and a vertical wedge filter is required to compensate for the vertical obliquity of the surface contour of the neck (see Fig. 7.25).

Wedge Filters

For an early (T_1) cord lesion treated by two anterior oblique fields, two 40° wedges with their thick ends close to each other, at a hinge angle of approximately 90°, give a balanced dose distribution.

In all other cases where two lateral opposed fields are used, two 20° wedges, one on either side of the neck, or more commonly a plain field (unwedged) on one side and a 40° wedge field on the opposite side are usually necessary to correct the horizontal irregular surface contour of the neck. The thick end of the wedge is placed anteriorly. If the neck is short, an additional 30° or 40° wedge is necessary, placed vertically on the unwedged side of the neck, as well as the wedge on the opposite side of the neck in the horizontal plane.

Dose, Fractionation, and Overall Time

It is critically important to adhere to a well-established optimum dose, time, and fractionation schedule which has been determined over a long period of clinical experience. Until we understand more clearly the relationship between dose and time, an established treatment regime which gives good results should not be replaced. Clinical experience in the past and contemporary studies indicate that increasing the overall treatment time beyond 3 weeks does not influence survival, morbidity, or the laryngectomy rates.

It should be stressed that especially for tumours of the head and neck region, accurate beam direction to a minimum volume is of paramount importance. The highest dose can then be delivered homogeneously to the treated volume without exceeding the normal tissue tolerance, and a high percentage of tumour control is achieved. In patients with laryngeal carcinoma, a necrosis rate of 3%–5% is acceptable and should be expected following radical radiotherapy. Failure to produce a small incidence of necrosis suggests inadequate dosage, which is associated with a lower cure rate.

Figure 7.25 demonstrates the incidence of recurrence and necrosis plotted against dose, the dose always being given in 16 fractions over 22 days (3 weeks) with a 4-MV linear accelerator. The recurrence rate of T_1 tumours is constant over the dose range 5250–5750 cGy, and this group has the

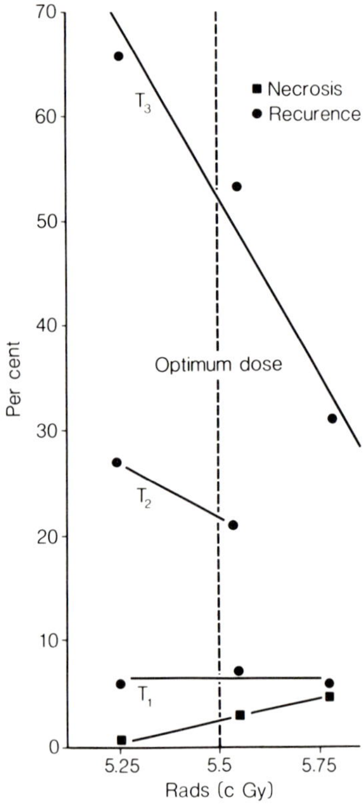

Fig. 7.25. Carcinoma of larynx—dose response curves.

least risk of necrosis. For T_{IS} and T_1 tumours, 5250 cGy is adequate for tumour control, but for more advanced lesions (T_{2-3}) the recurrence rate is significantly lower in the higher dose ranges. However, the optimum dose should be chosen by balancing the increased tumour control against the incidence of necrosis. In most situations with a treatment area of up to 35 cm^2, a dose of 5500 cGy in 16 fractions over 22 days is the optimum.

Radiation Reaction

A sequence of changes occurs in the tumour-bearing area and in the surrounding normal tissues during and immediately after radiation therapy which is often uncomfortable, but unavoidable. A frank discussion with the patient before starting treatment helps to allay fear, and good nursing care helps to minimise discomfort.

The time of onset and the duration of the reaction period depend on the dose, the overall time, and the fractionation regime, in addition to individual susceptibility to radiation. Following the start of a 5 days per week, 3-week course of treatment, there is a latent period of about 7–10 days before visible changes occur in the treated area. After a brief erythema, white or yellowish patches develop which slowly become confluent. At the same time the tumour begins to resolve, though restoration of normal contours does not take place till about 2 months after treatment, and in advanced cases may take longer. There is some oedema which, whilst usually not sufficient to cause concern, rarely develops to the point of causing obstruction, and when this happens usually indicates an ill-judged initial selection of patients.

The peak of the radiation reaction usually occurs at about the 12th treatment. Completion of the treatment to the prescribed radical dose does not usually enhance the reaction. In a small proportion of cases the reaction develops late, with very little fibrin visible by the end of treatment. Conversely, the radiation reaction may develop during the early part of the treatment. In either situation there may be a temptation to alter the prescribed dose, which should be resisted. Early and late reactions do develop in a small number of patients, and are related to the variations in individual susceptibility to radiation. The reaction in such situations should rarely be used as an indication for a change of dose.

The radiation reaction makes swallowing difficult and in most cases the voice becomes more hoarse. An antibiotic syrup is often helpful during the final week of treatment. Paracetamol mucilage about 20 min before each meal helps to make swallowing easier. The skin reaction in most cases does not need any treatment, but if moist desquamation does develop, the local application of a simple cream is soothing.

Subsequent Management

Follow-up examinations are best conducted by both radiotherapist and surgeon in a combined clinic. It is most important to watch for early tumour recurrence or persistent residual tumour because salvage surgery may still be possible. If indirect laryngoscopy is inadequate because of anatomical distortion or lack of cooperation of the patient, even after using a local anaesthetic spray, it is essential to carry out direct laryngoscopy without delay.

Careful palpation of the neck for lymph node metastases is equally important. If a soft mobile node is found, which is tender on palpation, it could well be an inflammatory lymphadenitis. If the node persists, however, even after a course of antibiotics, block dissection of the neck should be carried out without delay. If a node appears and disease is still present in the larynx, laryngectomy and a block dissection is indicated.

It is not uncommon after treatment to find persistent changes which lead to a suspicion of residual or recurrent disease. It is then tempting to take a biopsy, or even repeated biopsies, but in general the temptation should be resisted because of the real danger of precipitating necrosis in the irradiated tissues. Moreover, such biopsies frequently show no tumour, even when subsequent events show tumour to have been present. Under the circumstances, clinical experience is often of more value than a biopsy, and should take precedence in determining whether or not rescue surgery is necessary.

Complications

Necrosis of the laryngeal cartilages is the major complication, which occurs in about 3% of cases following well-planned beam-directed radiotherapy, especially if the tumour has infiltrated cartilage. The onset of perichondritis or necrosis may be immediate or delayed, and is marked by pain, local tenderness, and sometimes fever. If the symptoms are more than transient it may be safest to proceed with laryngectomy immediately, because a painful necrotic larynx never heals with conservative treatment, and underlying neoplasm is often present. Persistent laryngeal oedema may be a cause of concern after radiation therapy, but oedema by itself has little prognostic significance.

Palliative Management

Stridor, dysphagia, excessive salivation, and pain are the most unpleasant symptoms from advanced laryngeal cancer. The sensation of suffocation from airway obstruction is distressing to the patient and to the family, and should be avoided by timely tracheostomy. Any major surgical procedure at this terminal stage only adds further misery. Although radiotherapy may offer some palliation by reducing tumour mass and diminishing local pain, the small benefit is so often outweighed by the symptoms of sore throat and increasing dysphagia induced by the treatment that radiotherapy in such a situation is of no overall benefit and should be withheld. Similarly, any attempt at intense treatment using combination chemotherapy is probably not justified, but one or two injections of methotrexate (100 mg/m^2) at an interval of 3–4 weeks may be helpful without causing harm.

For dysphagia in the terminal stages of laryngeal cancer gastrostomy is sometimes recommended, but should be avoided if possible. It is very unpleasant for the patient, and by prolonging life for a little while may only give time for the patient to develop further unpleasant complications, such as severe pain.

Excessive salivation is also common in uncontrolled cancer of the larynx. Repeated mouth washes with 1% sodium bicarbonate and a liberal fluid intake help to aid expulsion of the viscid secretions. Humidifying the room is also of some benefit, and probanthine or a small dose of belladonna may be a useful addition.

Local pain, often due to involvement of cartilage, or pain referred to the ear from involvement of the glossopharyngeal nerve is common in advanced cases and needs appropriate analgesics. Aspirin or paracetamol in sufficient dosage and at frequent intervals may soon have to be replaced by stronger drugs such as physeptone and finally by morphia or heroin. The well-known Brompton cocktail is still useful, primarily because the patient can keep it at his bedside. Fear, depression, and anxiety are always present, and may be at least partially relieved by the addition of a tranquilliser such as diazepam or chlordiazepoxide. Lack of hygienic conditions in the mouth together with accumulated mucous secretions in or around the tumour may encourage infection and therefore increase pain, so that a course of broad-spectrum antibiotic may be helpful.

Nose and Nasal Sinuses

Clinical Features

The aetiology of the majority of malignant tumours of the nose and nasal sinuses remains unknown. There is good evidence to suggest that persons engaged in the manufacture or repair of leather footwear run a special risk of developing cancer of the nasal cavity or associated nasal sinuses. Although the carcinogen has not been isolated, the evidence points to the dust generated in processes connected with the preparation of leather in the footwear manufacture and repair trades. In most cases there is a long latent period up to 40 years. Adenocarcinoma of the nasal cavity and sinuses is a rare condition, but there is good evidence that workers in the furniture industry run a special risk of developing it. The hazard involves the inhalation of wood dust but here, too, a specific carcinogen has not been identified. The wood dusts mainly involved are those of oak and birch. The latent period following exposure is again about 40 years. Another industrial hazard is the processing of certain nickel-rich raw materials. The precise causal irritant has not been identified. In such cases the average duration of exposure to risk before diagnosis is 22 years.

Carcinoma of the Nose

Carcinomas of the nasal cavity and septum are rare. Before the lesion is accepted as arising primarily in the nose, the ethmoids, maxillary antrum, and postnasal spaces must be excluded as primary sites. Lesions involving the floor of the nasal cavity may arise primarily in the skin and less commonly from the hard palate. Histologically the common lesion is a squamous cell carcinoma but transitional cell carcinoma, adenocarcinoma, adenoid cystic carcinoma, and malignant melanoma all occur, together with rare lesions such as olfactory neuroblastoma. Clinically, having excluded a possible origin from nasal sinuses, the most critical feature is the posterior extent of the lesion. If there is doubt about this, resort should be made to examination under anaesthesia before planning treatment.

Treatment

Anteriorly situated lesions may be treated by a single megavoltage X-ray field, care being taken to avoid irradiating the eyes. This can be achieved by narrowing the field superiorly, thus producing a spade-shaped field. Using such an arrangement a dose of 5500 cGy in 15 fractions over 21 days is given, using a field 6×5 cm in size (Fig. 7.26). An alternative method is the use of two wedged fields

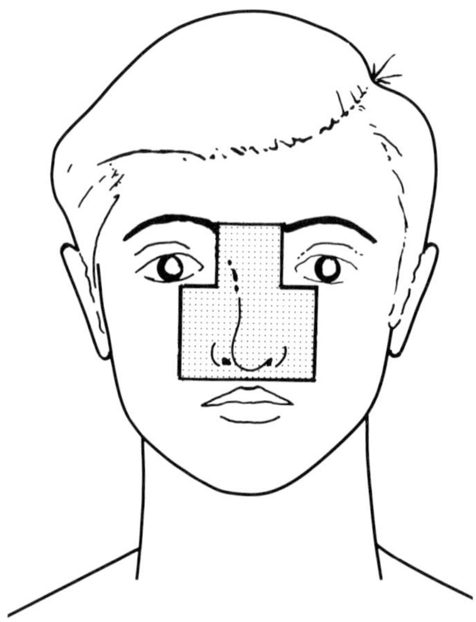

Fig. 7.26 Carcinoma of nasal cavity—single anterior field.

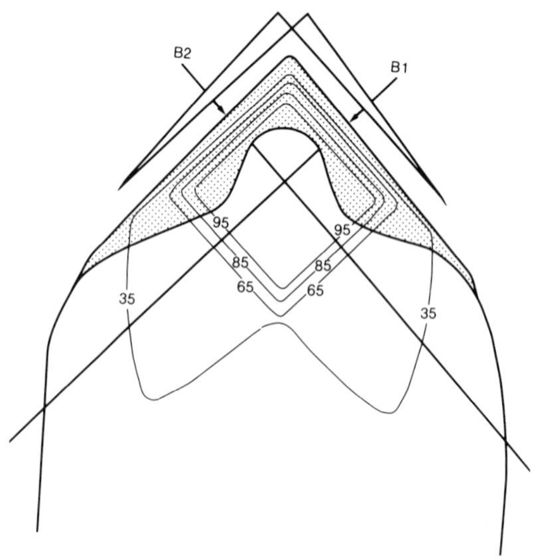

Fig. 7.27. Carcinoma of nasal cavity—wedge pair.

(Fig. 7.27), which is particularly suited to lesions arising from the lower part of the nose, septum, and vestibule. The field size used is 5×5 cm or less and the dose delivered is 5250–5500 cGy in 16 fractions over 21 days.

Maxillary Antrum and Ethmoid Sinuses

Carcinomas of the maxillary antrum and ethmoid sinuses are uncommon. Their maximum incidence occurs in patients between 55 and 75 years of age, with a mean age of 62 years. The male-to-female sex ratio of incidence is 1.5:1.

Histology

Over 80% of tumours are of epidermoid origin. The other principal histological types are adenocarcinoma, adenoid cystic carcinoma, malignant melanoma, lymphoma, and soft tissue sarcoma.

Lymph Drainage

Whilst it is generally accepted that the primary lymphatic drainage is to the retropharyngeal lymph nodes, in clinical practice the lymph nodes involved are those draining the tissues involved when the tumour has, in addition to the retropharyngeal nodes, extended beyond the anatomical boundaries of the primary site.

Clinical Presentation

The maxilla, in addition to forming the hard palate and upper alveoli, forms a large part of the floor of the orbit. The medial walls form the lateral walls of the nose. The ethmoid sinuses form the upper part of the nasal passages and part of the floor of the anterior cranial fossa. The clinical features of antral and ethmoidal carcinoma are determined by these anatomical boundaries and thus may be considered under the following four rubrics:

1) Nasal Cavity

There may be nasal obstruction due to tumour, with associated discharge which may be bloody. The nose may be broadened. Widening of the bridge of the nose with bulging in the inner canthus is a characteristic feature of ethmoidal involvement.

2) Cheek

With anterolateral extension of the tumour there will be bulging of the cheek and there may be involvement of the soft tissues and skin of the cheek. Asymmetry may be present and this is more obvious if the patient is viewed from behind with the neck extended. With gross involvement the normal folds of the face will be obliterated, with depression of the angle of the mouth. Anaesthesia of the skin may be present, usually in the distribution of the second division of the fifth cranial nerve.

3) Orbit

With involvement of the orbit, proptosis and displacement of the eye may result.

4) Mouth

There may be bulging of the hard palate with ulceration. When there has been considerable destruction of the palate, a probe can be passed with ease through the palate into the antrum. There may be filling of the alveolobuccal sulcus and an antro-oral fistula. If there is extension to the pterygoid fossa, trismus will be a feature.

Investigation

While careful clinical examination will indicate obvious extension, the full extent of the lesion will only be demonstrated by precise radiology. Wide-angle tomography (i.e. hypocycloidal or spiral) is an essential part of the investigation. CT scanning is complementary to, but affords no significant advantage over, good wide-angle tomography. Disease confined to the maxillary antrum alone is much less common than antro-ethmoidal involvement. It is rare to find less than two walls of the maxillary antrum involved. The demonstration of orbital involvement is of paramount importance in the planning of treatment.

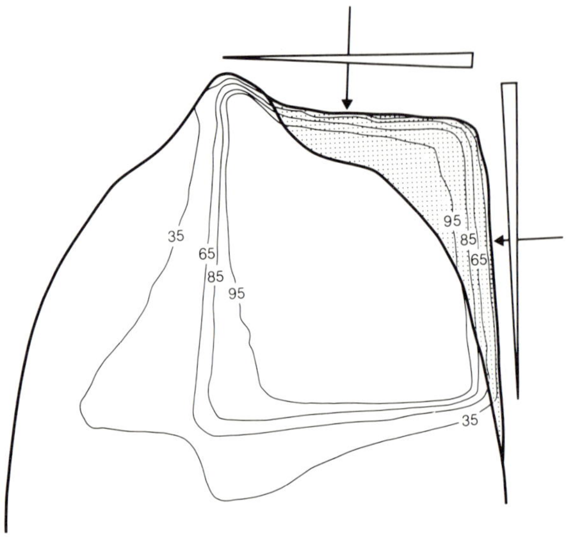

Fig. 7.28. Carcinoma of antrum—wedge pair.

Classification and Staging

There are at present no recommendations by the UICC for the classification and staging of tumours of the paranasal sinuses, a fact which underlines the difficulty of devising a wholly satisfactory system of staging.

Treatment Policy

The successful management of a patient with carcinoma of the nose and nasal sinuses depends on full cooperation between the ear, nose, and throat surgeon, the oral surgeon, and the radiotherapist. Each patient should be jointly assessed and the subsequent management agreed. The policy adopted is that radiotherapy is the principal method of treatment. The role of surgery may be summarised as (1) to provide adequate material for histological diagnosis, (2) to establish drainage, (3) to indicate, where necessary, the extent of the lesion, and (4) rarely to remove the bulk of the tumour.

Routine fenestration of the hard palate has not been practised at the Christie Hospital because it was felt that with modern radiotherapy it did not contribute significantly to management and was therefore not essential.

Treatment Technique

The main aims in planning treatment are to subtend an adequate volume, to avoid irradiating the contralateral eye, and to shield the eye on the affected side as far as possible. Except where age, general condition, or a very advanced or metastatic lesion preclude it, every attempt should be made to deliver a radical dose.

Antrum Without Involvement of the Orbit

A wedge pair of fields, anterior and lateral, are used. The superior edges of the fields pass just below the pupil of the eye, while the inferior limit will be dependent on the extent of involvement of the cheek. The standard use of a bite-block ensures that the tongue is kept out of the high-dose volume.

The medial extent of the treated volume should extend at least 0.5 cm across the midline. The posterior border of the lateral field will at least subtend the posterior wall of the antrum and may need to be extended if there is involvement of the pterygoid fossa. If there is any suggestion of soft tissue involvement of the cheek, wax build-up will be necessary to ensure full dosage on the skin of the cheek (Fig. 7.28).

The usual field size employed is 7×7 cm, and the volume subtended 7×7×7 cm. The dose delivered to this volume should be 5250–5500 cGy in 16 fractions over 21 days. When there is involvement of the orbit and ethmoid sinuses, this approach is not satisfactory.

Antrum and Ethmoid

An L-shaped plain anterior field may be used, subtending the ethmoid cells, the nose, and antrum, and sparing the eye. This dominant single-field approach has the disadvantage of a falling dose posteriorly. This is overcome by the use of a lateral parallel pair of steeply wedged fields (Fig. 7.29). The anterior edge of the lateral fields is positioned at the posterior wall of the orbit, thus sparing both eyes. Using this technique, it is mandatory to avoid exceeding a dose of 4500 cGy to the optic chiasma. To achieve this aim, the superior margin of the lateral fields is shaped to follow the line of the base of the skull by the use of lead shielding, wedge-shaped in a posteroanterior direction.

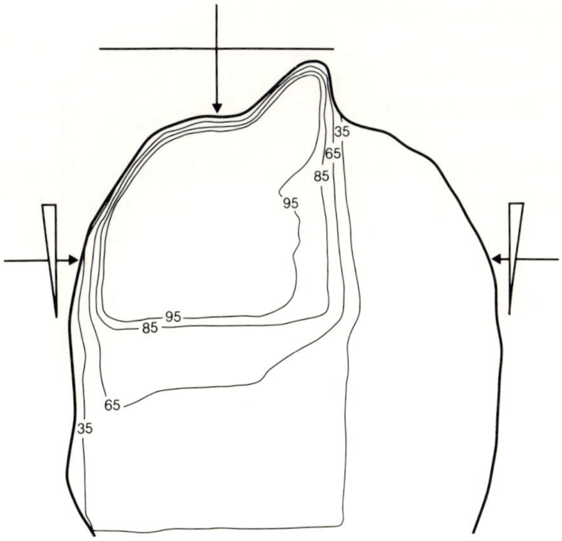

Fig. 7.29. Carcinoma of ethmoid and antrum—three-field technique.

Where there is evidence of orbital involvement, the homolateral eye cannot be spared. An open "peephole" 1.5 cm in diameter centred over the pupil and directed in the axis of the beam will spare the anterior segment of the eye from the full dose, while casting no shadow deep to the eye. Particular care should be taken to ensure full dosage at the surface of the inner canthus by the use of wax build-up.

The dose aimed at for a volume of 7×7×7 cm is 5250 cGy in 15 fractions over 21 days. As this treatment depends on a dominant anterior field, the dose applied to this field will have to be loaded to 5550 cGy, while the dose on the two lateral wedged fields is approximately 10% of this (see Fig. 7.29). The reaction from such a treatment is brisk. There will be dry desquamation of the skin of the cheek, which may proceed to some degree of moist desquamation, depending on the amount of build-up used. There will be a fibrinous reaction over the hard palate, alveolus, and buccal mucosa on the affected side. If the eye is irradiated, there will be some degree of conjunctivitis, but there should not be any significant reaction. The use of chloramphenicol eye-drops is recommended during and after treatment. The patient should be warned of epilation of the posterior scalp resulting from the exit beam from the anterior field.

Carcinoma of the Frontal and Sphenoid Sinuses

Primary tumours of the frontal and sphenoidal sinuses are exceptionally rare. Involvement of these sinuses is almost invariably the result of extension from advanced ethmoidal-antral lesions. Treatment planning follows the principles described for ethmoidal-antral lesions.

Palliation

For carcinoma of the nose and nasal sinuses, the optimum palliation is achieved by a full course of treatment as described. When this is not practicable, however, distressing symptoms may be relieved by a simple, single, anterior-field approach. The dose delivered will depend on the size of field necessary, but will be in the order of 3500 cGy in 8 fractions over 10 days.

Complications

Nasal Cavity

The principal problem is atrophic rhinitis and the persistent formation of crusts. If crusts are removed regularly within the first few months following irradiation, the subsequent development of crusts of any magnitude is unlikely.

Bone Necrosis

Bone necrosis following megavoltage X-ray therapy occurs in about 5% of cases but it is usually of a minor degree and only rarely is active intervention indicated.

Eye Complications

The major eye complications following megavoltage X-ray therapy for carcinoma of the antrum and ethmoid are cataract and blindness. Other sequelae are keratitis and persistent conjunctivitis. Unilateral blindness occurs in approximately 10% of cases. Bilateral blindness has been rarely observed, almost certainly the result of excessive dose to the optic chiasma.

Secondary Nodes

Involved cervical lymph nodes are usually associated with an uncontrolled primary lesion. The results from block dissection of the neck for secondary nodes from a primary antral lesion are so poor that it is rarely justified to submit the patient to this procedure. Secondary nodes should, therefore, be managed by an appropriate radiotherapeutic technique.

Results

The overall 5-year survival rate for carcinoma of the antrum and ethmoid sinuses is in the order of 30%. Lesions confined to the inferior half of the antrum have a better prognosis. Involvement of the orbit presages a poor prognosis as does the presence of involved cervical lymph nodes.

Non-odontogenic Tumours of the Jaw

The majority of tumours of the upper jaw arise in the nasal sinuses, while in the lower jaw, carcinoma of the alveolus is the common lesion.

Primary non-odontogenic tumours of the jaws are rare and are comprised of various histological types, the most frequent of which are fibrosarcoma, chondrosarcoma, osteosarcoma, angiosarcoma, histiocytic lymphoma (reticulum cell sarcoma), myeloma, and giant cell lesions.

The management of these lesions is discussed in Chaps. 14 and 15.

Tumours of the Middle Ear

Included in this group are:

1) carcinoma of the bony portion of the external auditory meatus
2) carcinoma of the middle ear
3) tumours of the glomus jugulare (chemodectoma)

Extensive carcinoma of the bony portion of the external auditory canal usually cannot be separated from carcinoma of the middle ear and as they have common clinical features, they will be considered together in the next section.

Carcinoma of the Middle Ear

Clinical Features

Over 80% of these lesions will be squamous cell carcinoma, the remainder will be composed of basal cell carcinoma, adenocarcinoma, malignant melanoma, adenoid cystic carcinoma and, in childhood, embryonal rhabdomyosarcoma.

The majority of patients with middle ear carcinoma have a long history of chronic suppurative middle-ear disease. As the tumour advances, destruction of the local tissues of the middle ear occurs with invasion of the adjacent bone. In spite of extensive bone involvement radiologically, the ossicles of the middle ear often appear intact. Symptomatically, there is increase in discharge, often bloody, associated with increasing pain. As the lesion advances, vertigo, facial nerve paralysis, and increasing pain result. These symptoms may be thought to be related to mastoiditis and only surgical exploration and biopsy will confirm the presence of malignancy.

The majority of these lesions will be advanced on presentation, with destruction of the petrous bone and involvement of the base of the skull in 60% of cases. The full extent of the lesion can only be demonstrated by good polytomography of the region, reinforced by CT scanning. In addition to these specialised investigations, particular note should be made of any soft tissue involvement in the mastoid or parotid areas, as this will obviously influence treatment planning.

Treatment Technique

The treatment of choice is megavoltage X-ray therapy. Preferably, pretreatment surgery should be limited to proving the diagnosis. Extensive surgery should be avoided because subsequent X-ray therapy is made more difficult and the chance of cure reduced, as well as causing a considerable increase in morbidity.

The aim of treatment will be to irradiate the known disease with an adequate margin of normal tissue. In practice, this will mean treating the whole petrous temporal bone as a minimum. To achieve this a very careful beam-directed technique is essential, following the principles previously described. The object is to subtend the required

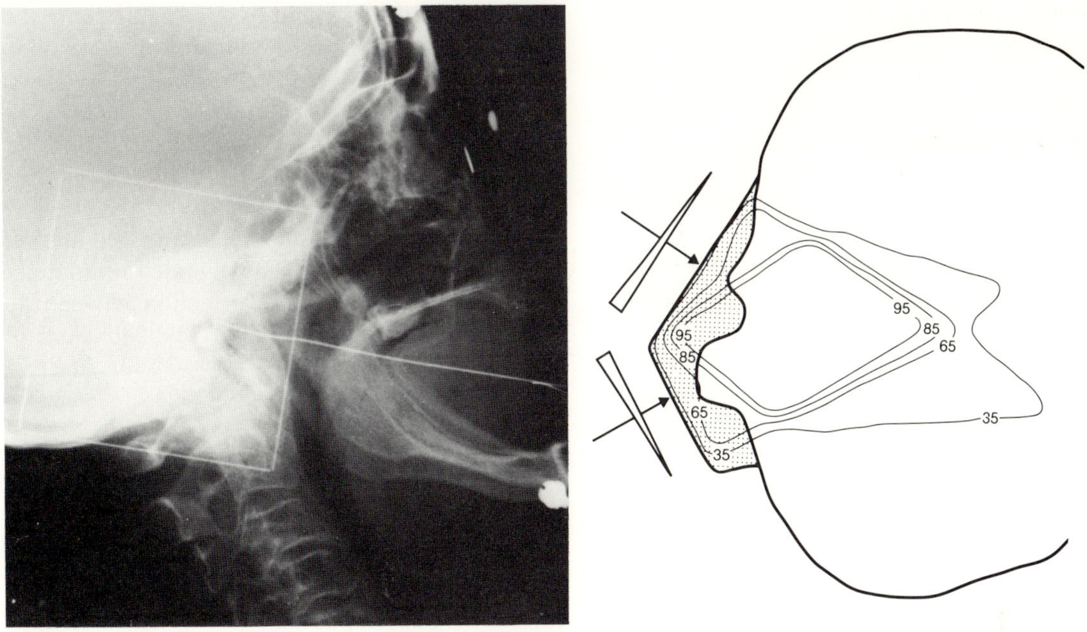

a b

Fig. 7.30. a Carcinoma of middle ear—verification radiograph. **b** Wedge pair technique.

treatment volume while avoiding excessive dose to the midbrain and also taking particular care to avoid irradiating the orbits with exit beams. The latter objective is secured by selecting an angled axis of treatment such that the beams exit below the floor of the orbit (Fig. 7.30).

The normal treatment plan involves the use of two steeply wedged fields so arranged as to produce a homogeneous volume of high dose which subtends the petrous bone. It is of advantage to have a skull available at this stage to orientate treatment planning. The common field sizes used are 5×5 cm and 5×6 cm, arranged to form a wedge pair as shown in Fig. 7.30. It will be necessary to use wax build-up over the external auditory meatus and over any adjacent soft tissue involvement. The dose delivered to such a volume will be 5500 cGy given in 16 fractions over 21 days. The dose will, of course, need to be adjusted according to the treatment volume selected. A radical treatment should be attempted wherever feasible because good palliation is rarely achieved with anything less. The reaction following treatment should not be troublesome provided that sepsis is controlled.

Subsequent surveillance should be at a joint radiotherapy and surgical clinic. Primary recurrence is rarely amenable to radical surgery, though useful palliation may be secured with cryosurgery.

Secondary spread to preauricular and upper deep cervical nodes is relatively uncommon and is usually associated with an uncontrolled primary lesion. Management will be influenced by the overall clinical situation.

The 5-year survival rate for carcinoma of the middle ear is approximately 30%.

Tumours of the Glomus Jugulare (Chemodectoma)

Clinical Features

This rare tumour arises from structures resembling carotid bodies near the jugular bulb and may arise at different sites within the ear. The tumour produces its effect by expansion and destruction of surrounding structures. Characteristically, there is a long natural history, the commonest symptoms being deafness, tinnitus, bleeding, vertigo, and pain. In the more extensive lesions, there may be multiple cranial nerve palsies. Metastases are very uncommon.

Diagnosis may be made clinically, usually as a result of the characteristic vascularity of these lesions. Biopsy may therefore be difficult but is usually attainable in the majority of cases.

Radiological investigation is as for a carcinoma of the middle ear.

Treatment Technique

The treatment of choice is by means of megavoltage X-ray therapy. The technique used is the same as for a carcinoma of the middle ear, but the dose delivered is lower, namely 4500 cGy given in 16 fractions over 21 days.

The response of these tumours to irradiation is slow, but there is often a rapid symptomatic improvement. Rarely, however, is there an improvement in cranial nerve palsies. The natural history of these tumours is such that very long-term surveillance is necessary before definitive views on prognosis can be expressed.

Tumours of the Thyroid Gland

Clinical Features

Primary thyroid cancer is rare and accounts for around 1% of all cancers in the United Kingdom. Optimum management results from close cooperation between pathologists, surgeons, radiotherapists, and nuclear medicine specialists, for the histology is diverse, and the course of the illness may be protracted over many years or prove rapidly fatal.

Epidemiology is controversial but previous radiation has been established as one of the aetiological factors. There is evidence that irradiation of the thymus gland in infancy increases the incidence of thyroid cancer in children; the incidence is related to the dose received. The adult thyroid gland is less susceptible to radiation. There is no evidence of an increased incidence of thyroid cancer in patients who have received radioactive iodine treatment for hyperthyroidism. Malignant tumours are rarely seen in hyperthyroid glands, but can coexist with chronic thyroiditis of the Hashimoto type.

Thyroid cancer is more than twice as common in women as in men. The peak age incidence is between 50 and 60 years, but the cancer can occur at any age from childhood to old age. Well-differentiated carcinomas are more frequent in the first five decades, but poorly differentiated tumours and malignant lymphomas predominate in later life.

Pathology

A classification of primary cancers, based on that of Woolner, can be a valuable guide to treatment and prognosis, as there is a correlation between the histological features and the clinical behaviour of thyroid malignancies.

Classification

(a) Well-differentiated adenocarcinoma
  1. papillary
  2. follicular

(b) Undifferentiated carcinoma
(c) Malignant lymphoma
(d) Medullary carcinoma
(e) Rare cancers

(a) *Well-differentiated adenocarcinoma*
All degrees of differentiation are seen from tumours that resemble normal thyroid tissue, even in a distant metastasis, to those showing some undifferentiated features.
  1. *Papillary carcinoma.* Although seen at all ages, tumours in children are usually of this type. They have a tendency to remain localised in the neck for a long period although frequently there is spread to the local lymph nodes. Distant metastases are less common. The primary tumour may be occult. It is often multifocal, particularly if nodes are present.
  2. *Follicular carcinoma.* The tumour may be very well-differentiated and encapsulated but the histological pattern is not constant. Hürthle cell carcinoma is included in this group. Invasion of the blood vessels and capsule, infiltration into the surrounding tissues, and less well-differentiated elements all indicate a more malignant tumour. There may be lymphatic spread, and haematogenous metastases are most frequent in bone.

(b) *Undifferentiated carcinoma (anaplastic carcinoma)*
This is usually a rapidly growing, highly malignant tumour composed of a disorderly

arrangement of cells showing frequent mitoses. The cell type variants include squamous cell, spindle cell, giant cell, and small cell carcinoma. Blood-borne spread is common, particularly to lung, bone, and liver. Small cell carcinoma may be difficult to distinguish from a poorly differentiated malignant lymphoma.

(c) *Malignant lymphoma*
The tumour types that occur primarily in the thyroid gland are usually histiocytic or lymphocytic lymphomas, although Hodgkin's disease and plasmocytoma have been found. Growth is usually quite rapid. Distant sites may be involved later in the course of the disease.

(d) *Medullary carcinoma*
This is derived from parafollicular C cells which secrete calcitonin. Spread into the mediastinum and lymph node metastases are common. Many are slow-growing tumours but spindle cells, frequent mitoses, areas of necrosis, and absence of calicification indicate more rapid progression. The majority of medullary carcinomas are sporadic but a few are familial. It may be asymptomatic in relatives and these should be investigated. There may be an association with phaeochromocytoma and other abnormalities such as mucosal fibromas. Humoral features such as diarrhoea and flushing are sometimes present. High levels of plasma calcitonin are found, but an increased concentration is not diagnostic of medullary carcinoma as this may occur in patients with non-thyroid tumours.

(e) *Rare cancers*
Although soft tissue sarcomas such as fibrosarcoma and haemangiosarcoma have been reported rarely in the thyroid gland, the majority of these tumours are now thought to be variants of undifferentiated carcinoma. Squamous cell carcinoma has also been reported.

The incidence of each histological type, stage of the disease, and age of the patients will vary according to the source of the material. The true figures will not be reflected in centres treating predominantly by surgery or in other centres using radiotherapy. It is inevitable that a large proportion of elderly patients and those with undifferentiated carcinoma, malignant lymphoma and late stages of differentiated carcinoma, will be referred to radiotherapists. Approximately 80% of primary thyroid malignancies are well-differentiated or undifferentiated carcinomas, 10%–15% malignant lymphomas and 5%–10% medullary carcinomas.

Mode of Presentation and Investigation

Thyroid cancer presents as follows:

1) Unsuspected histological finding after operation, or radiological evidence of an anterior mediastinal mass
2) Solitary thyroid nodule
3) Recent enlargement of a pre-existing goitre
4) Rapid enlargement of the thyroid gland with or without lymph nodes
5) Lymph node, or nodes, in the neck
6) Symptoms from distant metastases, usually in bone or lung

It may be difficult to establish a malignant diagnosis before operation. In addition to films of the chest and thoracic inlet, radiology includes anterior-posterior and lateral soft tissue views of the neck. A benign enlargement of the thyroid gland can cause deviation of the trachea and sometimes compression, but marked compression with obstructive symptoms is usually due to cancer. Tomographs of the larynx or trachea and barium swallow radiographs may help to distinguish a primary thyroid cancer from a cancer arising in an adjacent site. Skeletal films are indicated if symptoms suggest bone metastases.

Scanning of the thyroid gland as a diagnostic procedure is carried out 1 h after 80 MBq (2.16 mCi) sodium pertechnetate (^{99m}Tc) has been administered intravenously, or 24 h after 10 MBq (270 μCi) sodium iodide (^{131}I) orally. If there is greater radioactivity in a solitary thyroid nodule than in the remaining thyroid tissue, it is unlikely to be malignant since cancer cells are less efficient at taking up radioisotope than normal thyroid cells. A "cold" nodule may be malignant or result from reduced uptake in an inactive part of an adenoma, a cyst, or haemorrhage. Ultrasound and CT scanning may give additional information. Well-differentiated metastases from thyroid adenocarcinoma may take up radio-iodine, but usually only after the thyroid gland has been excised or destroyed by a therapeutic dose of iodine-131. However, if lymph node or bone metastases are present and carcinoma of the thyroid is suspected, it is worth scanning these sites, since uptake of radio-iodine in the metastases confirms the diagnosis, although lack of uptake does not exclude thyroid carcinoma. In the investigation of known thyroid cancers, non-functioning metastases in bone, liver, brain, and other organs may be detected by scanning after the appropriate radiopharmaceutical has been given. The diagnosis is established by histology. This is usually from the thyroid gland following exploration of the region, or from an excised lymph node. A needle biopsy is often possible when advanced disease in the neck prohibits open biopsy. Thyroid carcinoma and malignant lymphoma can coexist with Hashimoto's disease (lymphocytic thyroiditis). Tests for thyroid antibodies and thyroid function, liver function, and calcium and phosphate estimations are carried out in addition to a full blood count. Plasma calcitonin is measured by radioimmunoassay for medullary carcinoma.

Staging

Classification by TNM categories is usually impossible if surgery has been carried out before this has been done. No international stage grouping is at present recommended by UICC. The staging as practised at the Christie Hospital is given in the App. 2 and can be summarised as follows:

Stage	I	Mobile primary. No nodes
Stage	IIa	Mobile primary. Mobile unilateral or bilateral nodes
Stage	IIb	Small fixed primary and/or nodes, or small residue following surgery
Stage	IIIa	Large fixed primary and/or nodes, or residue exceeding 5 cm
Stage	IIIb	Extension into upper mediastinum
Stage	IV	Distant metastases present

Treatment Technique

Treatment of thyroid cancer must take into account the stage of the disease and the variation in behaviour of the different histological types (Table 7.5). For the radical treatment of patients with early well-differentiated carcinoma, surgery is the main therapeutic method for the primary tumour and regional lymph node metastases. This may be followed by radiotherapy for residual disease, or to ablate the remnants of the thyroid gland. As well as being essential replacement therapy, thyroid hormone may suppress the growth of potential cancer cells. Surgery is also recommended for medullary carcinoma as it does not respond well to radiation. Malignant lymphomas and a number of undifferentiated carcinomas are radiosensitive and treatment is by external irradiation. This may be very effective even when the tumour is large.

Surgery

This should be the treatment for stage I and IIa differentiated papillary, follicular, and medullary carcinoma unless other medical conditions contraindicate radical surgery. For a very small low-grade papillary carcinoma, the removal of the affected lobe, together with the isthmus and a thin portion from the opposite lobe, should be adequate if the patient is maintained in a euthyroid state with thyroid hormone. Total thyroidectomy is recommended for the other tumours in this group. A rim of normal thyroid tissue can be left on one side to protect the recurrent laryngeal nerve and parathyroid glands. Mobile nodes are dissected. X-ray treatment is given if the surgery has not eradicated all the tumour. Postoperative radio-iodine studies on patients with papillary or follicular carcinoma are carried out before replacement thyroid hormone is commenced.

In advanced cancers surgery is of limited value. Total thyroidectomy for operable local disease will enable functioning metastases to be treated immediately by radio-iodine, thus avoiding delay during radio-iodine ablation of bulky normal thyroid tissue. Partial removal of a tumour may be indicated to relieve tracheal obstruction before external radiation is given, and to provide material for histology as a guide to future management. Radiotherapy may have to be started for a rapidly growing tumour before a needle biopsy is taken. Biopsy can be done when obstructive symptoms regress but before the histological features are altered by the radiation. Tracheostomy may be a life-saving measure, but difficult or impossible with disease low in the neck. If the patient is to

Table 7.5. Treatment policy.

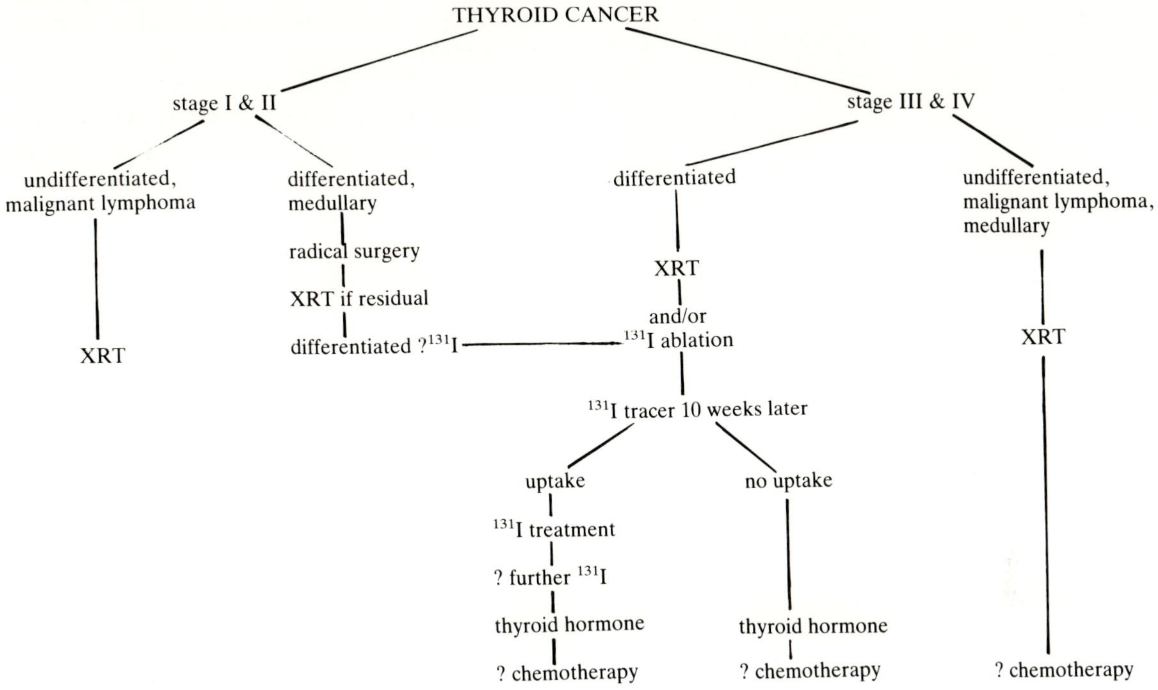

receive external radiation, a plastic tracheostomy tube is used. Other palliative surgical procedures are rarely necessary, but decompression for a metastasis in the spine causing or threatening paraplegia may prove worthwhile for patients with slow-growing tumours.

External Radiation

Radical Treatment

The technique employed depends on the type and extent of the primary growth and lymph node involvement. Beam-directed treatment is used for residual differentiated carcinomas requiring small-volume irradiation, but anterior and posterior parallel opposed fields are necessary when the tumour extends behind the plane of the spinal cord, into the upper cervical region or mediastinum, and for malignant lymphoma and anaplastic tumours. The treatment is given in 16 fractions over a period of three weeks.

Beam-directed Techniques

A cellulose acetate shell is made with the patient supine, in the treatment position, with the neck extended over a neck-rest. A lateral radiograph is taken showing the radio-opaque planning markers on the shell and a wire marker on the operation scar. Following a tracer dose of iodine-131, a scan of the neck is carried out with the patient wearing the shell. Residual thyroid tissue can thus be related to the shell markers before defining the treatment volume. Usually the vertical extent is from the hyoid bone down to 1–2 cm below the sternal notch, but there are individual variations. The posterior limit is parallel to the spinal cord and includes the anterior border of the vertebrae. Anteriorly the skin of the neck is included, but not the skin of the upper sternal region. These limits are marked on the lateral radiograph and a lateral verification film is taken. Vertical and horizontal contours are drawn through the central planes for treatment planning. The region of the scar and any superficial tumour requires full bolus with cellulose acetate or wax extending down to the level of the clavicles. Sparing of the skin is achieved by removing the cellulose acetate from the treatment fields above, below, and posterior to the bolus.

This information is recorded on the treatment plans.

A 2-field technique employs lateral fields angled downwards towards the chest with a vertical wedge filter inserted to compensate for this angle and the oblique incidence of the X-ray beams. A horizontal wedge is used to compensate for oblique incidence in the anteroposterior plane. As a safety measure a field is not wedged in two planes at the same time. The angle of the fields is chosen so as to irradiate the required volume with a vertical wedge in one beam only and a horizontal wedge in the other beam. The wedges are interchanged after eight of the 16 treatments have been given, in order to produce homogeneous irradiation. For 10×5 cm fields a tumour dose of 4500–4750 cGy is given in 3 weeks using 4-MV radiation. The calculations and dosage distribution are shown in Fig. 7.31. Beam direction is achieved by the use of an extended front pointer if access for a back pointer is not possible (Fig. 7.32). When a larger area requires bolus, both lateral fields are completely waxed up and the horizontal wedge is omitted.

A 3-field technique is used when the tumour is low in the neck or if the neck is short. An anterior field of the same width as the neck is added to two lateral angled-down fields to limit the full-dose zone. This is directed through the tumour centre. The jaw, shoulders, and chest wall produce such irregular contours that homogeneity is obtained by withdrawing each field to the furthest point of entry into the skin, and waxing the shell to this distance (Figure 7.33). Alternatively, skin sparing of the anterior chest wall is achieved by omitting the wax from the anterior field and inserting a vertical wedge into the beam. The tumour dose is 4500–4750 cGy in 3 weeks.

Occasionally, only the primary site is treated by an anterior and two anterolateral oblique wedged fields (Figure 7.34). A tumour dose of 5250 cGy in 3 weeks can be given for field lengths of 6–7 cm. Care must be taken to avoid irradiating the spinal cord with the oblique fields. The position of the cord is determined from the lateral marker radiograph and transferred to the contour before planning the treatment.

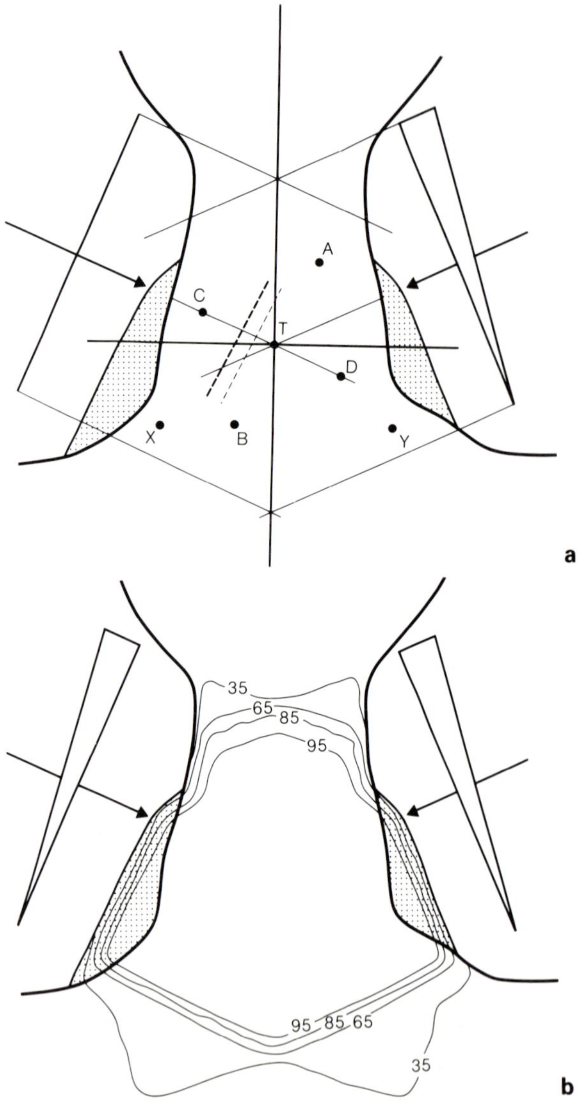

Fig. 7.31a,b. Carcinoma of thyroid—two-field technique. **a** Working diagram and calculation. **b** Vertical dose distribution.

10×5*W* (50° degree horizontal wedge)	10W×5 (45° vertical wedge)
Given dose 1320 cGy for treatments 1–8	Given dose 1320 cGy for treatments 1–8
plus	plus
10W×5 (45° vertical wedge)	10×5*W* (50° horizontal wedge)
Given dose 1320 cGy for treatments 9–16	Given dose 1320 cGy for treatments 9–16

Calculations

Fields of 10×5 cm with a 45° vertical wedge on left side but no wedge in vertical plane on right side. Tracings of the isodose curves are positioned at an angle to the verification plane so that the isodose curves are parallel after correcting for oblique incidence. The percentage depth dose is read off at points A, T and B along the direction of the curves, at points C and D, at right angles to these, and at points X and Y where the dose distribution will be uneven because of the wedge.

(*continued on next page*)

Fig. 7.31. Calculation (*continued*)

Fields for treatments 1–8	Percentage depth dose						
	A	T	B	C	D	X	Y
left 10W×5	86	86	83	70	104	70	127
right 10×5	85	85	85	96	74	92	64
	171	171	168	166	178	162	191

To obtain a homogeneous dose distribution the vertical wedge is changed to the right side after 8 treatments.

Fields for treatments 9–16	Percentage depth dose						
	A	T	B	C	D	X	Y
right 10W×5	72	85	103	96	75	125	68
left 10×5	95	85	74	78	92	64	92
	167	170	177	174	167	189	160
Total % depth dose	338	341	345	340	345	351	351

Taking the tumour dose as 341%=4500 cGy in 3 weeks then given dose to each field is 100%=1320 cGy
Maximum dose 351%=4640 cGy
Confirmation by computer: tumour dose 100%=4500 cGy
maximum dose 103%=4640 cGy
In the transverse plane a 50° wedge is required on 1 side to make the isodose curves parallel and this is changed over to the opposite side after 8 treatments.

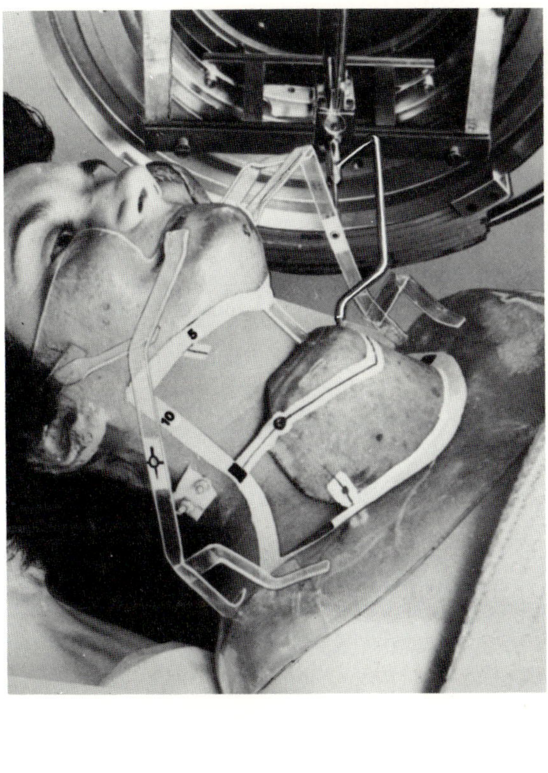

◁ **Fig. 7.32.** Carcinoma of thyroid. Patient in treatment position showing bolus, cut-out areas and extended front pointer.

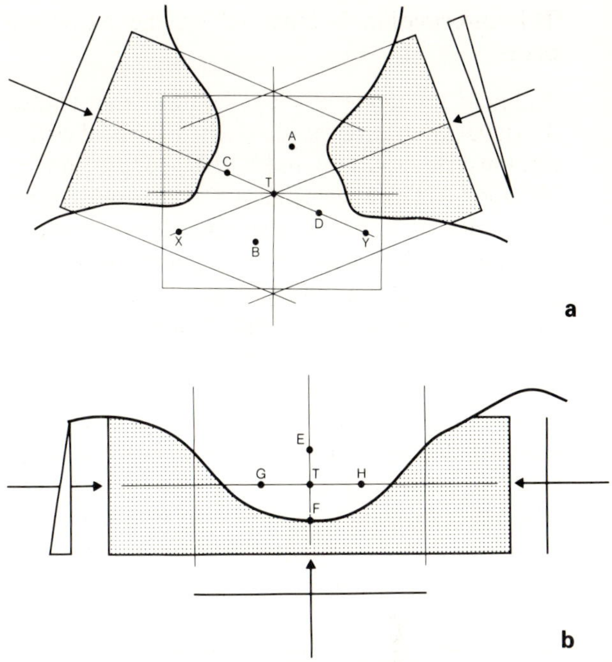

Fig. 7.33. Carcinoma of thyroid—three-field technique. **a** Vertical contour. **b** Horizontal contour.

Calculations
Vertical contour: the percentage depth dose from the lateral fields is calculated using a 45° vertical wedge on 1 side and changing this to the other side half way through the course of treatment.

Fields	Percentage depth dose						
	A	T	B	C	D	X	Y
left 9W×6	62	63	62	50	79	45	92
right 9×6	62	63	62	74	54	76	45
	124	126	124	124	133	121	137
left 9×6	71	63	56	55	70	45	74
right 9W×6	54	63	72	74	53	92	46
	125	126	128	129	123	137	120
Total	249	252	252	253	256	258	257

Horizontal contour: A 50° horizontal wedge is required in one lateral beam to compensate for the falling dose from the anterior field in the anterior-posterior direction. This is placed in the opposite beam from the lateral wedge.

(*continued on next page*)

Fig. 7.33. Calculation (*continued*)

Fields	Percentage depth dose G	T	H	E	F
left lateral 9×6	54	63	74	62	62
right lateral 9×6W	74	63	54	70	57
	128	126	128	132	119
				13/12	
anterior 9×11	92	92	92	86	98
anterior×13/12 (108%)	100	100	100	93	106
Total	228	226	228	225	225

As the gradient from highest to lowest depth dose is less from the anterior field than the combined lateral fields, homogeneity is obtained by increasing the contribution from the anterior field by this fraction.

If dose at tumour centre is 226% = 4750 cGy in 16 treatments then:
given dose to anterior field is 108% = 2250 cGy
given dose to each lateral field is 100% = 2080 cGy

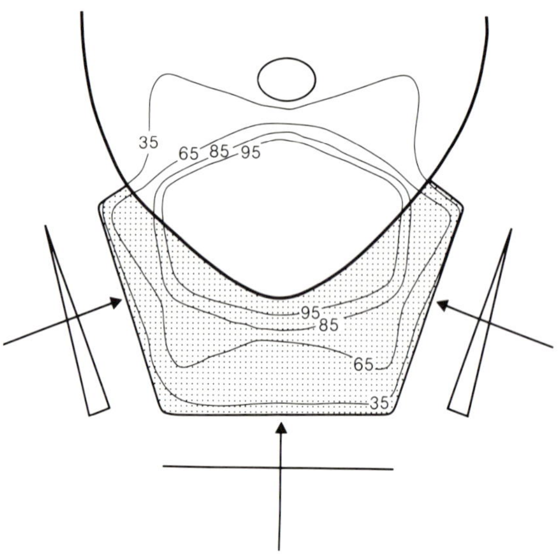

Fig. 7.34. Carcinoma of thyroid—three-field technique for treatment of primary site only.

Medium and Large Volume Irradiation

This is carried out by anterior and posterior fields using the 4-MV linear accelerator. The size of the fields and the tumour dose depend on the extent of the tumour. The normal practice is to treat the anterior field with the patient lying supine. If a foam pad is required under the head, this will increase the interfield distance. Full bolus is used over scars and tumour. The patient lies prone for treatment of the posterior field with the forehead supported on a foam pad. The lower corners of both fields are shielded with lead to protect the lung if they extend more than 3 cm below the sternal notch, and the centres and lower corners of the fields are tattooed on the skin. Alternatively, the posterior field can be treated through the grid part of the treatment couch with the patient remaining supine. When positioning the patient for the anterior field, the neck is extended to spare the mouth from irradiation and the lips are shielded if they are within the beams. The vertical line drawn on the neck and cheek at the upper limit of the fields is kept clearly visible throughout the course of treatment in order to reproduce the correct position and ensure parallel opposed fields. The tumour dose is calculated on the average of the central, minimum, and maximum interfield distances and is determined by the tolerance of the spinal cord and mucosa in relation to the length irradiated. For medium fields 12 cm long, 4000 cGy in 3 weeks can be given, but this must be reduced to 3250–3000 cGy in 3 weeks for field lengths of 20–25 cm.

Patients unable to lie down are treated in a special chair which is simple to fit on top of the treatment couch (Fig. 7.35). It has a strong, thin,

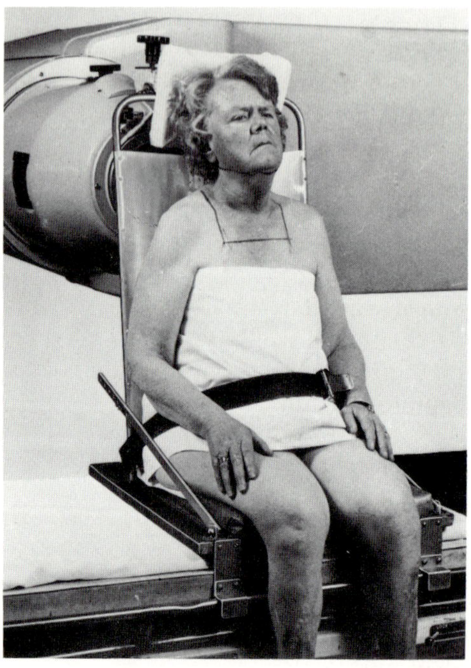

Fig. 7.35a. Treatment chair.

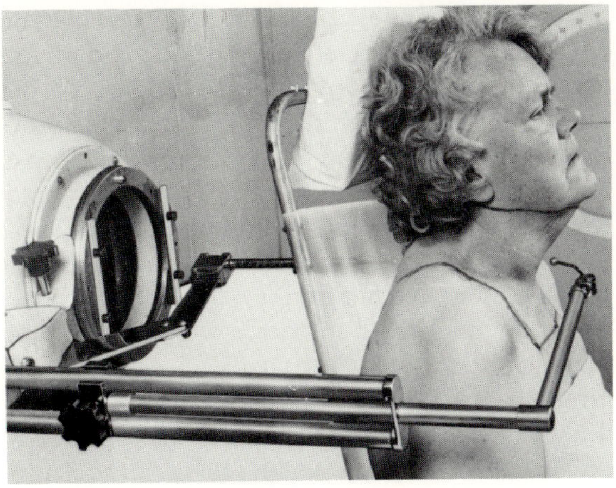

Fig. 7.35b. Carcinoma of the thyroid. Posterior field set up with front and back pointer.

flexible transparent back-rest and the posterior field can be treated through it. The fields are checked daily by the machine lights and by front and back pointers. Bolus is strapped on, leaving a hole around a tracheostomy opening if this is present. The tubular steel frame is outside the treatment area.

Late Radiation Effects in Normal Tissues

Several years after small-volume treatment, telangiectasia is seen where there has been full dose to the skin, and rarely a small area of skin necrosis. Fibrosis of the oesophagus may produce mild dysphagia but this can be controlled by careful bouginage. A rare but serious complication is fibrosis of the irradiated tissues around the trachea, causing respiratory obstruction. If this is too low for tracheostomy, the gradual narrowing of the trachea as the fibrosis proceeds over the years may eventually be the cause of death. When the upper mediastinum is included in the volume irradiated by larger fields, fibrosis of the lungs may be seen on the radiographs, but this rarely gives rise to symptoms.

Palliative Treatment

Palliative external radiation to the neck is by anterior and posterior parallel opposed fields, or by a single anterior field. The dose is 3000–3500 cGy for medium fields and 2500 cGy for large fields given in eight fractions over a period of 10 days. A small field can be treated with a single exposure of 1250–1500 cGy. Bone and other distant metastases are treated in a manner appropriate to their site.

Radio-iodine

Treatment by iodine-131 is only possible for functioning differentiated adenocarcinomas. About half of these tumours will take up iodine to some degree after all normal thyroid tissue has been eliminated, the follicular variety more often than the papillary type. The concentration is not always great enough to be of therapeutic value and therefore preliminary baseline measurements and scans are carried out 24 h after a 40-MBq (1.08-mCi) tracer dose of iodine-131. Treatment is given to all patients with stage III and IV disease if there is significant uptake. Absence of pick-up in tumour is common when normal thyroid tissue is present, and further tests are carried out 10 weeks after an ablation dose of iodine-131 to destroy it. Our standard ablation dose is at present 3500 MBq (95 mCi). Baseline measurements are also carried out on patients with stage I and II carcinomas with a view to ablating residual thyroid remnants following surgery, except in children and young adults. The biological half-life in different parts of the tumour may vary, and all the tumour may not take up radio-iodine at the same time. A therapeutic dose of 7000 MBq (190 mCi) is given if the average concentration is 0.1% per gram of functioning tumour at 24 h. This will give a radiation dose in the region of 6000 cGy, assuming a biological half-life of 3 days. It may be difficult to demonstrate uptake in multiple small deposits in the lung, but a therapeutic dose may be worth giving. Treatment can be repeated at intervals of 3–4 months on three or four occasions if there is adquate concentration. As part of the tumour is destroyed by the radiation, a different part may take up iodine-131 and respond to subsequent doses. When the efficacy of treatment is in doubt, borderline uptake may be increased by giving thyroid stimulating hormone (TSH), 10 international units intramuscularly daily for 3–5 days before the therapeutic dose of radio-iodine. It is important that a patient is not hypothyroid for longer than is necessary to carry out radio-iodine tests and treatment, since the tumour may be stimulated by the hypothyroidism. Thyroid hormone is therefore given in the intervals and triiodothyronine (liothyronine) is preferred to thyroxine, as its effect and its removal from the circulation are more rapid. Triiodothyronine is stopped 2 weeks before, and thyroxine 4 weeks before the tracer tests, as these would suppress the uptake of iodine in thyroid tissue. Thyroid hormone medication is recommenced a few days after treatment, when the residual radioactivity is no longer of therapeutic importance. When it is urgent to establish whether treatment with iodine-131 is possible, TSH may induce uptake even in the presence of circulating hormones.

A patient receiving a large dose of radio-iodine must be accommodated in a side room of the ward and toilet facilities arranged to dispose of the radioactive waste safely. For the first few days, medical examinations and nursing procedures are kept to a minimum and protective precautions are taken. Rubber gloves are worn when handling articles that may be radioactive or when cleaning contaminated areas. Only short visits by relatives are allowed, and children and pregnant women are not permitted. In accordance with the British Code of Practice, the patient is not discharged from hospital until the radioactivity has fallen to at least 555 MBq (15 mCi) if public transport is to be used, or 1110 MBq (30 mCi) if private transport is available. This is delayed if there are young children at home. The room is checked with a Geiger counter and contaminated articles are kept in a special store until they are innocuous.

Radiation Effects

Radio-iodine therapy is contraindicated in pregnancy as it may cause abortion or radiation damage to the foetus. Side effects otherwise are usually mild. Treatment may induce nausea and vomiting within a few hours of administration and antiemetics are given if there are symptoms. Suitable receptacles are provided to avoid contamination should vomiting occur. When there is a substantial part of the normal thyroid gland present, the neck may become swollen and painful for a few days because of radiation thyroiditis. This usually settles spontaneously, but if it is severe, oral or parenteral steroids, in addition to analgesics, will give relief. Erythema and epilation can occur from superficial metastases and occasionally the salivary glands are painful. Hypothyroidism is inevitable if replacement thyroid hormone therapy is withheld. A temporary fall in the blood count may be observed but aplastic anaemia is very rare. The risk of anaemia or leukaemia is greatest in patients with multiple bone metastases who have had very large total quantities of iodine-131 of over 37 GBq (1 Ci), and for whom there is no other means of controlling the thyroid cancer. Radiation fibrosis of the lungs has been reported following similar treatment for miliary lung metastases. These dosage levels are exceptional, as most tumours fail to take up iodine before they are reached. There may be temporary disturbance of gonad function. Young patients who have had radio-iodine treatment should be warned about the radiation before they consider having a family but there is at present no evidence that the incidence of infertility or abnormal births is significantly different from that found in the general population.

Thyroid Hormone

This may be necessary as replacement of normal physiological requirements but, in addition, it is known that well-differentiated adenocarcinomas may be thyrotrophin-dependent. Thyroid hormone to normal tolerance should be given, in addition to any form of treatment for these tumours, since suppression of pituitary TSH may result in tumour regression. In adults 300 μg of thyroxine or 80 μg of triiodothyronine daily is the average dose required to maintain the euthyroid state following ablation. The optimum level is judged clinically and biochemically. Serum TSH estimations are carried out regularly to ensure that the dose is adequate to suppress it. Triiodothyronine is preferred when radio-iodine investigations and treatment are anticipated.

Chemotherapy

Cytotoxic drugs have been used in an attempt to control thyroid carcinomas of varied histology when other methods have failed. Only small numbers of patients have been treated in each centre and a wide range of drugs used either as single agents or in combination. The number responding and the duration of remission have as yet not been very encouraging. Chemotherapy for malignant lymphoma of the thyroid, as in other sites, will depend on the histology (see Chap. 14).

Treatment in Special Circumstances

Children

Tumours are most commonly papillary carcinomas and are more likely to be hormone-dependent than in adults. They tend to grow slowly. Unless there is extensive disease, external radiation and radio-iodine can be withheld to see whether residual tumour following surgery responds to thyroid hormone. If iodine-131 is given to small children, the adult dose is reduced. Prolonged follow-up should be maintained as recurrence can occur many years later.

Ectopic Thyroid Cancer

Thyroglossal duct tumours can be treated in a similar manner to those occurring in the thyroid gland. Lingual thyroid cancer is treated by external radiation to the primary site, keeping surgery in reserve should this fail. Radio-iodine ablation is indicated for differentiated adenocarcinoma and ^{131}I for subsequent treatment if it is taken up by residual tumour. Treatment of metastatic disease is in accordance with the policy for other thyroid cancers.

Rapidly Growing Cancers Causing Obstruction

X-ray treatment may have to be started before the histology is known, in the hope that the tumour is a malignant lymphoma or a radiosensitive carcinoma. It is important that a tumour-lethal dose is obtained rapidly and therefore the 3-week treatment course is reduced to an overall time of 10 days and the equivalent radiobiological dose given in eight fractions. Moderately large fields are required and the initial exposures must be large enough to give a chance of partial resolution. Treatment begins with an anterior field on an empiric basis giving 500 cGy for each exposure and after 2 or 3 days this is reviewed. The prescription is then amended to give the appropriate dose in the remaining fractions, and to balance the dose from the anterior and posterior fields if parallel fields are used. High-dose steroids have an anti-inflammatory effect and in severe cases these are given parenterally before the first X-ray treatment. This is repeated later if an emergency arises, but the patient is also given steroids orally, the dose being tailed off rapidly if obstructive symptoms recede.

Paraplegia

Paraplegia resulting from bone metastases in the spine, or backward extension of the carcinoma in the cervical region, is particularly distressing if the cancer is compatible with prolonged survival. Surgical decompression followed by X-ray therapy to radical dosage should be considered for patients with reasonable life expectancy. In addition, radio-iodine and hormone treatment may be relevant for those with differentiated carcinomas. There may be complete recovery of paraplegia and the outlook from this complication is significantly better than with most other malignancies.

Results and Prognosis

The wide variation of the cell types and their different behaviour patterns have a marked influence on survival. Many early differentiated carcinomas are curable and 70% of patients with stage I and II disease survive 10 years. Recurrence or the presence of distant metastases can be compatible with life for 10–15 years or more. Long-term follow-up is therefore necessary. The sex of the patient plays a minor role, but age has a significant effect on prognosis. Figure 7.36 shows the decreasing survival with age of patients with differentiated carcinoma, as calculated by the life table method described in Chap. 18. Less well-differentiated carcinomas and those with anaplastic areas within them are associated with poorer survival. A prognostic index based on the factors influencing prognosis has been devised by the EORTC Thyroid Cancer Group, but this has not yet been tested in a prospective study. As cancer can become more aggressive over the years, earlier detection and appropriate treatment of thyroid malignancy should give improved results. At the extreme end of the scale, approximately half of the patients with undifferentiated carcinoma are dead within 6 months, and two-thirds within a year of diagnosis. Those under the age of 40 do better than older age groups. Malignant lymphoma has a much better prognosis than undifferentiated carcinoma.

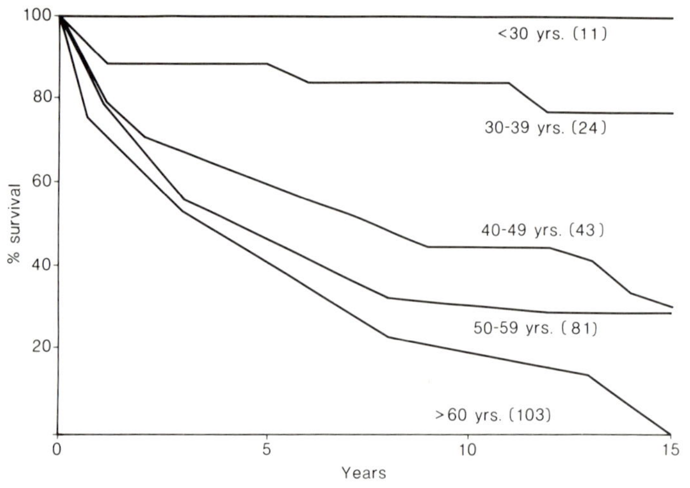

Fig. 7.36. Well differentiated carcinoma of thyroid. Survival related to age of patient at time of treatment (number of patients in each group in brackets).

Although X-ray therapy to the neck may be indicated for either condition, cytotoxic drugs may be successful in controlling disseminated lymphoreticular disease but not carcinoma. The diagnosis given by the histopathologist is therefore important for correct management. Medullary carcinoma has a long natural course and a 10-year survival of 60%–70% can be expected following treatment.

There is no doubt that iodine-131 treatment is very effective in the control of a small number of well-differentiated carcinomas. It is difficult to assess its value if it is given at the same time as other forms of treatment for disease in the neck, but when given for metastatic disease, the patients who had a good response to radio-iodine had a mean survival of over 8 years. This was twice as long as those with slight or no response, although there was iodine uptake in the metastases after ablation. All the patients received thyroid hormone except for temporary withdrawal of this before treatment.

Over the last few years radioimmunoassay techniques have made it possible to measure serum thyroglobulin. This provides a tumour marker for recurrent differentiated adenocarcinoma in patients who have had total removal of the thyroid gland. Immunotherapy using thyroglobulin as the immunising agent may be developed. Thyroid-stimulating antibodies have also been detected in the serum of thyroid cancer patients, but their role is at present unknown.

Tumours of the Salivary Glands

Clinical Features

The World Health Organisation has recommended the following histological typing of salivary gland tumours (1972):

Epithelial Tumours

A. *Adenomas*
   1. Pleomorphic adenoma (mixed tumour)
   2. Monomorphic adenomas
      (a) Adenolymphoma
      (b) Oxyphylic adenoma
      (c) Other types

B. *Mucoepidermoid tumour*

C. *Acinic cell tumour*

D. *Carcinomas*
   1. Adenoid cystic carcinoma
   2. Adenocarcinoma
   3. Epidermoid carcinoma
   4. Undifferentiated carcinoma (anaplastic)
   5. Carcinoma in pleomorphic adenoma (malignant mixed tumour)

   (ii) Non-epithelial tumours
   (iii) Unclassified tumours
   (iv) Allied conditions

From a radiotherapeutic point of view, the two most relevant lesions are pleomorphic adenoma and carcinoma.

Pleomorphic Adenoma

Histologically the pleomorphic adenoma has a heterogeneous appearance, the epithelial elements being interspaced between areas of mucoid, myxoid, and chondroid appearance. Areas of duct formation are seen as well as keratinisation and epithelial pearls. There is a wide variation in the proportion of the different elements present in these tumours, which accounts for the differing clinical consistency which may be present. It is essentially a benign tumour. Malignant change may occur in pleomorphic adenomas of long standing and the longer the history the more likely is this to occur.

Site

Over 90% of pleomorphic adenomas occur in the parotid salivary gland; the rest are almost equally divided between the submandibular salivary gland and the minor salivary glands.

Clinical Features

Pleomorphic adenomas are almost twice as common in women as men. The usual presentation is that of an asymptomatic lump in the parotid salivary gland, slowly increasing in size over many months or years.

Treatment Policy

Formerly, our managment of these tumours was to combine surgical enucleation with a radium needle implant which was carried out either at the completion of the enucleation or within a few weeks of surgery. However, with more careful surgery alone, either by local capsular dissection or superficial parotidectomy, the recurrence rate in previously untreated cases was reduced to less than 2%. In view of this, it was felt unjustified to carry out routine postoperative irradiation and accordingly follow-up only is now practised. The period of surveillance must, however, be prolonged since recurrence may occur many years after the initial treatment.

In those cases presenting with recurrence after surgery, further excision should be carried out combined with mandatory postoperative radiotherapy. The majority of recurrences following surgery are multifocal, so that it is essential to include the whole affected area with a wide margin; in addition the volume treated must be planned to include the deep lobe of the gland.

Treatment Technique

For superficial lesions, a radium needle implant is simple and effective. This may be a single-plane implant or more frequently a V-implant where the posterior needles run deep to the ascending ramus of the mandible. The V-plane implant is considered as a single-plane implant for the purpose of calculation. The dose aimed at is 6000 cGy at 0.5 cm in 7 days (Fig. 7.37).

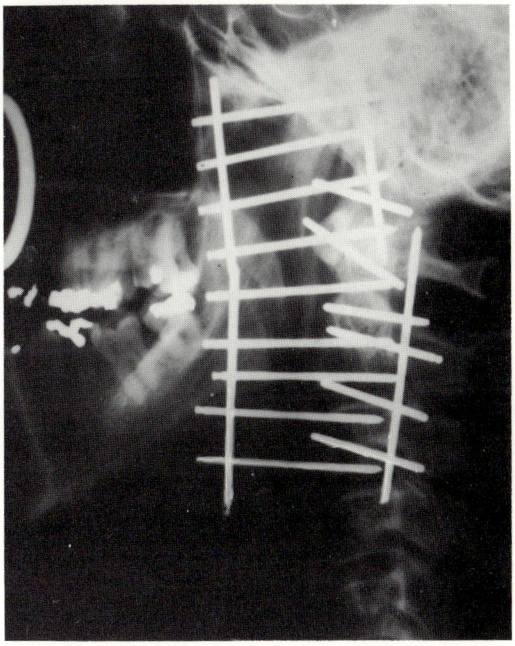

Fig. 7.37. Mixed salivary adenoma of parotid. V-plane radium needle implant.

Calculation.

Parotid. V-plane implant
Implanted area=44.5 cm^2
Dose required=6000 cGy
Approximate treatment time=168 h
mg h/1000 cGy=692
mg radium required=24.7 mg
Needles used 5×2 mg active length 3.0 cm
2×3 mg active length 4.5 cm
12×1 mg active length 3.0 cm
mg radium used=27.4 mg (including filtration correction)
Final treatment time=152 h

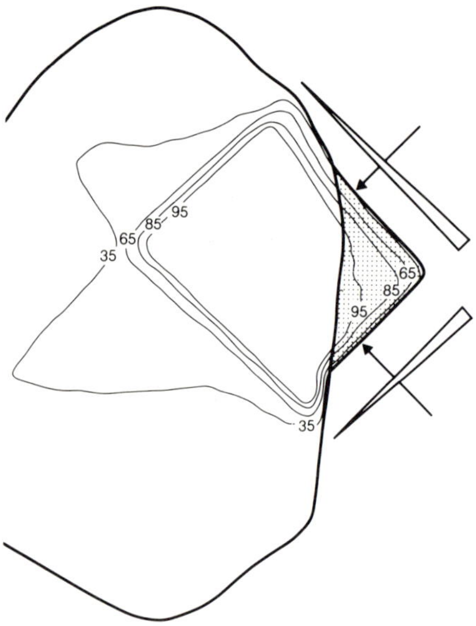

Fig. 7.38. Parotid tumour—wedge pair technique.

More frequently a megavoltage X-ray treatment will be performed, in view of the multifocal nature of recurrences and the need to subtend the deep lobe of the gland. This may be achieved by a wedge pair approach (Fig. 7.38) or by the use of a dominant lateral field subtended by two wedged fields (Fig. 7.39). In selecting the plane of the treatment, an inclined plane is preferred to avoid irradiating the eyes with the exit beams (Fig. 7.39). The dose aimed at is 5000 cGy in 15–16 fractions over 3 weeks.

Carcinoma

Clinical Features

The majority of these carcinomas occur in the parotid gland with few at other sites, the exception being adenoid cystic carcinoma where 50% occur in the minor salivary glands. Many of the patients with malignant tumours give a history of having had a swelling for many years. The sex incidence is generally equal, with a mean age of 57 years for all types. Six histopathological types commonly occur:

1) *Mucoepidermoid carcinoma*
   This histological diagnosis is made more frequently than previously and consequently mucoepidermoid carcinoma now represents about 25% of all malignant salivary tumours. It may be a low-grade tumour developing slowly over many years, particularly if arising in a minor salivary gland. It can, however, present as a relatively rapidly growing tumour with local invasion, cervical lymphadenopathy, and distant metastases.
2) *Acinic cell carcinoma*
   This is usually a low-grade tumour arising in the parotid gland. Involvement of the facial nerve is rare and metastases are uncommon. The prognosis is usually good.

a

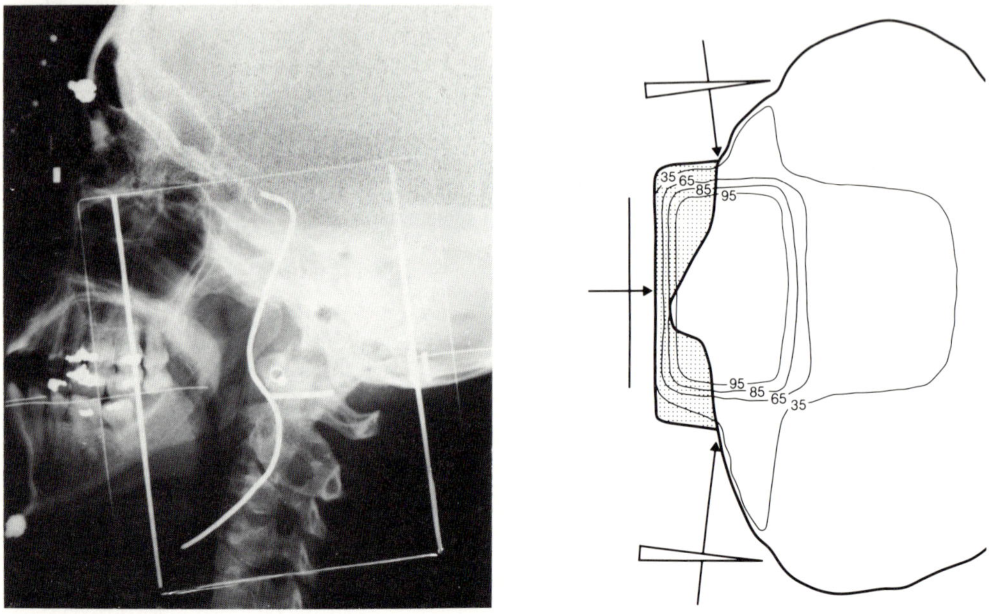

b

Fig. 7.39a,b. Parotid tumour. a Verification film in treatment axis. b Three-field technique.

3) *Malignant mixed salivary tumour*
   This is characteristically a slow-growing, locally invasive tumour. It may metastasise to lymph nodes as well as through the bloodstream.
4) *Adenocarcinoma*
   This is usually a highly malignant tumour frequently presenting with lymph node metastases.
5) *Epidermoid carcinoma*
   This is a rapidly growing tumour metastasising to lymph nodes early.
6) *Adenoid cystic carcinoma*
   Adenoid cystic carcinoma histologically has a characteristic cribriform appearance due to spaces between cellular areas, although some may be more solid. Approximately half occur in the major and half in the minor salivary glands. The growth of the tumour is by local invasion and by blood-borne metastases, particularly to the lungs. The degree of local invasion is often extensive with involvement of bone but without obvious radiological changes. Characteristically, it spreads via the perineural lymphatics. Lymph node metastases may occur, but these are much less common than distant metastases. It is a slow-growing tumour but the prognosis is ultimately poor.

Treatment Techniques

The treatment of malignant tumours of the major salivary glands requires a combination of surgery and radiotherapy. Wherever possible, surgery is used to excise the tumour locally as completely as possible, with sacrifice of branches of the facial nerve if needed on the grounds of infiltration by tumour. Radiotherapy by means of megavoltage X-ray therapy is commenced as soon as the wound is healed. In some cases the degree of local advancement of the tumour is such that excision is impracticable and then biopsy only is performed.

For the parotid gland, the volume to be irradiated must include the whole gland and the surgical scar with a wide margin, subtending a block of tissue of not less than 5 cm depth. Before planning treatment it is wise to have a soft tissue radiograph of the postnasal space, as this may demonstrate an unsuspected extension of tumour. The radiotherapy technique normally employed is as described above for pleomorphic adenoma.

Many of these tumours will present with involved cervical lymph nodes, which should, if possible, be included in the volume subtended. Elective neck irradiation has been advocated particularly with undifferentiated tumours, but this has not been our standard practice.

The dose to be delivered should be the same as for epidermoid carcinoma of the head and neck but will, of course, vary with the volume irradiated. Adenoid cystic carcinoma arising in the minor salivary glands presents a specific entity. The clinical features on presentation are such that a diagnosis may be confidently made. These tumours can be controlled adequately by radiotherapy alone and the initial role of surgery is a confirmatory biopsy. The presence of pulmonary metastases does not invalidate a radical treatment of the primary lesion since these metastases grow slowly and the patient may survive many years in spite of them. The volume to be irradiated must include a wide margin in view of the mode of local extension of this type of tumour.

The technique of megavoltage X-ray therapy to be employed will vary according to the site of origin of the tumour, i.e. mouth or antrum. The method used will be as described previously for these sites, the doses being the same as for a primary epidermoid carcinoma.

Carcinoma of the salivary glands may be treated by electrons rather than photons if a suitable energy of electrons is available. (The RBE for electrons is the same as megavoltage photons.) Fast neutron therapy has been claimed to be more effective than photons in the treatment of carcinoma of the salivary glands, but this has yet to be substantiated by controlled clinical trials.

Prognosis

The nature of salivary gland tumours is such that long-term follow-up is essential because late local recurrences occur, particularly with adenoid cystic carcinoma. The multiple types of histology and methods of presentation make comparison of treatment methods and prognosis difficult. The best prognosis is found with acinic cell and mucoepidermoid tumours. Anaplastic and epidermoid carcinomas of the salivary glands carry a poor prognosis.

8 Adult Central Nervous System

M. L. Sutton

Introduction

Historically, the adult central nervous system (CNS) was regarded as relatively immune to the effects of ionising radiation, and the recognition of the CNS as a radio-vulnerable structure occurred later than was the case for many other tissues. Increasingly precise knowledge of the time-dose-volume relationships for CNS tolerance has had two important consequences: (1) it has permitted the avoidance of catastrophic and usually lethal late effects in the brain and spinal cord when these tissues are unavoidably irradiated during the treatment of adjacent non-CNS tumours, and (2) it has encouraged referral for irradiation of certain technically benign lesions which, although compatible with prolonged survival, represent a continuing threat to the patient—for example arteriovenous malformations, pituitary adenomas, and some meningiomas. Many of these can now be controlled for very long periods following radiation doses consistent with the long-term functional integrity of the CNS.

Acute Effects

Large single doses of radiation cause "brain death" within hours (see Chap. 2). This is associated with widespread increase in vascular permeability and an increase in intracranial pressure. At the dose levels used in therapy at the Christie Hospital (230–375 cGy per fraction) the same phenomena probably occur to lesser degrees. For example, patients with raised intracranial pressure commonly used to complain of increased headache following their first few fractions of treatment; occasionally there was reduction of conscious level and worsening of focal neurological signs, sometimes culminating in death from pressure coning. These phenomena are rarely seen today, due to the liberal use of dexamethasone before and during radiation and to the provision of shunts.

Late Effects

As perhaps the most highly differentiated cell in the body, the adult neurone is incapable of division, and cannot, therefore, directly demonstrate radiation death. However, the neurones are dependent for their nutritional requirements and spatial interrelationships on the several types of glial tissues to be found in the CNS. The mature glial cells are now believed to represent part of a cell renewal system in which gradual cell loss is matched by equally slow replacement. This implies that mitosis occurs in a stem cell compartment, and explains why virtually all adult CNS malignancies arise not from neurones (which cannot divide), but from the supportive elements.

Late changes following CNS irradiation result from a mixture of two effects: (1) cellular depletion in the glial cell renewal systems, and (2) changes in the vasculature, namely diminution of the internal calibre of small arteries and arterioles, which may culminate in infarctive occlusions. Both effects may be expected to compromise the nutrition of the neurones proper, leading ultimately to their depletion, but the striking feature of radiation

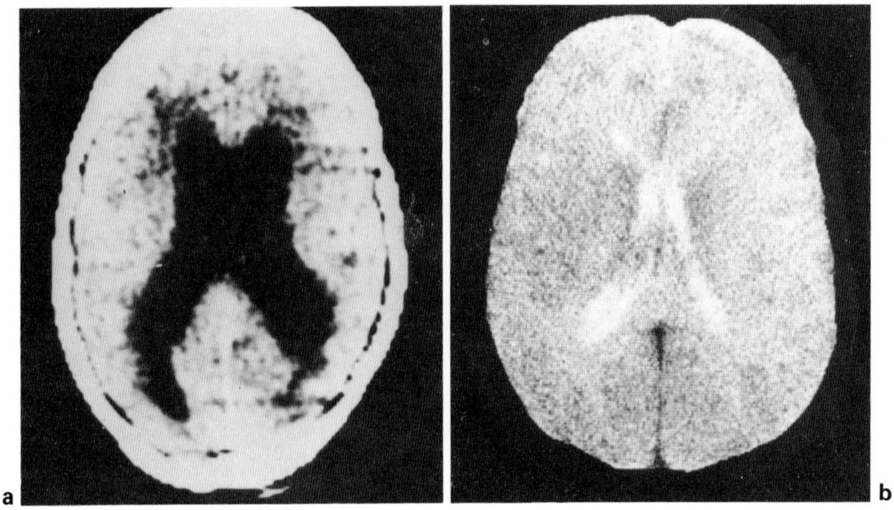

Fig. 8.1. **a** CT scan of brain irradiated 8 years previously by parallel opposed beams encompassing virtually the entire intracranial contents. Dose 3000 cGy in eight fractions over 11 days. **b** Normal unirradiated brain.

overdose near the upper limit of therapeutic dosage is demyelinisation proceeding to necrosis of the white matter. Midline structures (the midbrain, brain stem, and hypothalamus) are particularly vulnerable in this respect, and the consequences are lethal.

The brains of long-term (i.e. beyond 2–3 years) survivors of wide-field high-dose brain irradiation show generalised atrophy, with wide sulci and big symmetrically dilated ventricles. These changes are now regularly and safely demonstrated in life by CT scanning (Fig. 8.1). Provided that the mentation and sensorium of the patient were intact before irradiation, the atrophic appearances described do not seem associated with noticeable deterioration in the patient's intellectual status, but we have not carried out formal psychometry. The immature CNS is, however, likely to demonstrate failure of maturation; see Chap. 16.

CNS Lesions Important to the Radiotherapist

Supratentorial Gliomas

These tumours, which comprise roughly 1% of adult primary malignant neoplasms, have been classified into systems frequently of bewildering complexity. Whatever the histopathological merits of these orders of classification, we recommend a simpler, unpretentious approach to the problem, being content to regard these tumours as being either astrocytomas, oligodendrogliomas, ependymomas, or microgliomas (in decreasing order of incidence). The first two tumour types are *graded* 1–4 along the lines suggested by Kernohan, but ependymomas are usually described as being either well or poorly differentiated. Following tradition, the grade 4 astrocytomas are usually called "glioblastoma multiforme". Astrocytomas are much the commonest of this group of tumours, and unfortunately grades 3 and 4 are much more common than grades 1 and 2. The histological grading 1–4 implies not a discontinuous but an equally progressive tendency to increasing aggressiveness. In practice, grade 2 tumours behave much more like grade 1 tumours than like grade 3. Similarly, grade 3 tumours behave much more like grade 4 tumours than grade 2, although most patients who survive more than 2 years following irradiation had grade 3 rather than grade 4 tumours. Subtotal tumour resections provide adequate amounts of tumour for histological grading, but when the diagnosis is made on burr-hole aspiration biopsy, tumour heterogeneity may result in sampling errors, with the risk that the tumour may be assigned to a grade lower than that appropriate for the most aggressive part of the tumour, which dominates its clinical behaviour. The importance of uniformity in reporting the grades of these tumours is obvious, and this uniformity is readily achieved in a regional institute.

Like other supratentorial mass lesions, these tumours may present with (1) raised intracranial pressure, (2) epilepsy, (3) focal neurological signs, or (4) any combination of (1)–(3). Patients presenting with epilepsy and/or raised intracranial pressure alone generally respond to treatment much more satisfactorily than patients in whom focal neurological signs are prominent, and this tendency is true for each individual tumour type and grade. Thus the mode of presentation is an important factor in the selection of patients who should receive radiotherapy. Furthermore, even in doomed patients there is an important association between the quality of survival and its duration. Those who survive several years do not do so with the burden of crippling neurological deficits; many indeed return to their former employment in their previous capacity. In general, severe neurological disabilities are associated with the early death of the patient. However, this may not be the case when the neurological signs are in large part the consequences of oedema and/or distortion within the substance of the brain. In such cases marked improvement can occur with high doses of dexamethasone, demonstrating that the deficits are not due to irreversible destruction of neural tissue (Fig. 8.2). Similar improvement can occur following the aspiration of the contents of a cystic glioma (Fig. 8.3).

Many of this group of tumours are not amenable to even a subtotal resection, and this is particularly true of the glioblastomas, which tend to arise in eloquent cortical regions, particularly in the temporal and parietal lobes. Frontal tumours are usually astrocytomas grades 2 and 3, or oligodendrogliomas, while occipital gliomas of any type are relatively uncommon. Patients who have had subtotal resections before radiotherapy survive longer than patients whose gliomas are verified by closed biopsy only. Accordingly, patients who are in an eligible neurological state should not be accepted for irradiation until partial removal has been attempted. This is readily achieved in the polar gliomas, but it is sometimes forgotten that useful resections can be accomplished in more central tumours, particularly in the non-dominant temporal and parietal lobes. Subtotal resections confer benefit not solely by reducing the number of malignant cells within the cranium; they also provide an internal decompression, a "dead space" as it were, into which a recurrent tumour can grow against minimal resistance. For a while, this spares the adjacent normal brain the consequences of compression and distortion, and possibly of invasion also. The patients survive longer because an increase in intracranial

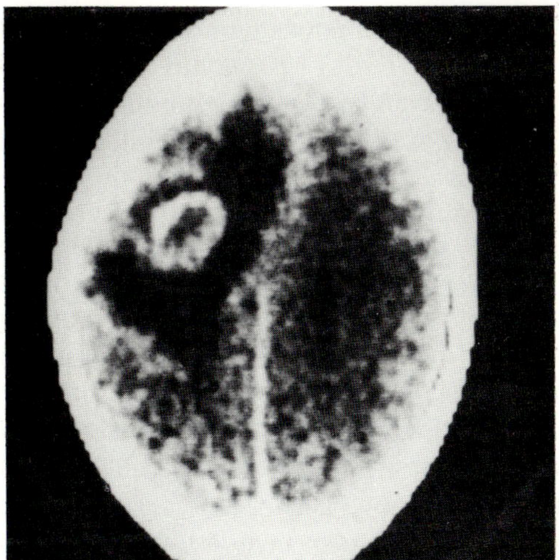

Fig. 8.2. CT scan of a small glioblastoma demonstrating ring enhancement with contrast and intense peritumoural oedema causing midline shift. Symptoms and signs of raised intracranial pressure and the patient's hemiparesis and dysphasia cleared almost completely with dexamethasone 16 mg daily.

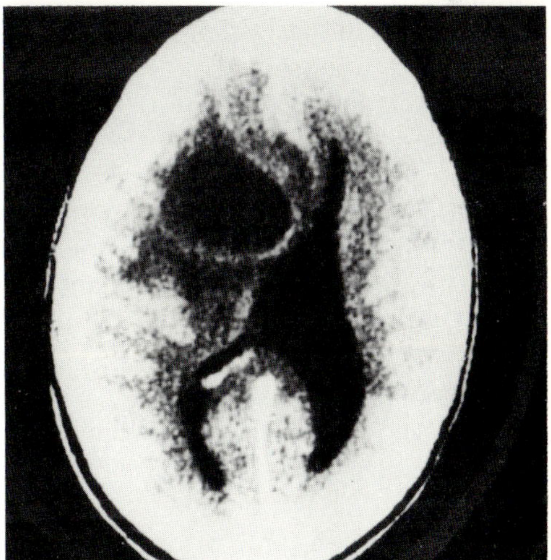

Fig. 8.3. CT scan of a frontotemporal glioma with a prominent cystic component. The patient's level of consciousness improved dramatically following aspiration of the contents of the cyst.

pressure is deferred and the quality of their survival is enhanced by the minimisation of neurological deficits arising from focal pressure effects on adjacent normally functioning brain. All supratentorial gliomas tend to be diffuse and infiltrating rather than discrete, and this is particularly so with the higher grades of astrocytoma and oligodendroglioma, which may transgress the midline grossly or microscopically. These considerations determine treatment techniques, but when death occurs, the terminal illness resembles a recapitulation and progression of the presenting illness, suggesting focal recurrence and indicating that the diffuseness of the gliomas is not the key to their lethality.

Treatment Policy

Patients with supratentorial gliomas require thoughtful assessment to determine (1) whether or not X-ray treatment is indicated, (2) the appropriate treatment volume, and (3) the optimum overall treatment time and dose.

Adequate X-ray treatment prolongs survival in virtually all patients with supratentorial gliomas, but its indiscriminate application is inappropriate. Many published survival curves for grade 3 and 4 astrocytomas, for example, show as their origin a percentage survival less than 100%, implying that a proportion of patients died before their X-ray treatment course was completed. We consider this largely to be due to the inclusion, in the various series, of patients who should not have been accepted for irradiation. The single criterion for determining whether or not a patient should be accepted for cerebral irradiation is the presenting level of neurological disability. Several other factors strongly influence the prognosis for both length and quality of survival (see below), but they are irrelevant to the decision to treat or not to treat.

Disability should not be assessed exclusively in physical terms, for cerebral lesions can cause profound disablement in intellectual, social, and emotional spheres also. When impairment of the higher functions of the cerebral cortex is due to the destruction of the relevant cerebral tissues, improvement is no more likely to occur than it is when marked sensorimotor signs are present. As noted above, severe disabilities in any sphere are associated with an early and practically inevitable death, and we do not regard as a legitimate aim of treatment the short-term prolongation of life for individuals who have become travesties of their former selves. These observations are particularly true of the higher-grade astrocytomas and oligodendrogliomas. (The lower grades of these gliomas have a much slower evolution of symptoms and signs, and are usually diagnosed and referred for treatment before gross neurological deficits have occurred). Before a patient is rejected as a potential recipient of radiotherapy, consideration should be given to the possibility that the apparent disabilities may be due to factors which are potentially reversible, and which may therefore be recoverable. Such factors include blocked shunts, untreated gross peritumoral oedema, postictal paralysis, inadvertent discontinuation of dexamethasone before referral (not uncommon), haematoma from burr-hole biopsy, or internal hydrocephalus from reversible kinking of the third and fourth ventricles by brain shifts.

The choice of the treatment volume depends on several factors, of which the most important is the grading of the tumour; all four main histological types, because of their diffuseness and tendency to infiltrate, require generous margins, and the higher the grade of the tumour the more generous the margins are required to be. So-called "whole brain" treatments are rarely required, and with truly polar lesions half-brain treatments are adequate, or even one-third brain treatments if the histological grade is low. High-grade lesions in the parietal or temporal regions require treatment of not less than two-thirds of the brain.

Rarely, apparently well-circumscribed low-grade tumours are seen which justify the use of multiple small fields and a beam-direction shell. Such tumours, whether amenable to resection or not, enlarge slowly, and many neurosurgeons prefer to defer radiotherapy until progression or postoperative recurrence is demonstrated on investigation, or until the early development of potentially disabling focal features.

Sometimes the stated grade of the tumour is clearly inappropriate to the rapidity of development of severe symptoms and signs. In such cases, the grading has almost invariably been on a burr-hole aspiration biopsy, and not upon material provided by formal resection.

Treatment Techniques

The majority of these tumours are treated with simple unwedged parallel pairs of beams. Such arrangements give surprisingly uniform dose distribution within the cranium, because the effect of reduced tissue attenuation of the beam over the doubly convex surface of the calvarium is approximately equally and oppositely balanced by the reduced scatter contribution of the "missing" tissue. Figure 8.4 demonstrates that there is indeed a zone of high dose close to the sagittal sinus, maximal in that portion of sensorimotor cortex devoted to the functions of the extremities of the lower limbs. Long-term survivors do not show paraparesis, reflecting the fact that this volume of higher dose is still within the radiation dose limits for cerebral cortex: the midline white-matter structures determine the dose tolerance limits for wide-field irradiation.

The low limit of the lateral field is usually one connecting the centre of the external auditory meatus to the outer tip of the eyebrow. Even temporal lesions presenting on the inferior or uncal aspects of the lobe are thereby adequately subtended. Lesions requiring wide-field treatments are sometimes inadvertently given fields larger than required to cover adequately the intracranial treatment volume. One late (and inconsequential) result of unnecessarily large fields is shown in Fig. 8.5; this patient at 3 years after irradiation has not regrown hair in a midline region of the scalp where the superior and anterior margins of the field were unnecessarily generous, resulting in a "hot spot" defined on the surface by the permanently epilated area. It is seldom necessary to check the treatment fields on a simulator, but because of differences in the shape of the calvarium it is prudent to check the field margins on the treatment machine using the beam-defining lights. When this is done, it sometimes appears that large volumes of brain are outside the treatment volume, but visualisation of the illuminated volume along its illuminated margin often reveals that the "missed" tissue is in fact only a very shallow inverted saucer of scalp and outer portions of skull. Most of this group of tumours are given 3000 cGy in eight fractions over 11 days, but some patients are considered to warrant more protracted fractionation and a higher cumulative dose. The longer treatment (3750–4000 cGy in 16 fractions over 20 or 21 days) appears to be associated with milder acute and late radiation sequelae in normal tissues, and permits the administration of a 250-cGy (one fraction) or occasionally a 500-cGy (two fractions) "boost" in the incident dose to the volume containing the radiologically evident tumour mass. The prognostically favourable features which are associated with eligibility for more protracted treatment are:

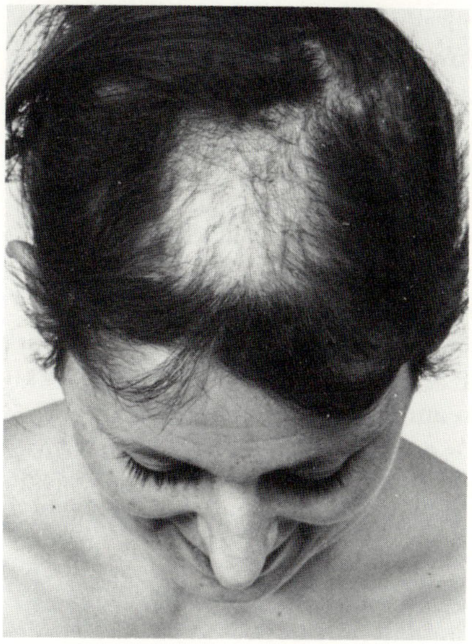

Fig. 8.5. Photograph showing adequate regrowth of hair following 3000 cGy in eight fractions, except in the midline anteriorly where a hot spot occurred.

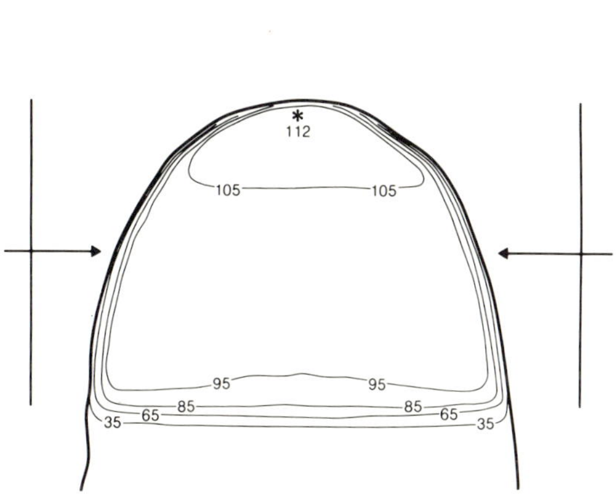

Fig. 8.4. Vertical contour showing relative hot spot in the parasagittal regions when whole brain irradiation is carried out using parallel opposing fields.

1) Absent or minimal focal neurological deficits
2) Previous successful attempt at subtotal resection

3) Relatively low treatment volume, i.e. neoplasms of low Kernohan grading
4) Patient age in the third, fourth, or fifth decade of life
5) Freedom from serious coincident illness

The sex of the patient and whether the lesion arises in the dominant or non-dominant hemisphere have no influence, provided all or most of features (1)–(5) above are present. At the Christie Hospital both 8- and 16-fraction treatments are carried out, treating only one field of the parallel pair daily. This results in a high dose-perfraction value, which may partly explain why the relatively "low" total doses recommended result in survival curves equal or superior to those obtained with 5–6 week regimes giving up to 6000 cGy (see Chap. 2). Because of the high dose-per-fraction rate in eight-fraction treatments, when pressure effects are prominent, the initial fraction is given from the side least involved by tumour, and such patients are never permitted to go home on the first weekend of their treatment, nor to receive treatment as out-patients. Dexamethasone, in addition to minimising the unfavourable effects of peritumoral oedema, also appears to attenuate the increase in oedema that occurs in the tumour itself following the first few fractions of treatment.

Both of the above treatment schedules are compatible with adequate restoration of the scalp hair (see Fig. 8.5), which occurs 2–4 months after completion of treatment. It is not necessary to shave the head before irradiation in order to protect the hair follicles from electron build-up caused in the hair when 4- or 8-MeV X-rays are used, but departments obliged to use cobalt-60 units for brain tumour treatments may find shaving a marginal advantage. (Strikingly uneven patterns of epilation are sometimes seen in patients who have had craniotomies, but this is not due to the fact that only one side of the head has been shaved before irradiation: the distribution of relatively conserved hair may be on the unoperated and unshaven side, and probably reflects protection of the hair follicles by relative hypoxia consequent upon postsurgical interference with the normal pattern of scalp blood flow.)

Infratentorial Gliomas in the Adult

Clinical Features

Adult infratentorial gliomas constitute less than 10% of the primary intracerebral neoplasms referred to the Christie Hospital. Ependymomas are easily the most common, followed by adult medulloblastomas and astrocytomas. The last mentioned are possibly more common in neurosurgical practice than the other two combined, but these tumours carry the relatively favourable prognosis associated with their juvenile counterparts and many or most are not referred for irradiation. Patients tend to be in early adulthood in all three tumour types, although ependymomas can occur in middle age. Ependymomas and medulloblastomas tend to arise in the midline and in general present at a stage when cerebellar signs are less advanced than is the case in childhood. The signs and symptoms of non-communicating hydrocephalus are more prominent than those of cerebellar dysfunction. Astrocytomas, conversely, usually arise in the cerebellar hemispheres, and unilateral disorders of coordination tend to precede the onset of raised pressure. Ependymomas arising in the adult posterior fossa are less likely to disseminate across the neuraxis than in children, and the same is probably true of the adult medulloblastomas; cerebellar astrocytomas almost never demonstrate this tendency.

Virtually all adult ependymomas and medulloblastomas are referred for radiotherapy following surgery, as total removal is rarely possible, particularly in the region of the fourth ventricle.

Treatment Policy and Techniques

As discussed later in this chapter, our experience of whole CNS irradiation in the adult has not been satisfactory. At present most of these patients are treated by a parallel pair of radiation beams directed with generous margins across the posterior fossa. Most patients can be treated brow-down, and the provision of a wedge on one field minimises dose heterogeneity from the curvature of the back of the head and upper neck (Fig. 8.6). Approximately one third of these patients have tumour volumes small enough to justify the use of a beam-direction shell. Midline tumours, particu-

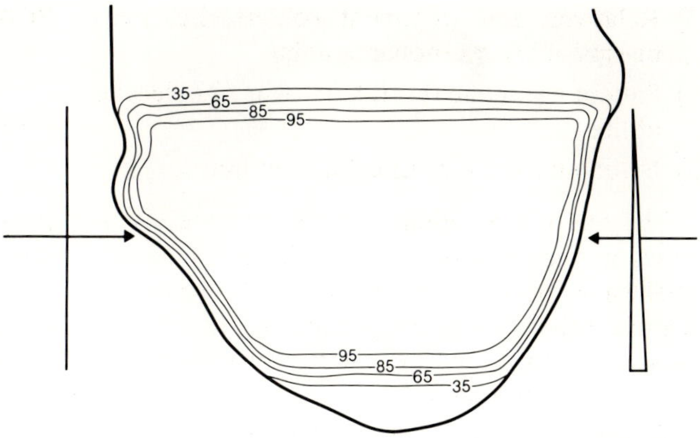

Fig. 8.6. Plan of a posterior fossa treatment using one open and one wedged field. Field sizes 7×7 cm. Tumour dose 4250 cGy, given doses 2560 cGy. Photon energy 4 MeV. 38° wedge. 16 fractions in 3 weeks.

larly astrocytomas, invite the use of wedge pair treatments (Fig. 8.7).

Whatever technique is employed, two considerations are remembered when the treatment volume is being assessed:

1) As its name suggests, the tentorium cerebelli is indeed tent-shaped and a verification field which has, as its upper margin, a line from the posterior clinoids to the internal occipital protuberance will not cover the contents of the normal posterior fossa, let alone one containing tumour.
2) Many patients have had posterior decompressions, and the usually substantial bone defect permits herniation of the posterior fossa contents postero-inferiorly, even when ventricular shunts are present.

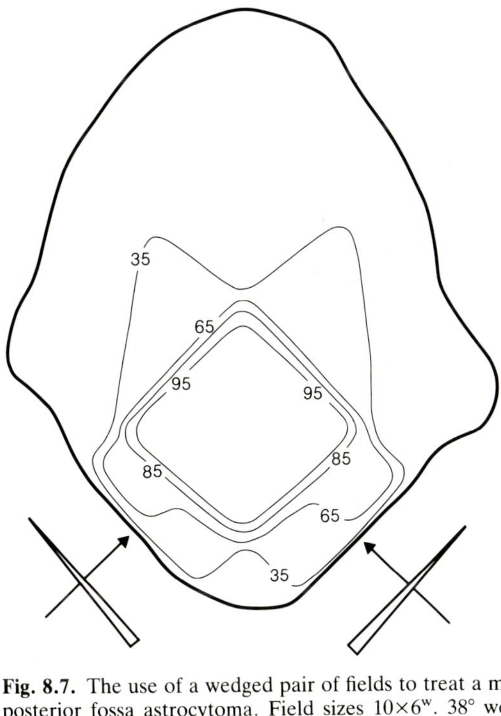

Fig. 8.7. The use of a wedged pair of fields to treat a midline posterior fossa astrocytoma. Field sizes 10×6^{w}. 38° wedges. Tumour dose 4250 cGy, given doses 2780 cGy. Photon energy 4 MeV.

Pituitary Tumours

These tumours, of which a small proportion are not technically benign, present as (1) endocrine overactivity; (2) mass effects (pressure, distortion); (3) endocrine underactivity; (4) any combination of the above. We have experienced a sustained and apparently continuing increase in the number of patients annually referred for X-ray therapy for pituitary tumours, because neurosurgeons now acknowledge that:

1) "Complete resections" are often incomplete.
2) Routine postoperative X-ray therapy dramatically and safely reduces the long-term incidence of recurrence.
3) Many past "radiation failures" were undoubtedly simply geographic misses, which historically led to an under-appreciation of the ability of X-ray therapy to control these tumours (Fig. 8.8).

Present delineative techniques, especially CT scanning and contrast cisternography, are less unpleasant and less hazardous than their predecessors, angiography and air encephalography. Accordingly, they are employed more freely, and they indicate that pituitary adenomas can be unexpectedly extensive. Modern delineative tech-

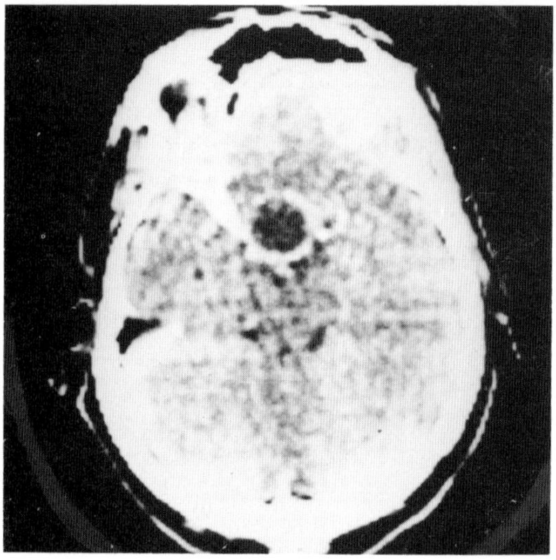

Fig. 8.8. CT scan of a pituitary adenoma with two cystic components. A rotation treatment of this adenoma with the field sizes based on radiographic appearances on lateral films alone would have led to parts of this tumour being outside the high-dose volume.

niques are also more accurate than their antecedents and, in the case of CAT scanning, can safely be employed postoperatively. These considerations have led to the changes in neurosurgical attitudes noted above. They also make comparisons of the results of present treatments with the results of historical material even more invalid than is usually the case.

The increase in annual case load of pituitary adenomas has been accompanied by an equally marked trend towards earlier diagnosis. The expansion of clinical services in endocrinology and infertility, with facilities for the reliable radioimmunoassay of pituitary-derived hormones, is responsible for this development. These radioimmunoassay methods are also responsible for the realisation that apparently satisfactory resections of adenomas are frequently incomplete.

The traditional classification of anterior pituitary tumours into chromophobe, eosinophilic, basophilic, and mixed, is obsolete. (Tumours of the posterior pituitary are very rare.) Eighty per cent of the adenomas of the anterior pituitary are hormonally active, since many of the chromophobe adenomas which were previously regarded as being metabolically inert are now known to secrete prolactin inappropriately in both sexes. No attempt is made to "stage" pituitary tumours on any of the several systems presently adopted by many neurosurgeons, which are based on a confusion of anatomical extent and histological grading. The staging proposals of Sheline are attractive in that they harmonise with the familiar TNM system, but prognosis for quality and duration of life is determined more by the metabolic and neurological state of the patient, at the time of referral, than by a pre-operative radiological assessment of the volume and direction of extension of disease. Accurate delineation of the volume of residual disease has precedence over the assignment of the tumour to an arbitrarily defined pre-operative category.

Mass effects are dealt with first, since they are common to all expanding or invasive pituitary tumours.

Mass effects These are compression, distortion, and/or invasion of the following adjacent structures which are in decreasing order of involvement:

1) Optic chiasma nerves and tracts (resulting in visual field defects)
2) Posterior pituitary (resulting in diabetes insipidus)
3) Hypothalmus (resulting in disorders of appetite, sleep, or libido)
4) Third ventricle (resulting in obstructive hydrocephalus)
5) Invasion of the sphenoid sinus and/or nasopharynx, which may result in cerebrospinal fluid (CSF) rhinorrhoea and meningitis (Fig. 8.9). Involvement of the sphenoid sinus, although unusual, seems to be becoming more common, especially in patients who have had a transphenoidal resection not followed by routine postoperative X-ray therapy.

Most patients presenting with mass effects have prolactinomas or metabolically inert "chromophobe" adenomas; patients with acromegaly and Cushing's and Nelson's syndromes now rarely have pressure effects. When pressure effects are prominent the resection is nearly always judged to be incomplete by the neurosurgeon, and serum prolactin levels often confirm this to be the case, either immediately after operation or some months later. All cases operated upon by virtue of pressure effects should receive radical postoperative X-ray therapy. Even when surgery has not been performed (by reason of unfitness or refusal)

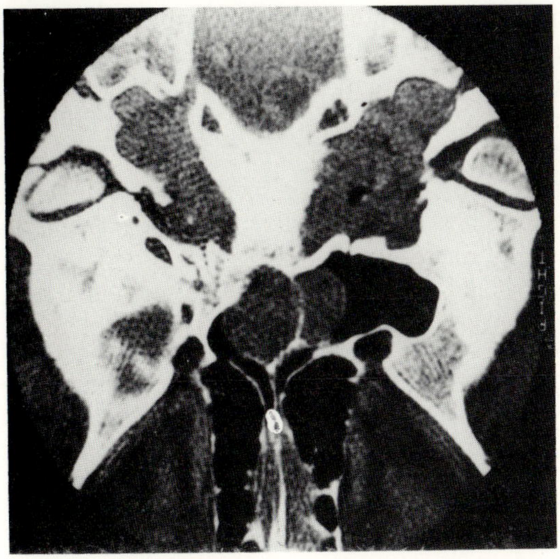

Fig. 8.9. A bilobulate pituitary adenoma involving the sphenoid sinus.

mass effects including headache may improve within a very few weeks of radiotherapy, whereas hormonal responses invariably take many months or even years to become maximal. Serial CAT scans show that pituitary adenomas involute very slowly following radiotherapy, so that the early improvement in mass effects presumably reflects the sensitivity of the CNS to small but critical changes in pressure or distortion.

Hormonal Tumour Effects Historically most adenomas were "chromophobe" and presented as pituitary failure with mass effects. Since the development of the appropriate assays, many of these tumours are now recognised as "prolactinomas".

Prolactin-Producing Tumours In the elderly these may be very large on presentation, but in younger patients diagnosis is increasingly commonly made when the tumour is in a microadenomatous stage. In the female they present with amenorrhoea, and in both sexes they can present with loss of libido, hypogonadism, mastalgia, and galactorrhoea. Transethmoidal resection of a microadenoma can be curative, but sometimes the microadenoma cannot be found. Postoperative serum prolactin levels may demonstrate persistence or recurrence of active neoplasm, and these patients are accepted for postoperative irradiation; patients in whom the serum prolactin level falls to normal and remains so are not accepted for X-ray treatment. Big prolactinomas often have mass effects necessitating a subfrontal resection that is virtually always incomplete. Provided that the neurosurgeon can achieve satisfactory decompression, the resection can be conservative, provided that radiation is later to be given. Following X-ray treatment, up to 5 years may pass before the serum prolactin returns to normal or ceases to decline: the belief that prolactinomas are "radioresistant" is erroneous. This is also shown by the fact that mass effects in undecompressed patients regularly show quite rapid improvement following X-ray therapy. Visual field defects, for example, can disappear after a small but obviously very critical reduction in tumour bulk: this is consistent with the observation that prolactin levels take several years to return to normal or near-normal values, as this depends on the total involution of an adenoma with a very small growth fraction. Female microadenomas, induced or unmasked by the use of hormonal methods of contraception, rarely require radiotherapy, since treatment with bromocryptine is usually effective in causing their apparently complete involution.

Acromegaly and Giantism Adenomas causing these conditions constitute something less than 10% of our pituitary tumours. Newly diagnosed giantism is exceedingly rare, and many acromegalics are now diagnosed because of the appearance noted when they present with apparently non-acromegalic symptoms. Visual field defects are now uncommon, so that acromegalics are consequently more often referred for radiotherapy without the benefit of previous surgery than are hyperprolactinaemic patients. Uncontrolled acromegaly approximately halves the patient's life expectancy at the age of diagnosis, and 50% of such patients will die before the age of 50. In subtotally resected cases, and in unoperated cases, 2 years often pass before serum growth hormone levels approach the normal range, and further falls gradually occur for up to 10 years following irradiation. The patient is treated with bromocryptine during the "lag time" between irradiation and the achievement of serum growth hormone levels consistent with freedom from:

1) Symptoms, such as hyperhidrosis, dysarthria, carpel tunnel syndrome, headache
2) Signs, such as hypertension and cardiomegaly
3) Abnormal and potentially lethal biochemical

disturbances, such as diabetes or hypercalcaemia

The duration of treatment with bromocryptine can only be determined by periodic withdrawals of the drug and subsequent clinical, biochemical, and hormonal evaluations. Some acromegalic symptoms, for example the discomfort of premature and accelerated osteoarthrosis, never improve. Headache, when present, usually greatly improves. Few virgin acromegalics who are given X-ray therapy subsequently require surgery. There is poor correlation between the pre-irradiation growth hormone levels and their response at 2 years after irradiation. This is expected, since the clinical severity of acromegaly correlates more with plasma somatomedin levels than with growth hormone levels. In about a quarter of acromegalics, hyperprolactinaemia is also found.

Cushing's Syndrome A handful of new pituitary-dependent cases are seen every year. Bilateral adrenalectomy, a major and hazardous procedure in a metabolically ill patient, is obsolescent, especially since metyrapone, aminoglutethimide, and OPDD now provide the means for adequate metabolic control during the 12–24 months which must elapse following radiotherapy before serum ACTH levels fall. Approximately two-thirds of all treated patients respond satisfactorily. Yttrium-90 implantation for Cushing's syndrome has been abandoned, as it has for acromegaly.

Nelson's Syndrome This condition, a legacy of adrenalectomies performed in the past for the control of Cushing's syndrome, is still occasionally seen. Over 50% of Christie Hospital cases are referred for X-ray therapy without previous surgical pituitary interference. These cases rarely have mass effects or hypopituitarism, since virtually all are under continued medical supervision following their adrenalectomies and are accordingly diagnosed before such eventualities occur. Although no conscious attempt has been made to prevent the development of this syndrome in adrenalectomised patients who had pituitary-dependent Cushing's syndrome, we have no single case in whom Nelson's syndrome has developed following pituitary irradiation for Cushing's syndrome: post-irradiation serum ACTH levels pursue a leisurely downward course, the dynamics of which cannot at present be confidently stated. No irradiated patient has subsequently developed mass effects.

Craniopharyngiomas

In the adult, the clinical evolution of these usually "benign" abnormalities often proves to have been even more insidious than it is in childhood. Frequently the antecedent history extends over many years or even decades, and the legitimacy of X-ray treatment in the management of these rare tumours in the adult is impossible to assess. We accept adult cases for irradiation on the grounds that:

1) X-ray treatment frequently inhibits reaccumulation of fluid in previously aspirated truly benign cystic lesions.
2) Because of their suprasellar situation, few of the histologically more aggressive variants of this lesion can be adequately resected.
3) The radiation tolerance for the adjacent normal CNS is known with sufficient precision for X-ray treatment to be carried out without more than a small (but unquantifiable) risk to the patient.

Craniopharyngiomas not infrequently interfere with the normal mechanisms inhibiting the release of prolactin from the anterior pituitary, and can be mistaken for prolactinomas. In such cases the serum prolactin levels will provide an extremely unreliable guide to the state of the lesion after treatment.

When it is available, the histology of suprasellar cysts invariably indicates an origin from squamous tissue; accordingly, higher radiation doses are given than are necessary for the control of pituitary adenomas. In the adult, the optic chiasma is commonly outside the high-dose treatment volume or in its penumbra, and these circumstances reinforce confidence in giving these tumours doses of 4250–4500 cGy in 16 fractions over 21 days, depending on the volume. The radiotherapy techniques are very similar to those exploited in the treatment of pituitary tumours, but because the prescribed dose is higher, we almost invariably construct a mould room shell, particularly when the visual fields are already compromised.

Sometimes these lesions are aggressive both

clinically and histologically at presentation, or occasionally become so after usually a long period of non-interventional clinical and radiological supervision: such tumours require bigger treatment volumes, and their surrounding tissues tolerate lower radiation doses than do their truly benign counterparts. These tumours are to a degree radioresponsive, demonstrated after radiotherapy by the cessation of the progression of their symptoms and signs, but improvement in established neurological abnormalities is rarely complete.

Arteriovenous Malformations

Clinical Features

Accessible examples of these benign but potentially lethal abnormalities are usually managed by microneurosurgical techniques, but many arteriovenous malformations (AVMs) are surgically inaccessible, and some arise in very eloquent neural territory. We now treat more AVMs annually than in the 1970s, and this is possibly because the widespread availability of non-invasive CAT head scanning has raised the detection rate for AVMs.

AVMs may present with one or any combination of the following features: headache (often suggestive of migraine, and sometimes classically migrainous), epilepsy, focal neurological signs, or as acute subarachnoid haemorrhage. The Sturge-Weber syndrome is rare, and the intracranial component is often immediately subjacent to the dura and therefore amenable to surgical treatment.

AVMs vary greatly in size, situation, vascularity, number of feeding vessels, and estimated rate of growth; their size and vascularity as demonstrated angiographically do not appear to influence the length of history or mode of presentation. All patients referred are accepted for radical irradiation since they are generally in good or reasonable neurological state. Those who present with focal neurological features have usually experienced a slow progression of their symptoms and signs, and have been diagnosed whilst still in an acceptable state functionally. Cases presenting as subarachnoid or intracerebral haemorrhage either make a good recovery, or are not referred for irradiation. AVMs presenting with epilepsy or headache have mild or fugitive focal signs only. Epilepsy and headache respond more readily to treatment than do focal neurological deficits, but prognosis for survival does not seem to be greatly different in the three groups. Mortality is highest in those patients who are referred following recovery from a bleed, and who have a second bleed within weeks or a few months of their X-ray treatment.

The antecedent history (except in cases presenting as intracerebral haemorrhage) often extends over many years, so that these lesions are only slowly progressive. Their rate of shrinkage following radical X-ray therapy is comparatively rapid; investigations have revealed substantial reduction in volume and vascularity in 50% of cases within 9–12 months of treatment. Serial investigations show that involution continues thereafter for up to 2 years. It is improper to subject treated patients who are utterly well to the slight but finite hazards of arteriography, so that very few of these lesions are now demonstrated to have completely disappeared angiographically. Historical material pre-dating the advent of CT offers ample evidence that all but the most extensive AVMs can be induced to disappear entirely, as assessed angiographically, and the subsequent clinical performance of these patients indicates that the disappearance is nearly always permanent. X-ray treatment fails to confer material symptomatic benefit in about 20% of patients who do have symptoms (those presenting in the recovered state following an intracerebral haemorrhage may have no symptoms at all). Angiography may be repeated in these patients, and usually shows no change from the pretreatment condition. The safest way of monitoring response in most patients is by performing serial CT brain scans with and without contrast enhancement, at intervals of 9–12 months. Digital subtraction angiography following intravenous contrast injection should prove to be a useful monitoring technique in the future.

Treatment Techniques

The site and size of the vascular abnormality determine the technique employed. These lesions are sometimes huge, involving brain on both sides of the falx and tentorium, and in such cases a simple parallel pair of X-ray beams is appropriate. Even when deeply situated, most AVMs are strictly unilateral, inviting the use of wedge-pair

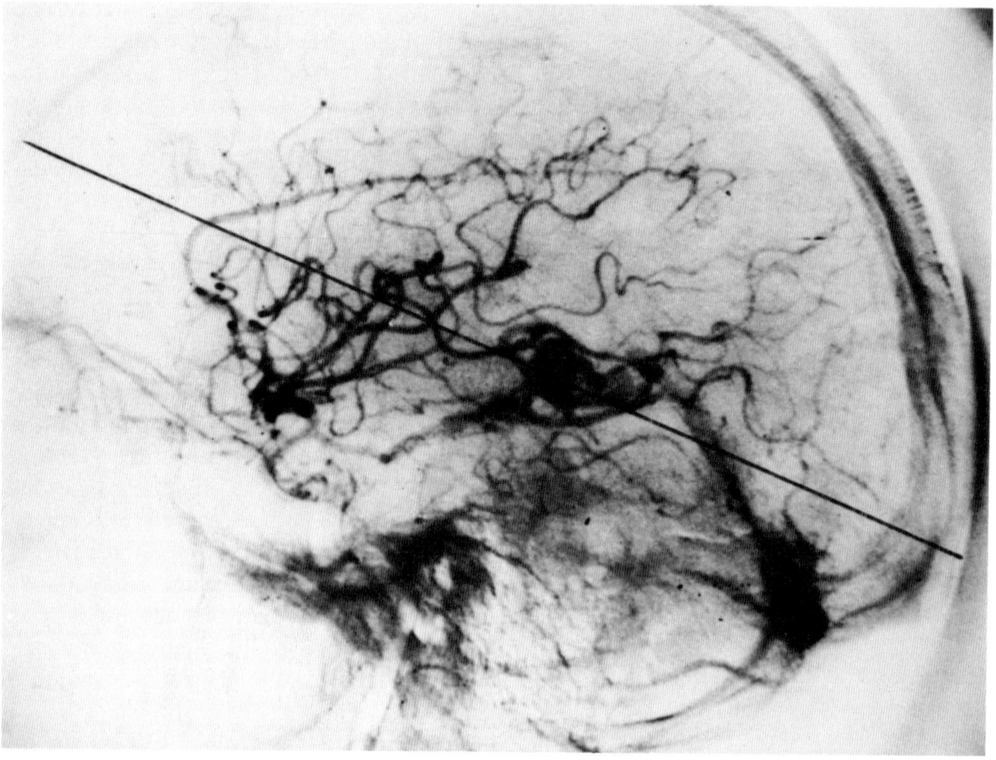

a

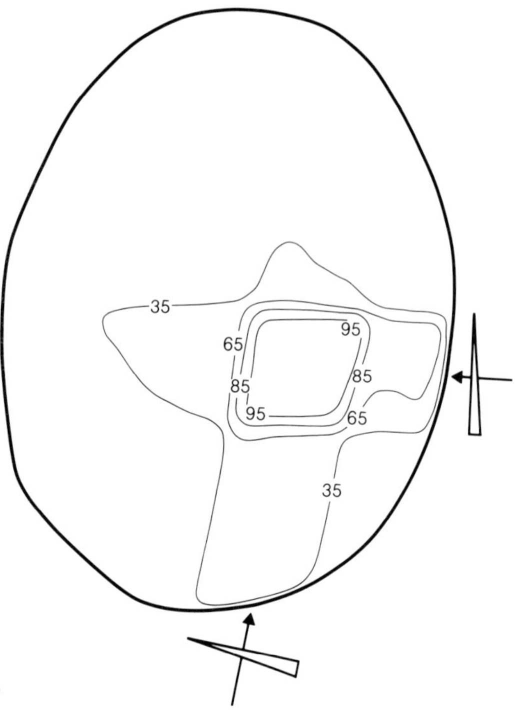

b

Fig. 8.10. a A small arteriovenous malformation situated deeply in the left temporal lobe. b Treatment plan for this lesion. Note that the treatment plane is chosen to exclude the orbit from the path of the posterior beam. Field sizes 4×4 cm. 46° wedges. Tumour dose 4500 cGy, given doses 3100 cGy. Photon energy 4 MeV. 16 fractions in 3 weeks.

field arrangements (Fig. 8.10). Wax bolus is almost never required. The convexity of the cranium can be overcome by the use of more steeply angled wedges, as in Fig. 8.11, which illustrates a vertical wedge pair to treat a triangular AVM in one occipital lobe close to the midline.

For treatment planning purposes, lateral and anteroposterior angiograms are greatly superior to CT scans; with judicious choice of the distance between the patient's head and the X-ray film when the localisation and verification films are taken, these films will have a magnification identical to that present in the delineative angiograms supplied by the neurosurgeon or neurologist. This makes very accurate localisation of the target volume a simple task. Only very small margins are required around the volume occupied by an AVM, since there is no invasive element in their enlargement; it is the *capillary* component of these malformaties that is radiosensitive and no effort should be made to encompass in the treatment volume those dilated arteries, arterioles, veins, and sinuses which may appear on irrelevant phases of the angiogram. Over 85% of

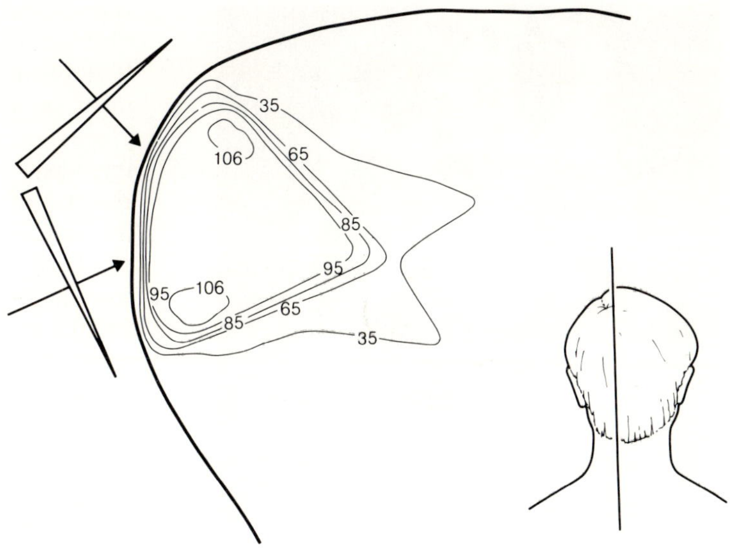

Fig. 8.11. Vertical contour demonstrating treatment of an AVM with a wedged pair of fields, designed to create a triangular cross-section corresponding to the shape of the AVM. Field sizes 7×6^{w}. 53° wedges. Tumour dose 4000 cGy, given doses 2120 cGy. Photon energy 4 MeV. 16 fractions in 3 weeks.

our AVMs are treated with small fields and a beam direction mould. Very small lesions in the cortical substance are given 4500 cGy in 16 fractions (occasionally 15 fractions, if a three-field technique is employed) over 3 weeks. Larger lesions, up to volumes of 300–350 cm^3, are given 4250 cGy; very large lesions involving perhaps a third to a half of the intracranial volume are given 4000 cGy in 3 weeks.

The medical supervision of patients undergoing X-ray therapy for an AVM is the responsibility of the radiotherapist. The patient is advised to avoid extreme physical activity for at least 9 months after treatment, and special care should be taken to avoid blows to the head. Coincident arterial hypertension is sought and, when found, corrected. Currently even normotensive patients are given slow-release adrenergic blocking agents for at least 6 months. If bleeding has not occurred within 12 months of treatment, it is unlikely to do so. This contrasts with the 4% annual cumulative rate of subarachnoid haemorrhage in untreated lesions.

Meningiomas

Clinical Features

Spinal meningiomas are nearly always amenable to total surgical removal, and rarely possess the invasive qualities more commonly seen in their intracranial counterparts. Accordingly, at the Christie Hospital, X-ray treatments of spinal meningiomas are seldom required, but when the need does arise the techniques employed are similar to those described for the treatment of intrinsic spinal tumours (described later in this chapter).

Five to ten per cent of the intracranial meningiomas diagnosed in neurosurgical and neurological departments are referred for consideration of X-ray therapy. The grounds for referral, in decreasing order of acceptability are:

1) Histological or operative evidence of "malignancy" or invasion, usually of bone, less frequently of CNS tissue itself
2) Neurosurgical assessment that resection has been incomplete
3) Pre-operative (angiographic) or operative recognition that the tumour is highly angioblastic (see below)
4) A second or even third operation for a technically benign meningioma which has thereby demonstrated its potential for local recurrence
5) Presence of a surgically inaccessible tumour, for example, one arising at the clivus or torcula (Fig. 8.12)
6) Radiological demonstration of recurrence in a meningioma which previously appeared to have been completely resected, in circum-

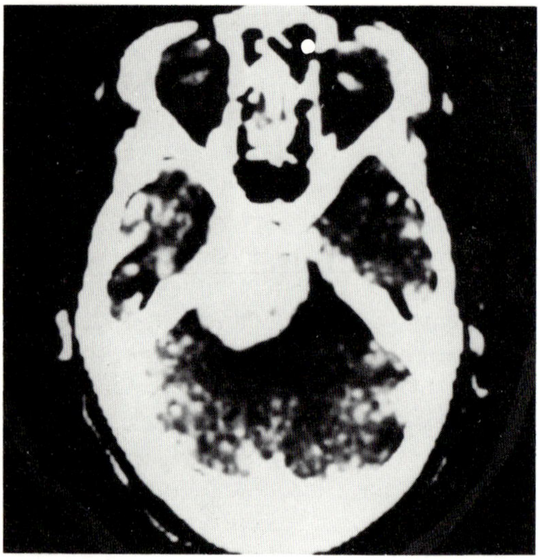

Fig. 8.12. A clivus meningioma not considered amenable to surgical removal.

stances where the neurosurgeon considers re-exploration unacceptably hazardous

7) Presence of a meningioma in a patient not considered fit for a major neurosurgical procedure, such patients usually being elderly and in poor general (and neurological) condition

Patients referred for grounds (5) and (7) above will not often have histological verification of the nature of their radiologically demonstrated tumours.

Patients referred for reason (2) have comprised virtually 75% of Christie Hospital meningioma treatments in the decade 1971–1980. Meningiomas arise at certain favoured sites (parasagittal, sphenoid wing, falx cerebri, calvarial concavity, sella, parasellar and suprasellar regions at the site of old skull fractures, and the basal meninges), and most are at least partly accessible to modern neurosurgical approaches. In this group, the commonest sites of residual tumour are

1) One or both sides of the sagittal sinus
2) The cavernous sinus
3) The sella turcica and adjacent parasellar structures
4) The falx cerebri (where multiple tumours and/or satellite deposits are not rare)
5) Any site where the meningioma has adopted a tendency to grow *en plaque*.

Very slowly growing meningiomas may invade the sagittal sinus and ultimately cause complete obstruction to blood flow. In such cases their leisurely progression permits the gradual development of adequate collateral routes for venous escape, so that large parts of the sinus and its impinging or invading meningioma can be safely resected in continuity. If, conversely, the wall of the sinus is involved by tumour, without occlusion of its lumen, sagittal sinus resection carries considerable risk of cerebral venous infarction, and the neurosurgeon will prudently elect to leave residual disease in the sagittal and parasagittal regions. Frequently meningiomas involving the cavernous sinus and/or investing the internal carotid artery are also amenable only to subtotal resection.

Treatment Policy and Techniques

Postoperative Treatments In this context, "postoperative" is taken to mean that a substantial proportion of the tumour has been resected, and the term does not refer to those cases where a non-resective procedure has been carried out, for instance a decompressive posterior fossa craniectomy or a ventriculo-atrial by-pass. Because these patients have been considered suitable for major neurosurgical intervention, they are usually in good general and neurological condition. In the first few postoperative weeks the majority have experienced gratifying recovery from their previous disabilities, are suitable for radical beam-directed X-ray therapy, and are capable of cooperating during this treatment. Most of these patients require a mould room shell, since the volume of residual disease is usually small.

Three main factors determine the target volume in patients with known or suspected meningiomatous residua:

1) The nature of the tumour itself. Most grow slowly and displace and compress the adjacent central nervous tissues rather than destroying and invading them. When such a manifestly non-invasive tumour is considered residual, it is usually only its site of origin which requires irradiation, as is commonly the case with parasagittal tumours (see also Fig. 8.17).
2) The degree of histological atypia noted in the surgical specimen. Tumours showing invasive features should be given more generous mar-

gins than their truly benign counterparts, for which only very modest clearances are required. "Malignant" meningiomas are sometimes encountered, and in such cases it is considered prudent to irradiate the whole of the volume occupied pre-operatively by the tumour, allowing generous margins.

3) The neurosurgical assessment of extent of disease. Ideally this should consist of marked posteroanterior and lateral skull films, or marked tracings

Pre-operative Treatments Very large meningiomas are sometimes referred for "pre-operative" radiotherapy in the hope that shrinkage following treatment will subsequently permit a less heroic surgical procedure than would otherwise have been required. In practice, these patients seem scarcely ever to come to their projected operations and such treatments are generally unrewarding.

Some meningiomas are intensely angioblastic, a fact which may have been demonstrated preoperatively by angiography but which is sometimes an unexpected operative finding. Attempts at the resection of such tumours usually fail, since there are great problems with haemostasis. The cranium should be closed with the tumour undisturbed or at most biopsied, and the patient subjected to radical X-ray therapy. After 6–9 months, angiography usually demonstrates a markedly reduced tumour blood-flow, and the residual mass may then be safely and successfully excised. The reduction in tumour volume obtained by X-ray therapy in angioblastic meningiomas can be impressive (which is rarely the case in ordinary meningiomas) and in those patients free of significant symptoms or signs, the neurosurgeon may elect to defer the planned resection until such times as serial investigations reveal renewed tumour activity. This renewal of activity may never occur (as is commonly the case with radically irradiated "ordinary" meningiomas).

Tumours Arising in the Spinal Canal

Clinical Features

Primary tumours affecting the spinal cord are uncommon. Many spinal meningiomas can be completely resected, and referral for postoperative radiation is rare. Primary astrocytomas of the cord are usually judged to be of low-grade malignancy on the basis of the slow evolution of their presenting symptoms and signs, but a definite histological report is often lacking, even when a conscientious attempt at biopsy has been made. When myelography and subsequent operative inspection confirm the presence of a fusiform swelling of the spinal cord, it is thought reasonable to accept the patient for irradiation, provided that there are no other explanations for the swelling, for instance a syrinx or a history of previous high-dose irradiation of the affected segment of cord. In both histologically unverified and verified astrocytomas of the cord, the treated length of cord should generously exceed the apparent rostral and caudal extent of disease, whatever technique is used. Before radiation is given, decompressive laminectomy should be performed over as much as is practical of the apparently affected segment. This laminectomy may result in rapid improvement in symptoms and signs, presumably due to improved local blood perfusion, but deterioration can also result, even when direct manipulation of the cord has been minimal. In such cases, high doses of dexamethasone are usually given, rarely with significant or lasting benefit. Direct visualisation of the cord also permits the identification of unsuspected AVMs.

Ependymomas arise most commonly in the lower regions of the spinal canal (Fig. 8.13), often in relation to the nerve roots of the cauda equina. In this situation they can be associated with the presence of very large amounts of abnormal CSF protein, which can even cause osmotically produced raised intracranial pressure with papil-

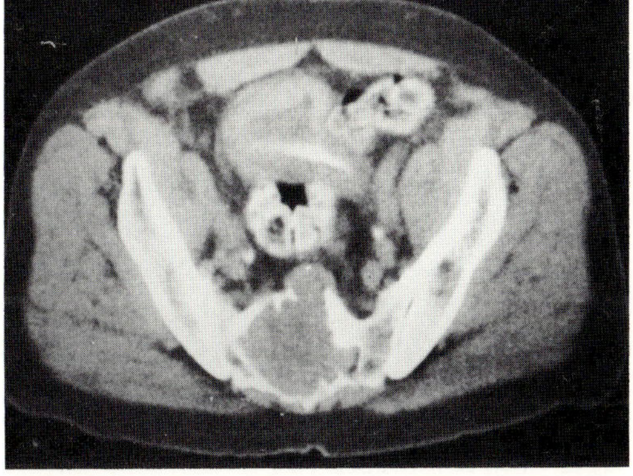

Fig. 8.13. CT scan of a massive ependymoma arising in the sacral canal and eroding forward into the presacral space.

loedema. For ependymomas the treated segment should include a generous rostral margin, and extend in continuity to the lowest limit of the spinal canal. Because of the lumbar lordosis and the presence of the buttock convexities at the sacral end of the fields, it may be worth constructing a mould to treat this region. As the cauda equina is essentially part of the peripheral nervous system, regeneration is possible, so that considerable improvement in function can occur. AVMs of the spinal cord are appropriately treated with minimal margins (1 cm or less) around the extent of the lesion, where this is accurately known.

Treatment Techniques

In palliative situations, or when the patient is severely incapacitated neurologically (in practice the two are often synonymous), a single straight-on megavoltage field is suitable, particularly when it can be delivered to the supine patient from an under-couch source. If under-couch simulation facilities are absent, and the localisation screening or radigraph is taken from the front of the supine patient, the indicated upper and lower limits of the field are marginally further from the field centre than will be the case when the treatment is actually given from the back of the patient; this is because the spinal column is closer to the patient's back than to his front. Provided that the screening or check radiograph confirms that the correct segment of cord is generously included in the middle of the field, the precise location of the upper and lower margins is unimportant.

Inhomogeneity of dose from single-field treatments of cord arise as much from the varying depth of the cord itself as from the fall-off dose across the dimensions of the spinal canal. Sometimes the former effect can be minimised by a 5°–10° inclination of the treatment head. A disadvantage of direct field treatments is that they cause upper aerodigestive tract mucositis when the cervical spine is treated, and gastro-intestinal disturbance when the lower thoracic and lumbar cord is treated. These side-effects can be avoided or minimised by techniques designed for radical treatments at the various different levels of cord (see for example Fig. 8.14). It is unnecessary to bring the tumour dose up to the skin scar surface when postoperative treatment is given for primary tumours of the cord or meninges. (However, when operation for spinal cord compression reveals a neoplastic cause which might contaminate the wound, for instance myeloma or metastatic carcinoma, then the whole extent of the wound in depth can be treated by adding a strip of wax bolus along the scar.) When mould room shells are employed, tumour localisation and verification proceed in the standard fashion. If a "free" set-up is to be employed for a radical treatment, the patient is supported prone on sandbags so positioned as to minimise the natural curvature of the spine in the involved area, and to bring the spine parallel to the top of the treatment couch. Posteroanterior and lateral marker radiographs are taken (1) to verify the correct localisation and size of the treatment field(s) and (2) to determine the correct pin-height for the two lateral wedge fields, and to verify that the spine is horizontal. Treatment planning is carried out on a life-size outline of the patient taken across the centre of the field (Fig. 8.14). Once the posterior pin-height is known, it can be checked that the distances d_1 and d_2 (which are usually identical) do indeed correspond to the appropriate FSDs read directly from the front pointers in their angled treatment positions. Small (approx. 0.96–0.98) depth-dose corrections are applied in dose calculation arising from the change in FSD. The table below is a guide to the doses that normal spinal cord will tolerate; it is derived from experience gained when normal spinal cord is unavoidably irradiated during the treatment of adjacent neoplasms not directly involving the cord. There is no clear evidence that the tolerance of diseased cord is significantly lower; at the suggested doses radiation myelitis is a rare event,

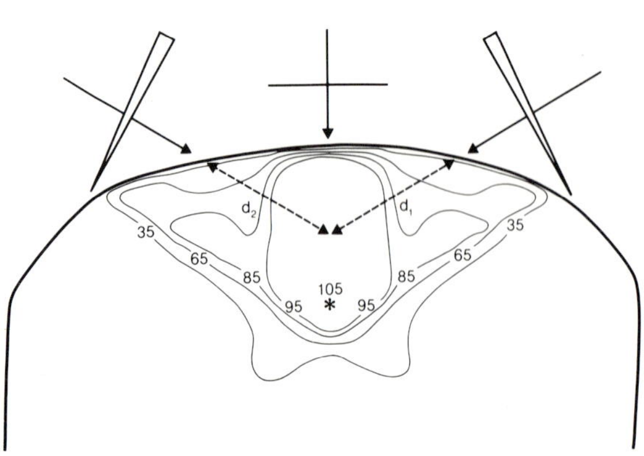

Fig. 8.14. Plan of "free set-up" treatment for a lumbosacral ependymoma; the anteroposterior dimension of the high-dose volume is several times that of the neural canal, to accommodate the varying depth of the canal from the skin throughout this region.

so that the doses given for spinal cord tumours may justifiably be higher.

Length of cord (cm)	15 fractions in 3 weeks (cGy)	8 fractions in 11 days (cGy)
<7.5	5000	4250
7.5–15.0	4250	3500
>15	3250	2500

Beam Direction in the CNS

Mould room preparation is essential for the adequate treatment of small intracranial lesions, and multiple-field techniques can be exploited to contend with any situation, however complex the technical difficulties in treating the necessary volume appear to be. In this aspect of neuro-oncology it is essential that neurological colleagues are schooled to understand clearly that the delineative information which they provide to the radiotherapist is crucial to satisfactory treatment. The task of representing the tumour volume dimensions on clearly marked anteroposterior and lateral radiographs, or tracings thereof, is commonly left to a junior member of the neurosurgical or neurological team, whereas in fact this task is sufficiently important to warrant the time and consideration of the neurosurgeon himself. The information presented to the radiotherapist should be a synthesis of knowledge from all available sources, i.e. clinical examination, radiological investigation, and not least, the operative findings. Intelligently to draw this information together is not a task for the inexperienced. A close professional relationship with the referring neurosurgeon encourages him to understand the technical limitations as well as the possibilities of small-volume high-dose treatments. Marked radiographs are superior to tracings, but when the latter are used, as many identifiable landmarks as possible should be indicated on the tracing. Ordinarily these will include the outlines of the pituitary fossa, the frontal air sinuses, the external auditory meatus, the floors of the anterior cranial fossa, the internal occipital protuberance, and any burr-holes or skull defects resulting from neurosurgery. Additionally, the positions of dural clips should be marked, but it must be remembered that the position of these clips is solely of use in orientating the tracings to the localisation and verification films: neurosurgical clips are haemostatic devices and are *not* intended to indicate the site of residual disease. Many of the lesions suitable for beam-directed X-ray treatment are histologically benign, so that the target volume often need be only marginally larger than the volume of the lesion itself. Minimisation of the target volume permits a combination of relatively high radiation dose with minimum risk of late sequelae. This avoidance of late radiation effects is nowhere more imperative than in the CNS. Because treatment volumes are kept as small as possible, accuracy and reproducibility in treatment set-up are essential. For most lesions, either an anterior two-thirds or a posterior two-thirds head shell is adequate. Occasionally a whole head shell is required, and this can be split obliquely to produce a shell suitable for treatment of a unilateral lesion in the temporoparietal region (Fig. 8.15). In treatment planning, ordinary principles of beam direction apply, but where possible "expendable" regions of the brain near the brunt of incident dosage when multiple fields are used. For example, when the sellar or suprasellar regions are irradiated, the provision of wedges on both the lateral fields produces a strong anteroposterior gradient in dose and to balance this equally and oppositely the anterior field

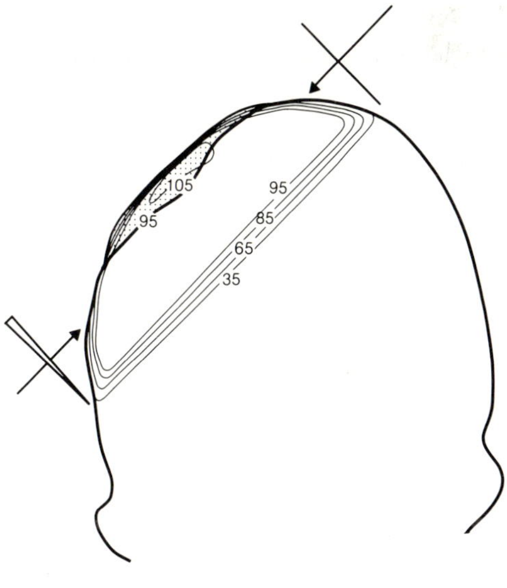

Fig. 8.15. A tangential pair of fields used in the treatment of a partly resected convexity meningioma. A small amount of wax has been added to the shell to fill in the depression caused by permanent removal of the bone flap. Field sizes 4.5×8 cm. Tumour dose 4500 cGy, given doses 2870 cGy. Wedge 38°. Photon energy 4 MeV. 16 fractions in 3 weeks.

requires a higher incident dose than the two lateral fields, commonly 60%–70% higher. In this way the relatively inessential mesial aspects of the frontal lobes bear a higher dose than the more vital temporal lobes. For lesions above the tentorium cerebelli, three-field treatments are more commonly appropriate than wedged pairs of beams. Lesions requiring more than three beams are very seldom encountered. When three fields are used the radiation dose to the hair follicles in all fields is usually sufficiently low to permit adequate regrowth of hair. This is frequently not the case when wedged pairs of beams are used—a marginal consideration when treating, for instance, a benign lesion in a young patient. It is rarely necessary to use build-up or bolus in CNS treatment, but it is sometimes useful in reducing dose heterogeneity over oblique doubly convex surfaces. Figure 8.16 shows the shell used to treat an extensive glioma of the right optic nerve which was involving the chiasm. The contralateral eye has been spared by skewing the parallel pair component away from the lateral, and the high-dose volume has been minimised by shielding the corners of the superior field. The critical structures in CNS treatments are the eyes, the optic chiasm, and the midline structures of the midbrain, and whenever possible these structures should not be irradiated. Particular attention should be given to avoiding inadvertent irradiation of the contralateral eye when unilateral wedge-pair treatments are used horizontally; the posterior of the two beams may exit through the opposite eye if the treatment plane is not sufficiently divergent from the anatomical coronal plane.

Previous neurosurgical intervention can sometimes significantly alter the near-symmetry of the normal calvarium. Usually this takes the form of a shallower contour on the operated side—as when a bone flap is not replaced at the end of the operation. Occasionally the operated side is 1–2 cm wider than the unoperated side, as when the subfrontal approach to a pituitary adenoma has been necessitated by marked suprasellar extension. Under these circumstances there is occasionally the possibility that geographical misses or near-misses will occur, due to failure to appreciate that the midline structures are not in fact along the middle axis of the treatment plan contour. Conversely, parts of critical midline structures may needlessly be included within the high-dose volume.

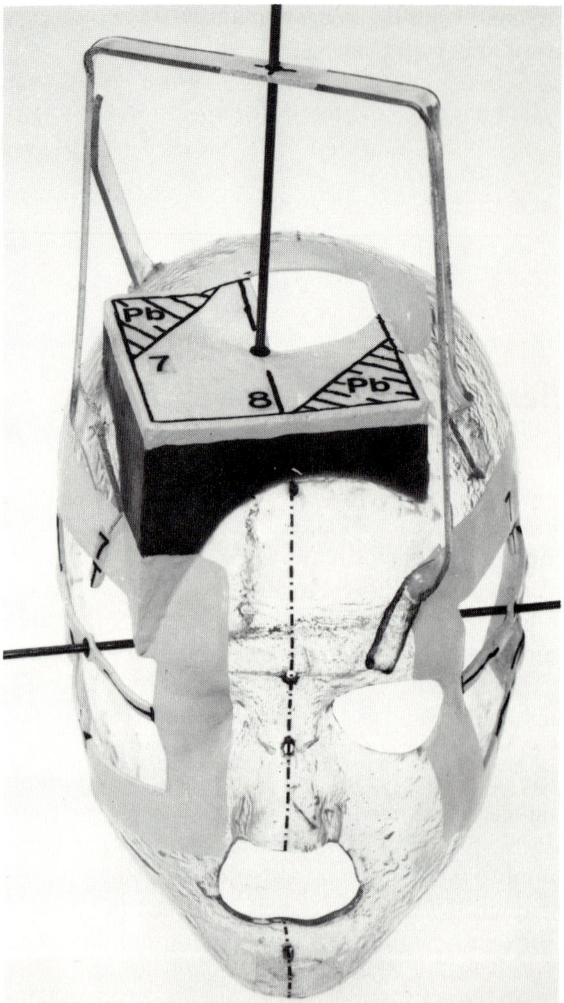

Fig. 8.16. Beam direction shell for a three-field treatment of a large optic nerve glioma. The skewed lateral fields are wedged vertically to create a dose gradient exactly balanced by the superior field.

Patients are sometimes referred for postoperative irradiation upon whom it is the intention to carry out a second operation some time after the irradiation has been completed. For example, it may be the intention to replace a bone flap that has been left out, or to insert a metallic or acrylic prosthesis, or to complete the resection of a lesion considered too intensely vascular at the first resection attempt. Under these circumstances it is usually possible to devise a treatment technique which relatively spares the skin and subcutaneous tissues through which the later incisions are to be made. Most CNS lesions require multiple fields, but occasionally single-field treatments with electrons are appropriate, for instance when treating a convexity meningioma that is growing *en plaque*. Areas up to 10×10 cm can be given 4500 cGy without build-up or beam scattering: epilation is complete and permanent. Figures 8.17–8.20 illustrate typical beam-directed CNS treatments.

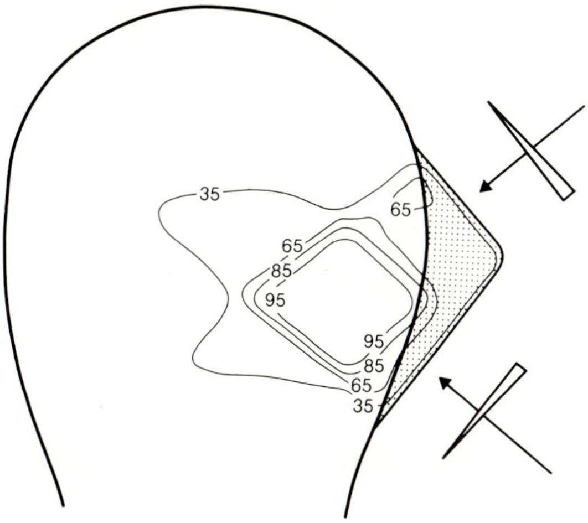

Fig. 8.17. Vertical contour of a field arrangement treating a small post-operative residium of a meningioma investing the vein of Labbé. Complete resection would have seriously imperilled the patient's ability to write. Field sizes $4.5^{w}\times5$ cm. Tumour dose 4250 cGy, given doses 2590 cGy. 46° wedges. 15 fractions in 3 weeks. Photon energy 4 MeV.

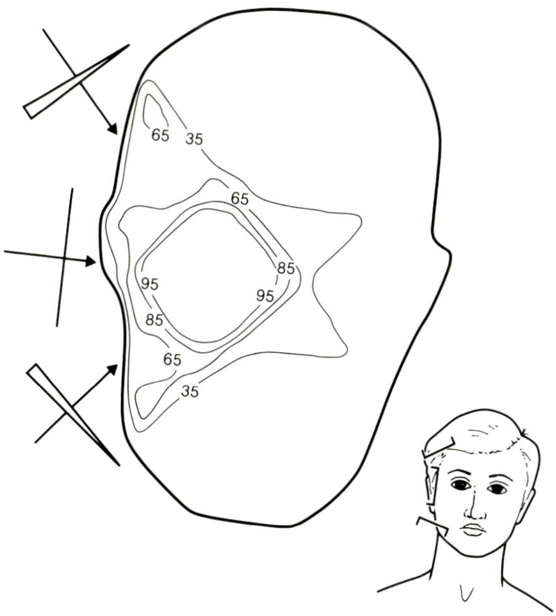

Fig. 8.18. A three-field treatment for a meningioma eroding the floor of the middle cranial fossa. Field sizes 6×6 cm. Tumour dose 4250 cGy, given doses 2240 cGy wedged fields, 1120 cGy open field. 53° wedges. 15 fractions in 3 weeks. Photon energy 4 MeV.

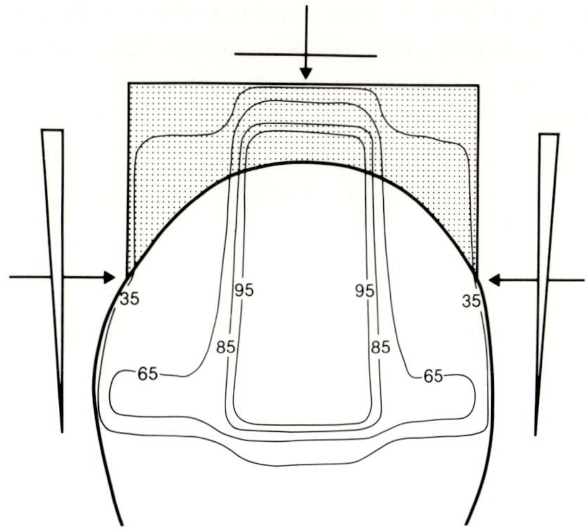

Fig. 8.19. In this example, the entire falx was covered on both sides with multiple deposits of a meningioma, which was involving the skin at the scar of the previous attempt at resection. Wax bolus has been used to bring the tumour dose up to the skin. Lateral field sizes 10×8.5^{w}, superior field size 5×8.5. Tumour dose 4250 cGy. Given dose lateral fields 1450 cGy, superior field 2680 cGy. 44° wedges. 15 fractions over 3 weeks. Photon energy 4 MeV.

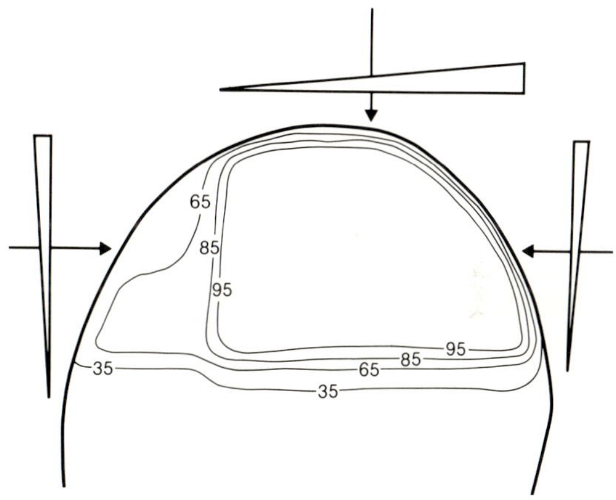

Fig. 8.20. This huge and very slowly growing meningioma had displaced the adjacent brain, of which there was very little in the high-dose volume; consequently the tumour dose was unusually high for a CNS treatment of this volume. Posterior field 8×10^{w} (15° wedge), opposed fields 8×7^{w} (38° wedges). Tumour dose 4000 cGy, all given doses 1650 cGy. 15 fractions in 3 weeks. Photon energy 4 MeV.

Whole CNS Irradiation in Adults

Clinical Features

The irradiation, in continuity, of the neuraxis, has been advocated for adult medulloblastomas, pineal germinomas and ependymomas, particularly when they occur in the posterior fossa. Our approach is determined by the following considerations:

1) The biological radiation dose required is considerably higher than that historically required for eradication of occult cerebrospinal disease in acute lymphoblastic leukaemia.

2) Whatever technique is employed (see below) overall treatment time is often increased by an early, profound, and persistent fall in the short-lived circulating formed elements of the blood, the white cells and the platelets. This is true even in young healthy subjects who have received no previous chemotherapy. When bone marrow collapse occurs it is neither prudent nor defensible to adhere to the originally planned treatment schedule, so that repeated and often quite lengthy gaps occur during which the marrow is allowed to recover and during which the effective biological dose to the putative and known CNS disease progressively falls. In approximately one third of cases the treatment has to be abandoned before the desired number of centigrays has been delivered to the patient, irrespective of the overall time taken to achieve the final dose.

3) All suggested techniques recognise that the site of bulk disease requires, and will tolerate, a higher dose of radiation than can be given to the whole neuraxis. If the site of bulk disease is indeed a potential source of CSF-borne seedlings, then the sooner it is sterilised the less the risk of seeding will be. In practice this dictates that the primary site is irradiated first to a dose well within its tolerance, and that subsequently it receives sufficient additional irradiation to take it close to its tolerance, in daily increments small enough to be tolerated by the whole neuraxis, with which it is irradiated in continuity. Clearly, when this second phase of irradiation is subject to interruption and even abrogation for haematological reasons, the primary site of disease will receive less than its optimum dose in biological terms. It is not practical to continue irradiation of the bulk disease during these interruptions, hoping to "catch up" with the neuraxial treatment later, because this necessitates subsequent shielding of the primary site and reintroduces the problems of junctions and their potential over- and under-dosage.

4) The development, after radiation, of CSF-borne deposits at sites remote from the bulk disease is rarely seen in the absence of an obvious failure to control disease at the primary site. This is not simply the result of low biological dose to the primary occurring for the reasons detailed in the preceding paragraph, for the same is generally true when only the primary site is irradiated (and moreover irradiated to tolerance levels).

In summary, neuraxial irradiation in the adult is often time-consuming, impractical and frequently fails to achieve its aims, both in completion of the prescribed treatment and in the results anticipated from it. For these reasons it has become our policy to restrict attempts at whole CNS treatments to patients in whom some or all of the circumstances listed below apply. (The situation in infants and children is demonstrably different, and it is conceded that the distinction between child and adult is arbitrary; in our material the age of 16 is used). CNS treatment in an adult is indicated when:

1) Investigations or operative findings indicate that two or more foci of disease already exist
2) The neurosurgeon considers that fragments of viable tumour have been lost into the CSF during surgery
3) The tumour morphology indicates an aggressive variant of the disease
4) The site of origin of the disease is in the posterior fossa

Treatment Techniques

Attempts to transpose the technically practicable "medulloblastoma treatment" (see Chap. 16) from the childhood to the adult situation have often been unsuccessful, always for haematological reasons. Haematologically active bone marrow is less widely distributed in the adult, and is so disposed as to fall almost entirely into the angled steeply wedged beams of the spinal component of the treatment. All of the vertebral column and most of the ribs and large flat bones of the pelvis either fall within the target volume or are within the exit paths of the two beams. When an attempt is made to give 3000 cGy in 4 weeks to the spinal column, the cumulative dose, for instance to the ileal marrow, is around 800 cGy—considerably above the LD50 for single-dose haematologic death. This is very significant, since marrow stem cells have small shoulders on their cell survival curves, so that the sparing effects of fractionation are minimised (see Chap. 2). The proliferative dynamics of the stressed marrow do of course modify the overall response, and must be responsible for the fact that some patients can endure the prescribed course of treatment without haematological catastrophe.

No wholly satisfactory megavoltage alternative to the "medulloblastoma treatment" has been devised. The orthovoltage treatment described in earlier publications from this hospital is practical and may still be used in circumstances where lack of resources make its employment necessary. For the present, we retain the wax box for the second-stage lateral parallel-pair treatment of the head and upper cervical spine (see Chap. 16). The spine is treated under-couch, using the same shifting-junction technique where the head and spine fields abut. Where possible the spine is treated as a single field, but whether this is possible or not depends on the length of the patient's spine and the FSD attainable in the under-couch mode. The FSD should be as great as possible, since this minimises to some extent the dose gradient across the spinal canal, but single-field spinal treatments are inherently inhomogeneous due to the normal dorsal kyphosis and lumbar lordosis. A long FSD also increases the likelihood of encompassing the whole spinal canal in one field. When this is not possible, because of limitations imposed by the available equipment, two or more fields are used, their junctions being staggered in exactly the same fashion as in the wedge pair used in children. In the adult the lowest extent of the CSF-containing space is at the second part of the sacrum, and heavy lead shielding is positioned to interrupt the lowest beam some 3 cm below this level: as in the childhood medulloblastoma treatment, this lower-limit lead shield remains at the same level throughout treatment irrespective of the stage of staggering of the craniospinal and (any) spinospinal junctions. Although this technique does not irradiate the functioning marrow in the ribs or the lateral halves of the pelvis, the vertebral column, much of the sacrum, and all of the sternum receive irradiation, and haematological problems during treatment are quite common.

Management of Raised Intracranial Pressure and Cerebral Oedema

Many patients with primary and secondary brain tumours have raised intracranial pressure (ICP) before, during, or after their X-ray treatment; it is commonly associated with the presence of cerebral oedema, which is sometimes very marked in degree and extent. This is especially so in the case of high-grade intrinsic (glial) tumours of the cerebral hemispheres (see Fig. 8.2). Benign tumours, for example sphenoid wing meningiomas, can also cause intense peritumoral oedema, but in general, tumours not invading the brain substance cause little or no oedema.

Excess brain extracellular fluid localises preferentially, but not exclusively, in the white matter, and often requires treatment in its own right, as it can greatly contribute to the severity of focal brain malfunction, and is itself often a major cause of raised ICP. Secondary effects, such as midline shift and kinking or obliteration of the CSF pathways may be responsible for additional deterioration in the clinical state of the patient.

All new patients referred for treatment to this Institute have recently had diagnostic CT brain scans, and most who have undergone craniotomy also have postoperative CT scans available at the time of referral. CT brain scans provide good indications of the degree and extent of cerebral oedema and patients with significant oedema have nearly always been started on dexamethasone before referral for radiotherapy, and have commonly experienced a diminution in their symptoms and signs. The acknowledged deleterious side-effects of prolonged high-dose glucocorticoids can lead to premature and precipitate attempts to reduce the steroid dosage. This commonly occurs in the interval between neurosurgery and the start of the course of radiotherapy.

The effects of steroids on peritumoral oedema are usually swift, and increase of the dose usually restores the improvement within 24–48 h. So predictable is this phenomenon that when it does not occur it may be thought that tumour extension rather than oedema has been the cause of the deterioration, and there may be a temptation, on these grounds alone, not to proceed with irradiation. In such cases a CT scan may demonstrate that this inference is wrong; it may show for example that there is displacement and occlusion of the third or fourth ventricle, causing an internal hydrocephalus that is virtually self-perpetuating. In such a "steroid-resistant" case, acute brain shrinkage achieved with intravenous mannitol infusions can result in dramatically rapid improvement.

Raised ICP tends to perpetuate cerebral oedema. In order to maintain brain perfusion against increased resistance, an accommodation takes place in the intracranial vasculature such that the arteriolar resistance to blood flow is reduced. This effectively increases the pressure at the arteriolar end of the cerebral capillaries, favouring the formation of extracellular fluid (Starling's law). This is a general effect, occurring throughout the vascular territory, and is not limited to the volume of the tumour and its environs. Most of the excess extracellular fluid is formed where the capillary vasculature is most abundant, i.e. in the grey matter, but the fluid subsequently localises predominantly in the white matter, which is relatively less vascular. This means that most of the excess fluid becomes situated in regions where it is relatively inaccessible to the osmotic effects of intravascular agents such as mannitol and glycerol.

In patients who do not have shunts, dexamethasone is our most frequently used agent for the control of cerebral oedema. It is commonly stated that the effects of dexamethasone are maximal in the dose range of 16–20 mg daily, and that higher doses are pointless. This is most certainly not the case, and patients with severe oedema problems may initially require 40 or even 50 mg daily. Attendant on such high doses is the penalty of increased incidence and severity of serious side-effects, but once improvement has been achieved, it is usually possible fairly rapidly to reduce the dosage to below 20 mg per day. Where even very large doses of dexamethasone fail to produce the desired fall in ICP, the use of hypertonic mannitol should be considered, provided that the cardiovascular condition of the patient permits. The aim is rapidly to achieve a high serum concentration of the sugar, which does not readily pass the intact blood-brain barrier, so that the brain experiences a disproportionately large share of the generalised dehydration induced by the osmotic diuresis. It is often sufficient to give 500–1000 ml of 20% mannitol by intravenous infusion in 30–45 min on one occasion to gain control over the ICP. If possible, repeat infusions should be at an interval of some days, since there is a danger of mannitol accumulating in the tumour owing to a disturbance of the blood-brain barrier in that vicinity. As mannitol is cleared rapidly from the blood by the kidneys, accumulation of mannitol in the tumour may actually increase tumour oedema because of the reversed osmotic gradient.

Once the acute threat to the patient has been overcome, and the prescribed course of cerebral irradiation has been carried out, it is commonly found that raised pressure and oedema remain problems for many weeks thereafter. In this context it should be remembered that the analgesics given for headache should not be those that cause depression of the respiratory centre. Increased arterial pCO_2 results in increased brain-blood flow, which in turn raises the ICP still higher. During this period patients should be given the smallest dose of dexamethasone consistent with maintenance of their improvement. Patients can rapidly become cushingoid on even "modest" doses of dexamethasone, and in this circumstance other manoeuvres of marginal effectiveness may permit further reduction of the steroid dose. In this category are:

1) Daily administration of a diuretic. (Although steroids can shift salt and water out of the brain, their net effect on the patient as a whole is to cause salt and water retention.) Acetazolamide is a mild diuretic most commonly used in glaucoma for its effect in reducing the rate of formation of aqueous fluid. It has a similar effect on the rate of CSF production, and is well tolerated. If no benefit is evident, it is worth changing to frusemide.

2) Some patients can be persuaded to drink glycerol, 30–50 ml four times a day, to produce a mild osmotic pull on the brain fluid.

9 Lung and Oesophagus

E. Sherrah-Davies

Lung

Introduction

It is sad to reflect that the incidence of primary cancer of the lung in Great Britain has continued to increase, and that at the same time there has been no real improvement in the cure rates. The most that can be said is that the criteria for attempts at radical treatment, whether by surgery or by radiation, are better defined, primarily through the realisation that patients who have disease which has spread to the mediastinum are, in general, not curable. Assessment of this spread is now much more reliable, thanks to better radiological techniques (especially transverse axial tomography and the arrival of the CT scanner) and the now prevalent use of mediastinoscopy. As a result, many of the larger surgical units now quote a reduction of the thoracotomy-only rate to less than 10%, and an increase in the 5-year survival rate of patients having a resection of up to 50%. Similarly it is known that radiation cannot cure lung cancer once it has spread to nodes. Radical X-ray treatment of patients who have demonstrable hilar or mediastinal node involvement produces a 5-year survival rate of a few per cent, and even these survivors tend to die in the sixth or seventh years of recurrent disease, suggesting that they are probably the patients with slow-growing tumours. By contrast, if the disease is "early", in the sense that as far as can be demonstrated, it is limited to the lung, a 5-year survival of the order of 30% can be obtained by radical radiotherapy. These apparently improved survival figures are only obtained of course by better selection of patients, and it is probable that the absolute numbers of patients cured have not changed significantly. Expressed as a proportion of the total number of patients diagnosed as having lung cancer, the cured group is tiny.

Most patients already have advanced disease when first diagnosed, and it is not difficult to guess why this should be so. Although squamous cell cancers of the lung are probably not intrinsically different in their behaviour and curability from their counterparts in the mouth or skin, being derived from the stomodeum, and therefore ectodermal, they can by comparison grow much larger before they give rise to noticeable symptoms. At the same time many a patient with a cough from a tumour developing in the main bronchus has been told that his chest X-ray is normal, because the tumour is hidden in the mediastinal shadow or merges with the hilar structures and is not recognised till a later X-ray shows the "sudden" appearance of a hilar mass. In addition, the loose tissue structure of the lung, with its rich blood and lymph supply and constant movement, presumably facilitates metastatic spread. For these reasons in most patients the disease is not diagnosed until the primary tumour is huge (compared with curable, smaller, squamous cell cancers of the mouth and skin), and moreover has already metastasised widely, so that the prognosis is already hopeless.

The vast majority of lung cancers are therefore only suitable for palliation, and the degree of palliation is usually of a lower order than we sometimes like to think. Distressing symptoms can often be ameliorated or removed, but survival is usually not increased significantly by our treatment, and most patients die within a year of diagnosis. The introduction of megavoltage machinery merely made treatment easier for both radiotherapist and patient, and hopes of better results were not substantiated. Neither has chemotherapy yet fulfilled its early promise. No cures by chemotherapy have yet been reported, and though it is undoubtedly often useful in the management of the late case, with the passage of time chemotherapy could well prove more limited in value than is sometimes claimed, unless more effective drugs are developed.

It is natural to think of instituting some method of screening the population mostly at risk, in order to detect changes at an earlier stage of development. It seems to be tacitly agreed that screening methods so far known (mass radiography, sputum cytology, and possibly fibre-optic bronchoscopy) are likely to give a poor return, and would certainly be inordinately expensive. The recognition of air pollution as a major problem, and the attempts being made to deal with it, may help. Anti-smoking propaganda seems to have had little or no value, and it is unlikely that human nature will change and the public will stop smoking en masse. It also seems unlikely that any government will ever attempt to ban cigarettes when the tobacco tax is so lucrative. In short, the outlook at the moment is indeed pessimistic and one can only hope that some unexpected avenue of advance will appear soon.

Clinical Findings

A lung cancer is occasionally discovered in a symptomless patient who has had a routine chest X-ray in his employment, or after an injury. On close questioning, however, most of these patients do have a cough, regarded as a smoker's cough or as chronic bronchitis. Cough is the earliest symptom for most patients. It is only when the first haemoptysis comes, or when dyspnoea becomes noticeable, that the patient asks for advice. Less commonly a series of "colds" or unexplained chest infections may lead to a suspicion of an underlying abnormality, though presentation as a classical case of unresolved pneumonia is no longer common, presumably because antibiotics are prescribed so freely.

Some patients present with pain due to chest wall invasion from a peripheral carcinoma, either in the rib cage or at the apex of the lung. Because the tumour is peripheral, symptoms referable to the lungs may be absent. It is also not uncommon for patients to present with pain due to a metastasis in bone, often in the spine, and the primary lesion in the lung is discovered later.

Rarely, symptoms referable to the chest may be minimal, or the patient does not pay attention to them, so that the tumour has spread widely by the time the patient presents with symptoms of a late complication such as superior vena caval obstruction, brain metastases, or dysphagia.

Clinical examination of the patient may reveal no discernible abnormality in an early case, but there are usually some localising signs in the chest of secondary changes such as collapse, infection, or an effusion. There may be localised tenderness or swelling if a peripheral tumour has invaded the chest wall, and an apical tumour may present as a Pancoast's syndrome. In particular, the medial corners of both supraclavicular fossae should be palpated carefully. Unlike the upper part of the neck, it is rare to find a palpable node at these sites which does not contain disease, and such a node should be regarded as a metastasis unless proved otherwise by biopsy. The only exception to this is in cases of obstruction of the superior vena cava (SVC), when multiple soft nodes, distended by fluid, are often found in the supraclavicular fossae and the axillae.

The abdomen must always be examined. It is interesting that herniorrhaphy scars are common, presumably associated with a long history of coughing, and scars of operations for duodenal ulcer are also more common than would be expected. A palpable liver edge in an elderly man may not be significant, but a hard or irregular liver, especially in association with nausea or anorexia, is highly suggestive of hepatic metastases. It is not uncommon to find a central epigastric mass of nodes, probably involved by retrograde spread from the posterior mediastinum.

If the pulse is irregular, an attempt should be made to ascertain if it is of long standing and a sign of known cardiac disease, or whether it is of recent origin. If the latter, it is an extremely bad prognostic sign, since it may well reflect cardiac upset due to direct invasion of the heart or pericardium by carcinoma. Such cases should be treated symptomatically in the simplest possible way.

The general condition of the patient is, as always, an important guide to management. If the general condition is poor, and especially if there is much weight loss or anorexia, advanced metastatic disease should be suspected rather than intercurrent disease or poor living conditions. At the same time, the presence of one of the more unusual manifestations of lung cancer, such as a neuropathy, a myopathy, or inappropriate hormone secretion, does not necessarily mean that the patient has widespread disease, and the treatment of these conditions is essentially the treatment of the lung cancer.

Pathology

The most common primary tumour of the lung is the squamous cell carcinoma, in all its varieties from well differentiated to undifferentiated or oat cell patterns. Pleomorphism is characteristic, and is probably a result of the inherent tendency of bronchial epithelium towards metaplasia. In contrast to squamous tumours at other sites, undifferentiated types predominate. Adenocarcinomas usually have the typical mucus-secreting glandular structure, and tend to be found more often at peripheral sites.

The so-called alveolar-cell or bronchiolar-cell variant is rare, and tends to spread widely and diffusely through the lung parenchyma without forming one dense primary mass, so that a chest X-ray may show a diffuse mottling which soon spreads from one lobe to involve the whole lung or both lungs. The disease is characterised clinically by gross dyspnoea and copious expectoration. Surgery is contraindicated, and X-ray treatment, sometimes attempted in desperation, is useless. The prognosis is always hopeless, and only symptomatic treatment is possible.

All other primary lung cancers are very rare, are mostly mesenchymal (e.g. fibrosarcoma, angiosarcoma), and should be dealt with surgically if practicable. The mesothelioma is not of course a tumour of the lung, but of the pleura, and its association with exposure to some kinds of asbestos fibres (notably crocidolite) has been firmly established. When first diagnosed, the disease is almost always diffuse, with more than one pleural opacity, so that surgery is rarely feasible, and radiation treatment is of limited value. The tumour is not sensitive to radiation, and little if any resolution occurs.

The peculiarities of the local anatomy are probably largely responsible for the high incidence of metastases from lung cancers, in addition to the fact of late diagnosis. It has been estimated that about 80% of patients when first seen will already have metastases in the hilar or mediastinal glands, and 60% will have venous spread, if the primary tumour is near the hilum. The percentages are lower if the primary tumour is peripheral. The incidence of metastases also partly depends on the histology, oat cell tumours in particular being notorious for their rapid spread. Whether this is entirely due to their rapid growth rate, compared with differentiated tumours, or whether they have in addition some intrinsic tendency to metastasise freely, is not known.

Investigation and Diagnosis

Radiological investigations, by routine chest films, show the majority of peripheral, mid-zone, and large hilar tumours. A penetrated anteroposterior film should be taken with the standard posteroanterior and lateral films. Not uncommonly, however, these films may not show a tumour near the origin of a main bronchus because it is buried in the mediastinal shadows, though there may be distortion of the bronchus or carina to be seen in the penetrated film. An apical tumour may also be missed if it appears as a thin apical cap.

The size and extent of the primary tumour is often not well defined by the standard films, and special films may help, such as oblique views or tomograms of a tumour invading the chest wall, particularly at the apex.

The mediastinum is best explored by tomography. Coronal tomograms may be sufficient to define a hilar tumour and show or suggest involvement of mediastinal nodes by distortion or splaying of the main bronchi, or broadening of the carina. In many cases, however, mediastinal nodes may be involved though not yet big enough to distort the anatomy, and in such cases transverse axial tomography is invaluable. It can clearly show the increased density of nodes under the carina, behind the heart, even when the presence of such nodes has not even been suspected from all other films. The technique has not so far been widely used, but now that CT scanners are becoming generally available the precision and quality of radiology of the mediastinum should improve. Radiology is also essential of course for demonstrating bone metastases, and isotope scans can often show soft tissue metastases, especially in the brain and liver. A barium swallow is occasionally useful to show pressure on the oesophagus by mediastinal nodes, or rarely, direct involvement of the oesophageal wall by neoplasm. Angiography of the mediastinum, and venography for SVC obstruction, are procedures which are neither useful nor necessary.

Bronchoscopy should be carried out in most cases, since it can be a good guide to the extent of tumour spread and can provide histological evidence. Modern fibre-optic bronchoscopes can reach much further into the lungs than the old rigid tubes, and it is even possible to take a brush biopsy of a peripheral tumour in the upper lobe. Such technical expertise should be exploited fully.

The larynx should first be inspected. Loss of movement of a vocal cord, usually the left, suggests a recurrent laryngeal nerve palsy, often due to malignant nodes under the aortic arch. The trachea or main bronchi may be indented or distorted by the pressure of adjacent nodes, and similarly the carina may be broadened. If the primary tumour can be reached, a biopsy should be taken to confirm the diagnosis. If the patient has dysphagia it may be convenient to perform an oesophagoscopy as well, since bulging or ulceration of the oesophageal wall confirms extensive invasion of the posterior mediastinum by tumour.

Sputum cytology can be useful, in that two or three clear-cut reports of the presence of malignant cells may save an ill patient an anaesthetic and a bronchoscopy. It may also help to confirm neoplasia in those patients who have a tumour too peripheral for bronchoscopic biopsy. It must be remembered, however, that the smears need expert interpretation and that a few cases may be falsely reported either negative or positive.

Pleural biopsy is usually useless, but malignant cells can sometimes be found in a pleural effusion.

Scalene node biopsy has been recommended as a routine procedure before thoracotomy, so that those patients whose biopsies show the presence of tumour can be spared useless major surgery. It seems that if the scalene pad of fat containing the nodes is excised from those patients whose nodes are not palpable, and the specimen is serially sectioned, many specimens (50% in one series) will show microscopic evidence of carcinoma. Whilst the technique is not practicable in most hospitals, it is common practice to excise a palpable supraclavicular node, because such nodes are almost always diseased, the diagnosis of cancer is usually confirmed, and extrathoracic spread of disease is confirmed at the same time.

Mediastinoscopy has come into general use as a relatively easy way of exploring the superior mediastinum for malignant nodes. If any are found, surgery is contraindicated.

Open biopsy of skin nodules or palpable supraclavicular nodes is useful for confirming the diagnosis in a late case.

Drill biopsy or needle biopsy of a lung tumour is practicable if the tumour is peripheral, and is possible for mid-zone tumours. It should not be used for central tumours because of the obvious hazards. It is now rarely used, partly because present-day fibre-optic bronchoscopes are so versatile, and partly because the complications, though uncommon, can be serious. These include tension pneumothorax, especially if the needle penetrates an emphysematous bulla, and seeding of neoplasm along the needle track. Other methods of obtaining histology are much to be preferred.

To summarise, these investigations should not only provide a histological diagnosis, but they should also define the limits of tumour spread with as much precision as possible.

Staging

The classification of the extent of spread of a cancer by stages, or by the TNM system, is useful for many cancers because it is a good guide to management and to prognosis. For lung cancer, both the UICC system and the slightly simplified American version are too complicated and detailed to be practical, and do not seem to have won general acceptance.

It is a fact of radiotherapy experience that about a third of patients who have a lung cancer which has not demonstrably spread beyond the lung can be cured by radical X-ray treatment alone. Most of the remaining two-thirds of this group are presumably lost because their cancer had in fact spread beyond the lung when the decision was made to treat radically, though this could not be demonstrated at the time. Once the cancer has spread beyond the lung, the cure rate is almost nil, and radical treatment with protracted fractionation to a high dose becomes an unnecessary burden for the patient and a waste of a bed and of machine time for the hospital.

The two groups are so distinct that a simple classification of lung cancers into early and late stages seems appropriate, as far as radiotherapy is concerned. The early stage (E) denotes a cancer limited to the lung which may be curable, and for which radical X-ray treatment should be given. The late stage (L) denotes a cancer which has spread beyond the lung, is almost certainly incurable, and for which only palliative treatment is indicated.

Radical Treatment

It must be clearly understood that the above classification is only useful to radiotherapists, who should never compete with surgeons for the treatment of the early case. There are two reasons for this:

1) If the cancer in confined to a lobe or a lung, surgery can remove it with finality, even if it is not small, whereas this is not always true for radiation. For example, even small squamous cancers of the skin are not invariably cured by irradiation, sometimes because of technical errors (wrong dose, geographic miss) and sometimes because of inherent "resistance" factors which we do not fully understand, such as the effect of hypoxia. Cancers of the lung are often relatively large and are often beginning to cavitate, so that factors such as hypoxia assume greater importance. It is understandable how, when the treated volume must be relatively large and perhaps respiratory function is poor and could be further restricted by post-radiation fibrosis, an inadequate dose may be prescribed. It is also easier to miss the tumour geographically when it is deep in the chest rather than on the body surface, especially since the lung is constantly moving with respiration.
2) Surgery can often remove involved hilar nodes and some mediastinal nodes as well, and can thus cure some patients with limited node involvement.

All patients thought to have an early cancer should therefore have the benefit of a surgical opinion. Radical X-ray treatment should only be given if surgery is not feasible, for example if the general condition is too poor, if respiratory function is much reduced, if the patient has associated disease such as a bad heart, or if he is too old or refuses surgery. This does mean of course that the radiotherapist tends to be given old or poor quality patients, and this is another quite significant factor which holds down our cure rates.

The histology of the tumour should not affect the decision as to whether to treat radically, with intent to cure, in the way described in this chapter. There is such confusion of thought on this point that, though it has already been discussed in Chap. 5, some further comment will not be out of place here.

In the first place, tumour sensitivity is sometimes loosely equated with curability, whereas sensitivity and curability are words which, if used precisely according to their dictionary definition, describe separate aspects of tumour behaviour. A sensitive tumour is one which disappears quickly when treated, relative to a resistant tumour. Curable tumours are those which experience shows are capable of being cured, as opposed to liposarcomas or glioblastomas, which are very rarely or never cured. Seminoma happens to be sensitive and curable. Cystic basal cell carcinoma is resistant, sometimes taking up to a year to disappear, but is curable. Sometimes a tumour such as a malignant melanoma is found to be sensitive, but is not cured. Undifferentiated and oat cell carcinomas of the lung can be very sensitive indeed, but they are also locally curable as often as differentiated tumours, and derive their sinister reputation entirely from their rapid growth and the associated high incidence of metastases.

Secondly, it seems to be sometimes assumed that a sensitive tumour needs rather less than tolerance dose for cure. This may or may not be so, but no one doubts that cure is dose-dependent, and it therefore seems quite wrong deliberately to give a curable tumour less than the maximum dose the tissues will tolerate. The point chosen on the dose-response curve where there is the maximum number of cures for the minimum number of necroses seems to be fairly critical, and a small drop in dose from this point leads to a sharp fall in the cure rate because the curve is steep.

A patient may have a tumour which seems to be

limited to the lung in so far as all investigations fail to show evidence of spread to mediastinal nodes or elsewhere, although we know from experience that quite a high proportion of such tumours (probably about two thirds) will in fact have already metastasised. When such a tumour is known to be of the undifferentiated or oat cell variety, it is often said that not only should the primary tumour be irradiated, but also the adjacent hilum and mediastinum, on the grounds that the regional lymph nodes are especially likely to be involved. This policy means, however, that a much larger volume of tissue has to be treated than would be the case if treatment were limited to the primary lesion, with a corresponding and significant reduction in the dose that can be given. This reduced dose must decrease the chance of cure to some extent.

If the nodes in such a case were in fact involved, and if it is accepted that cure of involved nodes is either rare or non-existent, then the treatment is merely palliative in effect. But if the nodes were not involved, the reduced dose to the primary tumour would mean a reduced chance of cure, which would not be the case if the primary tumour only had been treated to a higher dose. This is an example of the important basic principle that a tumour of limited volume should be treated in the smallest volume of tissue that is practicable, with avoidance of neighbouring tissues, so that the highest possible dose can be given. For the situation described, the difference in techniques could mean the difference between cure and death. In addition, if only the primary tumour is treated, and the nodes are in fact involved, nothing is lost because the treatment becomes palliative, and the mediastinum can be treated at a later date if necessary.

The correctness of this principle, in the case of lung cancer, is probably borne out by the fact that of the 10-year survivors at the Christie Hospital (admittedly few in number), more than a third had radical X-ray treatment to a localised undifferentiated or oat cell carcinoma. It is reasonable to presume that at least some of these patients would not have been cured if treated with a lower dose to a larger volume. In summary, the decision as to whether the treatment should be curative in intent, or palliative, should depend primarily on the stage, and not on the histology.

In practice, most cases thought at first sight to be suitable for radical treatment have to be excluded because it soon becomes obvious on investigation that gland masses are present in the mediastinum or hilum. In a few cases where the tumour is not near the hilum, and the mediastinum and hilum appear to be free from disease, the decision is easy. There is a third large group of patients having the common hilar tumour where the mediastinum is clear but the primary tumour itself is sufficiently irregular or knobbly in outline, especially on its medial aspect, to make one suspect a combination shadow made up of the primary tumour plus associated hilar glands, rather than a tumour whose growth has been irregularly constrained by the complex anatomy into having a lobulated margin. However, because certainty is not possible, such patients are usually given the benefit of the doubt and treated radically, and it is from this group of patients that most failures are derived.

The criteria for radical X-ray treatment can now be listed as follows:

1) Surgery has been rejected.
2) As far as can be demonstrated, disease is confined to the lung.
3) The tumour must not be larger than about 5 cm in diameter, or alternatively the field size must not be greater than about 8×8 cm. This criterion merely emphasises the empirical fact that cure of larger tumours is very rare in practice, presumably partly because such big tumours have almost certainly metastasised, and partly because a volume larger than 8×8×8 cm necessitates a reduction in dose. The commonest field size is about 7×7 cm, since most tumours are not found when small. Though this size is near the upper limit for a beam-directed technique, it is of interest to note that it is similar to that which has to be used for many bladder tumours.
4) The patient's general condition must be reasonably good, and in particular there must be no cardiac arrhythmia of recent and unexplained origin.
5) Histological proof should be obtained if possible. If this is not practicable, for example for a peripheral coin lesion in an old man, it is better to assume malignancy than to wait to see if the diagnosis is supported by tumour growth. More than 95% of coin lesions, especially in men past middle age, prove to be malignant rather than benign lesions such as harmartomas or other rarities.

Pre-operative and Postoperative X-ray Treatment

It is reasonable to suppose that X-ray treatment, given to tolerance doses before or after ablative surgery, may improve cure rates. It is said that pre-operative treatment will shrink the primary tumour to some extent at least, and may therefore make surgery easier in some cases. By killing some malignant cells and reducing the vitality of others, it may theoretically also diminish the likelihood of metastatic spread, especially from the tumour embolism which can occur by manipulation of the lung during surgery. It can also be argued of course that if surgical removal is made easier by previous X-ray treatment, it must be because the tumour was adherent to structures outside the lung, in which case the disease was advanced and not likely to be surgically curable anyway; and the possibility of tumour embolism is now usually minimised by ligation of the pulmonary veins early in the operative procedure.

Postoperative X-ray treatment has been given to the hilum and adjacent mediastinum after lobectomy or pneumonectomy in the hope that it might clear up microscopic or very small foci of residual disease.

Both these techniques have been tried by many radiotherapy centres in the past. Whatever theory might predict, it is now clear that they do not, in practice, improve the cure rates. They merely add a useless and protracted burden, and sometimes additional complications, to a patient already undergoing the stress of a major operation, and they should therefore be abandoned.

Techniques

The techniques described below will deal with most situations. A linear accelerator in the range of 4–8 MeV is the most appropriate machine. Telecobalt units are marginally inferior because of their slightly lower depth dose and greater penumbra, but are adequate for all but the largest of patients. Kilovoltage machines can be used, as they have been in the past, but are much inferior, in that six or even eight fields may be needed to give enough dose at the tumour, and the total volume dose to the normal lung tissue is great enough to be of concern.

A CT scanner is not necessary. It is of far greater value in the estimation of the limits of spread of the disease than in treatment planning, and though its use for treatment planning is elegant in the extreme, and mathematically precise, it must be remembered that to make full use of these qualities, other details of treatment must match this degree of precision. For example, it is only too easy to plan a treatment on a cut taken just above or below the equator of a spherical tumour, so that the chosen field-size may be inadequate to encompass the slightly greater width at the equator. The daily "setting-up" of the patient on the treatment couch, with or without a shell, must be accurate and sufficiently reproducible to justify the closer tolerances on the margin allowed round the tumour which may be suggested by the video display. The CT scanner has not been in use for long enough at the Christie Hospital to be able properly to evaluate its contribution to treatment planning.

For tumours at or near the hilum, the time-tested three-field technique is eminently satisfactory. It is simple to set up, calculate, and prescribe, and does not need a beam-direction shell (see Fig. 9.1).

The posteroanterior chest film is used to estimate the centre of the tumour in relation to the anterior rib cage and midline, and the field size. A simple ruler which has enlarged "centimetre" spacing to compensate for magnification is useful for estimating distances on the film. With the patient in the supine treatment position, a skin mark is made over the estimated centre of the tumour, and a diagnostic film is taken centred on this mark. The field edges can be outlined with wire taped to the skin, or if a simulator is available, the field can be delineated using the simulator's field-marker bars. A verification film is then taken and the skin mark adjusted if necessary, continuing the sequence until localisation is exact.

For increased accuracy it is useful finally to take two extra films, one after full inspiration and another after full expiration. Patients vary greatly in the range of tumour movement with respiration. In a tranquil patient with emphysema and limited chest movement, there may be only 0.5 cm of movement up and down (cranially and caudally), but a nervous patient with good lungs may show up to 2 cm of movment. This may have to be allowed for when deciding on the length of the field, so that the field will at all times subtend the tumour, whatever the depth of respiration.

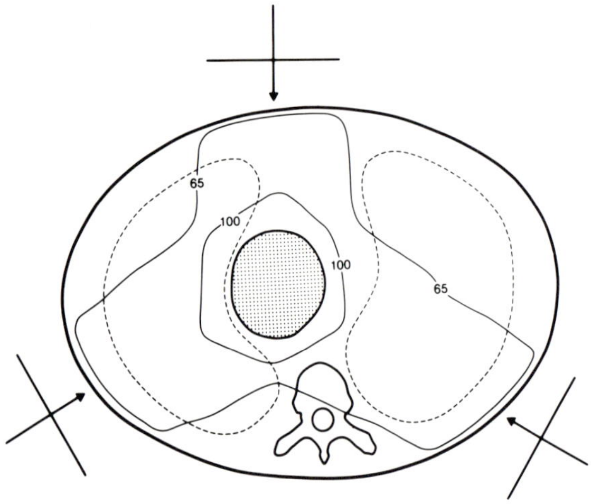

Fig. 9.1. Carcinoma of lung—3-field technique.

The depth of the centre of the tumour from the anterior skin mark is then measured by using an ordinary ruler on the lateral chest film, then measuring the depth of the whole chest at that level on the film. This gives a ratio which can be multiplied by the real chest depth, as measured using calipers with the patient in the supine treatment position, to give the true depth of the tumour centre.

The patient is now turned over to the prone treatment position, and a skin mark placed on the back and checked in the same way till it is accurate. It will be found that, for the anterior mark, the bony landmarks give a good guide and the first guess is often exact, or nearly so, whereas the posterior mark is usually only right the first time by luck.

With the patient still in the prone position, and with the simulator or treatment machine set up with its frontal pointer vertical and on the skin mark, the machine head is now rotated 60°, first to one side and then to the other. In each lateral oblique position a skin mark is made and the source-skin distance measured. If, for example, the machine is usually set up for 100-cm FSD, the FSD for the 60° mark on the same side as the tumour might be, say, 88 cm, whereas on the side furthest from the tumour it might be 83 cm.

Depth doses are now obtained for the three fields from the relevant tables. That for the front field is read directly from the 100-cm FSD table, whereas those for the two posterior oblique fields have to be corrected for the reduced FSD. It is convenient in practice to prepare a table of depth doses for common field sizes (say, 5×5 to 9×9 cm) and common FSDs (say, 70 to 95 cm) for this technique, so that calculations do not have to be made afresh for every patient, time is saved, and there is less risk of error. Jaw settings on the machine also have to be changed proportionately to the change in FSD.

It is usually worthwhile to make a correction to the depth dose, as read from the tables, to take into account the increased transmission of energy through air-filled lung. Because that section of lung between the chest wall and the tumour is often wedge-shaped (sometimes grossly and irregularly so), the ideal would be to use a "taken-back" wedge, contoured specifically for each beam to compensate for the shape of the section of lung plus any obliquity of the skin surface. In practice, this would be very time-consuming and is not warranted by the small increase in homogeneity of dose it would afford.

If, therefore, there is little or no aerated lung in the path of most of the beam, as is often the case for the anterior field, no correction is made. For the posterior fields a rough correction is usually made, the magnitude of which depends on the energy of the beam and the approximate average thickness of aerated lung traversed by the central axis of the beam. The figures used are based on calculations verified by measurements in a simulated phantom, and also by direct measurement on a few patients during treatment who had a miniature ionisation chamber passed endotracheally into the centre of the treatment field. For every 5 cm of air-filled lung, tumour depth doses should be increased by 10% (8 MeV), 15% (4 MeV), or 20% (telecobalt). For greater or lesser thicknesses of lung, these figures can be changed in simple proportion.

Because the three fields are symmetrically placed at 120°, equal contributions of dose at the tumour centre will give a homogeneous dose throughout the treated volume. Prescription of dose is therefore simple, since no balancing is necessary.

Long use of this technique has shown that for field sizes up to 8×8 cm, 5250 cGy given in 15 daily treatments (five fractions a week for 3 weeks) is optimum. If the field size exceeds 8×8 cm, or if the patient is sufficiently diabetic to need more than diet for control, the dose should be reduced to 5000 cGy. Very rarely, a small tumour is found which can be subtended by fields of 5×5 or 6×5 cm, in which case a dose of 5500 cGy can be given.

A rotation technique may also be used, either with megavoltage or telecobalt machines, though it is slightly less attractive because almost the whole of both lungs in the treatment plane is irradiated (Fig. 9.2).

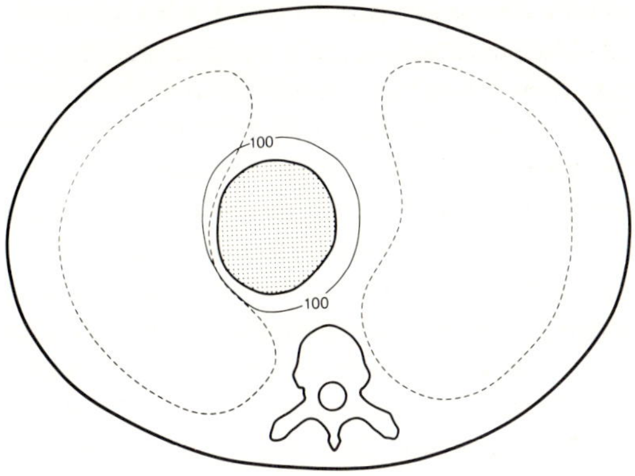

Fig. 9.2. Carcinoma of lung—rotation technique.

A small tumour at the periphery of the lung can sometimes be treated using a simple wedge pair. Such tumours often lie laterally, so that the patient can lie on the side of the normal lung, with the arm on the diseased side elevated, the hand being placed comfortably under the head. A shell is then made which is long enough to be held in place by the lower rib margin inferiorly and the shoulder and upper third of the arm superiorly. Anteriorly and posteriorly it must cross the midline for stability (Fig. 9.3).

The majority of peripheral tumours are too big, and lie too deep, for a wedge pair to give sufficient depth dose, and an additional plain field between the separated wedges must be used. It is worth noting that if such a larger tumour has already invaded one or two adjacent ribs, radical treatment may still be worth while, since cure has occasionally been obtained (Fig. 9.4).

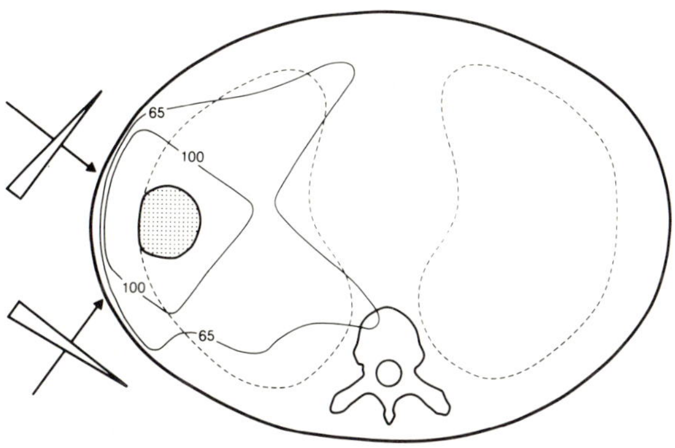

Fig. 9.3. Carcinoma at periphery of lung—wedge pair technique.

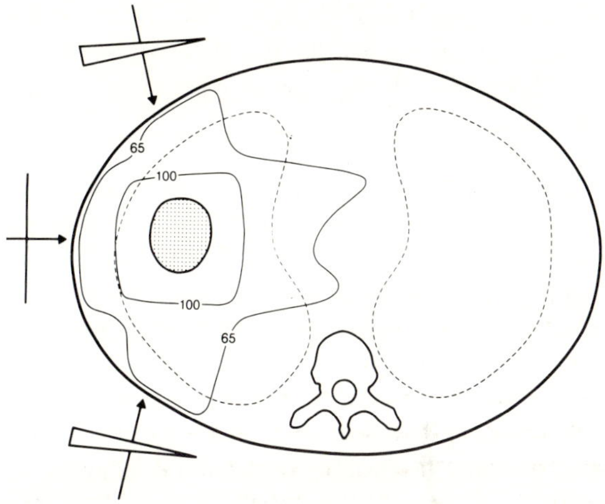

Fig. 9.4. Carcinoma at periphery of lung—3-field technique using wedges.

Uncommonly, a patient may present with a small tumour in the mid-zone at about the level of the clavicle, or just below, and none of the above techniques is suitable. For this site, a simple parallel pair of fields may be best.

Again uncommonly, a tumour may be found to lie in the posterior gutter, near to and perhaps almost touching a vertebral body, but without demonstrable involvement of the bone. Such a case needs a special plan, and the nearest field to the tumour will be dominant and therefore carry a high dose, whilst other fields are supplementary. It may be found that the placing of the medial edge of this dominant beam is critical in its relationship to the spinal cord. However accurately the beam direction is done, it is possible for a restless patient to rotate slightly from a perfectly flat prone position, so that he rotates his spinal cord into the beam. A suitable block of lead, well-seated on the treatment shell at the margin of the beam, will in such circumstances move with the patient sufficiently to protect the cord.

General Management

It is best to admit the patient to hospital for a radical course of treatment, if only to avoid the stress of daily journeys and conserve energy. Antibiotics should be given at the first sign of infection, preferably after isolating the organism and testing its sensitivity to common antibiotics, though a dirty sputum by itself does not warrant treatment. Postural drainage can be very helpful if there is much sputum. Any anaemia should be diagnosed and corrected if possible, and the pulse should be watched for any significant change.

Complications

Since most lung cancers, especially those near the hilum, are bound to cause some degree of obstruction with distal stasis and infection, and since many cancers cavitate early in their growth, it is quite remarkable that the development of a pyogenic abscess is so rare. When this does occur, conservative treatment using antibiotics and postural drainage is usually sufficient to enable the patient to finish his treatment, after which the abscess may disappear together with the cancer. Occasionally this process is hastened if a neoplastic abscess breaks into a bronchus, when the contents may be coughed up, and the patient feels better.

If the oesophagus has to be included in the treated volume, a radiation oesophagitis develops during the last week of treatment, and may persist for as long as 4 or 5 weeks if the treated segment has received the full tumour dose, though this is unusual. Most patients have either a transitory mild dysphagia for a week or so, or none at all. Mist. Paracetamol, taken about 20 min before each meal, helps swallowing by slightly anaesthetising the mucosa. The patient can be reassured that swallowing will soon become normal. It is exceedingly rare for subsequent oesophageal fibrosis to need dilatation.

It is worth noting that dysphagia which first appears later than 1 month after the completion of treatment cannot be due to the radiation reaction, though radiation is usually held responsible by those physicians unfamiliar with the effects of radiotherapy. Such dysphagia is always due to recurrent tumour in the posterior mediastinum and, apart from the timing, is often distinguishable from a radiation oesophagitis in that it tends to be felt as a mechanical obstruction rather than as soreness. Some patients, having had dysphagia because of the treatment, settle down, only to develop dysphagia a second time. The X-rays are always blamed, but again the tumour is responsible.

All tissues heal their insults by fibrosis, which is inevitable. It is nearly always possible to see some faint shadowing in the treated volume, and, especially when larger fields are used, the shadowing may be fairly well marked, and the associated late contraction may distort the anatomy. The shadows of fibrosis are not often dense, however, and usually shade off rapidly outside the treated volume. It is surprising, contrary to popular belief, how little the fibrosis seems to affect the patients; they rarely complain of increasing cough or dyspnoea, and once the fibrosis has matured the appearances on the X-ray films remain static.

A few patients seem to do very well after radical treatment, perhaps for several years, but over a period of a few months they subsequently become unwell, usually with increasing cough and dyspnoea, and serial chest films show a steady increase in the density, and later in the size, of the shadow of the "fibrosis". As in the case of the late onset of dysphagia, radiation is usually blamed, but it soon becomes obvious that the cancer has recurred. Late changes of this kind are always due to recurrence, and never to a simple increase in the density of the fibrosis: an exception to this rule has not been seen.

Very rarely indeed, a patient may develop what seems to be an excessive reaction to X-rays in the weeks following completion of treatment. Dyspnoea increases rapidly, and chest films show heavy shadowing radiating from both hila, which has been likened to a bat's wings. The patient dies after 2–3 months, and a post-mortem examination shows only an acute, diffuse, inflammatory reaction with a little early fibrosis. The cause is unknown, and may be allergic in nature. It is unlikely to be due to infection, whether opportunist or otherwise. Steroids and antibiotics proved useless in the few cases seen at this hospital.

Palliative X-ray Treatment

The palliation of patients with lung cancer is essentially synonymous with the palliation of symptoms, except in some cases where treatment may be expected to delay or prevent complications which are thought to be imminent, such as collapse of a lung or SVC obstruction. If a patient has no clamant symptoms or impending complications it may be best to do nothing, especially if the patient is old. X-ray treatment in such a situation leads to little or no benefit which is obvious to the patient, and when subsequent tumour spread produces symptoms such as bone pain, the patient and his relatives may even blame the treatment for his new trouble. Sooner or later, and usually sooner, a symptomless patient develops focal symptoms which can be relieved by treatment which the patient then appreciates. If there are no focal symptoms, but the general condition is deteriorating, chemotherapy may be indicated.

Most patients needing palliative X-ray treatment are ill and do not have long to live. It is therefore unkind to give long periods of fractionated treatment, especially if this necessitates admission to hospital, and the golden rule is to give the shortest possible treatment which experience shows will be effective. Over the last 40 years various treatment schedules, both long and short, have been compared at the Christie Hospital, and though the short schedules now in use may in some cases seem to be almost perfunctory by some standards, they have been found to be just as effective as the longer ones. Some common patterns of disease merit individual consideration.

Large Central Lesion with Symptoms

Symptoms referable to the lungs and mediastinum, such as dyspnoea from lung collapse, haemoptysis, dysphagia, and mediastinal pain, may diminish or clear up temporarily, though a cough almost always persists.

The primary tumour is usually near the hilum and has spread to the mediastinum, so that field sizes of the order of 12×10 cm or 15×10 cm may be needed. A simple parallel pair of fields, large enough to cover all obvious tumour, may be positioned and checked using diagnostic X-ray films with skin markers. If a machine is available with a head which can be rotated to point vertically upwards through the bed, and a panel in the bed can be replaced by a supporting grid of plastic strings, treatment planning is simpler and "setting-up" time shortened. Only the centre of the anterior field need be verified, and this field is treated with the patient supine. The head of the machine is then rotated 180°, so that alignment of the posterior field, through the grid, is automatically perfect, and skin sparing is achieved for both fields. Without the grid the bed acts as bolus and a skin reaction is produced, so that it is better to turn the patient to the prone position for treatment of the posterior field, which will have to be separately localised and verified.

Eight daily treatments are given over 10 days to a maximum *given* dose on each field of 3500 cGy, for field sizes up to 14 cm long, and proportionately less for longer fields. This gives about 3250 cGy tumour dose (using 4 MeV) for most patients. Dosage is limited by the tolerance of the spinal cord, and for diabetic or hypertensive patients the given dose should be curtailed by 250 cGy.

If the patient is in need of mediastinal treatment but is systemically ill, perhaps with distant metastases, the treatment can be shortened to four daily treatments, to a maximum given dose of 2750 cGy on each field.

Obstruction of Superior Vena Cava

Obstruction of the SVC by tumours in the superior mediastinum is common, and is usually due to the constricting pressure of involved nodes which surround the vein rather than from direct involvement by an adjacent primary tumour. Irradiation can give rapid and complete relief of both signs and symptoms, especially if obstruction has developed gradually and the patient is referred for X-ray treatment before it has become gross. The patient then usually dies from generalised disease without recurrence of the obstruction. Quite often, however, the patient arrives at the radiotherapy department with gross obstruction. In a few cases the condition has developed rapidly, perhaps overnight, and the presumption must be that incipient obstruction suddenly became complete by thrombosis. Anticoagulants may be given but do not usually help. X-ray treatment is rarely useful, and the patient soon succumbs.

Most patients arriving with a longer history of gross obstruction come either from their homes or from hospitals where it is not appreciated that X-ray treatment, if given when the obstruction is minimal, can probably avoid death by slow suffocation, which must surely be one of the most unpleasant modes of death. Given time, neoplasm in the superior mediastinal glands will grow by direct spread through the wall of the vena cava to reach the lumen which it will eventually block, whether aided by thrombosis or not. X-ray treatment cannot then be expected to help much, though it should be given because any improvement at all will be welcomed. Some patients may respond quite well, but with early relapse and death. Others respond not at all.

The average survival of all patients diagnosed as having SVC obstruction due to a lung carcinoma is of the order of 3–4 months. It is therefore a matter for wonder that in some hospitals such patients are sometimes given fractionated X-ray treatment over 4 or even 6 weeks. This represents a large proportion of the patient's remaining life-span, and seems difficult to justify. In the past, the Christie Hospital has tried many treatment techniques, ranging from a single treatment to 3 weeks' fractionated and beam-directed therapy. An analysis of the results showed that a single treatment given via a single anterior field produced the same results as any other method. If all cases of obstruction are grouped together, no attempt being made to subdivide them into categories such as minimal or gross, roughly 50% have complete remission and do not recur, 30% have partial or good immediate remission but recur, and 20% have little or no response.

Treatment is given by a 4- or 8-MeV linear accelerator using a single anterior field centred over the SVC, i.e. about 2 cm to the right of the midline. The exact centre may be adjusted to allow the width of the field to subtend the width of the neoplastic shadow which is often easily visible on the diagnostic films. The upper margin of the field lies at the suprasternal notch. Although the SVC is only about 5 cm long, it is usually advisable to make the field much longer, partly to subtend neoplasm at or near the hilum, and partly because one can do so with impunity. A typical field size would be 12×8 cm or slightly smaller, and the given dose 1500 cGy. If the field is bigger, and especially if it is longer than 12 cm, the dose should be reduced to 1250 cGy.

It is only of academic interest that if oedema and venous engorgement are limited to the head and neck and the arms, the site of pressure must be limited to that part of the SVC above the level of the azygos vein, whereas if a collateral venous circulation is developing round the lower chest wall, there must also be obstruction below the level of the azygos vein. In either case the whole volume of tissue in the vicinity of the vein should be treated, with a good margin inferiorly.

The patient should remain in hospital for one night because there is usually some increased oedema in the treated volume following the X-ray treatment, though it subsides within 24 h. Whilst not clinically noticeable in many cases, some patients feel temporarily worse and become more anxious, thereby increasing their dyspnoea and setting up a vicious circle of deterioration. The mainstay of treatment should be the administration of mild tranquillising drugs such as diazepam. Steroids are sometimes prescribed but should not be used routinely because there is evidence that they may give some protection from the effects of radiation. The patient can go home the day after treatment, and resolution usually takes about 2 weeks.

Chemotherapy is never indicated as the initial treatment for obstruction unless X-ray therapy is not available. Irradiation is simple to give, does not upset the patient systemically, and is much more certain in its local effects. It cannot be repeated, however, and recurrence of obstruction warrants a trial of chemotherapy.

Paraplegia

Paraplegia, though usually due to spinal metastases, may occur from subdural deposits in the absence of radiological evidence of bone involvement. In either case the extent of the metastatic disease is usually greater than the radiological or clinical evidence may indicate and it is wise to be generous with the field size. A single field of the order of 12 or 15 cm long by 7 cm wide is typical, placed to give a rather greater margin above the guessed centre of damage, or the sensory level, than below it. It may be possible to localise the field precisely if the patient has had a surgical decompression and the exact extent of the disease is known.

It is sometimes difficult to know how much treatment to give. If the patient is very ill and obviously does not have long to live, and the paraplegia has been established for many days, it is not justifiable to bring him into hospital for treatment. If such a patient has been sent to the radiotherapy department for an opinion however, it is worthwhile giving a single dose of 1250 cGy (megavoltage) as an out-patient since it can do no harm, and any improvement, however slight, will be appreciated. At the other end of the spectrum, a relatively fit patient, and especially those patients whose paraplegia has only been noticeable for 2 days or less, should be given fractionated treatment over 10 days to a given dose of about 3000–3500 cGy, depending on the length of the field. In general, the results of such treatment are not good and it is not usually worth while setting up a beam-directed treatment, especially if this means delay whilst a shell is made.

The most important single factor affecting prognosis is the time interval between the onset of the paraplegia and the beginning of X-ray treatment. An "early" paraplegia, that is, a paraplegia with a history of about 48 h or less, is one of the very few radiotherapy emergencies which warrant opening up the therapy department out of working hours, for the paraplegia can disappear completely. Even if the patient does not live long, he will then die without having experienced the miseries of this unpleasant complication.

Unfortunately, many patients are sent for treatment with a fully established paraplegia and a history of weeks' rather than days' duration. For these, little if any improvement can be expected.

Pancoast's Syndrome

Pancoast's syndrome due to an apical primary lung cancer is not uncommon, and like SVC obstruction, often presents to the radiotherapist as a fully developed syndrome with a fairly long history (averaging 6 months) of severe pain. The average survival after palliative X-ray treatment is of the order of 9 months, and almost all patients are dead within 2 years. Cure of such tumours by radiotherapy is known, but is a great rarity. Palliative treatment is almost always given in the hope of obtaining pain relief.

Routine chest films often show rib erosion, commonly in the region of the necks of the second and third ribs, but it is not usually appreciated that quite a high proportion of such cases (about 20%) also have erosion of the adjacent vertebrae, the extent of which can only be shown by special radiological investigation. It may be presumed that as with most cancers, spread occurs most readily along channels or planes of least mechanical resistance, and that at this site the direction of lymph drainage inwards along the neurovascular bundles and the pleura facilitates spread to the spine. In view of the high incidence of vertebral involvement, it is surprising that so few patients develop evidence of spinal cord damage. A paraplegia develops in about 5% of patients with Pancoast's syndrome, and can be shown radiologically or at post mortem to be due to cord damage from the tumour. This point is made explicitly because, as with so many complications arising after X-ray treatment has been given for malignant disease, the radiotherapist is sometimes held responsible. The onset of paraplegia is usually accompanied by a recrudescence of local signs and symptoms, and the patient dies within a few months, often with evidence of generalised disease.

The simplest treatment technique is that using a parallel pair of fields. From the centres of the fields upwards, the gap between the fields over the apex of the shoulder is filled by bolus to obtain homogeneity of dose. It is easiest to treat the patient supine, with accurate localisation and verification of the anterior field, then rotate the machine head through 180° and treat the posterior field through a "string" bed, as for palliative treatment of the mediastinum. Alternatively, the patient will have to be turned to the prone position and have the posterior field localised separately.

Field sizes of the order of 7×8 or 8×8 cm are usual. It is easy to decide where the upper, lower, and lateral margins should be placed, since the tumour limits are easily seen on the posteroanterior chest film. It is more difficult to decide where the medial edge should lie.

Because of the known direction of tumour spread, with frequent vertebral involvement, at least the lateral third of the vertebral bodies should be included in the treated volume. If the lateral margins of the vertebral bodies are known to be involved already then at least two-thirds of the width, if not the whole width of the spine should be included, though in this case the spinal cord is also included. This limits the dose to that of the spinal cord tolerance. For an 8-cm-long field, the tolerance dose of the cord is about 3500 cGy in eight treatments given over 10 days, or less if the patient is diabetic or hypertensive. If the cord is not included, the tissues will tolerate 4000 cGy in 10 days. The dose should certainly be kept as high as possible to give the best chance of obtaining at least some pain relief in this particularly intractable condition.

The results are poor, though those patients who have in the past been given a higher dose over 3 weeks fare no better. If those patients who are almost moribund when first seen are excluded, almost 50% of patients have complete pain relief, 20% have sufficient relief to be comfortable if they use analgesics, and 30% have little or no response.

Bone Metastases

Metastases in bone are best treated by single doses of megavoltage X-rays, giving 1250 or 1500 cGy to a typical medium-sized field of 15×7 cm, for example to the spine. Field sizes should be generous rather than otherwise, for metastases are usually bigger and more widespread than X-ray films indicate, and subsequent matching of fields to treat spread into adjacent areas can be awkward. For example, it is unwise to localise accurately a field which gives small margins round a single collapsed vertebra: a 12-cm-long field centred on the known disease would be better.

Superficial Nodules and Nodes

Skin nodules and superficial gland masses are most conveniently treated by single doses of 250-kV X-rays, giving 1000 or 1250 cGy according to site and size. It is worth noting two points about enlarged supraclavicular nodes. First, it is only rarely that neoplasm escapes from them by direct spread to involve local nerves and becomes the cause of local or referred pain. In most cases such pain is caused by involvement of the cervical vertebrae or other bones, or sometimes by an apical lung tumour, and superficial treatment of the nodes is then unlikely to relieve the pain. Second, quite large but soft nodes are often found in the supraclavicular fossae, and sometimes in the axillae, in patients with SVC obstruction. Associated obstruction of the lymphatic pathways causes massive distension of the nodes by fluid, and the nodes may disappear if the obstruction subsides after X-ray treatment. A biopsy of such nodes for diagnostic purposes is not likely to show histological changes of malignancy, and X-ray treatment of the nodes may be unnecessary.

Pleural Effusions

Pleural effusions, if small and symptomless, are best left alone. Some are transudates, and may clear up after the hilum and adjacent mediastinal area has been irradiated. If the effusion is large and causing gross dyspnoea, aspiration is helpful, though it may have to be repeated several times. Effusions persisting after X-ray treatment to the mediastinum, and refractory to repeated aspiration, sometimes respond to a single intrapleural injection of 60 mg bleomycin, and this may be repeated up to a maximum of three injections if necessary.

Brain Metastases

Metastases in the brain are sometimes worth irradiating if the patient's general condition is reasonably good. A parallel pair of lateral fields covering the whole brain above Reid's baseline is used to give a tumour dose of 3000 cGy in eight treatments. Clinical improvement can be rapid and complete but usually only lasts a few months. Prednisolone with simple chemotherapy may then give a further transitory improvement.

In conclusion, it is worth emphasising again that we could help more patients more effectively with our palliative treatment if it were not for our old arch-enemy delay. There are many situations, some described above, where prompt treatment can often completely abort a developing complication. The survival of the patient may not be increased significantly but extremes of misery can sometimes be avoided. Our duty to the patient thus includes education of our colleagues, not only general practitioners and nurses but also hospital doctors, both junior and senior. They may specialise in other fields and we must plead with them to send their patients to us earlier rather than later, because in our specialty delay is often detrimental.

Chemotherapy (See also Chap. 3)

No convincing evidence has yet been produced which might suggest that chemotherapy has a part to play in the management of a patient with an early lung cancer, whatever the histology, where the intention is to attempt cure either by ablative surgery or radical X-ray treatment. "Adjuvant" chemotherapy in such a situation is not only unhelpful, but is probably contraindicated. No-one has yet claimed that it can contribute to a cure, and at the same time it is bound to decrease the non-specific vitality or "resistance" of the patient to the stress of radical treatment, and potentiate infection, so that it may in this way even militate against cure. The hope that it might clear up micrometastases, residual after radical treatment of the primary tumour, has not been substantiated in practice.

Chemotherapy should certainly never be used as the sole treatment for an early cancer, for example because an opinion has been expressed that the patient is much too old for either surgery or X-ray treatment. Very old people can tolerate X-ray treatment to the lung surprisingly well, and a shortened treatment, with a slightly lower dose to allow for age, can sometimes be effective, without any upset to the patient.

For those patients with symptoms from localised foci of disease, such as SVC obstruction, bone metastases, or the common situation of a primary hilar mass plus mediastinal gland involvement, palliation by a simple X-ray technique remains the treatment of choice. There are usually no side-effects, and in particular, the general well-being of the patient is not assaulted. X-ray treatment is also more effective locally than chemotherapy, for all types of histology, and one can imagine this to be so because the tumour receives a relatively high "dose of energy", whereas the "dose of energy" reaching the tumour from drugs is relatively much less because of systemic dilution and the limitations on dosage because of toxicity.

Some patients are known to have advanced disease but are without major symptoms. These patients are best left alone to enjoy what brief symptom-free life remains to them, for they do not thank a doctor whose chemotherapy may make them feel worse when they can feel no obvious benefit in compensation. The situation is quite different from that pertaining in, say, Hodgkin's disease, where the benefit can be immeasurably greater. Chemotherapy is of most help to those patients who have no clamant focal symptoms, but whose general condition is beginning to deteriorate because of widespread disease. They begin to complain of serious weight loss, general lassitude, and anorexia, and may have diffuse, aching bone pains. Chemotherapy may also be helpful for those patients who have locally recurrent disease after X-ray treatment, for example recurrent SVC obstruction. If patients in these categories respond to drug treatment, the benefit is appreciated, and any toxic side-effects, if not too severe, are usually regarded as worthwhile.

The best and first choice of drug is undoubtedly a steroid in relatively high dosage, say prednisolone 10 mg three times a day. Even if used alone, many patients will respond, if only for a short time, by an increase in appetite, weight and vitality. They begin to feel better, and because of the steroid facies their friends tell them they are looking better, so that optimism returns and the downward trend is temporarily reversed.

This stage of the disease usually represents the last chance to help most patients, so that it is common practice to add a cytotoxic agent to the steroids. This can take the form of a single agent such as cyclophosphamide or methotrexate, and cyclophosphamide is probably the best choice as it is the least toxic and the safest. Given orally in a low dose of 50 mg twice or three times a day, the patient usually notices no side-effects, and blood counts only need to be done every 2 or 3 weeks, since a falling white cell count at this dosage is uncommon. The two drugs can be given for many months without obvious toxicity, and although the hair may loosen, baldness only occurs after about a year. Few patients live long enough for this to happen.

This regimen can be used irrespective of histology. Undifferentiated tumours, and particularly oat cell types, undoubtedly respond more quickly and more often than differentiated tumours, but they also tend to recur more quickly. Patients with differentiated tumours sometimes respond quite well, and at least should not be denied the possibility.

More effective drugs and drug regimes are available, and there is no doubt that combination chemotherapy can often produce longer remissions than a single agent with steroids, but always at a price. No regimen has yet been found which is outstandingly good enough to have found wide acceptance. It is a matter of fine judgement whether, in any individual case, the possibility of a longer (but always finite) remission justifies the increased toxicity of the more powerful combinations, even if the toxic episodes are arranged to be intermittent, for example by 2-weekly admissions to hospital for injections. It is the responsibility of specialised chemotherapy teams in cancer hospitals to undertake such experimental work, always in the hope of finding less toxic drugs, or combinations of drugs, which benefit the patient more. The hazards of such therapy are serious, and occasionally lethal, and highly specialised knowledge, equipment, and trained supporting staff must be available to deal with iatrogenic emergencies. Whilst a small incidence of lethal complications is acceptable from a treatment which carries a chance of cure, it is not acceptable for patients who are already near the end of their lives, and for whom one cannot even promise that the treatment will be beneficial. It should be obvious that such treatment must not be attempted other than in these special departments.

Oesophagus

Introduction

Carcinoma of the oesophagus is a relatively rare disease in Great Britain. In the post-war period till 1960, the incidence was remarkably constant at about 2300 cases a year. Since 1960, the incidence has slowly but steadily increased to 3700 in 1978. In 1950, the male-to-female ratio was 2:1, but there has been a bigger increase in the incidence in females than in males, so that the ratio now approaches equality. There must be a cause for these significant changes, though its nature is not known. There has certainly been a concomitant change of eating habits, in that the tremendous boom in foreign travel has encouraged an appreciation of foreign foods, and increased immigration has brought Indian, Chinese, and, to a lesser extent, Middle Eastern restaurants to almost every town and village in the country. There has also been a big increase in the supply of packaged foods, and therefore of the quantity of preservative chemicals consumed. Whether these changes are causally linked remains to be shown, but it is very tempting to assume a possible association.

Judging by the localised prevalence of the disease in parts of Africa, Iran, and the Far East, it is probable that some environmental factor will be found, perhaps in the local food or soil, which will account for these pockets of high incidence, but as yet there is no knowledge by which we can advise on prevention. Linhsien county, in the Honan province of China, probably has the highest incidence of oesophageal cancer in the world, and Chinese medical opinion blames the local diet. In particular, the Chinese identify carcinogenic nitrosamines and their nitrite precursors as important. It is interesting that in Linhsien chickens are also reported as having a high incidence of squamous cell carcinoma of the gullet, which suggests that the cause lies with the food rather than any genetic predisposition, and also presumably excludes alcohol and tobacco as significant aetiological factors, at least in that area.

Apart from food, many factors have been incriminated, such as alcohol, tobacco, and folate deficiency, which are probably of less importance. Leucoplakia is common in the oesophagus, but progression to malignancy is said to be rare. The Plummer-Vinsen (Paterson-Kelly) syndrome probably only applies to the postcricoid region, which is usually classified apart from the oesophagus proper. A hiatus hernia with a congenitally short oesophagus is undoubtedly sometimes associated with the development of oesophageal cancer.

The results of treatment are very poor. As with lung cancer, the disease starts in an inaccessible, hidden site, and symptoms are at first minimal and insufficient to frighten the patient into seeking medical advice immediately, so that by the time investigations begin the disease is advanced, radical treatment is not feasible, and palliation is mainly concerned with attempts at relieving the dysphagia. The average survival of this group of patients treated palliatively is about 6 months.

For those patients who have disease which is still sufficiently localised for either radical surgery or radical X-ray therapy to be attempted, the overall 5-year survival for either treatment method is of the order of 5%, though this can be increased to about 10% by better selection of patients. In addition, surgery is difficult and carries a very high postoperative mortality. Earlier diagnosis would presumably improve the survival rates, but it is difficult to see how this can be done other than by ensuring that all young doctors are taught to be acutely aware of the importance of early investigation of persistent dysphagia in elderly people. The disease is too uncommon for any known screening procedure to be economically feasible.

Pathology

Some 90% of oesophageal neoplasms are squamous cell in type, and are more often well-differentiated than undifferentiated. These are the tumours which radiotherapy can often palliate, and if they are small, can sometimes cure. At endoscopy, or in the operative specimen, the tumour can often be seen to conform to one of the four classical macroscopic types, and the classification is useful. Proliferative, cauliflower-like tumours, whose direction of growth is primarily inwards into the lumen, usually present early with obstruction or bleeding, and have the best prognosis. The nodular, indurated type tends to present later and more insidiously, and to spread outwards and penetrate the muscle coat to involve lymph nodes and adjacent structures early, so that it has the worst prognosis. The typical "malignant ulcer" with a fairly well defined circular or oval crater and raised edges is intermediate in direction of spread and prognosis. The annular type is a carcinoma that has had time to spread round the whole circumference of the lumen, so that it has also had time to spread widely outside the oesophagus. Obstructive symptoms are severe, and the prognosis is bad.

Multiple tumours are sometimes found, and are said to occur in 5%–10% of oesophageal cancers. The finding of one obvious lesion must therefore not preclude investigation of the whole length of the oesophagus.

About 10% of tumours are adenocarcinomas, arising in the lower third of the oesophagus at or near the cardia, from mucosal glands. Some of them are really gastric tumours which have spread upwards. Rarely an adenocarcinoma can arise elsewhere in the oesophagus from islands of gastric-type mucosa, but this type only forms about 1% of oesophageal cancers. Radiotherapy is not effective for adenocarcinomas, which will not be discussed further because their treatment is entirely surgical.

Sarcomas of the muscle and connective tissues are rare, and again their treatment is surgical. Malignant melanomas, sometimes multiple, may also occur.

Spread

The tumour first spreads submucosally, both directly and via the submucosal lymphatic plexus. This spread is usually extensive, so that a good margin must be taken above and below the obvious tumour when it is treated, whether by resection or by X-rays.

The oesophageal wall is then penetrated, and the tumour spreads to the local posterior mediastinal or cervical glands and to adjacent structures. The oesophageal wall is thin, and when infiltrated by friable neoplasm it is understandable that perforation by a bougie is notoriously easy. It is perhaps surprising that when such neoplasm resolves following X-ray treatment, the deficiency or weakness left in the oesophageal wall only rarely leads to a subsequent perforation, and in fact fibrosis sufficient to need dilatation is relatively frequent.

The incidence of involved local para-oesophageal nodes is very high. It has been estimated that if the macroscopic primary tumour is 5 cm or less in length, 50% of patients will already have metastases in the local nodes, and this figure rises to 90% for tumours longer than 5 cm. It is thus no wonder that cure rates are so low, for it is probable that once the nodes are involved both surgery and radiotherapy can rarely, if ever, be curative.

Which adjacent structures are involved by direct spread depends of course on the site of the tumour, and it is easy to memorise the possible secondary effects and complications (often lethal) of an oesophageal carcinoma by remembering the anatomical relationships.

A list can be made as follows of the main relationships (and the resulting complications in brackets).

> Posteriorly—vertebral bodies (pain, rarely paraplegia). From above downwards—trachea (fistula, lung infection); thyroid (abscess); great vessels and aorta (massive haemorrhage); left main bronchus (fistula and lung infection); pleura (empyema); pericardium (pericarditis); diaphragm and left lobe of liver (subphrenic abscess); mediastinum (mediastinitis, abscess); nerve palsies—phrenic, laryngeal.

The lymphatic drainage from the local glands follows the expected pathways. The glands at the root of the neck soon drain into the subclavian veins. The posterior mediastinal glands round the upper two-thirds of the oesophagus tend to drain upwards via the tracheobronchial nodes to the paratracheal nodes and thence to the veins, whereas the nodes round the lower thoracic and abdominal regions of the oesophagus drain mainly via the paracardial and left gastric nodes to the coeliac group, and thence to the cisterna chyli.

Blood spread is usually late. The liver and lungs become involved often, and other structures such as the brain and bones less often.

Clinical Features

The earliest symptom of oesophageal carcinoma, and often the only one for a long time, is dysphagia. At first the patient only notices a slightly abnormal sensation, sometimes intermittent, during the act of swallowing. Slowly and insidiously the sensation progresses to a definite feeling of obstruction so that the patient has to "swallow hard", and perhaps several times, before a firm bolus such as an unchewed lump of meat will pass. A bolus may plug the narrowed lumen temporarily and cause a violent fit of retching, coughing, and sometimes vomiting before it is released, upwards or downwards, and the patient learns to chew his food better, then to prepare only uniformly soft foods. Eventually even soft foods only pass with difficulty: the patient begins to live on fluids and to lose weight, until fluids can only be taken a sip at a time, and obstruction may finally become complete. It is usually said that patients cannot localise the site of the obstruction accurately, but some patients do so, especially if the tumour is in the upper half of the oesophagus.

Once obstruction is established, some dilatation of the oesophagus develops proximal to the tumour. The dilatation is never gross (partly because the walls near the tumour may be stiffened by tumour spread, and partly because the time scale is too short), but it may be sufficient to allow some mucus, food, and debris to accumulate. This material, which can be bloodstained, is sometimes regurgitated at times which are not necessarily related to meals. There may also be excessive reflex salivation, and the patient may describe his discomfort as "heartburn". These abnormalities may irritate the larynx and pharynx, so that a cough develops, which itself can lead to regurgitation, and the patient becomes increasingly miserable.

All other symptoms are due to spread of disease causing secondary complications such as lung infection, mediastinal or bone pain, hoarse voice, hiccup, and so on, and appear only when the disease is no longer confined to the oesophagus.

There are never any abnormal physical signs to be found until the disease is well advanced. Palpable nodes in the lower neck or supraclavicular fossa, a palpable irregular liver, or signs of infection in the lungs, pleura, or pericardium tell their tale clearly, often in conjunction with marked loss of weight, anaemia, and sometimes dehydration.

Diagnosis

After clinical suspicion is aroused, the diagnosis is made by radiology and endoscopy, which should not be delayed.

Plain films of the chest may show suspicious features such as lung infection, or a pleural effusion or empyema. The appearance of barium in the air passages, if a barium swallow has been done first, is highly suspicious of an oesophago-bronchial fistula.

The barium swallow is the key investigation. Typically, barium tends to be held up at the site of the tumour, where there is an irregular "rat-tail" filling defect. An ulcer crater or a neoplastic bulge into the lumen may be seen. There may be slight proximal dilatation of the oesophagus, and residual barium in the "rat tail" may be covered by a layer of frothy mucus. This is the picture of a well-developed tumour, however, and at an earlier stage of growth only a localised filling defect or irregularity of the mucosa may be shown, perhaps associated with what appears to be local spasm. Cardial growths may be suspected if the oesophagus empties rapidly and constantly into the stomach instead of in spurts, if the air bubble in the stomach is deformed, or if there is an increased thickness of tissue between the air bubble and the diaphragm. Associated conditions may come to light, such as a diverticulum containing a carcinoma, or a hiatus hernia which may itself be associated with a congenitally short oesophagus.

Transverse axial tomograms, whether taken by an X-ray machine or by a CT scan, are disappointingly unhelpful, though they may sometimes indicate the presence of a tumour mass which may be bigger than anticipated from the other films.

After radiological investigation, the patient must proceed to endoscopy. A bronchoscopy must not be omitted since it may give useful information. A paralysed vocal cord may be found. Pus in the bronchi may be associated with aspiration pneumonia or with a fistula. Infiltration of the trachea or left main bronchus by tumour may be seen, or a widened carina due to an underlying node mass.

At oesophagoscopy the tumour will probably be visualised, its characteristics noted, and a biopsy taken. The biopsy should never be omitted, for occasionally an inflamed benign stricture or benign tumour may mimic the appearance of a neoplasm, and the histology will also distinguish the radiotherapeutically treatable squamous cell carcinoma from the rarer neoplasms which can only be treated by surgery. Sometimes the surgeon may deem it possible partially to dilate the stricture, so giving the patient some temporary relief from the dysphagia, and perhaps an improved nutrition, especially if radical treatment is contemplated. The risk of perforation and mediastinitis is, however, not negligible. If on the other hand it is already obvious that the disease is advanced, the opportunity may be taken to insert one of the modern variants of a Souttar's tube.

A blood count may show anaemia, sometimes severe, and a high white count indicates infection. Specialised investigations may be helpful, such as an isotope liver scan, when trying to exclude metastases before embarking on radical treatment.

Staging

There is no generally accepted classification of the stages of progress of oesophageal carcinoma. Japan and North America have their own systems. The TNM classification cannot be usefully applied. For radiotherapists, and possibly for surgeons also, it is simplest to think of tumours under the headings of "early" and "late", as for lung cancer. An early tumour could be defined as one which is not more than about 5 cm long macroscopically, and has not yet spread either to adjacent structures or to distant parts as far as can be ascertained. All other tumours are late.

Treatment Policy

If the tumour is early, as defined above, an attempt should be made at radical treatment if the patient is not too old or unfit. In practice, this description limits radical treatment to very few patients, so that in this country few centres, whether surgical or radiotherapeutic, have an extensive experience of the disease, unlike Japan and China.

Surgical resection is a formidable procedure. There should be a margin of about 4–5 cm allowed beyond each end of the obvious tumour, so that a long piece of the oesophagus has to be removed. Recurrence of tumour at the anastomosis is common, especially if insufficient margins can be given. The oesophagus has no tough serosa like that of the bowel, anastomosis of oesophagus to bowel is difficult, and leaks occur.

The postoperative mortality is particularly high, and the more proximal the tumour, the higher the mortality. Excluding operations for adenocarcinoma of the lower third, the overall postoperative mortality is quoted as lying between 25% and 30%. However, because most patients are seen first by a surgeon, operation often becomes the treatment of choice for the early case. The results are admittedly poor, most patients dying by the end of the first year, and probably less than 10% of patients who have had a resection survive to 5 years.

If such patients are unfit or old or refuse operation, the radiotherapist may be consulted. If radical X-ray treatment is given, the results in terms of survival for this group of patients are much the same as the surgical results, in spite of the fact that one would expect them to be biased unfavourably because most of these patients are surgical exclusions. However, the complications of radiotherapy (fibrosis with stricture formation and occasional mediastinitis) are much less than those of surgery, and the immediate post-radiation mortality, mainly from mediastinitis, is only a few per cent. It would seem therefore that a case could be argued for treating all early cases by X-rays.

Preoperative and postoperative X-ray treatment have been given, but neither has been shown to be of any benefit. It is probable that radiotherapy could well increase the surgeon's difficulty if high doses are given, by jeopardising further the already precarious blood supply to the site of anastomosis.

Palliative surgery (a bypass operation, or excision when it is known that disease is left behind), is occasionally undertaken when a tumour is found to be inoperable at thoracotomy. It seems that it hardly ever proves to have been worthwhile, for the postoperative mortality is more than 30%, and the average survival is only about 6 months.

For the majority of patients who have disease

which is too advanced for radical treatment to be possible, increasing dysphagia and the threat of starvation demand some attempt at relief, especially if the patient is otherwise relatively symptomless. Local intubation is much the simplest method if the surgeon is able to dilate the stricture sufficiently for the stem to pass, and if the cup of the tube is held well enough by the stricture to prevent it passing through. A choice of several designs of tube is available. The procedure carries the risk of perforation (and therefore mediastinitis) during dilatation, and sometimes what seems to be a securely fitting tube is passed after only a few days or weeks, but a successful intubation allows the patient's nutrition and hydration to be well maintained by natural eating and drinking. As long as the tube stays in situ, it affords almost perfect palliation of the dysphagia, the only restriction being that lumpy food, which might block the tube, must be avoided.

If the stricture is so tight that only fluids can be swallowed, or if dilatation sufficient for local intubation is not possible, a thin nasogastric or oral tube should be passed. The oral route is much the best, for nasogastric tubes irritate the nasopharynx and can become most uncomfortable.

It is often difficult to decide whether to offer these patients palliative X-ray treatment, which is not without discomfort and risk. If a sufficient dose is given to anticipate good tumour resolution, there is bound to be some radiation oesophagitis, though patients seem to vary greatly in their response to the soreness on swallowing. Some patients merely confirm on questioning that they are aware of the soreness, whilst others find it distressing. Sometimes resolution of tumour opens up an incipient fistula, or a perforation into the mediastinum, and the radiotherapist may be blamed for a complication which would probably have been inevitable in any case, but delayed if no treatment had been given. On the other hand, palliative X-ray treatment can sometimes give a patient many months of relief before the disease overwhelms him.

It is probably best to limit palliative X-ray treatment to those patients whose general condition is still fairly good, who can still at least swallow fluids without difficulty, and who have no obvious metastases or complications which are likely to dominate the situation soon. Mediastinitis, fistula formation, and gross infective lung complications should be regarded as absolute contraindications.

Localised pain is best palliated by local X-ray treatment. Pain from the site of the primary tumour, whether from mediastinal invasion or direct spread to adjacent vertebrae, may be relieved by local X-ray treatment which can include the site of the obstruction and perhaps relieve dysphagia at the same time. Pain at other sites, especially if from a metastasis in bone, can usually be relieved by a single treatment.

There is general agreement that a gastrostomy should be avoided. Patients always dislike it greatly, and it is almost always possible to pass a very fine oral tube. If obstruction becomes absolute and an oral tube cannot be passed, then the patient's condition is becoming terminal and tranquillisers and morphia, expertly given, will provide comfort. Similarly, intravenous feeding is to be avoided.

There is no efficient chemotherapy for oesophageal cancer. However, there are a few patients who, having improved following radical or palliative X-ray treatment, pass into a phase where regrowth of tumour brings back dysphagia, whilst their general condition remains good. It is then worth trying prednisolone 30 mg daily with cyclophosphamide 100 or 150 mg daily, both in divided doses. This combination does no harm, and some patients will respond for a few months at most.

Radical X-ray Treatment Techniques

Kilovoltage X-rays can no longer be regarded as adequate for treating oesophageal cancer, and a linear accelerator or a cobalt source should be used.

A three-field technique, almost exactly as described for lung cancer, is probably the simplest and the best for tumours below, say, the level of the aortic arch. This part of the oesophagus lies approximately parallel to the bed when the patient lies supine or prone, and it is easy to put a cylinder of radiation round the tumour. The technique only differs from that for a lung cancer in the following respects:

First, localisation is mainly defined from the barium swallow films, though a CT scan can occasionally give extra information. Some surgeons will insert a metallic clip at oesophagoscopy which marks the proximal tumour limit. Verification is done by giving the patient thin barium to sip whilst a film is taken in the treatment position. Secondly, field size has to be of the order of 12–15 cm long by 5–6 cm wide. The 5-cm length limit for a radically treatable tumour is probably mandatory, for it is the only reliable guide we have to the extent of the disease. If the tumour is estimated to be small, say 3 cm in length, a 12-cm-long field will give the desired margins above and below. A 5-cm-long tumour will need fields of, say, 13 cm long, to an absolute maximum of 15 cm. Over 15 cm, radiation oesophagitis would be too severe, and the dose would have to be reduced. As regards width, 5 cm is adequate for most tumours, but presupposes accurate and repeatable setting up, and some radiotherapists may feel that 6 cm is safer, especially when it is borne in mind that the tumour may have spread laterally on either side of the oesophagus so that the tumour mass may be wider than can be guessed from the barium swallow. As in the case of bladder cancer, real precision of localisation is not possible, and localisation must remain an informed guess which includes compromise. The optimum dose is 5000 cGy in 15 fractions over 3 weeks, but should be reduced to 4750 cGy if the patient is diabetic or old.

A rotation technique can be used with the same size of treated volume and the same dose. It is slightly less attractive than the three-field technique because almost a whole body segment of lung tissue receives some irradiation, though more evenly diffused.

An oesophageal cancer at the root of the neck can be treated using a wedge pair separated by a plain field, all anterior, guided by a shell. The technique is similar to that used for a small carcinoma of the thyroid (see Chap. 7).

Treatment of a high intrathoracic neoplasm lying between the thoracic inlet and the aortic arch may need a variation of the wedge pair plus plain field technique. When the patient is supine, the oesophagus in this region lies at an angle to the bed, especially in a very round-shouldered patient, so that the long axis of the desired cylinder of radiation must also slope at the same angle. This is achieved by swinging the centre transverse plane of the three anterior fields downwards, till the plane is at right angles to the mean slope of the oesophagus. This manoeuvre usually leaves quite a large gap between the upper margins of the fields and the anterior chest wall, and the simplest way to correct the resulting oblique incidence is to fill the gap with wax, on which is marked the field outlines and centres, and the orientation for the two wedges. The thickness of the wax increases the effective depth of the tumour of course, and it then may be found that the slightly greater depth doses of an 8- or 10-MeV machine, compared with 4 MeV, are advantageous.

Palliative X-ray Treatment Techniques

For tumours of the lower two-thirds of the oesophagus, the three-field arrangement is best, giving a dose of 3500 or 3750 cGy in eight treatments over 10 days. The spinal cord is not irradiated, and the treatment cannot be blamed if the patient subsequently develops paraplegia.

For tumours above the level of the aortic arch, a parallel pair of fields will give as good palliation as any more sophisticated technique. In this case, however, the spinal cord is included in the treated volume, so that the dose has to be limited to 3500 cGy in 10 days for fields up to 12 cm long, and reduced to 3250 cGy for fields between 12 and 15 cm long.

There is probably some advantage in using somewhat shorter fields for palliative treatments. Margins can be less than with radical treatments, because one is only interested in treating the main bulk of obvious tumour in order to relieve dysphagia, and the shorter the length of the oesophagus which is treated, the more likely it is that the inevitable radiation oesophagitis will not be too troublesome.

Single treatments of 1250–1500 cGy, depending on field size, can be given to distant metastases in bone, nodes, or skin. They are just as effective in relieving symptoms as fractionated treatments.

General Management

It is most important to maintain, and often to improve, the patient's state of nutrition. For those who can swallow soft solids, meat can be minced and many solid foods homogenised in a kitchen mixer. A good dietician can be most helpful in ensuring that the diet is balanced and suitably prepared. If the patient can only swallow fluids, then broths, clear soups, and milk-based foods can be given temporarily if it is hoped that treatment will soon improve the situation. Several good proprietary preparations are available containing protein with added vitamins and minerals, and some of these are suitable for feeding via an oral or nasogastric tube. Hydration must be maintained, avoiding intravenous routes if possible. Paracetamol mucilage (10 ml) taken before meals may help the patient to swallow more easily during the radiation reaction.

Most patients become anaemic. If of slight degree, it may be that oral iron in fluid form will suffice for a time, but if the haemoglobin is less than 10 g a transfusion is desirable, especially before a patient begins a radical course of treatment.

All patients should have a 4-hourly chart kept of pulse, temperature, and respiration. A rising pulse rate can be the first sign of mediastinitis, to be followed by raised temperature and respiration rate. If X-ray treatment is being given, it must be stopped immediately, and an attempt made to pass a thin oral tube if the patient does not already have one. Nothing should be swallowed, and any post-nasal secretions or sputum must be expectorated. The only active treatment is by a broad-spectrum antibiotic. Occasionally a small perforation may close, probably plugged softly by growing tumour, and the symptoms and signs settle. No more X-ray treatment should be given, the patient should be fed by tube, and any symptoms other than dysphagia treated by drugs. More often the mediastinitis progresses to abscess formation and the patient becomes very ill. This situation should be regarded as terminal, and managed as such. It is not a kindness to attempt rescue by such measures as drainage of an abscess when destiny has decreed a hopeless prognosis.

Much the same principles apply to infection of the lungs. If the infection is due to aspiration, it may be treated with antibiotics and perhaps cleared up if the patient's general condition is good and the disease not too advanced. If, however, a fistula has formed, or the disease is advanced and the general condition is deteriorating rapidly, it may be best to do nothing.

Those few patients who do well after treatment may not need much help until the tumour recurs. Their quality of life can be good, and if nutrition is well maintained they can be comfortable and active, though they may always be conscious that swallowing is not quite normal. They may need occasional dilatation because of fibrosis, and may complain of unexpected and sudden regurgitation of food debris, especially at night. When it is obvious that their primary tumour is growing again, it is usual for distant metastases to declare themselves at about the same time, and they die soon afterwards.

Complications of X-ray Treatment

There is really only one complication due to X-ray treatment, and that is the inevitable fibrosis following healing of tumour in the treated volume. The extent of the fibrosis, and therefore the extent of the obstruction it may cause, is probably in direct relationship to the size of the original neoplasm. A small lesion occupying only a small part of the circumference of the lumen may well heal without causing noticeable obstruction, whereas at the other extreme, a large annular lesion will heal with an annular scar which is bound to cause at least some obstruction. Fortunately, such fibrous constrictions can usually be dilated by bougie well enough to keep the patient swallowing comfortably, though dilatation may need to be done regularly at intervals of a few months. The first dilatation is usually required at about 6–8 months after the X-ray treatment has finished, and it is not always possible to decide at endoscopy whether a simple stricture or recurrent tumour is present. It has been said that about 50% of radically treated patients will need subsequent dilatation for fibrosis, compared with 30% of patients who have had surgery and develop a stricture at the site of anastomosis.

The other complications which can occur during or soon after X-ray treatment are due to resolution of tumour which has already invaded nearby structures, and either weakened or partly destroyed them, so that as the tumour contracts and disappears the invaded tissue may give way. In this manner a perforation may occur, causing mediastinitis, a fistula into the air passages, or massive haemorrhage from one of the great vessels or the heart. These complications were probably inevitable in such patients and merely precipitated by the treatment, but they are usually lethal.

10 Breast

G. G. Ribeiro

Introduction

The treatment of malignant disease of the breast arouses more controversy and emotion than that of any other form of malignant disease.

Many clinical trials have been carried out and others are still in progress. In addition, research work continues in regard to other aspects of the disease, such as epidemiology, population screening, and endocrine factors; yet little is really known about the true biological nature of carcinoma of the breast. A vast amount of literature has accumulated on the treatment of "operable" carcinoma of the breast, but it is not proposed to discuss here the merits or demerits of the various suggested treatments. Instead this chapter will be confined to the practical management of carcinoma of the breast as seen from the point of view of radiotherapists. For this reason greater attention will be paid to the radiotherapy techniques as practised at the Christie Hospital.

Incidence and Mortality

The incidence of carcinoma of the breast remains highest in the female population of Western Europe, Canada, and the United States of America. In contrast, the incidence is very low in the female population of the East and Far East, particularly in Japan.

In England and Wales, approximately 20 000 women will develop carcinoma of the breast annually and 10 000 women will die from this cancer each year.

Pathology

A brief description will be given of the commoner types of primary carcinoma of the breast. For more detailed discussion of individual and rarer types of tumours, the reader is advised to consult textbooks on the pathology of tumours of the breast.

Intraductal Carcinoma

This type usually affects the larger ducts of the breast and in general the tumours tend to be localised to a particular part of the breast. Based on the histological appearances, various subtypes have been described, the most common being the papillary cribriform and comedo carcinoma. The latter is often visible on mammograms because of local calcification.

Lobular Carcinoma (Non-invasive)

This uncommon type affects the terminal ducts of the breast. It may also remain localised, but multifocal lesions have been described, and both breasts may be affected.

Infiltrating (Invasive) Duct Carcinoma

These tumours are by far the most common malignant lesions to be found in the breast. Histologically, the majority are described as scirrhous carcinomas, in view of their gritty consistency, which in turn is caused by the abundant proliferation of collagen tissue.

Infiltrating (Invasive) Lobular Carcinoma

The difference between this tumour and the scirrhous type is slight, but the former is more likely to be multifocal and bilateral.

Medullary Carcinoma

Although comprising only a small percentage of all breast malignancies, this group is important because the overall prognosis of patients with medullary carcinoma is considered to be better than that of patients with scirrhous carcinoma. Medullary carcinomas are often circumscribed and a particular feature is the intense infiltration of the whole tumour by lymphocytes.

Paget's Disease

In this condition the nipple and surrounding skin are affected by an exudate type of eczema which on histological examination reveals the characteristic Paget's cells. The skin is almost invariably associated at some time with an underlying carcinoma of the breast, which is invasive or intraductal in type. The breast carcinoma may not be palpable, but may be visible on a mammogram.

Miscellaneous

Very rarely, primary malignant carcinomas of the breast are mucin-producing carcinomas and adenoid cystic carcinomas. A wide variety of primary sarcomas of the breast have also been described, all of which are rare compared to the various carcinomas described above.

Spread

Direct Invasion

Usually this form of spread leads to ulceration of the skin of the breast. In its extreme form virtually all the skin of the chest wall is involved with tumour, a condition described as cancer *en cuirasse*. Blockage of the dermal lymphatics leads to thickening of the skin and pitting oedema clinically called *peau d'orange*.

Direct invasion can also extend through the thoracic cage and lead to involvement of the pleural cavity, causing effusions and eventually spreading to the lung parenchyma.

Lymphatic Spread

In general it may be stated that the larger the primary carcinoma of the breast the more likely it is that spread will have occurred to the regional lymph nodes. The majority of carcinomas are situated in the upper outer quadrant of the breast, so that the commonest site for lymph node involvement by tumour is the axillary nodes on the ipsilateral side. The other nodes likely to be involved are the internal mammary chain and the ipsilateral supraclavicular nodes. With widespread disease contralateral nodes may be invaded and become clinically palpable.

Haematogenous Spread

The majority of patients who die from carcinoma of the breast do so because of haematogenous spread. In the late stages of the disease an examination of the bone marrow will frequently show carcinoma cells within it. Virtually every organ in the body may be affected by the time death occurs, but the more common sites are the lungs, bones, and liver.

Clinical Examination

History

A detailed history is important in planning treatment for the individual patient and also to permit retrospective surveys at a later date. Symptoms and signs noted by the patient and their duration should be recorded. In particular, symptoms suggestive of distant metastases are important since more detailed investigations will be required. Examples would be pain in the vertebral axis which may be due to skeletal metastases, progressive dyspnoea due to lung metastases, or symptoms of raised intracranial pressure resulting from brain metastases. Also noted in the history are the patient's menstrual status, parity, and positive evidence of a family history of carcinoma of the breast.

Physical Examination

A detailed physical examination is necessary to permit accurate clinical staging, which in turn contributes to decisions on appropriate management.

The examination begins with inspection of the patient. The affected and normal breast are inspected for asymmetry and distortion of the nipples. Ulceration of the skin is noted, including *peau d'orange* in more advanced tumours. Paget's disease of the nipple is usually obvious, as is oedema of the arm or wasting of the muscles of the hand following involvement of the brachial plexus.

Visible and palpable nodules of tumour in the skin suggest widespread metastatic disease. Following inspection, palpation of the breasts should be carried out. Each quadrant of the breast is palpated in turn with particular care being given to the upper outer quadrant and axillary tail as the most common sites for malignant tumours in the breast. If a lump is found, the texture is noted and also whether it is fixed to the skin and/or deep fascia of the pectoral muscles. An estimate is made of the size of the tumour, preferably with measuring calipers. Any discharge from the nipple is also noted. Once the breast has been examined, attention is turned to the regional lymph node areas in a search for any enlargement of the nodes. Any abnormal increase in size is noted and also whether there is fixity of the nodes. The areas to be examined include the axilla, infraclavicular fossa, supraclavicular fossa, and parasternal regions. Examination of the abdomen is useful to exclude an enlarged liver or palpable abdominal masses arising from metastases in the para-aortic nodes or ovaries.

Clinical Staging

There are two main errors in clinical staging. Firstly, clinicians are inaccurate in their assessment of the size of the primary tumour, usually overestimating the true size. Secondly, in at least a third of cases, the clinical assessment is wrong as to whether the ipsilateral axillary nodes are involved by tumour or not. Given the facts that the size of the primary tumour and the node status are important prognostic factors, a combination of clinical and pathological staging would clearly be more accurate. Staging of carcinoma of the breast is therefore an important part of the clinical evaluation and a great help towards arriving at a decision on management for the individual. Use of a standard form of clinical staging allows the comparison of the results of treatment on a national and international basis.

At the Christie Hospital we use the UICC international staging for carcinoma of the breast first recommended in 1960 and published in 1968 (see App. 2).

Investigations

Before definitive operative treatment, distant metastases should be excluded as far as possible. A full blood count may reveal a simple anaemia in need of correction, or a leucoerythroblastic anaemia characteristic of bone marrow metastases. A biochemical profile is useful and abnormalities in the serum levels of calcium, alkaline phosphatase, and lactic dehydrogenase might suggest the necessity for further investigations to exclude bone and/or liver metastases. Also useful are the levels of the blood urea and blood sugar particularly in older patients and for those on treatment for other medical ailments. X-rays films of the chest should be taken, especially for those patients with operable carcinoma of the breast. Anteroposterior, lateral, and penetrated views should help to exclude gross metastases in the lungs, mediastinal nodes, and ribs.

In "early" operable cases of carcinoma of the breast, the number of positive findings revealed by a full skeletal survey are so few that it is difficult to justify such a time-consuming and costly procedure as a routine investigation. However, for patients with advanced disease, and particularly for those with bone pain, X-rays of the skeleton are mandatory. Isotope bone scans using a rectilinear scanner and a gamma camera can define small metastases which may remain undetected with conventional radiography. Bone scans are particulary useful for patients with advanced disease and symptoms but with apparently "negative" radiological findings.

The place of routine isotope bone scans for patients with early operable carcinoma of the breast has not yet been clearly defined and remains controversial.

Treatment Policy

In spite of a number of controlled clinical trials over the past three decades, little real progress has been made in reducing the mortality from carcinoma of the breast. Perhaps the results of trials in progress may be more helpful. In the mean time, however, it remains virtually impossible to formulate a definite treatment policy which is immune to criticism. It is therefore proposed to set out the guidelines used at the Christie Hospital, recognising that each case must always be treated on its own merits.

Surgery

In the past two decades the pattern of surgery for operable carcinoma of the breast has changed very considerably, at least in the United Kingdom. In clinical stage I cases the most common operation now performed is removal of the breast in toto, a simple mastectomy. The ipsilateral axilla may remain undissected or the nodes in the lower axilla may be sampled in continuity with the mastectomy in order to stage the patient more accurately. A few surgeons selectively carry out a wide excision of an early carcinoma and follow the operation with radical radiotherapy, although such a policy is more commonly followed because the patient has refused a mastectomy. Another operation which is gaining popularity especially among younger women is a subcutaneous mastectomy with immediate insertion of a Silastic implant. A radical mastectomy of the Patey type is more commonly done for patients with stage II carcinomas where palpably enlarged nodes suggest involvement of the ipsilateral axilla.

Whatever the operation chosen, we feel it is of paramount importance that every attempt should be made to eradicate the tumour locally, since there is nothing more depressing than a patient dying of uncontrolled, fungating local disease.

Though the operative approach to stage I and stage II carcinomas of the breast may depend on the personal preference of the surgeon, there is still general agreement on when not to operate. For example, it would be clearly pointless to subject a patient to a radical mastectomy if the carcinoma was already beyond the confines of the breast and/or axilla. A careful preoperative clinical assessment is thus essential to avoid ill-judged surgical intervention.

Radiotherapy

Carcinoma of the breast is only moderately sensitive to ionising radiation. For this reason, if radiotherapy is to be effective, high-dose radical therapy is essential. Because the therapy is radical, the risk of side effects in the short and long term is unavoidable whatever the technique used. If inadequate dosage is used, not only is the treatment useless but subsequent radical treatment to the area becomes virtually impossible. When the operative flaps are to be treated because of the possibility of residual disease, the delivered dose should be maximal in the skin. Such a dose will lead, more often than not, to moist desquamation of the skin. If megavoltage irradiation is used, adequate bolus is required to ensure full dosage at the skin surface. If it is decided that the postoperative flaps as well as the regional lymph nodes are to be treated in continuity, thought must be given to the level of dosage that can safely be given to this volume of tissue.

Hormone and Cytotoxic Therapy

These preparations are usually reserved for those patients with recurrent, metastatic, or inoperable disease. Approximately a third of all female patients with carcinoma of the breast will have tumours that will respond to endocrine therapy. At the moment, endocrine therapy is relatively easier to manage than cytotoxic drugs and it would therefore be a great advance if patients with hormone-sensitive tumours could be isolated from the other patients. Hormone receptor assays offer the first breakthrough in the right direction, but not all tumours are accessible to biopsy and a simpler test is also required.

Cytotoxic drugs can be very effective, particularly when used in combination. However, side effects can be severe, cumulative, and in some cases (such as alopecia) unacceptable to the patient. It is also difficult to continue cytotoxic drugs on a long-term basis. More recently trials have been in progress to assess the efficacy of using hormone and cytotoxic drugs as adjuvant therapy at the time of mastectomy to try to prevent distant metastases. The long-term results of these trials are not yet available.

Methods of Radiation Treatment

At the present time there is no perfect technique that can be used to cover the many situations under which patients are referred for radiotherapy. This is particularly so because of the differing forms of surgery now practised. Patients with carcinoma of the breast represent a substantial part of the workload of the Christie Hospital, so that the techniques we employ have to be practical both with regard to effectiveness and rapidity of execution. In addition, most of our patients are anxious to return to work as soon as possible so that the maximum overall time for radical treatment has been limited to 3 weeks (21 days). Even then, allowing for normal wound-healing and about 3 weeks for the radiation reaction to settle, the patient will still require at least 2 months off work from the time of mastectomy. What follows is a description of the radiotherapeutic techniques that have evolved at the Christie Hospital, bearing in mind the special factors mentioned above.

Kilovoltage Therapy: Quadrate Technique

This method treats the whole breast and axilla in one continuous volume by using X-rays generated at 250 kV or 300 kV. It is equally suitable for use in the postoperative patient and for the patient with the breast in situ. The fields are planned to include the breast and axilla in a single treatment zone. The region to be irradiated consists of the whole breast with its contained tumour or the postoperative flaps and also the lymphatic drainage area of the ipsilateral axilla up to the apex. The technique is particularly suited for patients with carcinoma of the axillary tail of the breast and/or enlarged glands in the lower axilla. Where the carcinoma has involved the skin of the chest wall, the obvious advantage of this technique is that the maximum dosage will be delivered to the skin by using kilovoltage X-rays. The main disadvantage is that the quadrate technique is a "freehand" method and, unless a lot of care is taken in carrying it out, considerable variation of dose will occur throughout the treated volume.

Irradiation of the total volume is achieved by three tangential fields each directed from the periphery to the centre of the volume. A posterior field supplements the dose to the apex of the axilla and an additional single field is directed to the ipsilateral supraclavicular fossa.

Each tangential field has to be directed so that the angulation of the beam is not too great, otherwise a large segment of lung will be irradiated. To help in deciding on the correct angle we use the device shown in Fig. 10.1. The flange *A* of the instrument is held flat against the face of the applicator as shown. The central rod *B*, which is graduated in centimetres, is moved forward until the vertical pin *C*, which is also graduated, is over the centre of the area to be irradiated. The central rod is now locked in position by a screw *D*. The axis of the central rod is parallel to the central axis of the X-ray beam. The vertical pin slides easily within the collar *E* in a direction at right angles to the central rod. The face of the applicator is then angled down towards the chest wall of the patient. The angle is correct when the vertical pin shows no more than 5 cm between the point of the skin of the patient and the collar *E* and 5 cm above the collar, as shown in Fig. 10.1b. With an applicator that is 10 cm deep in a vertical direction, this means that 5 cm of tissue will be treated and the remainder of the X-rays will pass through air (more precisely

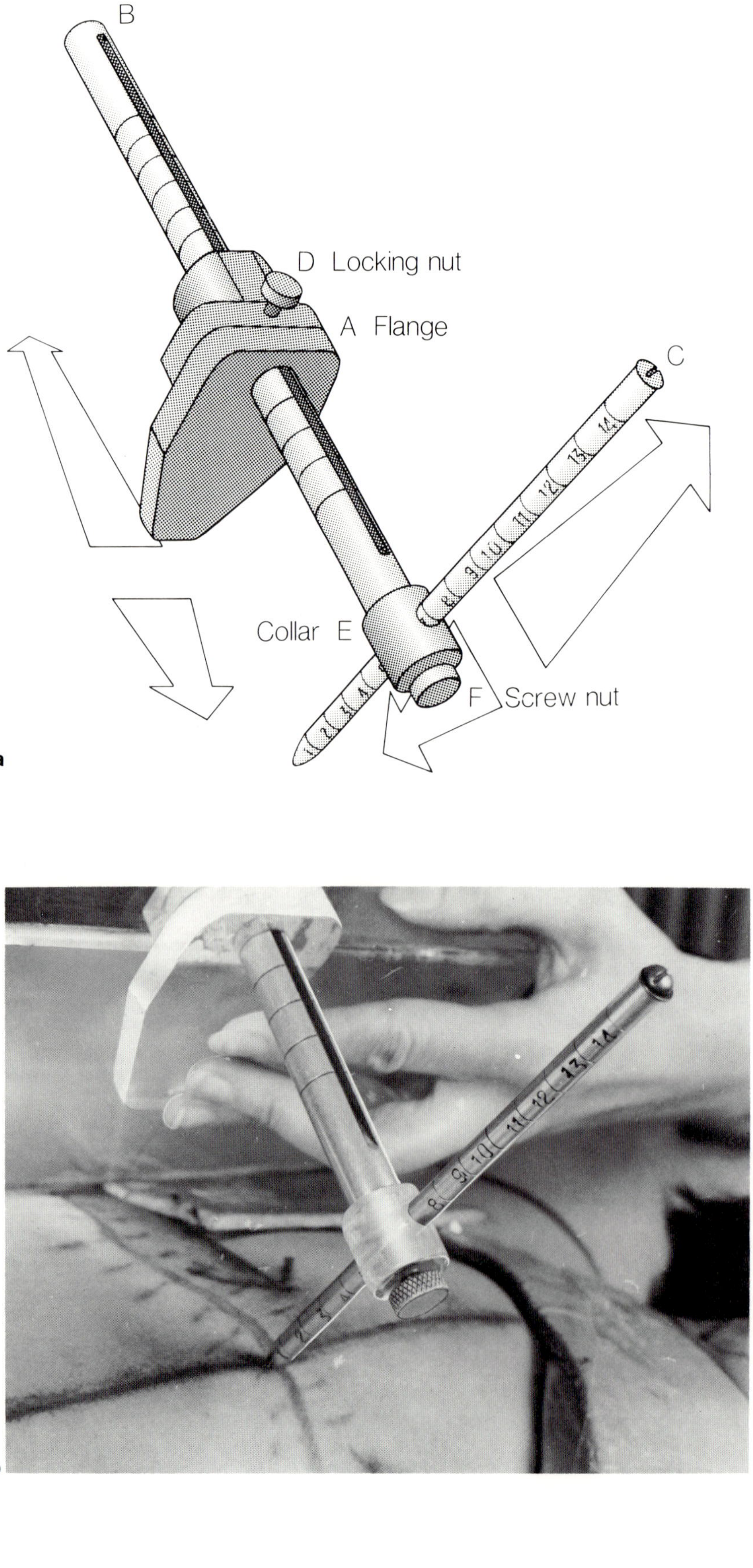

a

b

Fig. 10.1.

through bolus) above the skin. The tissue treated will include skin, subcutaneous tissue, the rib cage, and a minimal segment of lung in the postoperative situation. With the breast in situ, the vertical pin placed over the centre of the breast would, for example, show only 1 cm between the skin and the collar *E* and 9 cm above the collar, thus allowing 9 cm of breast, subcutaneous tissue and chest wall to be treated, as shown in Fig. 10.2.

The detailed set-up of the fields used is shown diagrammatically in Fig. 10.3 and is as follows:

Upper Medial Field

Depending on the width of the patient, an applicator 20×10 cm or 25×10 cm is placed so that its lower edge lies along a line which crosses the middle of the clavicle. The lateral end of the applicator is at the acromioclavicular joint and the medial end extends to a maximum of 5 cm beyond the midline. The focus-skin distance (FSD) is 50 cm to allow the applicator to clear the patient's head, which is extended and turned to the opposite side. There is no pillow under the head of the patient when this field is marked out and treated.

Lower Medial Field

The lower edge of an applicator 20×10 cm or 25×10 cm is placed along the costal margin below

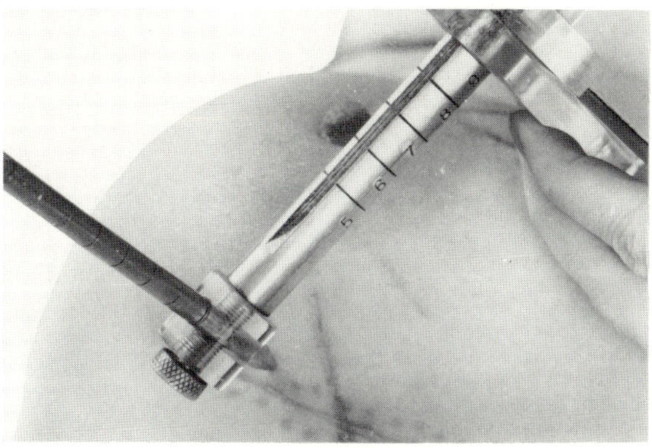

Fig. 10.2.

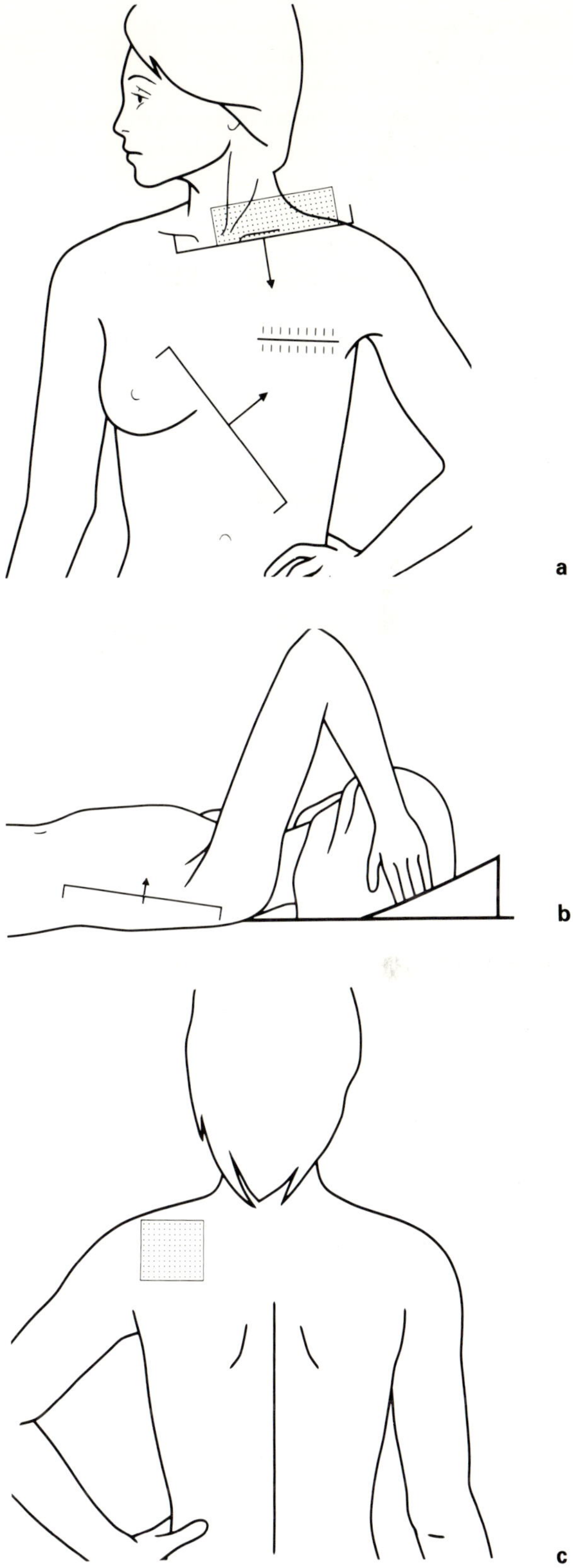

Fig. 10.3.

the breast so that it extends from a point opposite the medial end of the upper medial field, down to the flank at the continuation downwards of the line of the anterior axillary fold.

The gap between the medial ends of the upper medial and lower medial fields should not be less than 5 cm or more than 10 cm to avoid over- or under-irradiation of that area. The FSD is again 50 cm. The patient has a pillow under the head during the marking out and treatment of this field.

Lateral Field

The patient is moved from the centre to the edge of the couch, with the arm extended above the head, flexed at the elbow and with the palm of the hand on the occiput. (If the patient is unable to carry out this manoeuvre, it is not possible to employ the quadrate technique.) Depending on the size of the patient, the applicators required may be 25×10 cm, 25×12.5 cm or exceptionally 28×10.0 cm. The lower edge of the applicator lies along the posterior axillary fold from a point just above the axillary apex to a point level with the lateral end of the lower medial field, again leaving a gap of not less than 5 cm and not more than 10 cm. The patient has a pillow under the head during the marking out of this field.

Posterior Field

The patient sits upright in a chair during the marking out and treatment of this field. The central axis of the field is arranged so that its exit is at the coracoid process anteriorly. This field is used to supplement the dose at the apex of the axilla so that only a small applicator is required. Usually, an applicator 8 cm wide by 6 cm vertically is used, but for a small patient this may require to be reduced to a 6×6 cm applicator. Care should be taken that the upper edge of the beam does not overlap the supraclavicular field.

Supraclavicular Field

This field is strictly not part of the quadrate technique but is complementary to it. It is easiest to mark out immediately following the upper medial field. The patient has no pillow under the head and the head is turned to the opposite side. The lower edge of the field matches onto the upper medial field. The medial edge of the field is at the insertion of the sternomastoid muscle and the lateral end at the acromioclavicular joint. The majority of cases are covered by an applicator 12 cm long by 6 cm, but a smaller field size of 10×5 cm may be sufficient. To avoid any risk of overlapping on the skin, the edge of the medial field is shielded with lead while irradiating the supraclavicular field.

Treatment

Because of the tangential alignment of the applicators, scattering material must be placed in that part of the path of the tangential beam that does not pass through the tissue of the patient. With scattering material in use, the method of prescribing is then similar to that for an applicator firmly applied to the skin. For convenience, bolus bags containing unit-density material are used and during the treatment the whole area being irradiated is covered with bolus to the level of the upper edge of the applicator, as shown in Fig. 10.4. Prescription for the quadrate technique:

Upper medial field 20×10 cm at 50 cm FSD
Lower medial field 20×10 cm at 50 cm FSD
Lateral field 25×10 cm at 50 cm FSD
Upper medial to tumour=10 cm=36.5%
Lower medial to tumour=10 cm=36.5%
Lateral to tumour =10 cm=37.0%
Total=110%
Tumour dose=110%=3700 cGy in 15 treatments over 21 days
Given dose=100%=3360 cGy
Posterior field given dose=3000 cGy
Supraclavicular field given dose=3500 cGy

If the treatment time is reduced to eight treatments in 10 days then the doses are adjusted as follows:

Tumour dose=110%=3100 cGy in 8 treatments over 10 days
Given dose on the upper medial, lower medial, and lateral fields=100%=2800 cGy
Posterior field given dose=2500 cGy
Supraclavicular field given dose=3000 cGy

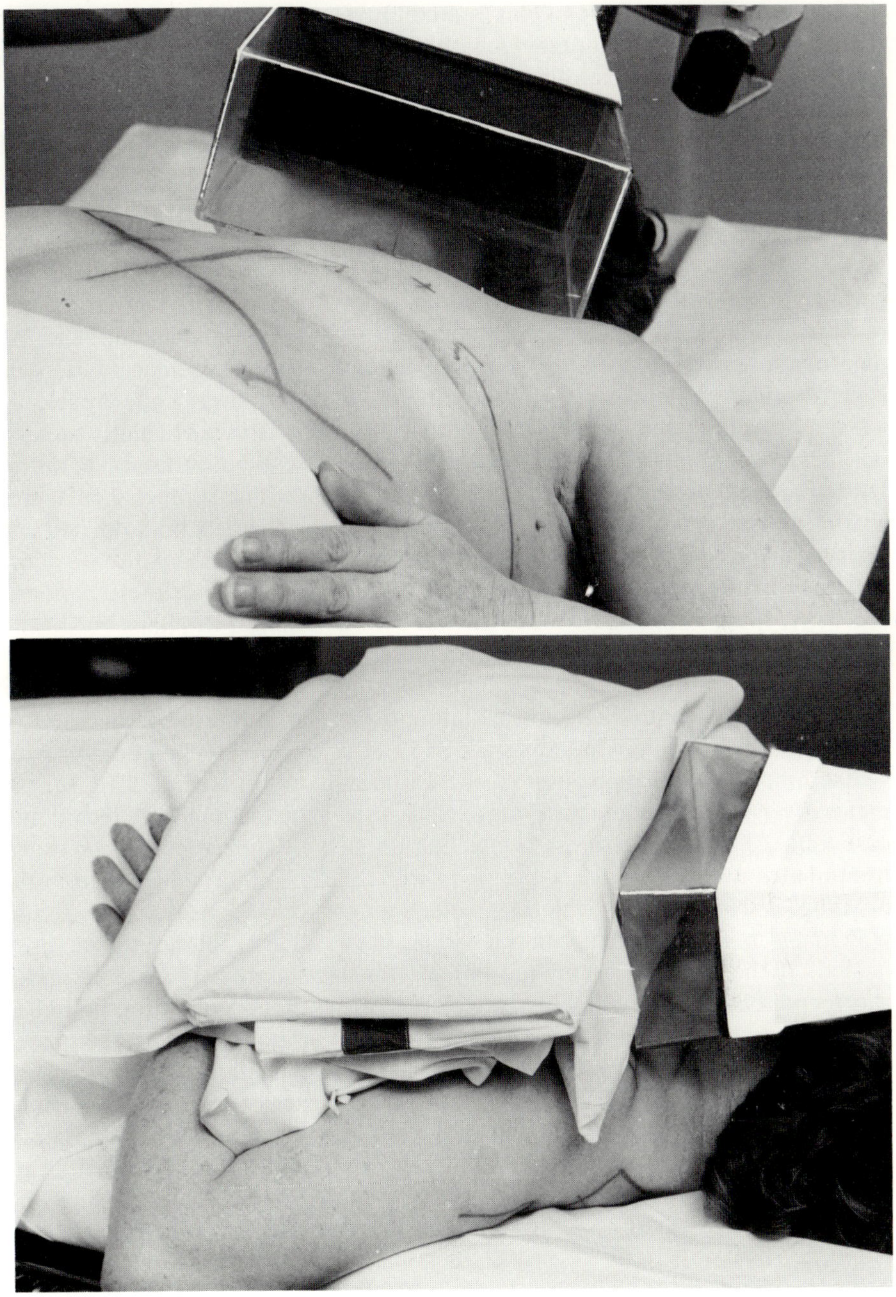

Fig. 10.4. a b

Side Effects

Acute Reactions

The effects of radical radiotherapy vary from patient to patient both in the severity and time of onset and for this reason it is necessary to monitor the reactions at least once a week. What follows is a description of the general side effects in the majority of patients after a 3-week course of radical radiotherapy by the quadrate technique. During the first seven treatments (of 15) there is usually no visible reaction in the skin. Very nervous patients may complain of nausea and insomnia and usually settle down with an antiemetic or mild tranquilliser. From the tenth treatment onwards the skin develops an erythematous reaction over the irradiated area. This is a confluent reaction but tends to get more severe in moist areas such as the axilla and the inframammary sulcus if a pendulous breast is present. The skin becomes very itchy. By the fifteenth treatment the axilla and the skin in the inframammary sulcus may develop moist desquamation and a soothing cream, which can be used whilst continuing irradiation, is 1% hydrocortisone cream. It is seldom necessary to curtail treatment because of unacceptable skin reactions. Some patients may volunteer a history of intolerance to ultra-violet radiation and, if there is no alternative to radiotherapy, they should be watched carefully with a view to modifying the dosage. In addition to the skin reaction, from the tenth treatment onwards, the patients complain of a sore throat and dysphagia as a result of a pharyngeal reaction. These symptoms can be relieved by the use of aspirin or paracetamol mucilage, 10 ml of which are taken 20 min before meals. Alternatively, some patients prefer a soluble aspirin gargle or lozenges with a mild anaesthetic incorporated. Both the skin and the pharyngeal reactions continue for a period of 2 weeks following the completion of the 15 treatments (over 21 days) before the symptoms begin to ease off. At 6 weeks from the completion of treatment most patients have no problems with the pharyngeal reaction and the skin reaction is beginning to settle and the moist areas have healed. If the quadrate technique is used for a shorter period of eight treatments over 10 days, the above reactions occur in the third week after the completion of treatment and the reactions may be more severe. Older or infirm patients can usually be treated over this shorter time but they need to be warned and possibly nursed through the reactions.

Late Reactions

Telangiectasia of the skin can occur within the irradiated area many years after the completion of treatment. The severity of the telangiectasia varies from patient to patient. A lot can be done to improve the cosmetic appearance in the supraclavicular area with special make-up.

Kilovoltage X-rays lead to a differential absorption in bone compared with other tissues and fractures of the ribs are a possibilcertain amount of fibrosis will occur in the apex of the lung on the treated side, but in our experience it has not been sufficient to cause symptoms.

Megavoltage Therapy—Peripheral Only

This technique has been designed for use with the 4-MV linear accelerator. It aims, by means of a single anterior field, to deliver a radical dose to the immediate lymph node drainage areas of the breast, including the axillary, infraclavicular, supraclavicular and parasternal regions (the peripheral node areas).

It is particularly suitable for the large patient with bulky disease in the axilla and/or infraclavicular and supraclavicular fossae. It is also useful for patients who have had a radical mastectomy and have residual disease at or beyond the apex of the axilla, since these patients do not require irradiation of the flaps but of the node areas only. This technique electively irradiates the parasternal nodes and is used postoperatively for the patients who had medially sited tumours. Finally, it is a useful technique for patients with limited arm movements and who therefore cannot be treated by the quadrate technique.

The patient lies on the treatment couch with the head turned away from the treated side. The arm on the treated side is slightly abducted and the hand is placed on the hip. Using the light beam, a square field is set up on the anterior chest wall on the side to be treated. The medial border runs parallel to and 2 cm beyond the contralateral parasternal border. The inferior border runs across to the lower border of the axilla. The superior margin takes in the supraclavicular fossa, and the lateral border runs vertically downwards from the acromioclavicular joint to meet with the inferior border.

The area to be irradiated is then marked out within this square, and the remainder of the area shielded during irradiation by means of lead blocks. The final area to be irradiated is shown in Fig. 10.5 and the details are as follows:

Using the same lateral border as the light beam, the parasternal portion of the field is marked out as a strip extending 12 cm distally from the suprasternal notch and 6 cm wide, 2 cm of the width extending into the contralateral side. From the superior edge of the medial border of the parasternal field a line runs down to the lower border of the axilla. The slope of this line will depend on the

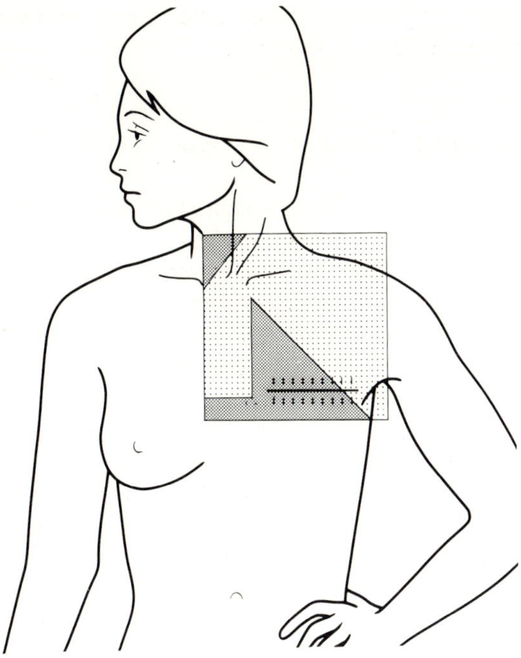

Fig. 10.5.

extent of disease present in the infraclavicular fossa, thus being sharply angulated in cases where no disease is palpable or in a more transverse position where substantial nodes are present. In the former case only the apex of the lung will be irradiated but in the latter case, of necessity, more of the lung will be included in the irradiated volume.

A Perspex tray is attached between the head of the machine and the patient and suitably shaped lead blocks are placed on the tray to shield the areas not being irradiated. In the usual case, this shielding would include most of the lung and the larynx. Very little of the head of the humerus is actually within the irradiated area, and we prefer not to shield it rather than run the risk of preventing irradiation of possible disease in the infraclavicular fossa. There is one important correction to be made before treatment. Post-mastectomy patients have marked curvature of their chest walls in two directions, from the midline towards the axilla and from the supraclavicular fossa towards the costal margin. If no correction were made for these circumstances then the surface dose would be non-uniform because of considerable variations in the source-skin distance (SSD) over the irradiated area. This non-uniformity is corrected by a step-wedge filter which modifies the intensity across the X-ray beam and gives a uniform dose at the surface of the skin. This correction is only exact for the "ideal" patient for which the wedge was designed, but it has been shown by measurements of the surface dose on a large number of patients that the correction gives a sufficiently uniform dose distribution for all the patients treated.

The breast wedge filter modifies the dose distribution in two dimensions normal to the X-ray beam. It is constructed of 20 sheets of hardboard cut to the required slope and glued together. The resulting wedge is not symmetrical (Fig. 10.6) and

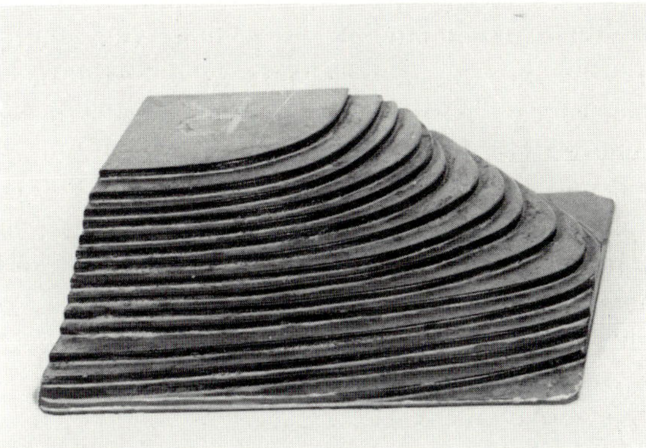

Fig. 10.6.

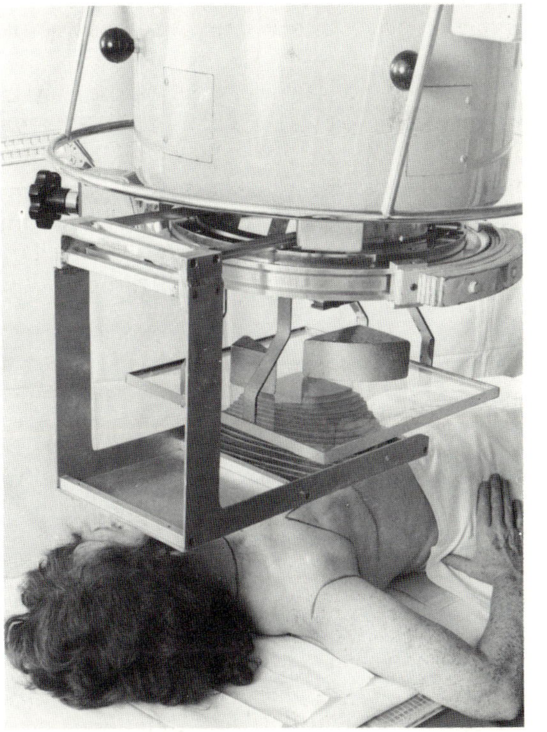

Fig. 10.7.

it is necessary to construct two wedges, one being the mirror image of the other, in order to treat the right and left chest walls of patients. These wedge filters are large, up to 30 cm^2, and up to 8 cm thick. The appropriate filter is located accurately in the beam axis by attaching it to the tray containing the lead blocks. Figure 10.7 shows the set-up with the area to be irradiated marked out, the lead tray and the breast wedge in position. The bolus has been left out of the figure for clarity. The average field size is an 18-cm square, to a maximum of a 20-cm square, with all the lead shielding considerably reducing the size of the actual irradiated area.

The dose delivered is 4000 cGy over 15 treatments in 3 weeks. The spinal cord irradiated within the parasternal field does not receive more than 2000 cGy even in the thinnest patient, and this dose is well within cord tolerance over the treatment time of 3 weeks. If the treatment time is reduced to 10 days the delivered dose is 3250 cGy in eight treatments over 10 days.

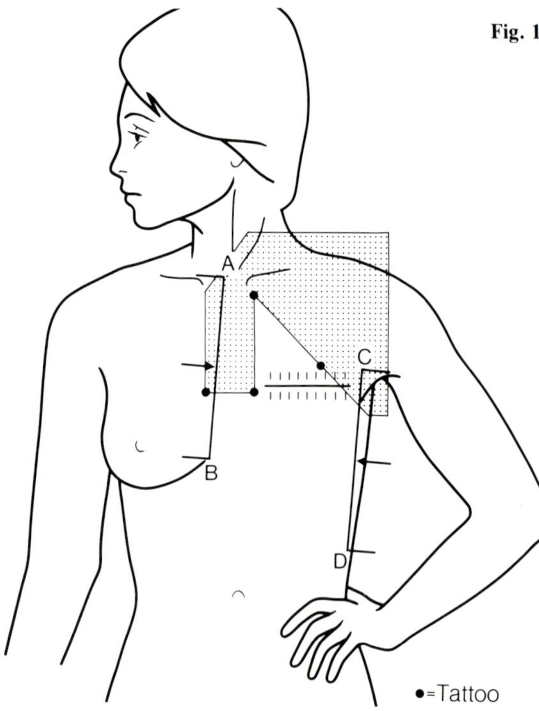

Fig. 10.8.

Side Effects

Acute Reactions

In the third week of a 3-week course of treatment, the skin within the irradiated area develops a confluent erythema which reaches its maximum just after completion of treatment and then begins to fade over the following 3 weeks. The only area which might develop moist desquamation is the skin in the axillary region. Eventually the skin reaction fades so completely that we recommend four small tattoo marks on the patient as shown in Fig. 10.8. If, in the future, addition radiation is required to the flaps, the original outline of the peripheral field can be redrawn with the help of the treatment chart and the tattoo marks. The patient is given 1% hydrocortisone cream to apply to the skin if symptoms develop during irradiation. A radiation reaction also arises in the pharynx and upper oesophagus and the patient usually complains of dysphagia during the third week of treatment. The symptoms can be relieved by aspirin or paracetamol mucilage given three times daily about 20 min before meals.

Late Reactions

Apart from apical fibrosis of the lung within the irradiated area, we are not aware of any other late side effects of the peripheral technique. The apical fibrosis is not sufficient, in the vast majority of cases, to cause any symptoms.

Peripheral (4 MV) plus Tangent Pair (300 kV)

The peripheral technique described above makes no attempt to treat the operative flaps, but should this be considered necessary it is possible to do so in a number of ways. One method is to apply a tangential pair of fields using 300-kV X-rays. The tangent pair consists of a medial and a lateral field. The applicator for the medial field is placed along the midline, with its superior edge high enough to take in the apex of the flaps left untreated by the peripheral field, while its distal end is at the medial end of the costal margin. The long axis of the applicator runs along *AB* as shown in Fig. 10.8. As this line is within the parasternal portion of the peripheral field, the latter should be leaded off when the medial tangent field is being irradiated.

The lateral tangential field is placed along *CD*. The superior edge should be high enough to take in the apex of the untreated flaps and the edge of the applicator then runs along the posterior axillary line. The superior part of the applicator overlaps into the axillary portion of the peripheral field, which should therefore be shielded with lead during treatment of the lateral tangent field.

The usual size of the applicators required is 20×10 cm, but for a small patient, 15×10 cm applicators will suffice. The fields are parallel to each other and the instrument designed to determine the angulations of the applicators for the quadrate technique is again used, to minimise the irradiation of the lung. The reference point used is a line midway between the two fields, and the distance from the applicator to the reference line is also used to determine the depth dose delivered from each field. The detailed prescription is as follows:

Fields

Anterior axilla, supraclavicular fossa, and parasternal
(peripheral area) 4 MV at 100 cm FSD

Set-up factors

Breast wedge filter
Full bolus 1 cm thick over treated area

Dosage

Given dose 4000 cGy in 15 treatments over 21 days
Maximum subcutaneous dose 4000 cGy

Tangent pair fields

300 kV at 50 cm FSD
Medial tangent—20×10 cm at 50 cm FSD
Lateral tangent—20×10 cm at 50 cm FSD

Dosage

Distance from medial tangent to centre of field=8 cm
% tumour dose=41%
Distance from lateral tanget to centre of field=41%
Distance from lateral tangent to centre of field=8 cm
% tumour dose=41%
Total tumour dose=82%=3000 cGy in 15 treatments over 21 days
Given dose to each field=100%=3660 cGy
Maximum skin dose at 16 cm=113%=4130 cGy

Peripheral plus Superficial Therapy

If the interfield distance between the tangent pair on 300 kV is more than 20 cm, the percentage depth dose at the centre of the treated area becomes too low. If the facility to treat with electrons is not available, an alternative method is to treat the operative flaps with low-voltage therapy machines, e.g. 100 kV. As shown in Fig. 10.9, the flaps are divided into single, conveniently small areas (*a,b,c,d*), each of which is treated separately. Treating the individual fields on separate days, each field is given a dose of 1500 cGy in a single exposure with 100 kV X-rays. The applicator sizes are 10–14 cm square and the area to be irradiated is outlined to the desired shape with lead. The FSD used is 30 cm.

The dose given produces a moist desquamation and quite marked telangiectasia as a late side effect.

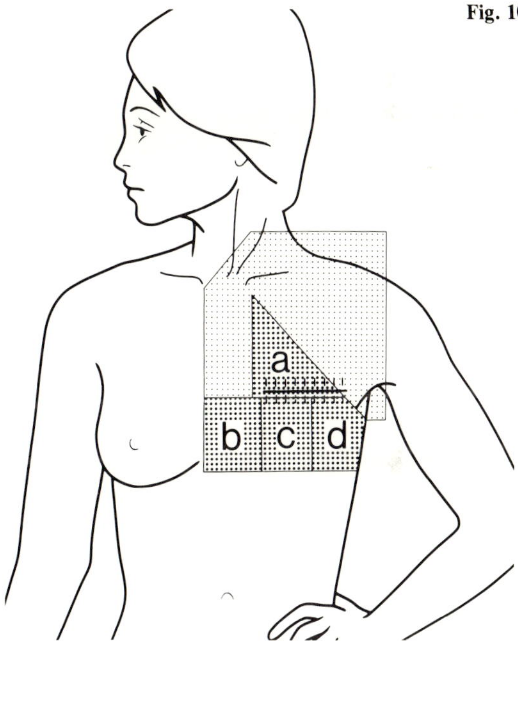

Fig. 10.9.

Modified Peripheral plus 8-MV Electrons

This technique aims to irradiate the axilla, the infraclavicular fossa and the supraclavicular fossa (but not the internal mammary nodes) with 4-MV X-rays and the operative flaps by a single matching field using 8-MV electrons. Using ultrasonic methods to measure post-mastectomy chest wall thickness we found that the mean thickness averaged over all patients is 1.7 cm. The maximum chest wall thickness in the midclavicular line averaged 1.9 cm. The maximum thickness measured anywhere on the chest wall in the simple mastectomy cases proves to be at the upper end of the anterior axillary line, the average thickness at that site being 3.1 cm.

These findings suggest that it is reasonable to include the thickest part of the upper chest wall in the area irradiated by 4-MV X-rays, while the remainder of the chest wall can be adequately treated by 8-MV electrons, since 90% of the given dose will be received by the tissue at a depth of 2 cm. It is best to start with the setting up of the electron field for the flaps, because it is essential to ensure a horizontal line at the upper edge of this area since this same line will form the lower border of the area to be irradiated by 4-MV X-rays. The superior edge of the applicator lies along a line which extends horizontally from the lower border of the axilla, medially along the second costal cartilage. The medial border of the field is along the midline of the patient. The patient's arm is abducted at right angles and the head turned to the opposite side. At present our electron applicator has an area of 22 cm^2 in order to accommodate the largest patients. When treating smaller patients, however, it will be necessary to shield the upper abdomen, and provided the medial border is at the midline of the patient the excess irradiated area laterally is then on the treatment couch and does not matter. The necessity for shielding could, of course, be obviated by having a series of smaller applicators.

The position of the patient and the treatment area are shown in Fig. 10.10. Built into the applicator for the electron beams there is a Perspex filter, 5 mm in thickness, with an increased thickness in the centre of the filter. This has the effect of bringing the dose up to the 90% isodose curve at the surface. It also has the effect of increasing the scattering towards the edges of the area being irradiated, thus creating a uniform distribution across the field. A series of measurements have been made during treatment, on individual patients, by placing thermoluminescent dosemeters within the irradiated area at the medial, lateral, and central positions. These measurements have confirmed the uniformity of the dose distribution. The subsequent even skin reaction has also provided further confirmation.

With the arm still abducted at right angles, a single anterior megavoltage X-ray field is used to irradiate the axilla, infraclavicular fossa and the supraclavicular fossa, the lower border of this field being the superior border of the electron field. The average field size used is 20 cm wide and 13 cm vertically. The medial border extends 1 cm beyond the midline of the patient. The larynx is shielded. It is not considered necessary to shield the humerus, and no attempt is made to avoid the spinal cord, as the length of cord actually irradiated is very small and the dose administered is well within the tolerance level.

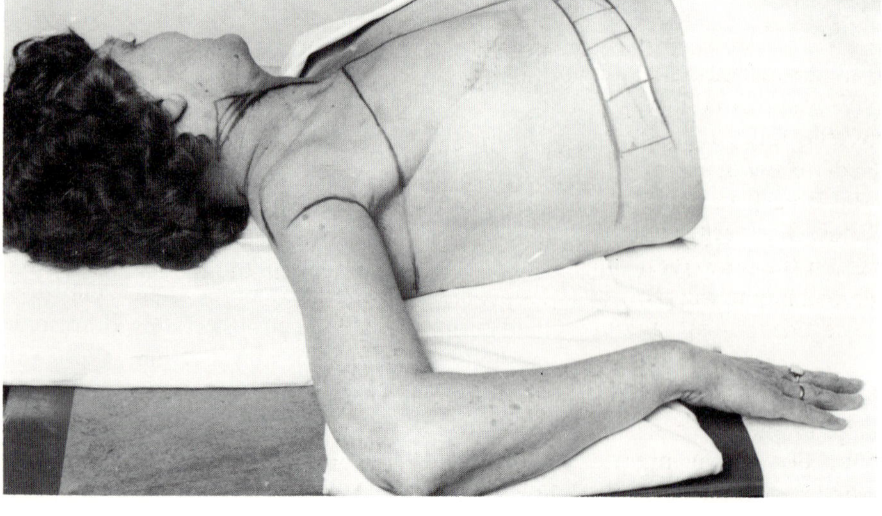

Fig. 10.10.

Anterior axilla, supra- and infraclavicular fossae
4-MV linear accelerator Field size 20×12 cm at 100 cm FSD
Full bolus Breast wedge filter
Given dose=4000 cGy in 15 treatments over 21 days
Maximum subcutaneous dose=4000 cGy

Anterior chest wall
8-MV electrons at 100 cm FSD
22 cm^2 applicator with lead shielding beyond the edges of the field as drawn on the patient
Given dose=4000 cGy in 15 treatments over 21 days

Criteria for the Use of Radiotherapy

What follows is a brief outline of the criteria we use for the selection of patients who would benefit from radiotherapy, and the types of technique that could be used in a given set of circumstances. It must be emphasised that our policies are under constant review because of changing patterns of surgical treatment and also in the light of results of clinical trials carried out at the Christie Hospital and elsewhere. Furthermore, because of the complex way carcinoma of the breast presents itself, any policy must remain flexible and ultimately each case is considered on its own merits. In view of these problems the most convenient way to consider our policy is to relate it to the various clinical stages of the disease. The staging used is that proposed by the UICC (see App. 2).

Stage I

1) If the patient has had an excision of the malignant lump with a wedge of surrounding tissue (lumpectomy, or tylectomy) the policy at present is to follow this surgery immediately with a course of radical radiotherapy to the breast and the ipsilateral regional lymph nodes. The technique we prefer is either the quadrate or the peripheral and tangent pair. With either technique we give an extra single dose of 500 cGy to the original tumour site.

2) Where only a simple mastectomy has been carried out, and if no enlarged nodes are clinically palpable in the axilla, we do not at present recommend routine postoperative irradiation, provided only that the patient can be kept on strict follow-up. During the first year the patient is seen every 2–3 months and the interval gradually increased over the next 4 years.

Because of the inaccuracy of clinical staging, up to a third of these patients are liable to develop recurrent disease in the operative flaps and lymph node drainage areas. Of the remaining two-thirds, the patients will either be cured or develop distant metastases. We feel therefore that a significant proportion of patients can be spared the added discomfort and morbidity of radiation by adopting a "watch" policy.

Should recurrence occur anywhere within the operative area the patient is then given radical radiotherapy to the operative flaps and regional node drainage areas. Techniques that could be used are the quadrate, the peripheral and tangent pair, or the modified peripheral and single electron field.

3) Patients who have had a radical mastectomy of the classical Halstead type or the Patey modification and whose lymph nodes are not involved with tumour do not require routine postoperative radiotherapy. The recurrence rate in the flaps following a radical mastectomy is very low (10%–15%) and by definition no recurrence should take place in the axilla if all the lymph nodes have been removed. A small proportion of patients may later develop enlarged nodes in the ipsilateral supraclavicular fossa and these patients could be treated by the peripheral technique alone. For those with recurrent disease in the flaps the choice of technique lies between the peripheral and tangent pair or the modified peripheral and single electron field.

In Stage I cases where the tumour is medially situated in the breast, we do not routinely advise radiotherapy to the internal mammary nodes, since the likelihood of involvement of these nodes is not as high as when the axilla is also known to be simultaneously involved. If radiation needs to be given to these patients at a later date for a parasternal and/or axillary recurrence, the peripheral technique alone could be used, leaving the flaps unirradiated.

Stage II

1) Included in this group are the patients who have had a simple mastectomy only but have been left

with palpable enlarged nodes in the axilla, and those who have had a simple mastectomy with removal of a variable number of nodes from the axilla, at least one of which has been shown to be involved with tumour histologically. In all these cases we would recommend radical postoperative radiotherapy. Suitable techniques would be the quadrate, the peripheral and tangent pair, or the modified peripheral and single electron field.

2) If a radical operation of the Halstead or Patey type has been done, and if less than three nodes from the lower axilla have been found to be involved histologically we would not recommend postoperative irradiation, provided close follow-up is maintained. Radical radiotherapy can be employed if and when local recurrence develops. However, if during a radical operation it is found that disease is present beyond the apex of the axilla, or if all the lymph nodes removed are massively involved with tumour, postoperative therapy should be given. The techniques are the same as those outlined in the previous paragraph.

Stage III

The borderline between operable and inoperable carcinoma of the breast varies with individual surgeons. However, we feel that the criteria determining operability should be fairly narrowly drawn, in which case the majority of stage III tumours as defined by the UICC staging are in fact inoperable and radical radiotherapy is the initial treatment of choice at present. In a small group of patients the tumour, though large, may be slowly growing, with a long history. Such tumours may be confined to the breast and with no obvious involvement of the axillary nodes. Following radical radiotherapy very considerable shrinkage of the tumour takes place and the residual tumour can later be excised. In these selected patients radiotherapy becomes preoperative, even though it is not planned as such. Suitable techniques for these cases are the quadrate or the peripheral and tangent pair. Occasionally the breast is so large that it becomes technically difficult to treat the patient. For these patients it is reasonable to ask a surgeon to remove the bulk of the tumour before starting elective radiotherapy.

Artificial Menopause

Between 1948 and 1955 a randomised clinical trial was carried out at the Christie Hospital on premenopausal women with operable carcinoma of the breast. All the patients had a standard radical mastectomy and immediately thereafter one group had an artificial menopause induced by radiation while the other group were followed up only (controls). The ovarian irradiation consisted of a single treatment using anterior and posterior opposed fields to the pelvis, 15 cm wide×10 cm vertically, and delivering a midpelvic dose of 450 cGy. The 15-year results of this trial show that prophylactic castration at this dose level did not significantly prolong the ultimate survival of the castrated group. There was, however, a statistically significant delay in the appearance of distant metastases in the irradiated group compared with the control group. The patients who appeared to benefit least from the procedure were those aged 40 years or less. The dose employed in this trial was insufficient to induce a menopause in 30% of these younger patients but even with the higher dose we now employ we doubt if an irradiation menopause can be said to be permanent and it would be preferable to carry out a bilateral oophorectomy in patients aged 40 years or less. Further analysis of the above trial also showed that if the results were to be judged on the survival rate there was no advantage in carrying out artificial castration, provided that the patients were carefully followed up and the appropriate hormone procedures vigorously applied when the patients developed recurrent or metastatic disease. At the present time, therefore, we do not recommend routine prophylactic castration at the time of mastectomy but reserve the procedure for those who develop recurrent or metastatic disease. We do, however, recommend the procedure for patients with inoperable stage III disease.

Technique

The true pelvis is covered by means of two parallel opposed fields, anteriorly and posteriorly. Each field is 15 cm wide and 10 cm vertically, centred 3 cm above the symphysis anteriorly. The centre of the posterior field is found by the pin and arc method, by rotating the tube head through 180°, and the patient can be treated through the grid without turning over. For those aged 40 years and under, the midpelvic dose aimed at is 1500 cGy in four exposures daily, using megavoltage X-rays. For patients aged over 40 years, the midpelvic dose is 500 cGy in a single exposure using megavoltage X-rays. We accept that some of the older patients may start menstruating again and require a further single treatment, but in our experience this is not more than 1% of the total number of patients irradiated. Before carrying out an artificial menopause, one should ascertain that the patient is not pregnant and that there is no known or obvious gynaecological abnormality present.

Recurrent Breast Carcinoma

Patients who have had surgery only for operable tumours may well develop recurrent disease in the chest wall and/or regional lymph nodes at some later time. It is worthwhile getting histological proof of recurrence whenever possible, particularly when the interval from mastectomy to first recurrence spans a number of years. Having proved a recurrence and excluded distant metastases, it is our policy at present to give full radical radiotherapy to the operative flaps and lymph node areas as would have been given on a "prophylactic" basis. Even when only a few nodules of tumour are present in the operative flaps, it is a mistake to limit the volume irradiated, because further skin nodules will soon appear in the operative flaps. A deliberate effort is thus made to cover the whole of the operative area and the adjacent lymph node areas even though the clinically obvious disease is confined to a smaller area. There are a few exceptions to this general rule. A patient who has had a radical mastectomy and whose flaps are so thin that the blood supply is precarious, or where a graft has been necessary, may present with disease in the supraclavicular nodes only. Such a patient could be treated by means of the peripheral technique alone, without irradiation of the flaps. A similar situation arises in old and frail patients who present with disease confined to the axilla or supraclavicular region. In these circumstances treatment can again be limited to the affected areas, leaving the flaps untreated.

Palliative Radiotherapy

Once metastatic disease is established, radiotherapy can be a simple and effective means of providing palliation of symptoms such as pain from bone metastases or bleeding and discharge from extensive ulceration from progressive disease in the chest wall. The relief of symptoms should not be replaced by discomfort from radiation reactions. For the latter reason the treatment volume is kept as small as possible, no attempt being made to take a wide margin or to cover other affected areas that are not causing symptoms. For the same reasons the doses delivered are such that they do not cause moist desquamation of the skin, though not so low that they are useless. Some patients may have disease that is too extensive to be covered by any acceptable radiation technique, while others will require a combination of radiotherapy and systemic chemotherapy of some sort. Some of the more common situations likely to be referred to a radiotherapist will be described below.

Massive Local Disease

Occasionally patients present with very large primary tumours and with distant metastases present. Such tumours may be too large to be totally encompassed by the usual techniques, but where the tumour has fungated through the skin causing discharge and bleeding it is worth attempting some palliative radiotherapy, both for relief of symptoms and to make nursing of the patient easier. The ulcerated portion of the tumour can be treated using a tangent pair of fields with either kilovoltage or megavoltage X-rays. An appropriate tumour dose for kilovoltage treatment is 2500 cGy in 10 days, or 3000 cGy for megavoltage treatment. For very old and frail patients a single field directed straight down onto the tumour may be used, giving a dose of 1250 cGy for kilovoltage or 1500 cGy for megavoltage X-rays. Involved nodes in the axilla or supraclavicular regions can be treated with small fields with megavoltage X-rays, the dose delivered being 1500 cGy in a single exposure or 3000 cGy over 10 days to the same size of field.

Skin Nodules

Provided it has not been previously used, local radiotherapy can be very useful in the control of bleeding and discharge resulting from the ulceration of skin nodules. Treatment is usually confined to a limited area and can be done with superficial X-ray therapy machines (60–100 kV). A maximum dose of 1500 cGy can be given in a single exposure for a field size of 10×10 cm or 12×10 cm.

Parasternal Node Metastases

Clinically these are only rarely encountered. They present as large ill-defining swellings to the side of the sternum, usually in the first three intercostal spaces. The skin over the swelling is often thickened and puckered and is not freely mobile because of attachment to the underlying tumour. The lesions can be adequately controlled by a single field varying in size from 12×10 cm to a maximum of 15×10 cm. The dose delivered using megavoltage X-rays is 3250 cGy in 10 days for the larger field and 3500 cGy for the smaller field. Bolus material must be used to ensure full dosage on the skin surface.

Bone Metastases

Radiotherapy to the site of bone metastases can lead to pain relief for prolonged periods. Once sclerosis of previously lytic metastatic disease has taken place there is the added bonus of a patient becoming mobile again. The majority of lesions can be treated with a single exposure of X-rays, with a single field, using megavoltage equipment. For a field of 10×8 cm the appropriate dose is 1500 cGy. Where a single vertebra is involved, and particularly if collapse is imminent, it is worth seeking a greater effect by a fractionated treatment. The treatment field should include at least one and preferably two of the adjacent vertebrae above and below the affected bone. The tumour dose for such a field size is 2500 cGy in eight treatments over 10 days with megavoltage X-rays. Large lytic metastases not infrequently occur in the upper end of the femur, eventually leading to a pathological fracture, so that these patients often present to the orthopaedic surgeon in the first instance. Where possible it is worth asking for internal fixation first, both to make transportation of the patient to the radiotherapy easier and also to hasten mobilisation of the patient. These lesions are best treated by means of a parallel opposed pair of fields, using megavoltage X-rays, to deliver a tumour dose of 2500 cGy in eight treatments over 10 days, or 1500 cGy in a single exposure if the clinical situation precludes a fractionated treatment. On occasion premenopausal women present with metastatic disease affecting the pelvic bones, preventing the patients from walking or standing for long because of pain. In these patients very good palliation can be achieved by irradiating the whole of the pelvis from the top of the iliac crests down to the level of the lesser trochanters. Two parallel opposed megavoltage beams are used, delivering a tumour dose of 2000 cGy in eight treatments over 10 days. This form of treatment causes little or no bowel upset, and in most cases achieves good pain relief. An added bonus is that this dose is sufficient to induce an artificial menopause, an important first step in the hormone management of premenopausal patients.

Brain Metastases

It is rare for brain metastases from carcinoma of the breast to be solitary. More commonly both hemispheres of the brain are involved and thus almost all of the brain needs to be treated. This is easily done with two lateral opposed fields using megavoltage X-rays, a common field size being 15×10 cm. The midplane dose is 3000 cGy in eight treatments over 10 days. Since the separation between the two lateral fields is seldom very great, the tumour dose is virtually homogeneous over the treated volume.

Metastases in the Choroid of the Eye

Very rarely the choroidal layer of the eye is the site of metastatic disease. These lesions are well worth treating with X-rays and this is carried out by means of a single field placed carefully over the lateral side of the orbit, in order to irradiate the retrolenticular area of the eye. The field size does not need to be more than 4×4 cm or at most 5×5 cm, and the dose delivered is 1250–1500 cGy in a single exposure using 300-kV X-rays or telecobalt therapy.

Endocrine Therapy for Advanced Carcinoma of the Breast

Patients with advanced carcinoma of the breast include those with tumours that are inoperable, recurrent following previous surgery and/or radiotherapy, and those who have metastatic disease. By definition, these patients are incurable, so that any therapy offered is aimed at palliation.

Endocrine therapy offers a very useful form of palliation because, with the newer drugs now available and with better methods of selection of patients for this form of therapy, control of the disease can be maintained for prolonged periods with minimal side effects. These patients can have a good quality of life, often into old age. A major advantage of endocrine therapy is the absence of bone marrow depression, and patients are thus spared both frequent blood counts and frequent visits to the clinic. Endocrine therapy rarely causes alopecia to the degree that some cytotoxic drugs do. The greatest disadvantage of endocrine therapy is that obvious therapeutic benefit is relatively slow to manifest itself and any individual drug requires a trial of at least 2 months before deciding whether it has been efficacious or not. Endocrine therapy is thus precluded in the face of rapidly advancing disease. The exact mechanism by which endocrine therapy works is still unknown. What is certain is that in a proportion of patients the alteration of the internal hormonal environment, whether by additive or by ablative endocrine therapy, will lead to objective measurable regression of disease for varying periods of time.

Hormone Receptor Assay

Within the last decade it has been shown that all steroid hormones have specific, high-affinity protein receptors in their target cells. Cytoplasmic receptors have been identified for several hormones by means of sophisticated radioimmunoassay methods. Whatever the biochemical method of assay, the test requires fresh tumour tissue; this is a major disadvantage, since not all metastatic carcinoma is necessarily accessible for biopsy. At the clinical research laboratories of the Christie Hospital we now routinely biopsy accessible tumour in patients with advanced or metastatic breast carcinoma and carry out hormone receptor assays on the material. It is as yet too early to make categoric statements, but the trends from our laboratories and those in Europe and America suggest that tumours which have hormone receptors present, particularly a high level of oestrogen receptors, are more likely to respond to hormone therapy and to regress, whereas those with an absence of receptors usually show no response to endocrine therapy and continue to progress. If these trends become established the tests would then become of great value in selecting patients for endocrine therapy, the remainder being managed by other forms of therapy.

Work is also being done to find out whether the hormone receptor status in the primary breast tumour is the same as that in subsequent metastases in the same patient. If the status is the same it would not be necessary to seek further material from the metastatic deposits and the patient could be treated on the basis of the result of the receptor assay done on the original primary tumour. Studies are also in progress to see if a more accurate prognosis can be given for any individual patient, by correlating the node status, the histological grading of the primary tumour, the hormone receptor status and the age of the patient.

Therapeutic Artificial Menopause

For those patients who are actively menstruating or less than 2 years past the natural menopause, therapeutic castration is still the first line of endocrine therapy for advanced carcinoma of the breast. It is possible that the results of studies now in progress may suggest an equally effective or superior form of initial therapy in the future. Usually an artificial menopause is induced by means of X-ray therapy, the techniques of which have been previously outlined, although we would suggest a surgical oophorectomy if the patient was under 40 years of age. Approximately 30% of premenopausal patients subjected to castration will benefit from the procedure and varying degrees of regression of disease will occur. However, our experience suggests that in young women, particularly those under 35 years of age, only a small percentage of tumours tend to respond to endocrine therapy. Among the factors contributing to this lack of response is the incidence in the younger women of tumours that are biologically more aggressive and with a higher proportion showing a negative hormone receptor status. Where there is no information on the hormone receptor status of the patient's tumour a response to an artificial menopause is a good indicator of the possible response to other forms of endocrine therapy used subsequently.

Androgens

Objective regression occurs in about 20% of patients treated with androgenic compounds. The response rate is low and in addition the side effects of these drugs can be unacceptable to young women. Nevertheless, androgen therapy is useful for patients with bone metastases as the dominant disease. Response to therapy leads to healing of bone metastases, pain relief and increased mobility of the patient.

The most effective of the androgens is probably testosterone propionate, but the major disadvantage is that the drug has to be given as an intramuscular injection in a dose of 100 mg three times a week, and the oily solution can be quite painful. Side effects, which come on rapidly, include hirsutism, weight gain, acne, deepening of the voice, and sometimes alopecia. An oral preparation with less virilising side effects is fluoxymesterone given in a dose of 5 mg three or four times daily. Another androgenic compound with less virilising side effects than testosterone is deca-durabolin. This is a long-acting preparation that is given by intramuscular injection in a dose of 50 mg every 3 weeks.

Oestrogens

Oestrogen therapy is reserved for postmenopausal patients, since there has been a suggestion that these drugs may cause enhancement of tumour growth in premenopausal women. The drug commonly used is diethylstilboestrol in a dosage of 15 mg daily, but regression of disease has been recorded at a dose level of only 3 mg daily. Side effects can be significant and are dose-related, including nausea, vomiting, vaginal bleeding, and hypercalcaemia. An objective regression rate of up to 50% has been noted following diethylstilboestrol therapy in women more than 10 years past the menopause. Another useful oestrogen preparation is ethinyl-oestradiol in a dosage of 0.5–2 mg daily. The side effects are similar to those of diethylstilboestrol though much less severe, and patients can tolerate the drug better.

Progestogens

The drug of which we have the most experience is norethisterone acetate. It is a potent progestogen and a possible mode of action is by a direct effect on the pituitary gland, suppressing the secretion of follicle-stimulating hormone and luteinising hormone. The drug is very well tolerated, but side effects can be significant in a small percentage of patients, requiring withdrawal of the drug. These side effects include nausea, vomiting, fluid retention, and vaginal bleeding. The dose commonly used by us is 10 mg three times daily.

Anti-oestrogens

The anti-oestrogenic Tamoxifen has now become one of the most common forms of additive therapy. There are a number of reasons for this popularity. Given the fact that the drug is as efficacious as any other hormone preparation in postmenopausal patients, the outstanding advantage of Tamoxifen is its singular lack of serious side-effects. Thus it is rare for the drug to be withdrawn during therapy. It can also be safely given to patients already on medication for heart disease or diabetes. Tamoxifen can also be used to treat premenopausal women with metastatic disease, although the objective regression rate is less than that obtained in postmenopausal women. Side effects of Tamoxifen include hot flushes, nausea, dizziness, and lassitude. If the patient has extensive bone metastases, hypercalcaemia can occur. In premenopausal women irregularity of menstruation is common during therapy; temporary amenorrhoea may take place, with permanent amenorrhoea in those women who are nearing the natural menopause.

Tamoxifen is given orally in doses of 20 mg or 40 mg daily. In recent studies it has been shown that the concentration of Tamoxifen is very slow to rise and eventually reaches a plateau in about 8 weeks from the start of therapy. This is also the time when clinical responses are manifest. By giving a "loading dose" of 160 mg (i.e. four doses of 40 mg) on day 1 we have been able to achieve a stable concentration of the drug in the serum in 8–10 days rather than 8 weeks. From day 2 onwards the patients are maintained on the usual dose of 20 mg daily. It is too early to know if this regime will lead to quicker and better responses. There has, however, been no increase in the side effects with this regime.

Ablative Endocrine Therapy

Major endocrine ablative therapy, such as bilateral adrenalectomy or hypophysectomy, is now seldom performed. The need for these operations has been partly obviated by the advent of better hormone preparations and also by the greatly increased use of combination chemotherapy following relapse from additive hormone therapy. Furthermore, except in very skilled hands, these operations carry an increased morbidity and mortality. Whether the operation of bilateral adrenalectomy or hypophysectomy is done depends on the local facilities for doing one or other of the operations, but so far as the likelihood of response is concerned the procedures can be considered roughly equivalent. The points in favour of bilateral adrenalectomy are: (1) it is much more certain that an adrenalectomy will be complete compared to a hypophysectomy, where the gland is more often incompletely removed or destroyed; and (2) during an adrenalectomy operation it is possible for the surgeon to look for macroscopic evidence of metastases in the liver, ovaries, or other abdominal organs.

We would still recommend bilateral adrenalectomy in the following special circumstances: (1) for women with very slowly progressing disease who, over a number of years, had obtained objective regression of disease in response to various additive hormone preparations; and (2) for very young women with rapidly progressing bone metastases only, where pain relief had not been obtained with analgesics or radiotherapy.

Patients with known liver or brain metastases would not be subjected to major ablative surgery, nor would those patients whose tumours lacked hormone receptors. With these exceptions, the very selected groups of patients—(1) and (2) above—might show an objective regression rate of 20%–30%. However, a number of patients who do not show measurable regression of their disease do nevertheless have significant relief of pain, often within 24 h of surgery. This relief of pain may continue for many months, and even at relapse the pain is not as severe as it was before the operation. The mechanism of the pain relief caused by major ablative surgery is unknown.

Breast Carcinoma Associated with Pregnancy

This is a rare combination and no one centre can accumulate a very large series, even over a long period. The patients can be divided into two groups: (1) those where the carcinoma was diagnosed during pregnancy or up to 1 year after childbirth (concurrent pregnancy group), and (2) those who became pregnant after completing treatment for primary carcinoma of the breast (subsequent pregnancy group).

Concurrent Pregnancy

Patients presenting with early carcinoma of the breast, in the first trimester of pregnancy, should be treated in the same manner as non-pregnant patients. There is no harm in letting the pregnancy continue unless it is against the express wishes of the patient and/or her husband. However, termination of pregnancy should be considered if adjuvant cytotoxic therapy is to be used following surgery because of possible damage to the foetus. There would appear to be no special risk attached to treating patients with carcinoma of the breast in the second half of the pregnancy. Patients with an early carcinoma can have definitive surgery performed, and the pregnancy allowed to continue if the delivery date is still some weeks away. If the carcinoma is found towards the end of pregnancy, an immediate simple mastectomy could be followed by radiotherapy after the birth of the child. Patients with stage III and stage IV disease, including the so-called lactational carcinoma, have such a poor prognosis that the pregnancy should be terminated and appropriate treatment instituted for carcinoma of the breast.

Subsequent Pregnancy

If survival of the subsequent pregnancy group is measured from the time of mastectomy, it is not significantly different from that of matched controls. Further, the longer the interval between mastectomy and subsequent pregnancy the better the survival, whatever the initial stage of the disease. However, if survival is measured from the start of pregnancy, there is a significant decrease of survival with increasing stage of the disease; 50% of stage II patients and all of stage III patients are dead within 7 years. Although the suggestions above are offered as a guide, in the end treatment has to be tailored to the individual patient in this very complex situation.

Carcinoma of the Male Breast

Disease in the male constitutes no more than 1% of all carcinoma of the breast. There is an increased incidence of carcinoma of the breast in males who have Klinefelter's syndrome. The median age at presentation is 65 years. The majority of patients who seek advice do so because of a painless lump in the breast, while the remainder either have pain or symptoms and signs relating to the nipple. Owing to the paucity of tissue in the male breast compared with the female breast, the tumours in the male tend to invade and fix quickly to the deeper structures, leading to inoperability and possible earlier dissemination. In our experience over the past 15 years there has been a statistically significant trend towards more patients presenting with clinical stage I disease and considerably fewer with stage IV disease.

The surgical attitudes towards carcinoma of the breast in males have followed those of the female counterpart, with a tendency in the last decade for operable tumours to be treated by a simple mastectomy followed by radiotherapy, rather than a radical mastectomy alone. Postoperative radiotherapy is given for the same reasons that apply to female carcinoma of the breast and the same techniques are employed. Most patients who develop recurrent and/or metastatic disease following a mastectomy do so within the first 2 years. For recurrent and metastatic disease, bilateral orchidectomy has commonly been recommended, but we have preferred additive hormone therapy first, reserving ablative surgery for patients with bone metastases.

In our series of patients treated with diethylstilboestrol, a response rate of 38% was obtained, with responses noted in skin, lymph nodes, and lungs, although no responses were noted in bone metastases. However, oestrogen therapy has a number of side effects which include nausea, vomiting, gynaecomastia of the remaining breast and the possibility of precipitating a cerebrovascular episode in these elderly patients.

The drug Tamoxifen, owing to its relative lack of serious side effects, is preferable to oestrogenic drugs as the hormone of choice. Although fewer patients with carcinoma of the breast in males have been treated with Tamoxifen, published reports so far suggest that it is just as efficacious in treating advanced disease in males as in females. The best reponses have occurred in soft tissue, lymph node, and lung metastases. From our past experience, we would still recommend bilateral orchidectomy and/or bilateral adrenalectomy for patients with bone metastases as the predominant feature. Too few male patients have been treated with cytotoxic drugs to draw valid conclusions.

The survival for stage I carcinoma of the male breast in our series is 60% at 10 years, after excluding non-malignant intercurrent deaths. Comparison with female patients with carcinoma of the breast of the same age and stage treated in the same manner and within the same period shows a survival rate which does not differ significantly between the two groups. However, in our experience once the axillary nodes are involved or with larger primary tumours (stage II and stage III), the male patients tend to have a worse survival, 10% at 10 years compared with 30% for females of the same age and stage of disease.

11 Female Genital Tract

M. P. Cole and R. D. Hunter

This chapter is concerned with cancers of the cervix uteri, the corpus uteri, the ovary, vulva, and vagina. Radiotherapy has an important place in the management of patients with cancers of the genital tract but the radiotherapist must collaborate closely with surgical colleagues, both gynaecological and urological. Each must appreciate the merits and limitations of surgery and radiation therapy, whether used alone or in combination, with curative intent or in a supportive role.

Cancer of the Cervix Uteri

Of all types and sites of malignant disease affecting the uterus, cancer of the cervix uteri is by far the most common. Its excellent response to radiation therapy, under favourable circumstances, justifies the detailed discussion which follows.

Pathological and Clinical Features

Histology

Histologically, the vast majority of cancers of the cervix are epidermal carcinomas. Adenocarcinoma occurs in about 5% of our cases, and very rarely a sarcoma, usually fibrosarcoma, is seen. (The latter, being radioresistant, is a surgical problem.) The epidermal carcinomas display all degrees of differentiation from the well-differentiated squamous cancer to the undifferentiated anaplastic variety. Adenocarcinoma, since it is of course the characteristic cancer of the corpus uteri, should be accepted as a primary cervical tumour only if it clearly arises from the cervical glandular epithelium. If it appears to arise from the isthmus or lower part of the body of the uterus, spreading distally to involve the cervix, it should be classified and treated as a carcinoma of the corpus uteri.

Presentation

Clinically, cancer of the cervix may present as a fungating proliferative tumour, an ulcerative lesion, or an endocervical lesion. The fungating proliferative tumour is often very vascular, friable, and may expand and project into the vagina without any involvement of the fornices. The ulcerative lesion may entirely destroy the cervix and spread into the fornices. Endocervical cancer often presents as a barrel-shaped enlargement of the cervix without any apparent involvement of the cervical mucosa. Only on dilatation of the cervical canal does it become obvious that the tumour occupies the cervix. Sometimes there may be a breach of the cervical mucosa or, less commonly, of the lateral fornix. The most common presenting symptom of carcinoma of the cervix is bleeding, sometimes preceded by a vaginal discharge. Though the bleeding may be induced by intercourse, the essential characteristic of this vaginal bleeding is its irregularity and sometimes it may be prolonged. More rarely the patient may present without any significant vaginal bleeding but complaining of pain in the buttock radiating down the back of the thigh. Sometimes the initial complaint is of bladder or rectal symptoms and these all point to an advanced stage of the disease and a consequently grave prognosis.

Examination and Investigation

After examination of the abdomen, and inguinal and supraclavicular lymph node areas, bimanual vaginal examination is performed. This will determine the extent of involvement of the cervix, fornices, and vagina, and also enlargement or impairment of the mobility of the uterus. Speculum examination of the vagina complements the digital findings. For an accurate assessment of the parametria a rectal examination is more informative than a vaginal examination, particularly with regard to the extent of disease at the pelvic side-wall and in the uterosacral ligaments. In addition, rectal examination will disclose involvement of the rectal mucosa by tumour. After a general clinical examination of the patient and a routine chest film, the following investigations are indicated:

Biopsy

In some cases the diagnosis of invasive carcinoma will have been established by cone biopsy following an abnormal cytological smear. More usually the clinical diagnosis is only too obvious, but a simple punch biopsy will provide histological proof of malignant disease.

Full Blood Count

If anaemia is present it may need to be corrected by blood transfusion and this is recommended whenever the haemoglobin falls below 10/100 ml. A significant leucocytosis suggests the presence of infection, which may require appropriate treatment.

Biochemical Profile

This may well give early or confirmatory evidence of impaired renal function.

Cystoscopy

Though this examination may not be rewarding in the early stages of cervical cancer, in the later stages of the disease cystoscopy is advisable, especially when any urinary symptoms are present. When the disease is advanced, frank ulceration of the bladder mucosa may be seen, or bullous oedema without breach of the mucosa. Malignant involvement of the bladder mucosa may well alter the entire plan of subsequent treatment.

Intravenous Pyelogram

In the later stages of the disease this investigation may reveal pressure on the ureter with varying degrees of hydroureter, while in the more advanced cases pyelography may disclose a non-functioning kidney. The finding of a hydroureter does not in itself preclude radical treatment, since pressure on the ureter may be reduced as treatment progresses.

Lymphangiogram

Evidence of involved lymph nodes on lymphography may help to determine the volume of tissue to be irradiated. Unfortunately, the absence of obviously involved lymph nodes does not preclude the presence of microscopic deposits in lymph nodes. The value of this investigation in planning treatment remains debatable.

CT Scan

Though not yet universally available, this type of investigation does have the potential for demonstrating the extent of the local disease and possibly also the presence of enlarged lymph nodes. The value of this investigation in the overall management of the disease awaits assessment.

Clinical Staging

The clinical staging referred to in this chapter is that accepted by the International Congress in Obstetrics and Gynaecology. It is based on a clinical examination without reference to lymphangiogram or CT scan.

Stage 0 Carcinoma in situ—intra-epithelial carcinoma.
Stage 1 Carcinoma strictly confined to the cervix.

Stage 2 Carcinoma extends beyond the cervix but does not reach the pelvic wall. Carcinoma involves the vagina but not the lower third.

Stage 3 The carcinoma has reached the pelvic wall (on rectal examination there is no cancer-free space between the tumour and the pelvic wall). The carcinoma involves the lower third of the vagina. All cases with hydronephrosis or non-functioning kidney.

Stage 4 The carcinoma involves the mucosa of the bladder or rectum or has extended beyond the true pelvis. (Bullous oedema only of the bladder does not make the disease stage 4.) Involvement of groin nodes. Distant metastases.

Subdivisions of the stages can be found in the UICC publication (UICC 1978).

Treatment

There can no longer be any doubt that radiotherapy plays a major role in the management of patients with carcinoma of the uterine cervix. The results of radiotherapy are at least comparable to those of Wertheim hysterectomy performed by skilled gynaecologists. The advantage of radiotherapy is that, with few exceptions, it is available for all patients, whereas there is inevitably some selection of patients for surgical treatment, even for those with the earliest stages of the disease. Treatment must be planned according to the extent of the disease, since this determines the volume of tissue to be irradiated. To this end, the three basic considerations in treatment planning may be briefly stated as follows:

1) The special anatomical features of the cervix, the ease with which radium can be placed within the uterus and the vagina, and the high level of tolerance of the vagina, cervix, and uterus to radiation, combine to make this an ideal site for intracavitary therapy. Indeed, it is difficult to envisage any satisfactory alternative method of radiation treatment, even by sophisticated megavoltage therapy.
2) Because of the falling gradient of radiation dose outwards from the central radium source towards the pelvic wall, it is necessary to supplement the dose laterally in the more advanced cases by some form of external radiation.
3) Carcinoma of the cervix metastasises to the pelvic lymph nodes (hypogastric and external iliac, common iliac, and presacral lymph nodes) and frequently even to para-aortic lymph nodes. The potential lymph node drainage area presents a considerable volume of tissue and any attempt to irradiate this *en bloc* with the primary tumour is destined to fail because of the impossibility of delivering to that volume a tumour-lethal dose without producing serious radiation damage to the normal tissues.

Radium Treatment

Soon after its discovery in 1898, radium was used in the treatment of cancer of the cervix and its curative value was quickly established. During the past decade radium has been replaced at some centres by other sources of radiation, such as radioactive cobalt or caesium, but the basic principles of radium treatment described in this chapter are equally applicable to the use of cobalt or caesium, with appropriate modifications. Remote after-loading techniques will be discussed later in this chapter with special reference to our own use of caesium. Intracavitary treatment for cancer of the cervix requires an intrauterine tube and vaginal applicators containing radium (Fig. 11.1). In the planning of radium treatment two facts are of prime importance: the volume of tissue to be irradiated and the tolerance of the relevant tissues to irradiation. Cervical cancer predominantly extends laterally through the paracervical tissues into the parametria. It also spreads upwards into the uterus and downwards into the vagina, but it does not so commonly spread anteriorly to involve the bladder or posteriorly into the rectum. Consequently, the volume of tissue to be irradiated is not a sphere but a pear-shape, flattened anteroposteriorly. What is required therefore, is a dose distribution which is trefoil in shape, providing maximal dosage towards the parametria laterally, as well as the uterus and vagina, but with minimal irradiation towards the bladder and rectum. As with any form of intracavitary radium treatment, the radiation distribution cannot be homogeneous, but falls from the central source outwards. It is therefore necessary to have some

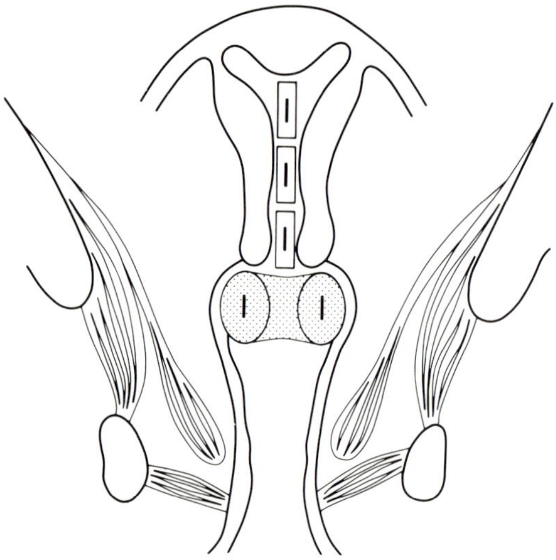

Fig. 11.1. Standard arrangement of Manchester uterine and vaginal applicators.

physically acceptable and clinically relevant point at which dosage can be expressed. In the case of cervix cancer this point is known as point *A*. It lies in the paracervical triangle and is defined as being 2 cm lateral to the central canal of the uterus and 2 cm proximal to the mucous membrane of the lateral fornix, in the axis of the uterus. A second dosage reference point, point *B*, is defined as being 3 cm lateral to point *A* and at the same level—5 cm from the midline (Fig. 11.2). The dose received at point *A* is in fact a measure of the dosage in the paracervical triangle. Experience has shown that while the cervix, uterus and vagina are remarkably tolerant to radiation, the tissues in the paracervical region are more vulnerable. Measurements of radium dosage at point *A* have been shown to correlate closely with the incidence of late normal-tissue damage in the pelvis, thus justifying the choice of this particular reference point for dosimetric purposes. The Manchester technique of radium treatment is designed to deliver a *pre-calculated* dose to point *A*, and the dose at each of the two points *A* will be equal when the uterus is in the normal central position, its axis midline, and the vaginal sources symmetrical. Any deviation from the normal position of the uterus, such as angulation to one side or the other, will inevitably produce unequal dosage at the two points *A*. However, detailed dose distributions have been calculated for a large consecutive series of patients, and in over 90% of cases the difference in dosage between the two points *A* was not greater than 10%. In short, by appropriate differential loading of radium in the intrauterine tubes and vaginal ovoids, an almost constant dose rate can be ensured at both points *A irrespective of the length of the intrauterine tube or the size of the vaginal ovoids*.

Intrauterine Tube (Fig. 11.3)

The cavity of the uterus varies in length and can accommodate one, two or three radium sources in line. The radium is enclosed in thin rubber tubes, the length of which is 2, 4, or 6 cm. Each

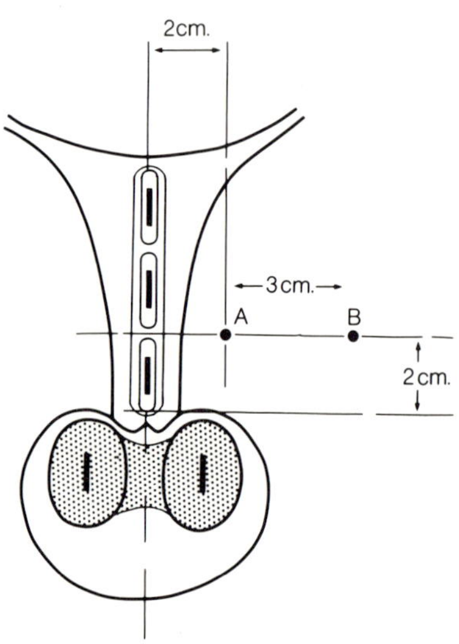

Fig. 11.2. Definition in ideal geometry of points *A* and *B*.

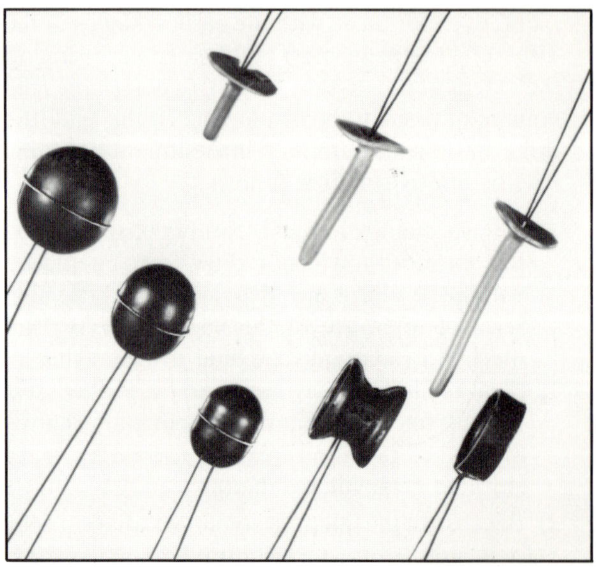

Fig. 11.3. Manchester uterine and vaginal radium applicators.

intrauterine tube has a flange at its distal end to ensure that the tube does not slip inside the uterus. The calibre of these intrauterine tubes is small in order to avoid excessive dilatation of the malignant cervix with the attendant risk of sepsis or possible dissemination of malignant cells.

Vaginal Ovoids (Fig. 11.3)

The vaginal applicators are made of rubber, ellipsoid in shape, and cored in their long axis to accommodate a radium tube of total length 2 cm and active length 1.3 cm. Three sizes of ovoids are available, the shortest diameters being 2 cm, 2.5 cm, and 3 cm for the small, medium, and large ovoids respectively. The ovoids are used in pairs and are held apart in the vagina either by a washer or a spacer. The washer produces a separation between the two ovoids of 0.1 cm, and the spacer a separation of 1.0 cm. The three sizes of ovoids were designed to fit the varying sizes of the vagina. The ovoids are placed in the lateral fornices at the level of the external os, as close as possible to the flange of the intrauterine tube. The largest acceptable size of paired ovoids is used in order to extend the tumour-lethal dosage in a lateral direction (Fig. 11.4). However, the mistake should not be made of using ovoids so large that they will not fit into the fornices, but lie in the vagina, leaving a gap between the ovoids and the flange of the intrauterine tube. This reduces the volume of adequately irradiated tissue. If it is impossible to place paired ovoids across the vault of the vagina, because of contraction of the vault or extension of tumour down the vaginal wall, the ovoids can be placed in tandem. Where the ovoids are placed in tandem the dose rate at point *A* for the standard ovoid loading is reduced by approximately 7.5%, and this may be compensated by a proportionate increase in the time of the radium treatment.

Differential Loading of Radium

Since the vaginal ovoids must vary in size for different patients, and the intrauterine tubes vary in length, the aim of ensuring a constant dose rate at point *A* can be achieved only by varying the amount of radium loaded into the different sizes of applicator. Moreover, while it might seem that the dose contribution to point *A* from the uterine tube should be similar to that for the ovoids, we have gradually come to regard a ratio of 1.8:1 from the uterine and vaginal sources as optimal.

To achieve a constant dose rate at point *A*, no matter what combination of intrauterine tubes and vaginal ovoids is used, and also to maintain the desirable ratio between the intrauterine and vaginal contributions, the relative loading—in terms of radiation "units"—is shown in Table 11.1. The precise amount of radium (or, of course, any appropriate radium substitute) which constitutes a "unit" must depend on the dose rate which suits the planned course of treatment. The radium "unit" which best suits our purpose is 2.5 mg (1-mm Pt filter). Expressed in total quantities of radium, the necessary radium loadings are shown in Table 11.2 along with the dose rates at point *A* in centigrays per hour.

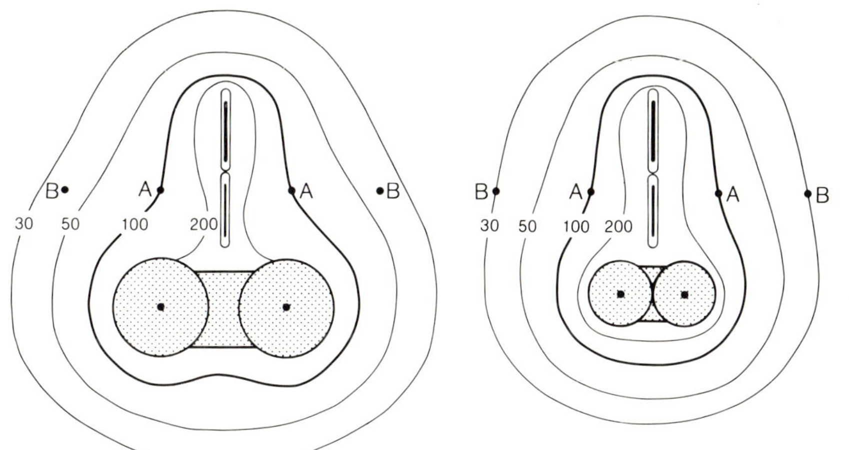

Fig. 11.4. A comparison of the different dose distributions achieved using standard applicators with (left) large ovoids and a spacer and (right) small ovoids and a washer. The dose rate at point *A* is unchanged.

Table 11.1 Differential loading of radium in tubes and ovoids in terms of units.

Intrauterine tube, counting from fundus to external os	Long	6 units, 4 units, 4 units
	Medium	6 units, 4 units
	Short	8 units (non-standard treatment)
Vaginal ovoids	Large	9 units
	Medium	8 units
	Small	7 units

Table 11.2. Radium content of intrauterine tubes and ovoids and dose rate at point A.

Intrauterine tube	Loaded	Dose rate (cGy/h)	
Long	15+10+10 mg	34.3	
Medium	15+10 mg	34.1	
Short	20 mg	27.3	
		Dose rate (cGy/h)	
Vaginal ovoids	Loaded	with spacer	with washer
Large	22.5 mg	18.3	18.9
Medium	20.0 mg	18.8	19.0
Small	17.5 mg	18.9	19.0

While differential loading of the large, medium, and small ovoids can ensure a near-constant dose rate at point *A*, this objective can only be achieved with the long and medium intrauterine tubes. The short intrauterine tube is rarely used in practice (for stump cancers or where the cervical canal cannot be found) and its 13% loss of radiation dosage is usually unavoidable.

Analysis of large numbers of our patients, over a period of four decades, has confirmed that using the Manchester radium technique the optimum dose level at point *A* is 7500–8000 cGy in 10 days. With a dose rate of 53.3 cGy/h, the optimum dose of 7500 cGy in 10 days can be achieved by two radium insertions of about 70 h each, with an interval of 4 days between the applications.

The cervix and vagina are relatively tolerant to radiation, unlike the normal tissues in the paracervical region. Whilst the latter, during a normal 10-day course of radium treatment, will receive the level of dosage as described at point *A* (7500 cGy), the dose on the wall of the uterus is estimated to be over 30 000 cGy. The dose on the vaginal vault will also be between 20 000 and 25 000 cGy. The rectum and bladder are much less tolerant to radiation and every effort is made to keep the dose delivered to these organs to less than that measured at point *A*.

Clinical Application of the Manchester Radium Technique

It is our standard practice to insert the radium with the anaesthetised patient in the knee-chest position (Fig. 11.5). The knee-chest position affords an excellent view of the cervix using a Sims' speculum and it is not necessary (and often impossible) to apply a volcellum forceps to the cervix. The cervical canal is found by gentle probing and is dilated only sufficiently to admit the slender intrauterine tube. The length of the canal is determined and the appropriate intrauterine tube selected and inserted. The diameter of the vault of the vagina is assessed and a pair of ovoids selected which will fit best into the fornices, being held apart transversely by a washer or spacer. The ovoids are then packed carefully in position, using moist gauze packing (with a radio-opaque strand throughout its length). Particular care is taken in packing the posterior fornix to increase the distance between the radium and the rectum. The packing is continued along the length of the vagina to a point just within the introitus. Before the radium insertion it is advantageous to insert into the bladder a selfretaining catheter which will remain in position throughout the radium treat-

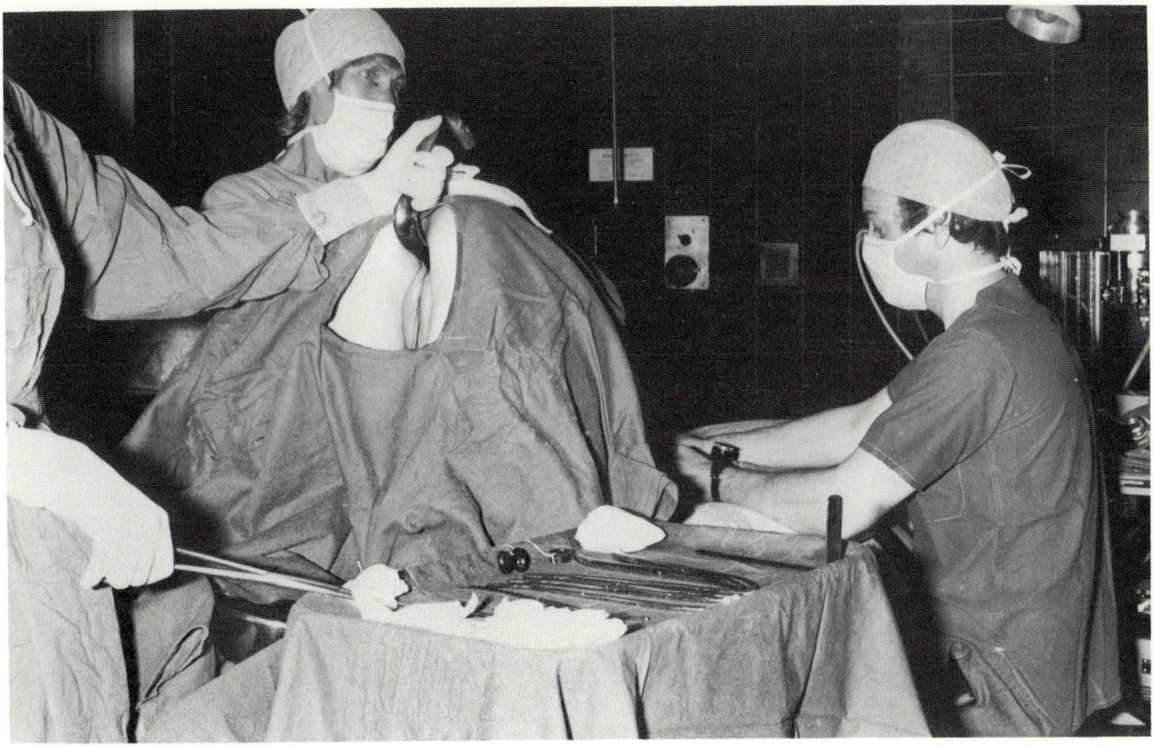

Fig. 11.5. Knee-chest position.

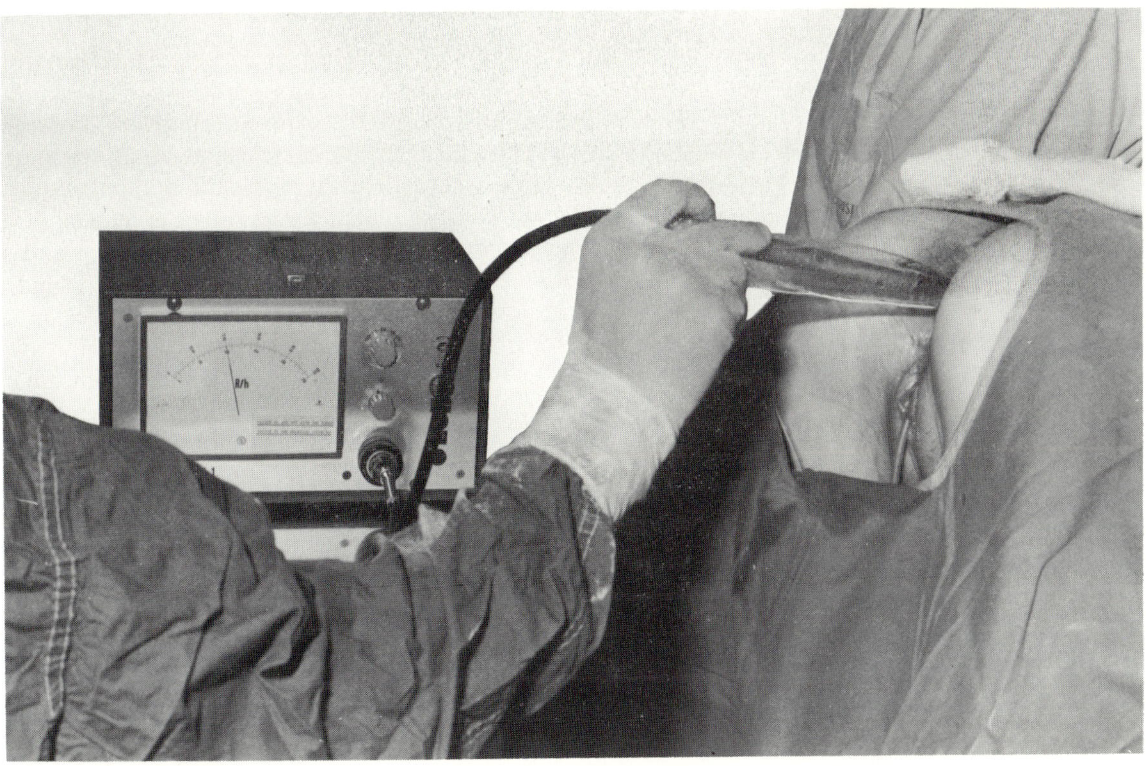

Fig. 11.6. Measurement of rectal dose.

ment. If a catheter is not inserted some patients who have difficulty in micturition may require a catheter to be passed in the ward, thus exposing nursing staff to unnecessary radiation. Before the patient leaves the knee-chest position a rectal probe carrying a scintillation counter can be inserted into the rectum to measure the dose rate on the rectal mucosa (Fig. 11.6). If this measurement is high, the vaginal packing should be removed and reintroduced until an acceptable reading is obtained. The total dose on the rectal mucosa from the two radium applications should not exceed 6250 cGy. Before the patient returns to the ward, anteroposterior and lateral radiographs should be taken as a check on the disposition of the radium applicators (Fig. 11.7). Placing a patient in the knee-chest position, as with any clinical manoeuvre, has advantages and disadvantages in practice and it is worth enumerating these here.

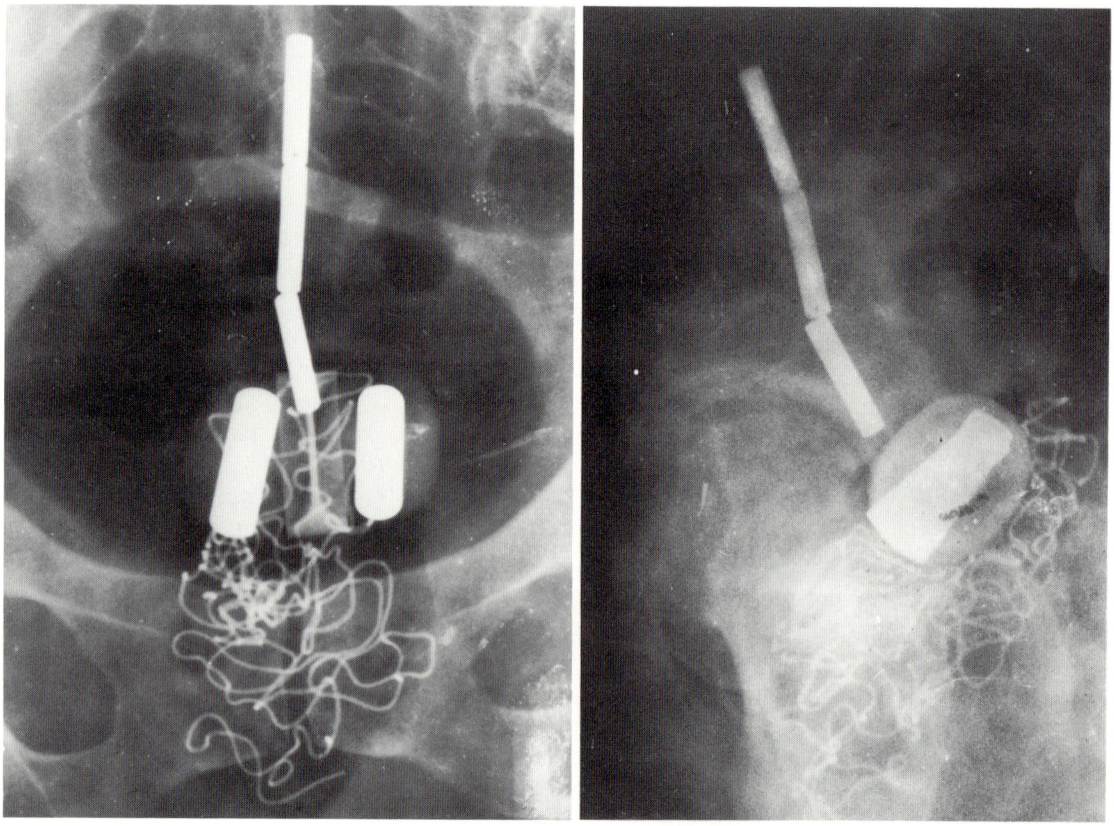

Fig. 11.7. AP and lateral radiographs of a standard radium insertion with good packing behind ovoids.

Advantages

1) Using only a Sims' speculum an excellent view is obtained of the cervix.
2) Once the intrauterine tube has been inserted into the cervical canal its own weight tends to keep it firmly in position.
3) If the uterus is mobile it will fall naturally into the anteverted position and firm packing of the vagina will not displace the uterus. This fact probably explains why the dose at the two points *A* rarely differs by more than 10%.
4) If the uterus should inadvertently be perforated while attempting to dilate the cervical canal the negative intra-abdominal pressure created by the knee-chest position results in an audible hiss of air passing into the abdomen. Treating in the lithotomy position gives no such clear sign of a perforation to the operator.
5) The posterior fornix can be easily packed to decrease the dose received by the rectal mucosa.

Disadvantages

1) In the knee-chest position it is not possible to carry out a bimanual examination to confirm, under anaesthesia, the stage of the disease as previously assessed in the conscious patient.
2) A full cystoscopic examination of the bladder cannot be carried out. Where such an examination is essential it should be done in the lithotomy position and the radium could be inserted at the same time.
3) It may not be possible to place a grossly obese patient in the knee-chest position, nor a patient with severe arthritis of the hip and/or knee joints.

In spite of all these considerations we have no doubt that under normal circumstances the advantages of the knee-chest position more than compensate for its disadvantages.

After-loading (R. D. Hunter)

With the introduction of artificial radionuclides it became obvious that radium was far from the ideal material for intracavitary therapy. The ideal radionuclide should produce only a single gamma ray spectrum with an energy of around 0.5 MV. Below this level attenuation, rather than the inverse square law, dictates tissue absorption and consequently influences dose distribution. At energies above 0.5 MV radiation protection becomes increasingly difficult and expensive. The nuclide should have a long half-life, be cheap and easily produced, preferably solid and with stable solid decay products. In particular it should have a high specific activity. The closest to the ideal for low-dose-rate intracavitary therapy at the present time is radioactive caesium (caesium-137) which, in spite of a relatively limited specific activity, allows treatment times approximating those used in the standard radium systems. Caesium-137 is a cheap by-product of nuclear fission. It is solid and its decay products are stable, its gamma emission is satisfactory at 0.6 MV and its half-life of 30.5 years is acceptable. Radioactive cobalt (cobalt-60) is the principal competitor of caesium-137 in remote after-loading systems. Though it is also solid and relatively cheap, its half-life of only 5.3 years requires more frequent replacement of decaying sources. The gamma emissions of cobalt-60 at 1.17 and 1.33 MV exceed those of caesium. In remote after-loading it is the high specific activity of cobalt-60 that determines its special role as a source of high-dose-rate gamma radiation.

The preloaded radium applicators described above give rise to significant levels of radiation exposure to the radiotherapists, to the radium technicians who prepare the applicators and maintain the radium sources, and not least to the nursing staff in the theatre and wards. The penetrating gamma radiation from radium is such that protective shielding in theatre is at best ineffective. This leads the radiotherapist to introduce the intrauterine tube and vaginal ovoids as swiftly as possible. Occasionally the resulting geometric relationship of these applicators may be so disturbed that there is no alternative to removing them and reintroducing them on another day. Sometimes the geometry of the applicators is less than perfect, but the radiotherapist may nevertheless decide to accept this rather than repeat the entire procedure at a later date. This requires experienced judgment—and the radiotherapist is sometimes in error.

These considerations gave rise to the concept of after-loading, where empty applicators are introduced, without the need for undue haste. After-loading applicators can be made from various plastic materials and metallic alloys. Whatever

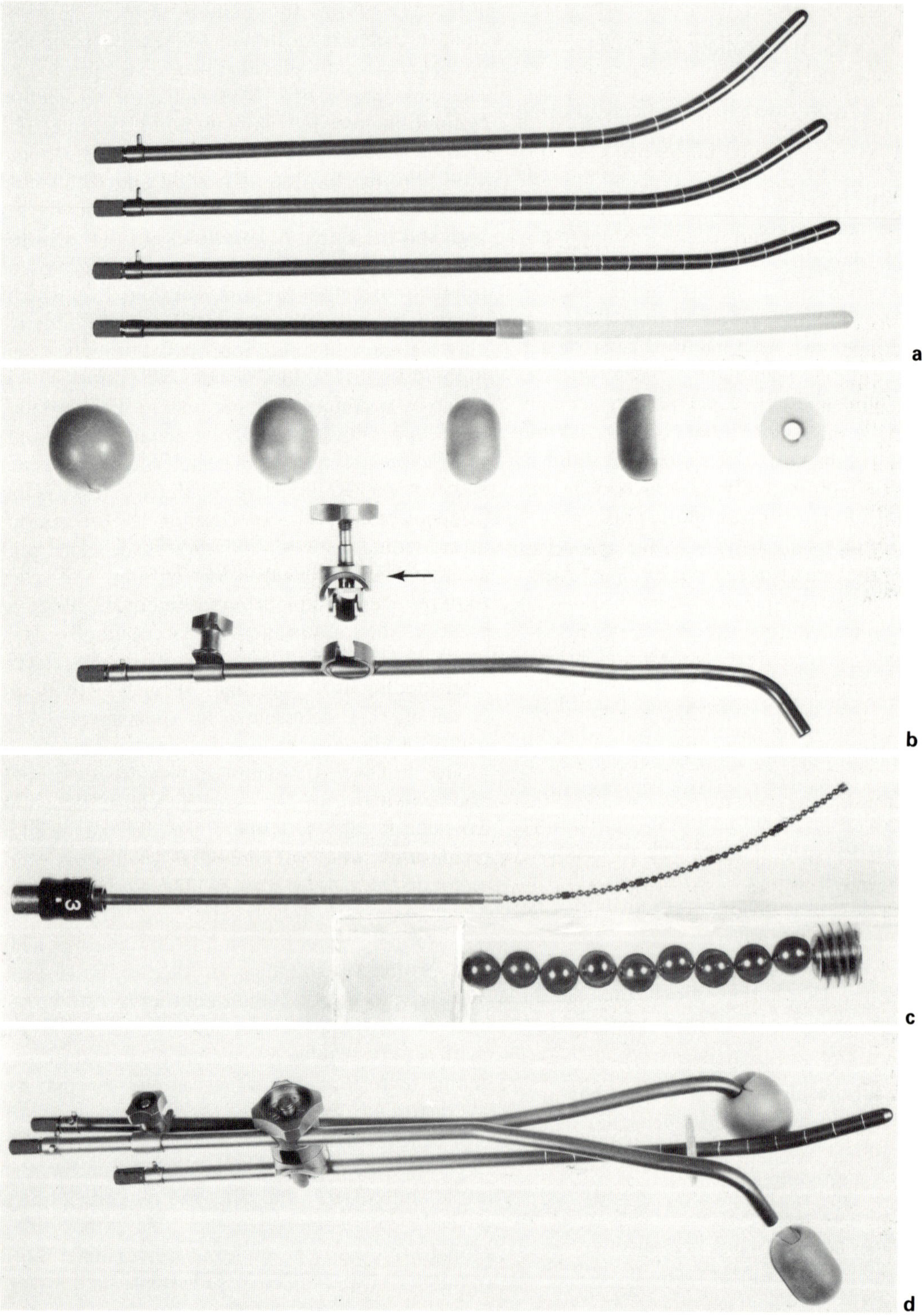

Fig. 11.8. Remote afterloading applicators. **a** Uterine applicators of different angles, graduated in centimetres. **b** Four standard ovoid sizes—large, medium, small and half—shown above a vaginal applicator. The clamp (arrowed) holds the three standard tubes together. **c** Manual insert for checking the position of individual sources after insertion of applicators. Enlargement of the tip shows line of pellets used to simulate active source. **d** The arrangement of applicators during treatment.

material is used for these small-calibre tubes they must be lightweight for the comfort of the patient and capable of easy sterilisation. They should not be adversely affected by exposure to gamma radiation and there should be minimal attenuation of gamma rays by the walls of the applicators. Only when the geometric relationship of these applicators is known to be ideal are the radioactive sources inserted into the applicators. Many after-loading techniques have been devised and in general they are described either as *manual* after-loading or *remote* after-loading. As the term suggests, manual after-loading involves the introduction of suitable applicators followed, after verifying the geometry, by the manual insertion of the radioactive material. Clearly, manual after-loading is advantageous to the *patient*—and to those working in theatre—but it does very little to reduce the radiation exposure of the nursing staff. This problem can only be overcome by remote after-loading, where after the dummy applicators have been placed in position, the radioactive sources are remotely introduced from a protective safe. Manufacturers have not been slow to devise a variety of sophisticated remote after-loading machines, each offering the radiotherapist a range of dosimetric options and in-built safety mechanisms. Not surprisingly, these machines have become increasingly expensive. As a result of this capital expense and the availability of a wide variety of artificial radionuclides, two general approaches to remote after-loading have developed during the past decade. The essential differences lie in the dose rates at which the equipment operates and the associated scheme of patient management. In high-dose-rate systems the applicators are introduced, usually under general anaesthetic, and then connected to the equipment while in the special treatment room. The selected sources are inserted by remote control from outside the room, and by using very high energy sources treatment can be accomplished in a few minutes. On completion of treatment the sources are retracted and the empty applicators are removed before the patient is returned to the ward. Experience with this high-dose-rate approach has shown that optimum results are only achieved by increasing the number of intracavitary treatments by a factor of three or four when compared with optimum radium fractionation.

This necessity to change dose, dose rate, and fractionation made the Christie Hospital reluctant to move so radically from a very successful low-dose-rate radium technique. A low-dose-rate remote after-loading system has been preferred, whose source strength and geometry allow radium-like fractionation and dose distributions to be maintained.

In this system the applicator (Fig. 11.8) is inserted under general anaesthesia in theatre and the conscious patient is then transferred to a shielded treatment room. The empty applicators are attached to the after-loading machine. Sources can be transferred by remote control from outside the room by the trained nursing staff.

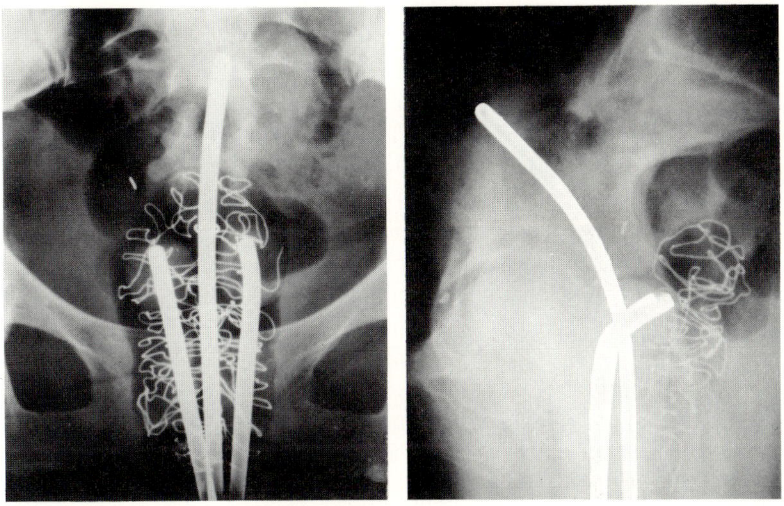

Fig. 11.9. AP and lateral radiographs of a patient with afterloading applicators in the correct position. A dead gold seed has been inserted in the right posterior lip of the cervix to act as a tissue marker.

Technique

In the theatre the patient is placed in the knee-chest position, as described previously for intracavitary radium therapy. The central canal is found and dilated gently to permit the introduction of an intrauterine tube which will carry a line source of caesium-137. Uterine cavity lengths of 2–8 cm can be accommodated (in 1.0-cm intervals) and the tubes also provide for a variety of angulations (Fig. 11.8a). During the procedure an inert gold seed marker is inserted into the cervix. A flange is placed on the uterine tube at the level of the cervix. This allows the position of the tube relative to the cervix to be checked radiographically at any time during the subsequent treatment (Fig. 11.9). Standard-sized Manchester ovoids are used for the vaginal sources and are placed in the lateral fornices at the level of the flange. The relative positions of the uterine and vaginal applicators are controlled by a clamp which is attached to the three applicator tubes outside the introitus (Fig. 11.8b). Gauze packing, as with radium therapy, is placed firmly and carefully behind the ovoids and around the applicator tubes down to the level of the introitus. In the normal patient this is all that is required to ensure that the applicators remain in position, and we regard corsets or other external restraining devices as an unnecessary burden for the patient. Needless to say, these after-loading applicators can also be introduced with the patient in the lithotomy position, but the knee-chest position is preferred unless contraindicated. Before the patient leaves the theatre, anteroposterior and lateral radiographs are taken (as with radium) to check the relationship of the applicators to one another and to the gold seed marker in the cervix, and the adequacy of the gauze packing (Fig. 11.9).

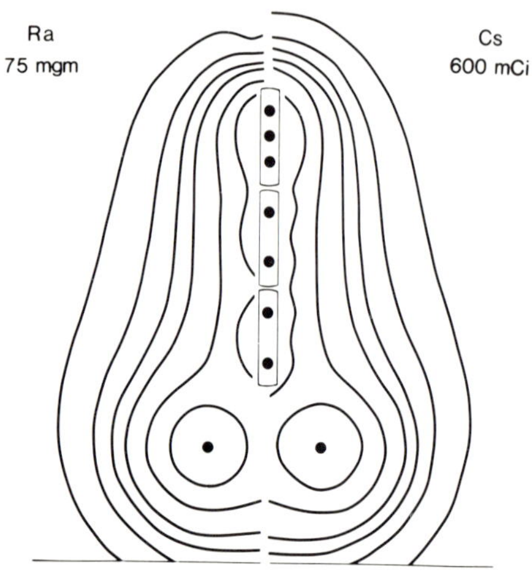

Fig. 11.10. A comparison of the calculated isodose distribution in a coronal plane from (left) ideal radium insertion utilising a long central tube and medium ovoids and (right) remote afterloaded caesium pellet loading pattern.

At the end of the procedure a direct assessment is made of the dose on the anterior rectal wall. Inserts mounted with caesium-137 pellets, in a distribution giving a rectal dose rate one quarter of that which will be achieved in the full treatment, are placed in the applicators. A rectal probe of sufficient sensitivity is then inserted in the rectum, as with radium, and an assessment of the dose rate at different parts in the rectum is made. This is not allowed to exceed two-thirds of the dose rate at point *A*.

In the treatment room the patient recovers fully from the anaesthetic before linking the intracavitary applicator tubes to the caesium-137 line sources in the protective safe. Our present remote after-loading system utilises caesium-137 as glass spheres incorporated in stainless steel spheres of 2.5 mm diameter. The maximum source strength is 40 mCi (1500 MBq). The treatment sources are constructed from a mixture of active and dummy spheres arranged in a line (Fig. 11.8c), and there is no difficulty in producing applicator loading patterns that will reproduce all standard Manchester dose distributions (e.g. Fig. 11.10). The source pattern construction takes place within the protected machine and the selected individual treatment "lines" are transferred to the intrauterine and vaginal applicator tubes by compressed air.

The safety and reliability of this two-way transfer of sources are of vital importance, and in practice angulations of even 90° can be negotiated satisfactorily. The patient is nursed on her back or side while attached to the equipment and movement is permitted under supervision. It is important to prevent traction on the air lines, since this could risk displacement. A marker system which identifies the position of the applicators relative to the patient's thigh is of considerable advantage to the nursing staff and is an added safeguard (Fig. 11.11).

During treatment, which may take 24 h, the control of the equipment is supervised by trained nursing staff. The system allows regular treatment interruption for nursing care, meals, etc., and there is total control of the position of the

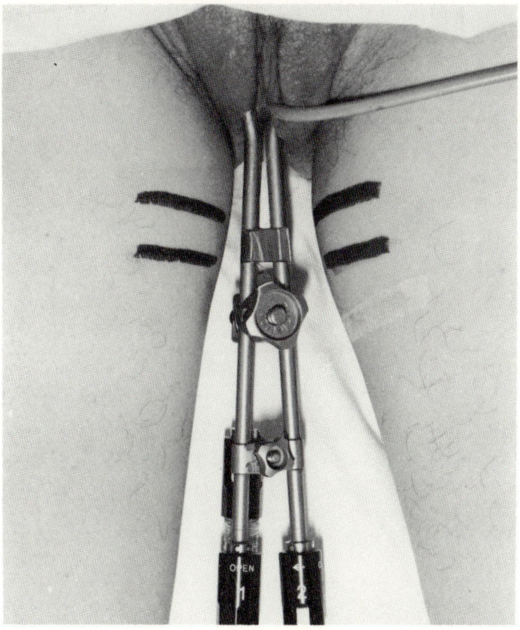

Fig. 11.11. Afterloading applicators emerging from the vagina. Their position relative to the thighs has been marked by drawing "tram lines" on the thighs and placing an adherent conspicuous tape around the applicators.

radioactive material from outside the room. A continuous record of interruptions and incidents is kept by the machine which ensures also that the patient has the correct treatment time before terminating treatment.

Dosage using this system, as with radium, is expressed at point *A*. The only significant difference between the low-dose-rate remote after-loading system presently in use and classical radium treatment is that the dose rate has been increased by a factor of 3.5. The implication of this dose rate increase is the subject of formal ongoing clinical trials.

Present clinical experience has shown that, whilst maintaining existing X-ray techniques and dosage, as well as the established intracavitary dose distribution and overall fractionation pattern, preloaded radium insertions can be safely replaced by remote after-loading caesium-137. This eliminates all the hazards of preloaded radium. If radium dose rates are also maintained, then treatment times and absolute doses would not, of course, need to be adjusted. The influence of dose rate on intracavitary dosage must ultimately await the outcome of prospective and randomised clinical trials with both low and high dose-rate techniques.

Experience with after-loading at dose rates three to four times those used in the Manchester radium system has confirmed the practical advantages of shorter treatment times, but a reduction in absolute dose must be made to allow for the increased biological effects of the higher-dose-rate treatment. Correction factors are still being investigated in ongoing clinical studies, but for the technique described above they appear to lie in the range 10%–20%.

X-ray Therapy

The isodose curves round the radium sources (Fig. 11.4) show a falling dose rate from the midline outwards towards the pelvic side wall. The central zone of the pelvis is adequately irradiated, but malignant disease in the outer two-thirds of the parametria almost certainly receives less than a tumour-lethal dose from the radium alone. X-ray treatment is therefore designed to extend the zone of effective irradiation to the lateral pelvic wall. This may be achieved by using either kilovoltage or megavoltage X-rays.

Parametrial X-ray Therapy

Kilovoltage This is essentially a beam-directed technique designed to give a supplementary dose of irradiation to the parametria. The X-ray dose is calculated at point *B* (Fig. 11.2) in the mid-pelvis. Anterior and posterior fields 12×10 cm are used with a 10×4 cm lead strip in the centre of the field in order to reduce the dose of radiation to the

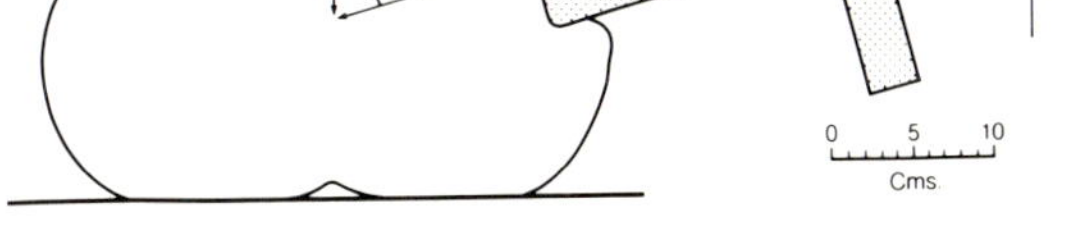

Fig. 11.12. Pin and arc technique used to set up kilovoltage parametrial treatment.

cervix. In addition, anterior oblique and posterior oblique fields are accurately directed towards point *B* using the pin and arc method of beam-direction (Fig. 11.12). This means that each point *B* is irradiated by four 10×4 cm beams of X-rays. The dose distribution achieved by this technique is shown in Fig. 11.13. Because of scattered radiation, some 50% of the dosage received at point *B* from this technique is also received at point *A* and for this reason the radium contribution to point *A* must be reduced to take account of the X-ray contribution at that site.

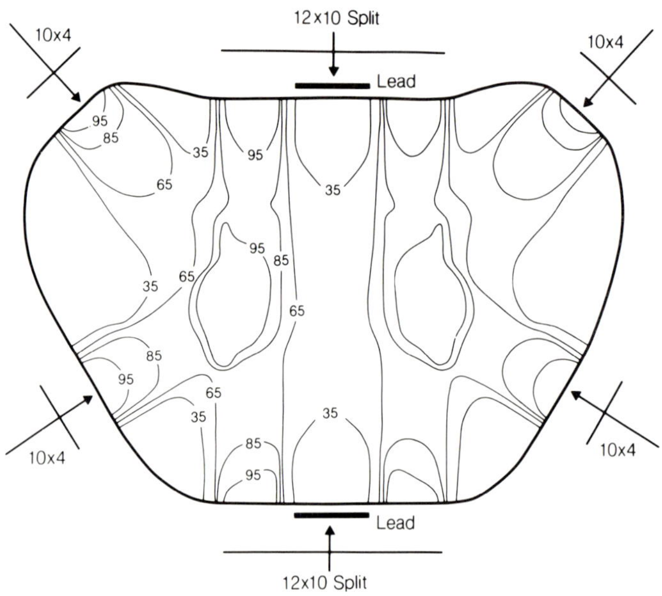

Fig. 11.13. Typical parametrial kV dose distribution.

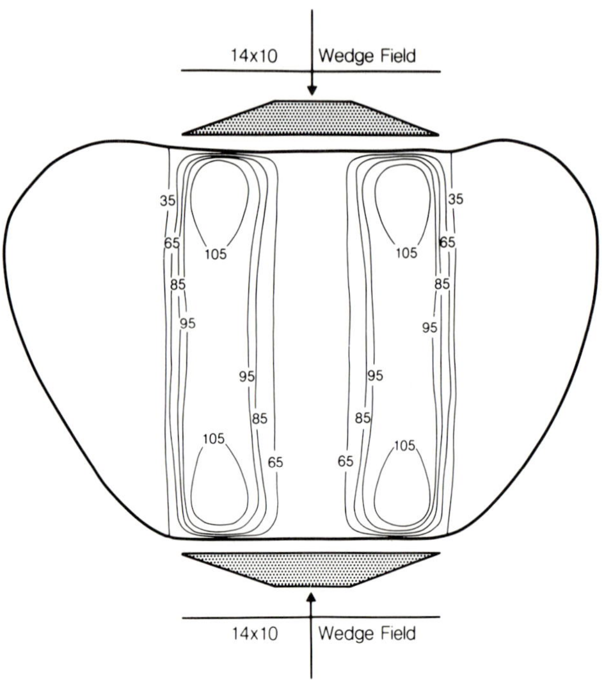

Fig. 11.14. Typical parametrial MV dose distribution using a special wedge filter.

Megavoltage With megavoltage X-rays it is possible to irradiate the parametria in a similar way but by a simpler method. By using an appropriate wedge filter incorporated in the head of the megavoltage machine and using anterior and posterior 14×10 cm fields, it is possible to create a dose distribution across the pelvis which gives 50% of the dose at point *A*, rising to 100% at point *B* (Fig. 11.14). For patients with stage 3 cancers of the cervix this megavoltage technique, combined with intracavitary radium, has given cure rates similar to those obtained with the kilovoltage technique and radium. In this context, therefore, megavoltage has not proved superior to kilovoltage therapy.

Hexagonal Technique It is often postulated that it is the failure to cure cancer in lymph nodes which is the main problem in treating cancer of the uterine cervix. Realising that the two previous methods of treatment were irradiating a length of only 10 cm in the pelvis and that this would include only a limited lymph node area (probably the obturator and a few hypogastric nodes) a further technique of X-ray treatment was designed. This method is planned to treat the whole pelvis and its lymph node drainage from the lowest extent of disease in the vagina to the level of the top of the fifth lumbar vertebra. It is a four-field technique, the shape of the anterior and posterior fields being hexagonal. The hexagonal shape is designed to cover the suspect volume but also to reduce where possible the total volume of tissue irradiated. The greatest width of the field is 19 cm, while the length ranges from 15 to 19 cm. The lateral fields are 10 to 11 cm wide and of the same length as the anterior and posterior fields (Fig. 11.15). For this treatment we have used the 8-MV linear accelerator. The centre of the pelvis is not shielded during this treatment and consequently the radium contribution must be significantly reduced. In spite of the careful thought given to the design of this technique it has not proved to be superior, in terms of survival rates of treated patients, to either of the two previously described X-ray techniques.

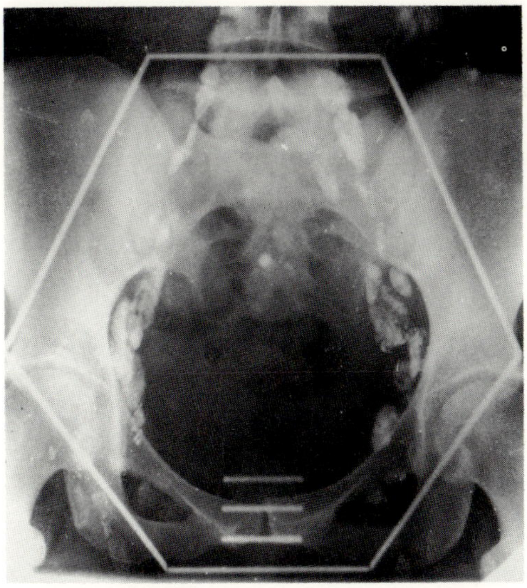

Fig. 11.15. Hexagonal technique anterior portal shown in a patient who has had a lower limb lymphangiogram.

Treatment Policy

Though the value of intracavitary radium therapy for cancer of the cervix is beyond doubt, the place of supplementary X-ray therapy has been debated widely. A randomised clinical trial was established at the Christie Hospital in Manchester from 1957 to 1964, designed to compare the results from radium alone with those from radium and supplementary X-ray therapy. This study was directed to the treatment of stage 1 and early stage 2 cases. Statistical analysis of the results of this clinical trial disclosed no significant difference between the two contrasted regimes. It remains, therefore, our considered opinion that it is sufficient to treat patients with stage 1 and early stage 2 cancers of the cervix with radium only. Patients with stage 2 cancers associated with more extensive invasion of the parametria, and all stage 3 patients, are treated by a combination of radium and supplementary X-ray therapy as described above. Our present policy of treatment, stage by stage, is briefly as follows:–

Stage 1 and 2a
Radium alone—7500 cGy at point *A* in two insertions in 10 days

Stage 2b and 3
Parametrial X-ray therapy and radium
(a) 3000 cGy at point *B* in 3 weeks (15 treatments), using 300 kV and pin and arc method
or (b) 3250 cGy at point *B* in 3 weeks (16 treatments) using 4-MV X-rays and wedge filter

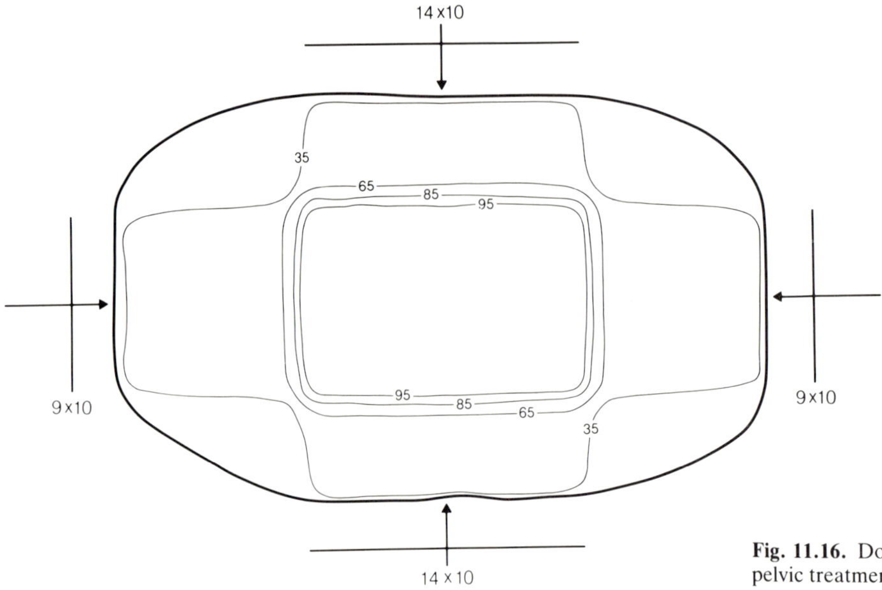

Fig. 11.16. Dose distribution from four field pelvic treatment.

In either case followed by radium, 6000 cGy at point *A* in two insertions in 10 days

Alternative for stage 3

Hexagonal four-field technique delivering 4000 cGy in 4 weeks (20 treatments) using 8-MV rays, followed by a single insertion delivering 3750 cGy at point *A*

Stage 4

Patients with stage 4 cancer of the cervix may present in a hopelessly advanced state with a rectovaginal or vesico-vaginal fistula. Any attempt at radiation treatment may only increase the size of the fistula and make the patient's condition more miserable. Even after palliative colostomy or diversion of the urinary tract it is often debatable whether radiotherapy should be considered at all.

One manifestation which deserves special mention is when a patient with a stage 4 cancer presents with anuria as a result of involvement of the ureters. Such a patient has a very poor prognosis and, especially in the elderly, it is often kindest to avoid treatment. Fortunately, death from uraemia is mercifully rapid. In young patients treatment must initially be directed to correcting the anuric state. This is best achieved by dialysis and as soon as possible thereafter the external irradiation is begun. If necessary dialysis may be repeated during the course of radiotherapy, preferably at the weekend. The object of treatment initially is to relieve the pressure on the ureters so that an adequate urinary output is established. If this is not achieved by the end of the course of X-ray therapy further intervention is unrewarding. Nephrostomy or ureterostomy is best avoided as it adds an unnecessary burden to a patient in an irretrievable situation. Some patients with a stage 4 cancer of the cervix, who are in good general condition, may derive reasonable palliation and even an occasional cure by radiation therapy—provided the disease is limited to the pelvis. Treatment in such cases is given to the whole pelvis using megavoltage therapy. This consists of two parallel opposed pairs of fields: (1) anteroposterior 14×10 cm and (2) lateral 9×10 cm or 10×10 cm. These deliver a combined mid-pelvis dose of 4750 cGy in 3 weeks (16 treatments). The dose distribution from this technique is shown in Fig. 11.16. The treatment is usually well tolerated, with only minor bowel upset, and there is usually sufficient tolerance for a short radium treatment at the completion of the X-ray therapy. Using an intrauterine tube and vaginal ovoids, 2500 cGy can be safely delivered to point *A* in 48 h. Unfortunately, in spite of the available tolerance for further radiation therapy, the vagina may be so contracted and the pelvic organs so distorted by tumour that a satisfactory intracavitary treatment may not be technically possible.

Complications During and Immediately Following Treatment

Haemorrhage

The predominant presenting sign of carcinoma of the cervix is vaginal bleeding. This may be continuous or intermittent with small or quite heavy losses. The resulting anaemia must be corrected, aiming to keep the level of the haemoglobin at not less than 10 g/100 ml. As treatment progresses, bleeding usually ceases, but if it is heavy it may be wise to interrupt the course of X-ray treatment and to proceed with the radium treatment, since this will more rapidly induce haemostasis. The X-ray treatment can be completed later.

Sepsis

Most cancers of the cervix are secondarily infected, but it is rare to have any serious pelvic infection such as a tubo-ovarian abscess—though such complications must be kept in mind. Pyometra may be encountered, especially on opening up the cervical canal of a patient with an endocervical cancer. If much fresh pus is evacuated it will be wise to postpone introducing radium for about a week. If pyrexia and signs of pelvic infection arise while the radium is in situ it is advisable to remove the radium, administer antibiotics, and only continue the radium treatment when all signs of the infection have subsided.

Perforation of the Uterus

Because tumour may occlude the external cervical os or penetrate the whole thickness of the uterus, the risk of perforation of the uterus is real when attempting to dilate the canal for insertion of the intrauterine tube. This is especially true when the vaginal cervix has been eroded and replaced by an infiltrating carcinoma. One of the advantages of the knee-chest position is that when perforation occurs air can be heard passing into the peritoneal cavity with an unmistakable hiss. In the lithotomy position this confirmatory hiss does not occur. Under these circumstances no intrauterine tube should be inserted into the uterus on that occasion but vaginal ovoids may safely be placed in position. A course of antibiotics is given and only rarely does a pelvic infection ensue from the perforation. On a subsequent occasion gentle probing will reveal the true canal and an intrauterine tube can be inserted. If it is not possible to complete the full radium treatment, alternative X-ray therapy or ablative surgery may have to be considered.

Proctitis

The rectal mucosa is not very tolerant to radiation but with careful packing of the vagina, to increase the distance between the radium and the anterior rectal wall, the dose to the rectum can be minimised. In addition, the use of a rectal probe carrying a scintillation counter is an added safeguard to assess the rectal dose before the patient leaves the operating theatre. If proctitis should develop—perhaps because of radium in a retroverted uterus, or a narrow vagina not permitting very satisfactory packing—it usually responds rapidly to retention enemas of prednisolone. In addition, mild aperients are prescribed to ensure the passage of a soft stool.

Small Bowel Symptoms

Small bowel symptoms—usually diarrhoea—are not often found with radium treatment alone, but can occur when the whole pelvis is irradiated by X-rays. They often subside with a temporary cessation of radiation and prescription of tincture of opium 5–15 ml, or a bowel sedative. Any excessive loss of fluid must be corrected by intravenous replacement. More serious symptoms can develop when a loop of bowel, bound down by adhesions in the pelvis, is irradiated and symptoms of subacute obstruction may develop. X-ray treatment has to be discontinued and it may not be possible to begin again. Though the subacute obstruction may well resolve with conservative management, surgical intervention for the cervical cancer may have to be considered.

Cystitis

Mild cystitis may develop at the completion of the radium treatment as a result of the indwelling catheter. It is wise to have specimens of urine examined at frequent intervals for bacterial growth and to prescribe an appropriate antibiotic. In addition, there will be some degree of radiation-induced cystitis producing some dysuria, but this subsides as a rule in about a week after treatment.

Menopause

All patients who are premenopausal at the time of treatment will have an induced early menopause because of the dose of radiation received by the ovaries. This should, of course, be fully explained to the patient before treatment. There is no contraindication to these patients subsequently having replacement hormone therapy for menopausal symptoms. Because of the risk of some contraction and adhesion of the vagina due to radiation it is advisable to instruct patients in the use of a plastic vaginal dilator for the first month or two until healing has taken place. If the patient later should develop dyspareunia, an oestrogen cream applied to the vagina may relieve symptoms.

Late Complications

Rectal Complications

Two kinds of rectal complications must be distinguished—(1) an intrinsic reaction and (2) an extrinsic reaction. An *intrinsic reaction* occurs at any time from 6 months to 6 years after treatment. It arises from localised high dosage received by the anterior rectal wall, probably because of unsatisfactory packing around the vaginal ovoids in the posterior fornix, or because of a fixed retroverted uterus. An intrinsic reaction produces an area of local ulceration on the anterior rectal wall with indurated edges and a central depressed area. Clinically this so resembles an adenocarcinoma that it has been called a "pseudo-carcinoma" of the rectum. The patient complains of pain on defecation, tenesmus, and bleeding. Healing takes place slowly but is helped by retention enemas of prednisolone and by mild aperients. In such cases there is clearly a risk of a rectovaginal fistula. Fortunately, this type of reaction is rarely seen today provided (1) careful packing of the posterior fornix increases the distance of the vaginal radium from the anterior rectal wall, (2) check radiographs of the radioactive sources in the uterus and vagina are taken at each insertion, and (3) rectal readings of the dose received at the anterior rectal wall are monitored and the radium repacked in position when the dose received on the mucosa is not below an accepted maximum level.

An *extrinsic reaction* is a late manifestation of an excessive dose of radiation to the pelvis. It is rarely seen today, since the levels of tissue tolerance within the pelvis have become firmly established. When it does occur, however, an extrinsic reaction is characterised by widespread induration and fibrosis of the parametrial tissues and is described as the "frozen pelvis". The excessive radiation produces widespread endarteritis obliterans of smaller vessels and thrombosis of some larger vessels. The consequent fibrosis may also lead to an annular stricture of the rectum. The patient complains of pain and difficulty in defecation, and colostomy may be required for the relief of rectal symptoms. The pelvic fibrosis may rarely cause progressive ureteric obstruction with the risk of renal failure.

Small Bowel Complications

Previous surgery may result in a loop of bowel being fixed in the pelvis by adhesions. Such a static loop of small bowel is especially vulnerable to high-dose irradiation and it may become fibrotic and stenosed and ultimately lead to intestinal obstruction requiring surgical intervention. Another possible feature of small bowel irradiation is the development of a malabsorption syndrome following high-dose radiation. The patient develops steatorrhoea and also a megaloblastic anaemia because of reduced vitamin B12 absorption from the damaged ileum. This is a rare complication, but it is a reminder that any deterioration of a patient's condition should not be too readily attributed to the malignant disease.

Bladder Complications

A variety of radiation changes can occur in the bladder and once again it is important not to attribute the resulting symptoms to malignant disease without adequate investigation. High localised dosage to the posterior wall of the bladder can lead to areas of avascular fibrosis and telangiectasis. The telangiectatic areas can occasionally bleed and sometimes this can be troublesome. A patient may often describe this bleeding as arising from the vagina but cystoscopy can readily establish the cause. No treatment may be necessary, though if the bleeding is persistent cystoscopic diathermy can be very effective. Apart from the rare formation of a bladder stone, phosphatic accretion in and around a fibrotic posterior bladder wall can be troublesome largely because of associated infection with repeated attacks of cystitis. These attacks usually respond readily to mild urinary antiseptics. A more disturbing late complication is the development of a vesicovaginal fistula, a rectovaginal fistula or even complex rectovesicovaginal fistulas. Should these complications be associated with malignant disease, as they often are, the only hope of successful management would lie in appropriate exenterative surgery. It is worth noting that when colostomy is planned, as for a benign rectovaginal fistula, a transverse colostomy is preferred in view of the previous irradiation to the pelvis. If a vesicovaginal fistula is entirely benign the question again arises as to possible closure of the fistula. This is rarely possible and creates considerable surgical problems. Ureteric transplant to an ileal conduit is the only truly effective method of treatment, following which the pelvic induration as the result of the fistula will settle rapidly. A similar approach may be required if a contracted bladder makes life miserable. Ureteric obstruction occurs almost entirely as a result of malignant disease in the pelvis, even though an extrinsic reaction with a "frozen pelvis" can on rare occasions create ureteric obstruction in the absence of malignant disease. The management of such a complication is an exercise in urological surgery. It may be possible to transplant one or both ureters, as necessary, performing a cystoplasty.

Pregnancy

Pregnancy complicating carcinoma of the cervix presents a difficult but fortunately not a common problem. In our experience most of these patients have been found to have relatively early cancers of the cervix in stage 1 or stage 2 at the time of the diagnosis. If the cancer first declares itself when the pregnancy is advanced, it is reasonable to await the certain viability of the child, provided it is only a few weeks, deliver by caesarian section, and proceed thereafter to the normal management of the cancer. At a substantially earlier stage in the pregnancy, however, there is no possibility of saving a viable foetus. The gynaecologist may, if the cancer is sufficiently early, combine termination of the pregnancy with a Wertheim hysterectomy. With somewhat later stages of the disease the termination of the pregnancy should be followed by a course of parametrial X-ray therapy (as described above) allowing the uterus to involute before proceeding to the intracavitary radiation. Sometimes the diagnosis is not made until the post-partum period, and in such cases the cancer should be treated according to the stage of the disease. Though this is a rare complication and few centres have sufficient cases to quote substantial results of treatment, we find that when identical stages are compared the survival rates for patients with carcinoma of the cervix complicated by pregnancy are similar to those treated without this complication.

Special Conditions

Cervical Stump Cancer

Fortunately, this is a rare condition since few women are now subjected to a subtotal supravaginal hysterectomy. Clinically these patients fall into two distinct groups: (1) *true* stump carcinoma, where the cancer develops at least one or more years after hysterectomy and (2) *coincident* stump carcinoma, where the cancer is diagnosed within 1 year of the hysterectomy and can be presumed to have been present but not diagnosed at the time of operation.

Patients with *true* stump carcinoma should be treated, as with a normal cancer of the cervix, by a combination of intracavitary radium and pelvic X-ray therapy. However, since there is no uterine body to carry radium, the best that can be achieved is to employ vaginal ovoids across the vault of the vagina and a small central tube within the cervical canal. In some cases even the smallest central tube cannot be accommodated and vaginal ovoids alone are used. Parametrial X-ray therapy is given, irrespective of the stage of the disease, thus increasing the total dose at point *A*.

Patients with *coincident* stump carcinoma present a different problem because, in all probability, the supravaginal hysterectomy will have cut through malignant tissue and tumour cells will doubtless have been spread into the pelvis. The prognosis is not good, but if the patient's general condition is satisfactory, treatment can be given by external megavoltage therapy as described for a stage 4 cancer of the cervix. On the grounds that tissue tolerance is decreased following surgery in such patients, we employ a mid-pelvic dose of 4250 cGy in 3 weeks. If the patient can tolerate it, the X-ray therapy should be followed by a short insertion of radium, using vaginal ovoids either alone or with a short central tube in the cervical canal.

Invasive Carcinoma Diagnosed in a Cone Biopsy

Cone biopsy, following an abnormal cervical smear, is being performed with increasing frequency and examination of the cone is disclosing more unsuspected cases of microinvasive carcinoma or true invasive carcinoma of the cervix. Though some gynaecologists will elect to treat the microinvasive carcinoma by a Wertheim hysterectomy, radiation therapy for microinvasive or truly invasive carcinoma of the cervix is a highly effective method of treatment. Radiation, however, should be postponed for a period of 4–5 weeks after the cone biopsy, to allow any postoperative infection to subside, and during treatment a broad-spectrum antibiotic should be administered. Occasionally some difficulty is encountered in dilating the cervix after cone biopsy, but usually it is a straightforward procedure. If, however, the difficulty is insurmountable and precludes an optimal intracavitary radium treatment, alternative surgical treatment must be considered for such a curable lesion.

Recurrences After Radiotherapy

It is unusual for recurrence to be found centrally in the pelvis in early cases of cancer of the cervix. When this does occur surgery must be considered—a Wertheim hysterectomy or an anterior or posterior exenteration. More commonly, the patient who is not cured presents with pain which is typical in site and distribution. This pain usually arises in the buttock and radiates down the back of the thigh. On pelvic examination no disease may be palpable. X-ray of the pelvis or the lumbar spine may show an area of bone erosion, but only after symptoms have been present for a long period (Fig. 11.17). A lymphangiogram may indicate involvement of the lymph nodes (Fig. 11.18), or a further intravenous pyelogram may reveal a hydroureter not present before treatment. Alternatively, the patient may present with an oedematous leg caused by venous or lymphatic obstruction, again resulting from pressure from involved lymph nodes. The symptoms of pain and/or oedema of the leg usually preclude any useful surgical intervention. Palliative X-ray therapy may be given for malignant lymph nodes not included in the previously irradiated area and this may produce some temporary relief of symptoms.

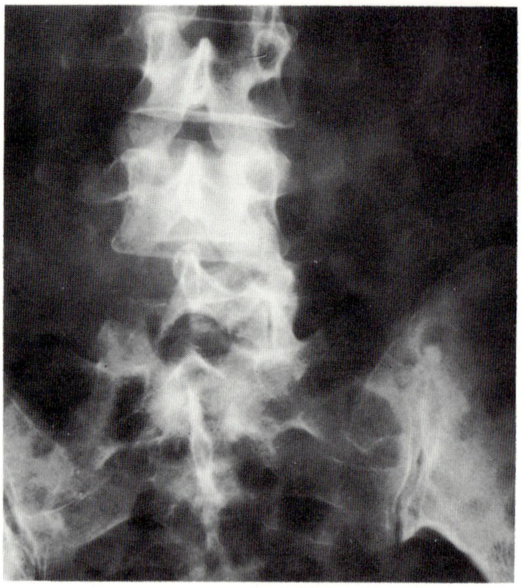

Fig. 11.17. AP radiograph of lower lumbar spine. The right side of the body of L5 and its transverse process have been eroded by metastatic nodal disease.

Adenocarcinoma of the Cervix

When the diagnosis is shown to be an adenocarcinoma arising in the cervix (and not an extension from adenocarcinoma of the corpus) the patient is treated by the same techniques as for squamous cell carcinoma and with the same prospects of curability. Papillary adenocarcinoma of the cervix, arising in the young patient, is an exception to this rule and is preferably treated by surgery.

Chemotherapy

Carcinoma of the cervix is a very unpromising tumour so far as cytotoxic chemotherapy is concerned. Bleomycin, methotrexate, and cyclophosphamide have all been tried but with very

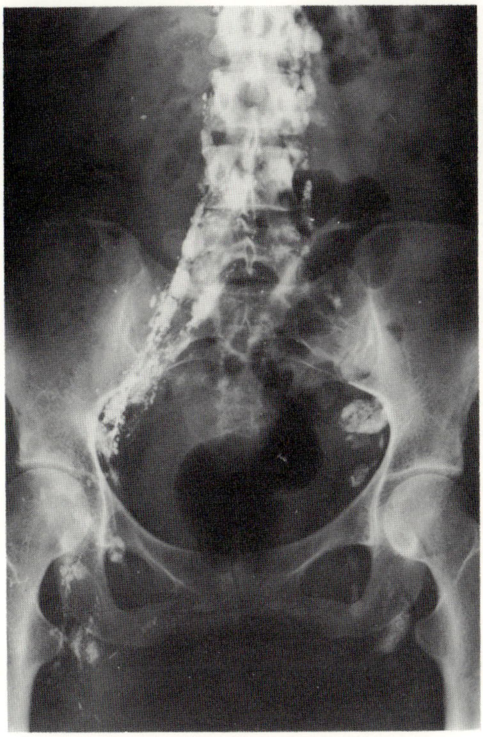

Fig. 11.18. Lower limb lymphangiogram showing malignant enlargement of left sided pelvic lymph nodes.

limited benefit. If the histology reveals adenocarcinoma there may be some value in using progesterone compounds as with adenocarcinoma of the corpus uteri.

Relief of Pain

In the advanced case of cancer of the cervix pain can be severe. Adequate analgesic drugs must be given regularly—for example, every 4 h—if the patient is to be kept entirely free of pain continuously. Morphia or morphine-like drugs will doubtless be required and should not be withheld. If the patient with pain is in good general condition and if the pain is unilateral, intrathecal injections of alcohol or tractotomy should be considered.

Results

The results of radiation therapy for cancer of the cervix are good and from our own experience should provide 5-year survival rates of at least 80% for stage 1 cases, 55% for stage 2, 35% for stage 3 and perhaps even 5% for those patients assessed as having stage 4 cervical cancer.

Cancer of the Corpus Uteri

In contrast to cancer of the cervix, cancer of the corpus uteri is more common in the older woman, usually of postmenopausal age. Though this cancer occurs frequently in multiparous women, the nulliparous woman is at a higher risk of developing this type of tumour.

Pathological and Clinical Features

Cancer of the uterine body is predominantly adenocarcinoma and ranges from the well-differentiated to the completely undifferentiated type of tumour. In some cases squamous metaplasia of part of the tumour occurs, giving rise to the so-called adenoacanthoma. Less frequently a sarcoma may arise from the uterine musculature, and very infrequently the uterus is the site of a mesodermal tumour. Adenocarcinoma of the body of the uterus may be papilliferous in character, filling the uterine cavity, and papilliferous material may even protrude through the cervical os. The tumour may infiltrate through the musculature of the uterine body to involve its peritoneal surface. The natural spread of this disease differs in some important ways from that of cancer of the uterine cervix. With the latter, the spread of tumour is predominantly in a lateral direction into the parametria and thereafter to the pelvic lymph nodes. Cancer of the body of the uterus tends to spread downwards to involve the cervix, and by lymphatic permeation down the vaginal wall, presenting as isolated nodules. The tumour may also spread to involve one or both ovaries, and may also metastasise to the hypogastric, external iliac, common iliac, presacral, and para-aortic lymph nodes. Blood-borne metastasis to the lung is more common with cancer of the body of the uterus than with cancer of the cervix. The common presenting symptom is postmenopausal bleeding and the diagnosis is established by a diagnostic curettage.

It is of special interest that adenocarcinoma of the corpus uteri arises with some frequency in women who are obese, diabetic, and hypertensive.

Staging

Stage 1 The carcinoma is confined to the corpus, including the isthmus.

Stage 2 The carcinoma has involved the corpus and the cervix but has not extended out-side the uterus.

Stage 3 The carcinoma has extended outside the uterus but not outside the true pelvis.

Stage 4 The carcinoma has extended outside the true pelvis or has obviously involved the mucosa of the bladder and/or the rectum. A bullous oedema as such does not permit a case to be allotted to stage 4.

For subdivisions of the stages, reference can be made to UICC (1978).

Treatment

When cancer of the uterine body is confined to the uterus it is probably equally amenable to treatment by surgery or by irradiation. In view, however, of the possibility of involvement of one or both ovaries, the treatment of choice for this type of cancer is panhysterectomy. In addition to panhysterectomy, some gynaecologists favour either preoperative or postoperative irradiation. The arguments in favour of preoperative irradiation rest on (1) the notion that rupture of the uterus at the time of operation will be decreased by the effects of irradiation, (2) the hope that any malignant cells dispersed locally or into the circulation at the time of operation will not be viable malignant cells, and this being so (3) the hope that the incidence of vault recurrence will be diminished. As yet, however, there is no well-documented clinical trial to establish the value of preoperative irradiation for corpus cancer—though it is extensively practised in many centres. Postoperative irradiation is discussed below.

Many circumstances arise where the gynaecologist considers panhysterectomy unwise—for example, gross obesity and hypertension (as mentioned above) or a variety of other clinical problems which make surgery inadvisable. Such a decision is made more readily acceptable by the fact that radiotherapy can, and does, cure a substantial number of patients with corpus cancer and, stage for stage, compares very favourably with surgery in terms of overall survival rates. The predominant method of approach for this kind of cancer is by intracavitary radium therapy. There are, however, some important differences from the treatment described above for cancer of the uterine cervix. For corpus cancer it is essential to include in the high-dose volume of radiation the whole of the endometrial cavity up to the fundus of the uterus, the muscular wall of the uterus, the cervix, and also a cuff of vagina. Though here, as with cervical cancer, the treatment depends on radiation sources in an intrauterine tube and vaginal ovoids, the likelihood of enlargement of the uterine body requires an extension of the available lengths of the intrauterine tubes—ranging from 6 to 12 cm long. The intrauterine tube used at the Christie Hospital for corpus cancer is made of plastic and has a diameter of 6 mm.

The amount of radium in the applicators is as follows:

Intrauterine tubes radium (mg) from fundus to cervix

30,15, 10, 15, 10, 10
30,10, 5,10,10
30,15,10,10
30,10,10

Ovoids large, 22.5 mg
medium, 20.0 mg
small, 17.5 mg

In order to extend the dose axially as far as possible at the fundal end of the uterine tube, the radium source at that end contains 30 mg and also has its fundal end thickness reduced to a total of 1 mm of platinum. The fundal end of the plastic uterine tube is also kept to minimal thickness (about 1 mm). Care must be taken to ensure that a sufficiently long uterine tube is employed so that its tip is in contact with the uterine fundus, even if this should mean that the cervical end of the tube projects through the cervical opening and lies between the vaginal ovoids. It will be recalled that for cancer of the uterine cervix a trefoil isodose shape was sought, but for cancer of the corpus uteri the stated dose is the mean value over the curved surface of a 4-cm-diameter cylinder coaxial with the uterine radium. Because of the shape of the isodose curve for the prescribed loading, the dose at point *A* is typically about 7% lower than this stated dose (Fig. 11.19).

The technique for inserting the intracavitary radium is very similar to that for cancer of the

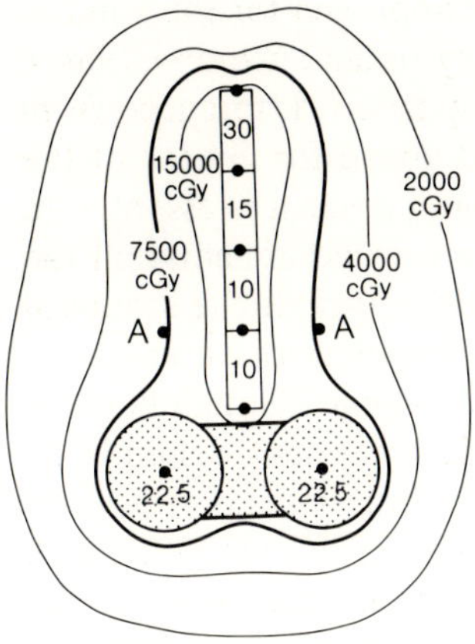

Fig. 11.19. Typical coronal dose distribution from an ideal radium insertion using an 8 cm uterine tandem and large ovoids.

uterine cervix, but the os requires to be dilated slightly wider to accommodate the greater diameter of this intrauterine tube. Because there is no flange on the intrauterine tube it is allowed to protrude slightly from the os. A pair of ovoids are selected which will best fit into the vaginal fornices. The radium is carefully packed in position, paying particular attention to the posterior fornix to reduce the radiation dose to the rectum. If tumour has already spread along the vaginal wall, the ovoids may be placed in tandem, thus extending the high-dose volume distally down the vagina. This, of course, will reduce the dose at point *A* by a small percentage and the time of the radium application will have to be adjusted to correct for this loss of dosage. A dose of 7500 cGy over the curved surface of a 4-cm-diameter cylinder is delivered in 10 days. This is achieved by two radium applications of 55 h each (subject to any necessary corrections, as with ovoids used in tandem).

Preoperative Radiotherapy

When it is planned to follow the radium therapy by a panhysterectomy the dosage is reduced to 6500 cGy in order to minimise the radiation reaction while at the same time ensuring the delivery of a dose of radiation approaching curative levels. This is important lest the intended surgery be abandoned for any reason. It is also important that the surgeon should not be tempted to accept less than radical surgery by relying on the preoperative irradiation.

Postoperative Radiotherapy

Postoperative radiotherapy is often requested as a prophylactic measure to prevent recurrence in the vault of the vagina. The incidence of postoperative vault recurrence is about 10%–15% in most published reports. It is usually sufficient to treat the vault with a pair of vaginal ovoids containing the appropriate amount of radium, as used in the treatment of carcinoma of the cervix. A single application of 96 h is given. In this treatment it is the local effect of the radium that is required, accepting that the amount of radiation extending into the parametria is low. A similar treatment can be used for very small vaginal recurrences, provided the malignant infiltration is minimal.

If examination of the postoperative specimen shows extensive infiltration of the myometrium or secondary tumour in the ovaries, it is clearly inappropriate to treat the patient with vaginal ovoids alone. Instead the four-field pelvic technique as used for stage 4 carcinoma of the cervix is indicated. After panhysterectomy the tissues are less tolerant to radiation and the mid-pelvic dose aimed at should be 4250 cGy in 3 weeks.

Recurrence

Post-radiation Recurrence

If the initial treatment has been by radium and the tumour recurs in the uterus, further radiation therapy is contraindicated and radical surgery must be considered, if feasible.

Postoperative Recurrence

If the initial treatment has been by surgery and a recurrence develops in the pelvis, the four-field pelvic technique described above can be used. In some cases an isolated metastasis may occur in the lower third of the vagina, particularly in relationship to the external urethral meatus. An isolated metastasis of this kind may be successfully treated by a radium needle implant or radioactive gold grain implant (see Chap. 12).

Hormone Dependence

Adenocarcinoma of the corpus uteri may be hormone-dependent and respond to progesterone compounds. Because of this, some gynaecologists prescribe a progesterone compound before surgery and/or postoperatively, and maintain the patient on this hormone for a prolonged period. Where lung metastases have occurred it may be possible to induce regression in these by progesterone hormones. Progesterone compounds are usually prescribed either as depot-progesterone intramuscularly or orally as high-dose medroxyprogesterone acetate.

Carcinoma of the Vagina

Pathological and Clinical Features

Vaginal cancer is relatively rare and occurs more commonly in postmenopausal women. The tumour is usually a squamous cell carcinoma with varying degrees of differentiation. Adenocarcinoma of the vagina is also rare and it is always important to exclude a primary adenocarcinoma of the uterus. It is now well-established, however, that some young girls can develop a primary adenocarcinoma of the vagina if they were exposed to stilboestrol in utero. In such cases the stilboestrol had been prescribed for a threatened abortion in the mother. Young girls at risk after this exposure to stilboestrol should be kept under observation by a gynaecologist. In childhood the sarcoma botyroides can occur but is discussed with other childhood malignant disease in Chap. 16.

The common presenting symptom of vaginal cancer is bleeding and dyspareunia. Dysuria and frequency may result from extension of tumour to the bladder while painful defecation may indicate rectal involvement. Further advancement of the disease may result in vesicovaginal and/or rectovaginal fistula. This may result in incontinence of urine and/or faeces.

Staging

The clinical staging of vaginal cancer is briefly as follows:

Stage 1 Tumour limited to the vaginal wall
Stage 2 Tumour involving the subvaginal tissue but without extension to the pelvic wall
Stage 3 Tumour with extension to the pelvic wall
Stage 4 Tumour involving the mucosa of the bladder and/or rectum and/or extension beyond the true pelvis

Treatment

Primary squamous cell carcinoma of the vagina can be treated either by surgery or by radiotherapy. Because of the close proximity of the vagina to the rectum and the bladder an adequate surgical clearance of the tumour in depth, as well as in area, will in all probability necessitate anterior, posterior, or total exenteration. For this reason radiation treatment of the vaginal cancer should be considered seriously as an alternative to surgery. Such extensive salvage surgery can reasonably be kept in reserve—and, of course, constantly kept in mind during the follow-up period. If the cancer is confined to the upper third of the vagina it is feasible to treat it in the same manner as a stage 2 or 3 cancer of the uterine cervix with vaginal involvement. Intrauterine and intravaginal radium is used, extending the radiation dose laterally into the parametria with supplementary X-ray therapy where this is deemed necessary. When the cancer is situated in the middle or lower third of the vagina it is more appropriate to treat it by beam-directed X-ray therapy. The extent of the tumour is defined by examination under anaesthesia. At this time the limits of the tumour are demarcated by the insertion of inert gold grains. Localisation radiographs (anteroposterior and lateral) are obtained as in the method described for cancer of the bladder (Chap. 12). The procedure localises the tumour with reference to its depth from the anterior skin as well as its size in all planes. A three-field technique is used, consisting of a symmetrical arrangement of one anterior and two posterior fields (Fig. 11.20). Using megavoltage X-rays and fields not exceeding 10×10 cm, a total tumour dose of 4750 cGy is given in 15 treatments over 3 weeks. In the very advanced cancer of the vagina, where bleeding is a problem and where there is no possibility of cure, the insertion of a vaginal sorbo containing radium sources may

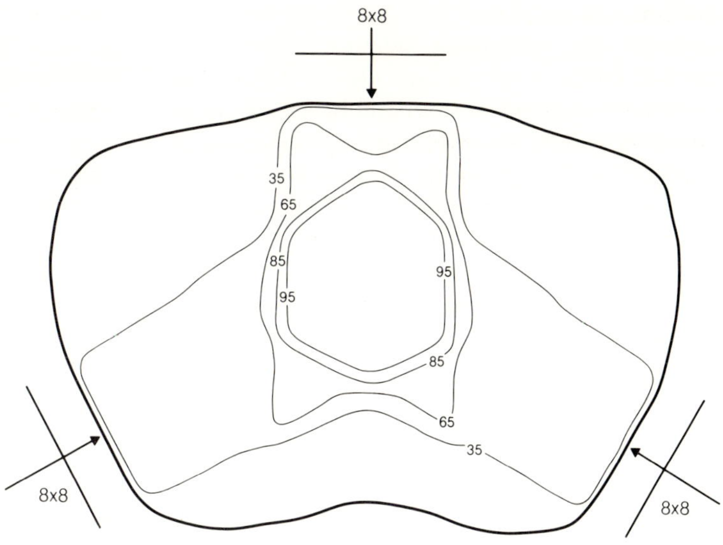

Fig. 11.20. Three field isocentric field arrangement useful in carcinoma of vagina.

produce haemostasis. The vaginal sorbo consists of a sponge rubber cylinder 2.4 cm in diameter, containing a central rubber tube with three or four 10-mg radium tubes in line. The sorbo is inserted into the length of the vagina without any packing and is stitched in position at its distal end. A dose of 7500 cGy is given on the surface of the sorbo in one insertion (Fig. 11.21). For the young girl with a primary adenocarcinoma of the vagina, surgery is the treatment of choice, even though this may require anterior, posterior, or total exenteration. Following surgery the gynaecologist can later consider the reconstruction of a vagina, if the patient remains free of disease. Though radiotherapy could be considered, as for squamous cell carcinoma in the older patient, surgery is preferred for two reasons: (1) the adenocarcinoma in the young girl is not likely to be radiosensitive, and (2) high-dose radiation would be required and, if this did prove curative, such high dosage of radiation in the pelvis might in 30–40 years' time become the site of sarcomatous changes or at least present problems from fibrosis in the bladder or rectum.

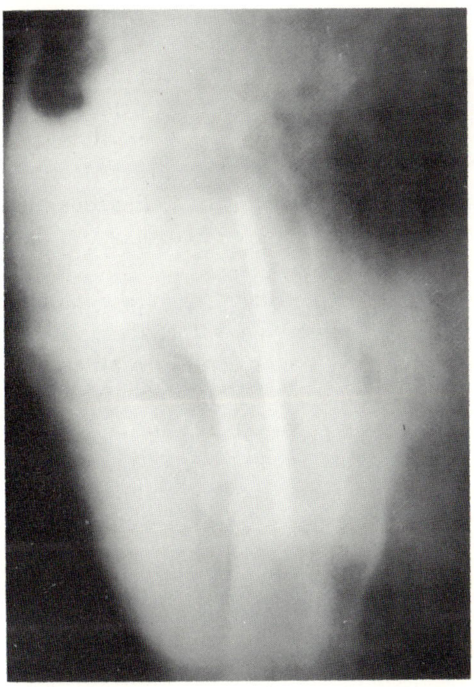

Fig. 11.21. Lateral radiograph with vaginal sorbo in position.

Procidentia and Cancer of the Vagina

Sometimes an elderly patient presents with a procidentia and an extensive carcinoma of the vagina. Usually no surgical treatment is contemplated either because of the age of the patient or because of the extension of the tumour to the limits of the procidentia. If the procidentia cannot be reduced, radiotherapy—by external irradiation—is more likely to render the situation worse, with a painful ulcerated reaction and irradiation of small bowel within the procidentia. Such a patient is better left untreated, apart from symptomatic management. If the procidentia can be satisfactorily reduced, intrauterine and vaginal radium may at least produce relief by controlling discharge and bleeding and it may indeed cure the cancer. In addition, the subsequent radiation fibrosis may prevent further descent of the uterus. The vaginal radium sources will very probably require to be placed in tandem to cover the extent of the vaginal cancer. In an elderly frail patient it is reasonable to give a single application of radium therapy, delivering a dose of 5250 cGy at point *A*.

Cancer of the Vulva

This is a comparatively rare condition, again occurring predominantly in the postmenopausal woman. Unfortunately, it is often in an advanced stage before the patient seeks medical care.

Pathological and Clinical Features

The commonest histological type is squamous cell carcinoma, though basal cell and intra-epidermal carcinomas occur, as does malignant melanoma. Adenocarcinoma can arise in Bartholin's gland or in sweat glands. Leucoplakia may precede the squamous cell carcinoma and probably accounts for the multifocal nature of the tumour. The presenting feature is usually ulceration or swelling of the labium, though this may be preceded by vulval pruritus where leucoplakia has been present. The tumour may be confined to the vulva or extend into the vagina. The tumour may spread posteriorly to involve the anus or anteriorly to the clitoris or even the mons pubis. The urethra may also be involved in the extension of tumour. Secondary spread occurs commonly to the inguinal and femoral lymph nodes and even to pelvic lymph nodes when the disease is extensive.

Treatment

The optimum treatment for squamous cell cancer of the vulva is surgery—usually radical vulvectomy and block dissection of the inguinal and femoral lymph nodes. Sometimes the lesser operation of simple vulvectomy is preferred in the elderly frail patient. The vulva is not very tolerant of radiation, so that radiotherapy is reserved either for local recurrence following surgery or for those whose age and general condition preclude surgery. Radiotherapy may, however, be preferred for the lesion in the posterior third of the vulva, encroaching towards the anus, where surgery is likely to jeopardise the anal sphincter. In this situation a radium needle implant, as either a single-plane or a two-plane implant (Figs. 11.22 and 11.23) may be acceptable as an alternative to surgery. If a two-plane implant is required to cover the extent of the disease, one plane is implanted in each labium, care being taken to ensure that the two planes of radium are as parallel and as close to one another as possible. Each needle should be stitched in place individually. A tumour dose of 5250 cGy at 0.5 cm, in 7 days from a single-plane implant should be achieved. Where a two-plane implant is used, a minimum dose of 5000 cGy is given in 7 days, measured at the midpoint between the planes of radium. Permanent gold seed or grain implants (gold-198) are single-plane implants and are feasible only for small lesions not more than 1.0 cm thick.

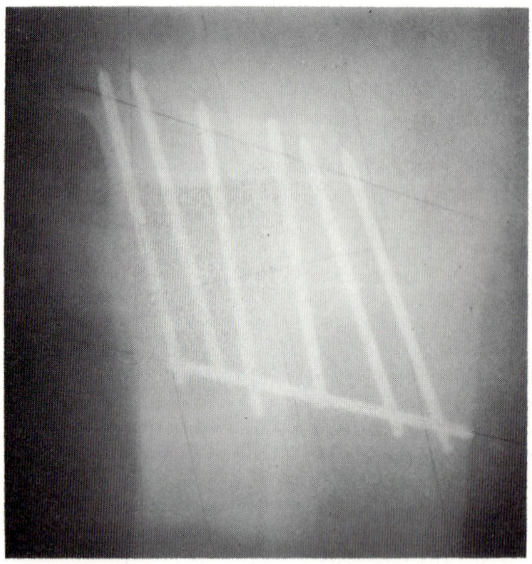

Fig. 11.22. Vulva. Single-plane implant.
Implanted area=23.6 cm^2
Dose required=5500 cGy
Approximate treatment=168 h
mg h/1000 cGy=443
mg radium required=14.5 mg
Needles used 3×3 mg active length 4.5 cm
4×1.5 mg active length 4.5 cm
Total mg radium used=14.55 mg (including filtration correction)
Final treatment time=167 h

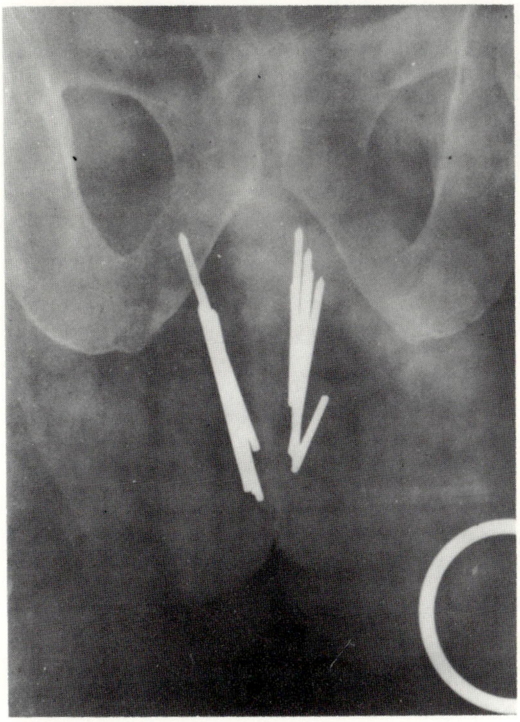

Fig. 11.23. Vulva. Two-plane implant.
Implant area=16.3 cm^2
Dose required=5250 cGy
Approximate treatment time=168 h
mg h/1000 cGy=345
2-plane separation factor=1.65
mg radium required=17.79 mg
Needles used 10×1.5 mg active length 4.5 cm
2×3 mg active length 4.5 cm
Total mg radium used=20.37 mg (including filtration correction)
Final treatment time=147 h

Postoperative Recurrence

A postoperative recurrence in the vulval area should be considered for further local excision if at all possible, because the tissue tolerance to radiation in the operation site is poor, there is much scar tissue, and the anatomy is distorted. Occasionally there is no possibility of further surgery and radiotherapy must then be considered, though each implant must be individualised and the final decision on the type of implant to be carried out is made at examination under anaesthesia. If the recurrence is limited, a radium needle or gold grain implant may be feasible. For lesions—either postoperative or new—extending beyond the limits of interstitial irradiation and yet still occupying a reasonable volume, resort may be made to beam-directed megavoltage therapy. The technique used is as described for the treatment of a bladder carcinoma. A certain amount of build-up is necessary to extend the tumour dose to the surface. The reaction following this treatment is brisk and with a treatment volume of 7×7×7 cm the tumour dose delivered should not exceed 4500 cGy in 15 or 16 exposures over 21 days. Electron therapy would not appear to have any significant advantage over megavoltage therapy, except for small lesions which can be treated by medium-energy electrons (8–10 MV). Very rarely will patients with advanced vulval cancer achieve any useful palliation from radiotherapy and it is better withheld.

Lymph Node Metastases

Secondary mobile inguinal nodes are best managed by block dissection of the groin (see Chap. 17).

Cancer of the Ovary

Cancer of the ovary is one of the common causes of death among women. It has a low cure rate because the disease is often extensive before it is diagnosed.

Pathological and Clinical Features

There is a wide variety of tumours affecting the ovary, with varying degrees of malignancy—the papillary cystadenocarcinoma, the pseudomucinous cystadenocarcinoma, the solid ovarian adenocarcinoma, the dysgerminoma occurring in the young girl, the feminising granulosa-cell tumour, the masculinising arrhenoblastoma; teratoma also occurs, and the ovary is a common site for secondary tumours.

An ovarian tumour may be quite large before symptoms develop. The patient may seek medical care only when she becomes aware of an increase in girth, because of the enlarging tumour itself or the associated ascites. In some cases acute symptoms may develop, as with torsion or rupture of the ovarian tumour. Postmenopausal bleeding can occur in association with a granulosa-cell tumour, while virilising signs are seen with the rare arrhenoblastoma. Clinical examination of the patient will often reveal either unilateral or bilateral ovarian swellings. Laparotomy will establish the diagnosis, the extent of the disease and the histological type. The disease may be limited to one ovary, sometimes both, and local spread can occur to the pelvic side wall, uterus, and omentum. Secondary peritoneal deposits may be present. Lymph node involvement may be found in the hypogastric, iliac, and para-aortic nodes and even in the left supraclavicular region. Ascites is common and sometimes pleural effusions are also present. Secondary deposits may occur in the liver.

Staging

The clinical staging for ovarian tumours is briefly as follows:

Stage 1 Tumour limited to ovaries
Stage 2 Tumour involving one or both ovaries with pelvic extension
Stage 3 Tumour involving one or both ovaries with extension to small bowel or omentum, limited to the true pelvis, or intraperitoneal metastases beyond the true pelvis, or positive retroperitoneal nodes or both
Stage 4 Spread to distant organs

Treatment

Surgery is the primary treatment for ovarian cancer. Indeed, the patient is unlikely to be referred to the radiotherapist until at least a laparotomy has been performed. When a patient reaches the radiotherapist she presents in one of the following categories, which will be discussed in turn.

1) The tumour has been completely removed by hysterectomy and bilateral salpingo-oophorectomy.
2) The tumour has been removed as completely as possible but some "adhesions" were encountered between the tumour and the pelvic wall or pelvic organs.
3) Though the tumour was completely removed, the cyst ruptured at the time of operation, spilling its fluid contents into the abdominal cavity.
4) The ovarian tumour was completely removed, but many peritoneal deposits were observed by the surgeon.
5) The laparotomy was limited to confirming the diagnosis because a fixed unresectable ovarian tumour was found with evidence of widespread abdominal disease.

Category 1

When the tumour is considered to have been entirely cleared by operation it seems reasonable not to subject the patient to radiotherapy. Some gynaecologists may elect to treat the patient with adjuvant chemotherapy but this also may not be necessary.

Categories 2 and 3

Where there is known to be residual tumour in the pelvis, or the possibility of pelvic disease because of the ruptured tumour, a course of pelvic X-ray therapy should be considered. This radiation therapy should be delayed for 5–6 weeks after the laparotomy to allow adequate healing and recovery from the operation. The four-field megavoltage technique described previously for stage 4 carcinoma of the cervix can be employed, delivering a mid-pelvis dose of 4250 cGy in 3 weeks (16 treatments). No supplementary radium treatment is given in such cases as this is not likely to be effective, the area at risk being at the periphery of the irradiated area rather than centrally in the uterine zone.

Category 4

When the patient presents with multiple peritoneal deposits, but is in good general condition, the choice of treatment lies between chemotherapy and whole abdominal X-ray therapy. The problem with irradiating the whole abdomen is the need to shield the kidneys for part of the X-ray treatment (to avoid the risk of radiation nephritis), with the consequent danger of shielding tumour at the same time. Because of this difficulty it may therefore be wise to treat the patient initially with chemotherapy, reserving X-ray therapy until the patient is no longer responding to chemotherapy. Whole abdominal X-ray therapy, using megavoltage X-rays, irradiates the whole abdomen from the xiphisternum to the vulva and including the inguinal lymph node drainage. Laterally, the field extends to the limits of the peritoneal cavity. The field size may be of the order of 40×25 cm. Anterior and posterior fields are employed to give a mid-tumour dose of 3000 cGy in 4 weeks (20 treatments). The kidneys are identified by an intravenous pyelogram and it is our practice to shield both kidneys after 2000 cGy. This treatment may produce some temporary nausea and diarrhoea but in our experience it is rare to have to interrupt treatment for these symptoms. If the white cell count falls below 2.5×10^9/l or the platelet count below 75.0×10^9/l, treatment is temporarily discontinued. Careful observation of the blood count is especially important if the patient has had previous chemotherapy. In such cases the leucocyte and platelet counts fall more quickly and more substantially than in the patient who has not had chemotherapy.

Category 5

In patients who have had only a diagnostic laparotomy, the disease is so widespread that there is little prospect of any useful remission with X-ray therapy. If, in the light of all the clinical features, chemotherapy is employed and if there is a worthwhile reduction in tumour masses, the possibility of following this with X-ray therapy can be considered, to try to reduce the masses still further. When significant tumour resolution has been achieved, some gynaecologists undertake a "second look" laparatomy in the hope of being able to remove tumour masses and perhaps prolong the period of chemotherapeutic control.

Chemotherapy See Chap. 3

Cancer of the Fallopian Tube

This is an extremely rare cancer and the diagnosis is seldom made before operation. It is generally an adenocarcinoma. The presenting symptom is often a blood-stained discharge or frank bleeding. The management of the patient with this condition is surgical. X-ray therapy may be given postoperatively if the clearance of the tumour has not been complete, as described for ovarian tumours.

Reference

UICC (1978) TNM classification of malignant tumours, 3rd edn. UICC, Geneva

12 Genitourinary Tract

R. C. S. Pointon

Renal Tumours

The three principal tumours are:

1) Renal carcinoma
2) Carcinoma of the renal pelvis
3) Wilms' tumour

Wilms' tumour is considered in Chap. 16.

Renal Carcinoma

This is the commonest renal tumour. It occurs most frequently in the fifth and sixth decades of life but may occur in young adults. The lesion is commoner in males, the sex incidence being 3:1. It is believed that renal carcinoma arises from the renal tubules. Three cellular types are described—clear cell carcinoma, granular cell carcinoma, and spindle cell carcinoma. The tumour extends locally and may replace the whole kidney. There is no true capsule between the tumour and the renal parenchyma. In advanced lesions the tumour extends through the kidney into the perirenal structures. It may extend via the regional lymphatics and involve the retroperitoneal nodes.

Invasion of the renal vein and inferior vena cava is common. Blood-borne metastases are frequent; the most commonly involved sites are the lung, liver, and bone.

Clinical Presentation

The most common symptoms are haematuria, pain in the loin, and presence of a mass. Occasionally metastatic disease may be the presenting feature. Among the less common findings associated with carcinoma of the kidney are polycythaemia, pyrexia, and hypercalcaemia. Investigations will include intravenous pyelography, ultrasound studies and CT scanning. Renal angiography may be indicated.

Treatment

The treatment of renal carcinoma is essentially surgical, i.e. nephrectomy. Routine postoperative radiotherapy is not indicated. Where the tumour is inoperable or where only incomplete removal was possible, postoperative X-ray therapy to the renal bed is indicated. Localisation of the volume to be irradiated is facilitated if the surgeon leaves clips or similar radio-opaque markers at the limits of the known disease.

Method A simple parallel pair of megavoltage X-ray fields is used. The volume treated will include the known disease with a substantial margin. The tumour dose aimed at using 4- or 8-MV X-rays is 3500–3750 cGy in 16 exposures over 21 days. Cognizance of the length of spinal cord subtended must be taken in selecting the tumour dose. The response to irradiation of renal carcinoma is not entirely predictable, as there is a wide range of sensitivity.

Metastases Spontaneous resolution of metastases following nephrectomy has been observed but is not a common phenomenon. Bone metastases may be very vascular and pulsation and a bruit are commonly observed. Useful palliation may be obtained from a single exposure of X-rays to a focal lesion, giving a skin dose of 1250–1500 cGy.

Systemic Treatment Cytotoxic drugs have been disappointing in the treatment of renal carcinoma and no particular regime can be recommended at present. Hormone therapy using medroxyprogesterone (Provera) gives a modest level of objective response.

Carcinoma of the Renal Pelvis

Carcinoma of the renal pelvis is one manifestation of urothelial malignancy and is often associated with lesions in the bladder. It may precede or follow the development of a bladder lesion, often with a considerable time interval. The treatment of transitional cell carcinoma of the renal pelvis is normally by nephro-ureterectomy. Routine post-operative X-ray therapy is not indicated. Inoperable or residual disease is treated by radiation as described for renal carcinoma. Occasionally a patient presents with bladder tumours, having had a carcinoma of the renal pelvis treated by nephrectomy only. In such circumstances, the residual ureter must be removed before treatment of the bladder lesion is instituted.

Carcinoma of the Ureter

Tumours of the ureter are usually part of a multifocal disease involving the urothelium. Primary carcinoma of the ureter is a very rare lesion and is usually a transitional cell carcinoma. The treatment is surgical except when the lower end of the ureter is involved, when it is treated as for a primary carcinoma of the bladder. Postoperative radiotherapy is usually not indicated except when surgical clearance is inadequate. The technique used will be similar to that employed for residual renal carcinoma following surgery.

Bladder

Successful treatment of the patient with carcinoma of the bladder can only be obtained when there is the closest cooperation between urologist and radiotherapist. Ideally, the patient should be jointly assessed and a common treatment policy decided upon. Surgery and radiotherapy remain the only curative methods of treatment and their respective places in the management of the disease is a joint decision by surgeon and radiotherapist.

Clinical Features

Epithelial tumours of the bladder present a wide range of biological behaviour. At one end of the scale are papillary tumours of low-grade malignancy and at the other, solid grossly anaplastic tumours with loss of transitional epithelial characteristics. The recognition that the degree of infiltration of the bladder wall by tumour is the most significant feature forms the basis of clinical staging.

This, together with an appreciation of the natural history of bladder tumours and their mode of spread, permits the development of an ordered treatment policy.

To establish the precise extent and nature of the tumour, the necessary preliminary investigations of each case are as follows:

1) *General Assessment*. The patient's general condition and fitness for treatment should be assessed. Routine examinations should include a full blood count, blood profile, and chest X-ray.
2) *Urine Examination*. This should include microscopy and culture. Exfoliative cytology may be of value in diagnosis.
3) *Intravenous Urogram*. Renal pelvic and ureteric tumours may accompany a vesical lesion and their presence should be excluded. Evidence of renal function should be noted, together with the presence of obstructive changes. The cystogram may demonstrate a filling defect and indicate the size and position of the tumour. The radiographs provide a limited skeletal survey which may demonstrate the presence of osseous metastases.
4) *Cystoscopy*. This should be carried out under general anaesthesia. The number, size, and appearance of the tumours and the nature of the surrounding mucosa should be assessed.
5) *Biopsy*. At the time of cystoscopy, biopsy or transurethral resection of the tumour should be carried out.

6) *Examination Under Anaesthesia.* Careful bimanual examination under anaesthesia to determine the size of the tumour and the degree of invasion of the bladder wall, is essential for pretreatment staging.
7) *Other Imaging Techniques.* Ultrasonic examination of the pelvis may be of value in the assessment of the degree of invasion of the bladder wall. CT scanning may provide further information on the degree of infiltration of the bladder wall and perivesical tissues. It can be a valuable aid to treatment planning and to the assessment of response to treatment.

Classification of Malignant Tumours of the Bladder (TNM 1978)

The classification applies only to epithelial tumours.

T **—Primary tumour**

Tis —Pre-invasive carcinoma (carcinoma in situ): "Flat tumour".

Ta —Papillary non-invasive carcinoma.

T0 —No evidence of primary tumour.

T1 —On bimanual examination a freely mobile mass may be felt: this should not be felt after complete transurethral resection of the lesion
and/or
Microscopically, the tumour does not invade beyond the lamina propria.

T2 —On bimanual examination there is induration of the bladder wall which is mobile. There is no residual induration after complete transurethral resection of the lesion
and/or
There is microscopic invasion of superficial muscle.

T3 —On bimanual examination induration or a nodular mobile mass is palpable in the bladder wall which persists after transurethral resection of the exophytic portion of the lesion
and/or
There is microscopic invasion of deep muscle or of extension through the bladder wall.
T3a Invasion of deep muscle.
T3b Invasion through the bladder wall.

T4 —Tumour fixed or extending to neighbouring structures
and/or
There is microscopic evidence of such involvement.
T4a Tumour infiltrating the prostate, uterus, or vagina.
T4b Tumour fixed to the pelvic wall and/or abdominal wall.

N **—Regional and juxta-regional lymph nodes**

N0 —No evidence of regional lymph node involvement.

N1 —Single homolateral regional.

N2 —Contra- or bilateral/multiple regional.

N3 —Fixed regional.

N4 —Juxta-regional.

M **—Distant metastases**

M0 —No evidence of distant metastases.

M1 —Evidence of distant metastases.

Clinical Assessment

Accurate clinical assessment and classification is essential for planning treatment, for evaluation of treatment methods, and to provide precise information for the comparison of results of treatment. The principal factors to be considered are:

1) Stage
2) Multiplicity of tumours
3) Gross macroscopic type

Stage

The stage of the primary lesion is the most important single factor. The distribution of the stage of the disease seen at any one centre will depend on the referable pattern. The majority of patients referred for radiotherapy will have infiltrative lesions and thus not represent the true stage incidence of the disease.

Multiplicity

Multiple tumours are most frequently found where the lesion is T1 or confined to the mucosa.

Infiltrative tumours are single in the majority of cases and predominantly so where deep invasion has occurred. Thus in T3 stages the lesion is solitary in over 90% of cases.

Macroscopic Type

The macroscopic appearance of bladder tumours falls into the following main groups:

1) Papillary
2) Nodular
3) Papillary plus nodular
4) Ulcerative

The majority of superficial tumours are papillary, in contrast to infiltrative tumours, which most frequently will be nodular. In addition, the state of the surrounding mucosa should be carefully inspected with respect to its stability. The presence of diverticula or any other anomaly should be noted. Obstruction to urinary outflow due to tumour or prostatic enlargement, if discovered, should be corrected before X-ray therapy is commenced. Where there are multiple tumours the prostatic urethra should be examined carefully to exclude further deposits of tumour. At the completion of the examination, biopsies of relevant areas should be taken.

Examination Under Anaesthesia

Of equal importance to the cystoscopic examination is the examination under anaesthesia per vaginam and per rectum. Careful palpation with the patient fully relaxed will indicate the degree of infiltration of the bladder wall and its relationship to neighbouring structures. The information so secured will permit staging of the primary tumour and the formulation of treatment policy.

Intravenous Urogram

The presence of obstruction of the upper urinary tract is directly related to the stage of the tumour on presentation. In over 90% of T1 lesions, normal upper urinary tracts will be found. This may be contrasted to T3 lesions, where half the patients have evidence of obstructive uropathy with a non-functioning kidney. The presence of a non-functioning kidney carries a poor, but not hopeless, prognosis. The return of function following a successful course of X-ray therapy is uncommon.

Histology

As has already been mentioned, tumours of the urinary bladder, while almost entirely epithelial in origin, present a wide range of biological behaviour. At one extreme the tumour may be composed of transitional epithelium of normal thickness and cellular appearance; at the other, there may be gross anaplasia with complete loss of transitional epithelial characteristics. There may be papillary tumours which, following treatment, remain controlled, yet some tumours of the same type and histology demonstrate aggressive features with early vascular invasion and early recurrence(s).

Treatment Policy

The decision on treatment policy for the individual case should be carried out jointly by surgeon and radiotherapist. It is clearly desirable that the policy adopted should permit of continuity, so that proper evaluation and comparison of treatment methods may be made.

Stage T1 Tumours

Surgery is the treatment of choice in the management of the majority of these lesions. Where multiple lesions develop, such that they cannot be controlled by endoscopic means, frequently cystectomy is required. Where cystectomy is contraindicated as a result of age or general condition, radical X-ray therapy should be given.

Invasive Carcinoma of the Bladder T2 T3

At the present, radical megavoltage X-ray therapy with salvage cystectomy remains as effective a method of treatment for invasive carcinoma of the bladder T2 T3 as any other. It moreover has the advantage that the majority of survivors will keep their bladders. The selection of this method of treatment is also influenced by the fact that many of the patients are over 70 years of age and are unfit for elective surgery.

Pelvic Fixation T4

The prognosis for this stage is poor and no significant difference in results can be demonstrated, whether the patient is treated radically or palliatively. Palliation is the principal aim in the management of this lesion, without the production of an arduous reaction. This aim may be achieved by the use of an abbreviated course of external therapy.

Radiotherapy Methods

The principal radiotherapeutic methods used are:

1) Interstitial implantation
2) Radical X-ray therapy (3 weeks)
3) Palliative X-ray therapy (10 days)

Interstitial Implantation This method of treatment is only suitable for single small localised T1 and T2 lesions. The tumour should not exceed 4 cm in diameter and not have infiltrated deep into the muscle coat of the bladder. It is a well tolerated form of treatment with little morbidity.

Radical Megavoltage X-ray Therapy The indications for this form of treatment are:

1) T1 tumours which cannot be controlled by endoscopic means and where other forms of surgery are contraindicated
2) Infiltrative carcinoma of the bladder, T2 and T3; also tumours which have infiltrated the muscle coat or have extended into the perivesical tissues and remain mobile
3) Some T4a tumours which may be contained in a reasonable volume

Palliative Megavoltage X-ray Therapy The commonest indications for this form of treatment are:

1) Where the tumour has infiltrated to such a degree as to be fixed in the pelvis (T4)
2) For patients with less advanced tumours unsuitable for radical treatment by virtue of age and general condition

Interstitial Irradiation

The treatment of small superficial carcinoma of the bladder by means of interstitial irradiation has declined very considerably. The principal reasons for this decline have been the introduction of better endoscopic instruments and the appreciation that for infiltrating lesions, equal results may be obtained by well planned external irradiation, affording as it does a greater margin of safety.

Interstitial irradiation has a place in the treatment of solitary superficial lesions (T1, T2) not greater than 4 cm in diameter. It is of particular value in the aged patient who might not tolerate a radical course of X-ray therapy.

The principle of bladder implants is a single-plane implant. This is carried out at open operation and a good exposure is essential. The tumour should be examined carefully and in particular the degree of infiltration of the bladder wall assessed. If there is any doubt about the suitability of the lesion for implant, it is wiser to mark the tumour using gold seeds, close the bladder and subsequently resort to external beam therapy. If the lesion is suitable for implant, any exuberant tissue should be removed by diathermy and the implant performed, treating the tumour together with a margin of 1–5 cm of normal tissue.

Permanent implants have the advantage that once the implant has been carried out, the bladder may be closed completely. This form of implant only will be described, as the use of a removable implant has been discarded (although it remains a practised alternative).

Permanent Implants These are carried out using either ^{198}Au seeds or ^{198}Au grains. The desired dose delivered should be between 6000 and 6500 cGy. The technique has the inherent disadvantages of permanent implants—it lacks precise physical control, in that the implant cannot be altered or the time adjusted. It is of considerable advantage to have available in the theatre a table showing the number of megabecquerels required for a variety of doses and areas (Appendix 1). From the strength of the sources available, the number of sources required is easily calculated. The distribution of the sources follows the dosage rules with two thirds of the sources distributed around the periphery and one third in the middle. Figure 12.1 illustrates gold seed and gold grain implants.

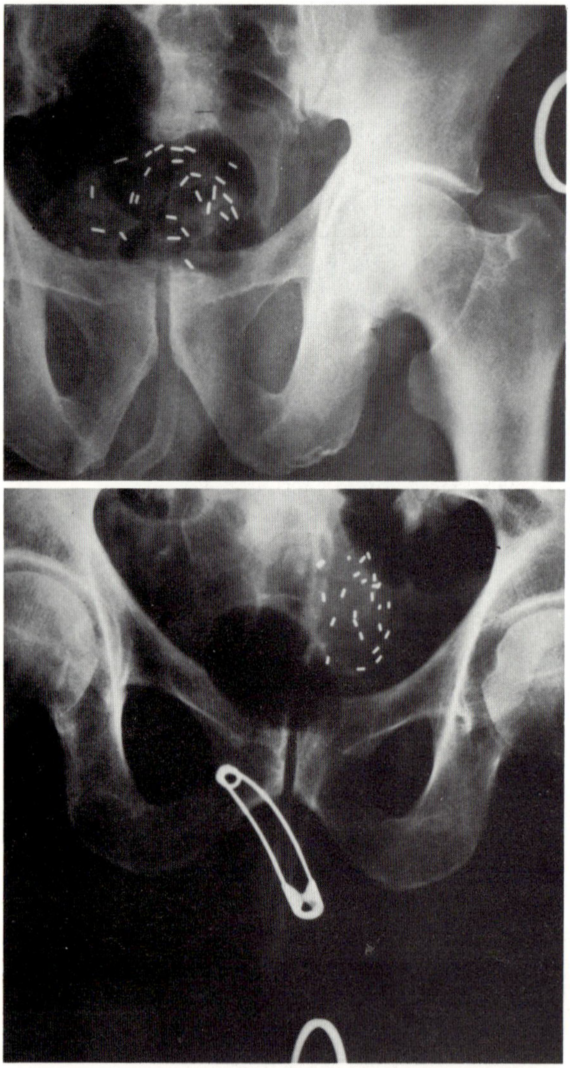

a

b

Fig. 12.1a,b. Carcinoma of the bladder. **a** Gold seed implant. **b** Gold grain implant.

Radical Megavoltage X-ray Treatment

A radical course of X-ray treatment for carcinoma of the bladder should be planned in methodical steps:

1) A good description of the cystoscopic findings is essential with particular reference to the size, type of tumour, number of tumours present, site of tumour relative to the normal anatomy, i.e. to the bladder neck or to the ureteric orifices. Additional helpful information will refer to the condition of the mucosa adjacent to the tumour and to the presence of diverticula.
2) The findings of the examination under anaesthetic are of equal importance. Where there is an obviously palpable lesion, the direction and nature of extent should be noted.
3) The intravenous pyelograms should be studied with reference to obstructive uropathy. The bladder films may demonstrate an obvious filling defect.
4) The tumour must be localised. The principal aids to localisation are:
   i) The insertion of gold markers via the cytoscope at the margins of the tumour. This, however, may be difficult and requires some degree of expertise if it is to be of value. The obvious advantage of this technique is that it permits verification radiographs to confirm the accuracy of localisation.
   ii) Cystograms remain the most commonly used means of localisation and will be discussed later in depth. Verification by standard radiographs and CT scanning have confirmed the value of cystography as a simple and accurate method of localisation.
   iii) A simulator with an opaque medium in the bladder is a perfectly satisfactory means of localisation but has no advantage over good cystograms. In a busy department it is relatively time consuming and does not permit the depth of study obtainable with cystogram films.
   iv) CT scanning and treatment planning is an elegant method of localisation and verification. Studies have indicated that it has no significant advantage over cystograms except in those circumstances where the cystoscopic findings are unsatisfactory.

Irrespective of the method employed, it is essential to recognise clot retention, which may produce misleading images.

Before treatment is started, any urinary infection should be treated and anaemia corrected. If there is obstruction to urinary flow, either by tumour at the bladder neck or by prostatic enlargement, this should be dealt with by perurethral resection before treatment is commenced. Generally it is undesirable to treat a patient with a catheter in situ.

Bladder tumours are of limited radiosensitivity and the principle of "small volume, high dose" is adhered to; the volume irradiated is reduced to the minimum which will include the lesion with a modest margin. No attempt is made to treat the

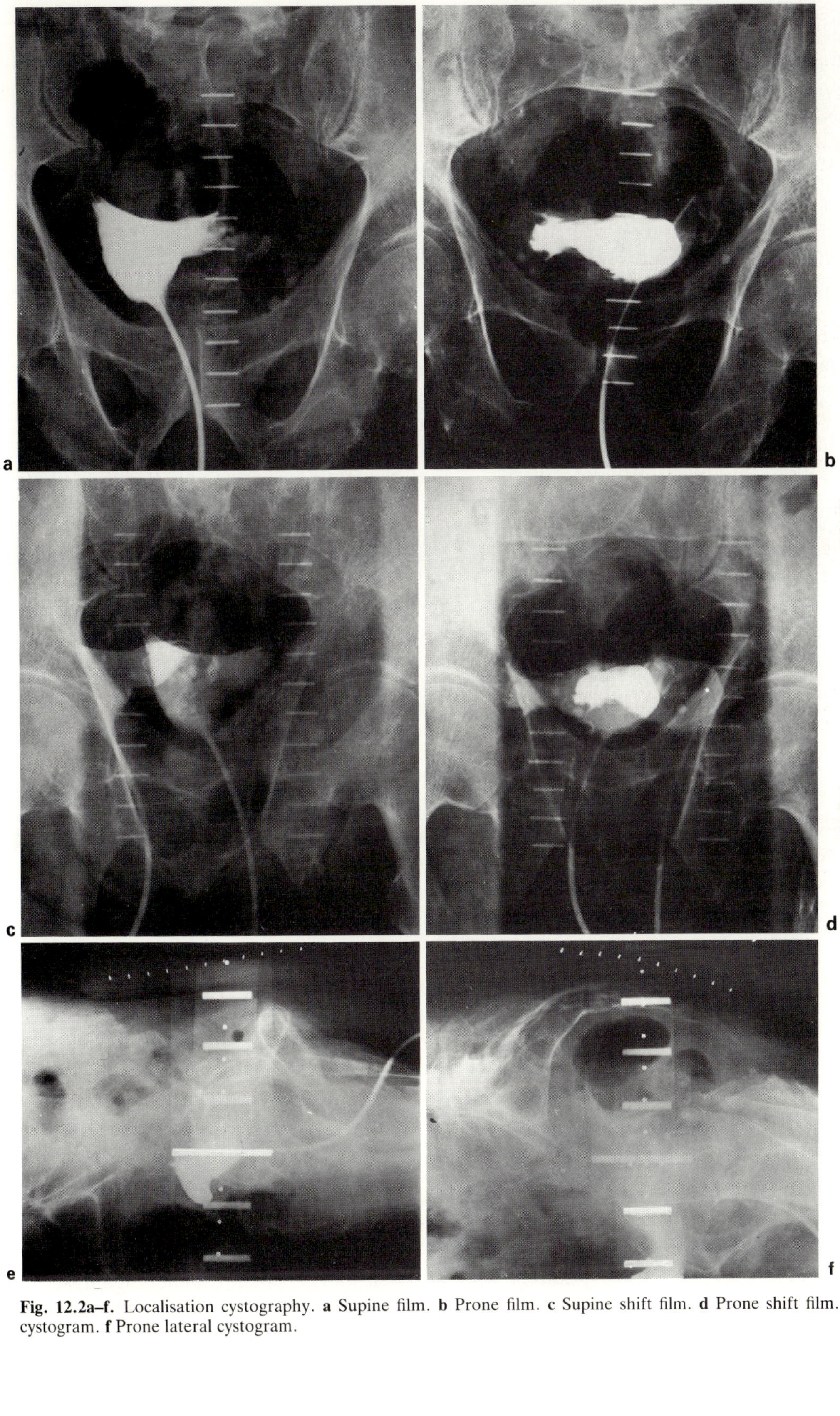

Fig. 12.2a–f. Localisation cystography. **a** Supine film. **b** Prone film. **c** Supine shift film. **d** Prone shift film. **e** Supine lateral cystogram. **f** Prone lateral cystogram.

whole bladder except when there are multiple tumours involving much of the surface of the organ. No deliberate attempt is made to subtend the regional lymph nodes within the treatment volume. This restriction of the treatment volume requires accurate localisation and precise beam direction.

Localisation Cystograms Localisation or marker cystograms are made using a weak solution of barium and an opaque catheter. The method used is as follows:

An anterior ladder 10 cm in length with lead strips at 1-cm intervals is taped to the abdominal wall with the lowest two or three marker strips overlying the symphysis pubis. The position of the ladder is carefully marked on the skin.

Two lateral posts are positioned on either side of the patient, one with lead strips and the other with lead spheres at 2-cm intervals from the table top. The 10 cm level is distinguished by two lead spheres on one marker and a long strip on the other. The posts with the spheres is on the film side of the patient and the post with bars is on the tube side.

The patient is catheterised and the bladder emptied. Then 20 ml of the barium suspension is instilled. Three radiographs are taken at 100 cm focus-to-film distance with the patient prone:

1) A straight anteroposterior radiograph
2) An anteroposterior film at the same focus-to-film distance, with two exposures on the same film, the tube being moved first 10 cm to one side, then an equal distance to the other side of the midline
3) A lateral radiograph taken with a horizontal beam centred on the 10-cm mark above the table top.

The whole procedure is then repeated with the patient prone, with the skin ladder taped to the skin overlying the sacrum. The resulting six films (Fig. 12.2) allow the depth of the catheter as it enters the bladder and the tumour from the skin surfaces to be measured exactly.

Megavoltage Techniques The appropriate field size to subtend the tumour with an adequate margin is selected and is then drawn on the films, with correction for magnification. The localisation of the tumour in terms of depth from the appropriate points on the anterior and posterior skin surfaces is as described above. With this precise information the isocentric rotation property of the machine ensures accurate beam direction.

The selection of the appropriate megavoltage technique to be used will be influenced by the properties of the apparatus available and the specific features of the individual case. The following three techniques have been found to be sufficiently versatile to treat the majority of patients with bladder tumours:

1) *Three-Field Technique, 4 or 8 MV* (Fig. 12.3). This method uses a three-field symmetrical arrangement with one anterior and two posterior oblique fields. The anterior and posterior pin heights are determined from the localisation cystogram or equivalent. Beam direction for the posterior fields is by virtue of the isocentric rotation of the machine. The disadvantage of this method is that the patient has to be treated in the prone position on most machines. Accordingly, this technique has largely been superseded by the two techniques described below. It however has some advantages if it is desired to treat the whole bladder.

2) *Three-Field Wedge Technique, 4 or 8 MV* (Fig. 12.4). This is preferred when the tumour lies not more than 7 cm deep. It employs a central anterior field coupled with two wedged anterior oblique fields and thus the patient is treated supine. With these fixed field techniques it is normal to treat the anterior field at an FSD of 100 cm—the FSDs for the oblique fields are determined by using a telescopic Perspex

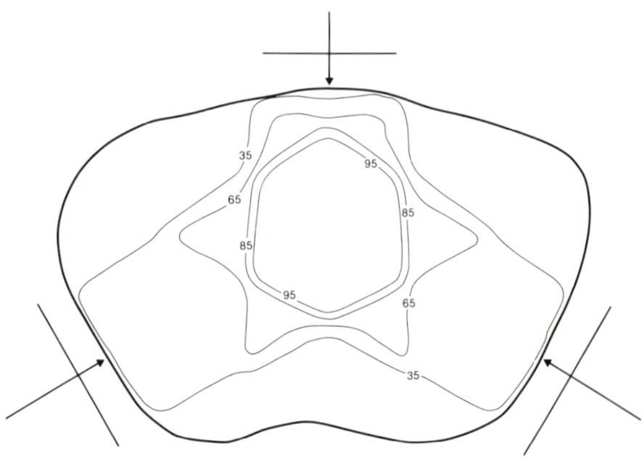

Fig. 12.3 Carcinoma of the bladder. Three-field technique, 8-MV.

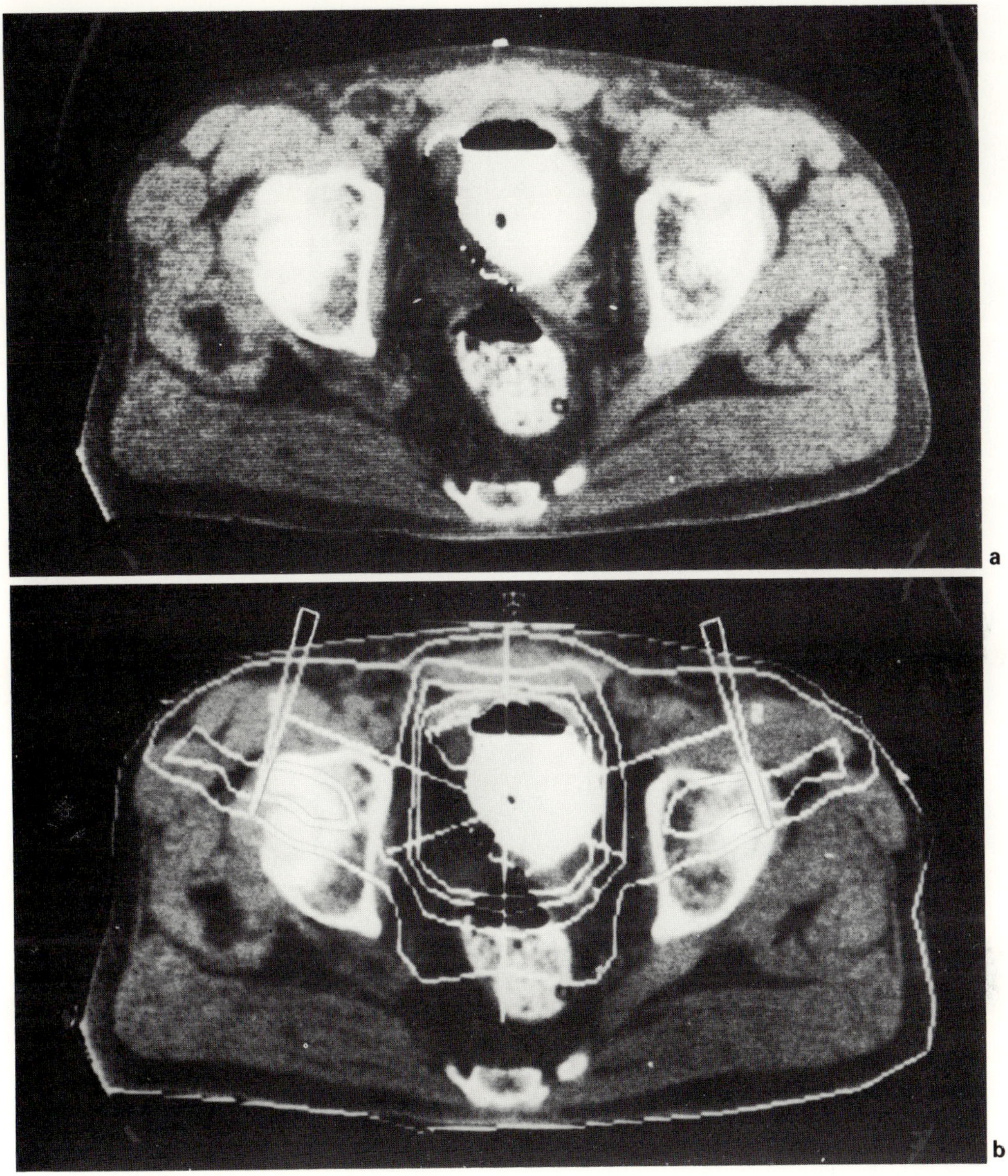

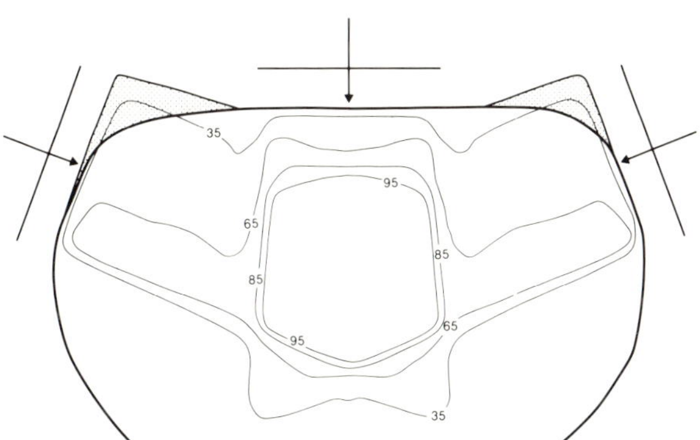

Fig. 12.4a–c. Three-field wedge technique, 8-MV.

applicator carrying an FSD scale. The appropriate depth-dose correction for a shorter FSD must be made using the formula described in Chap. 1.

3) *Rotation Technique, 4 or 8 MV* (Fig. 12.5). Where this facility is available, this technique has the advantage of ease in setting up and gives comparable dose distributions to those obtained with fixed-field techniques. Standard practice is to treat in two arcs of 140°–150° using a wedge filter to improve the dose distribution.

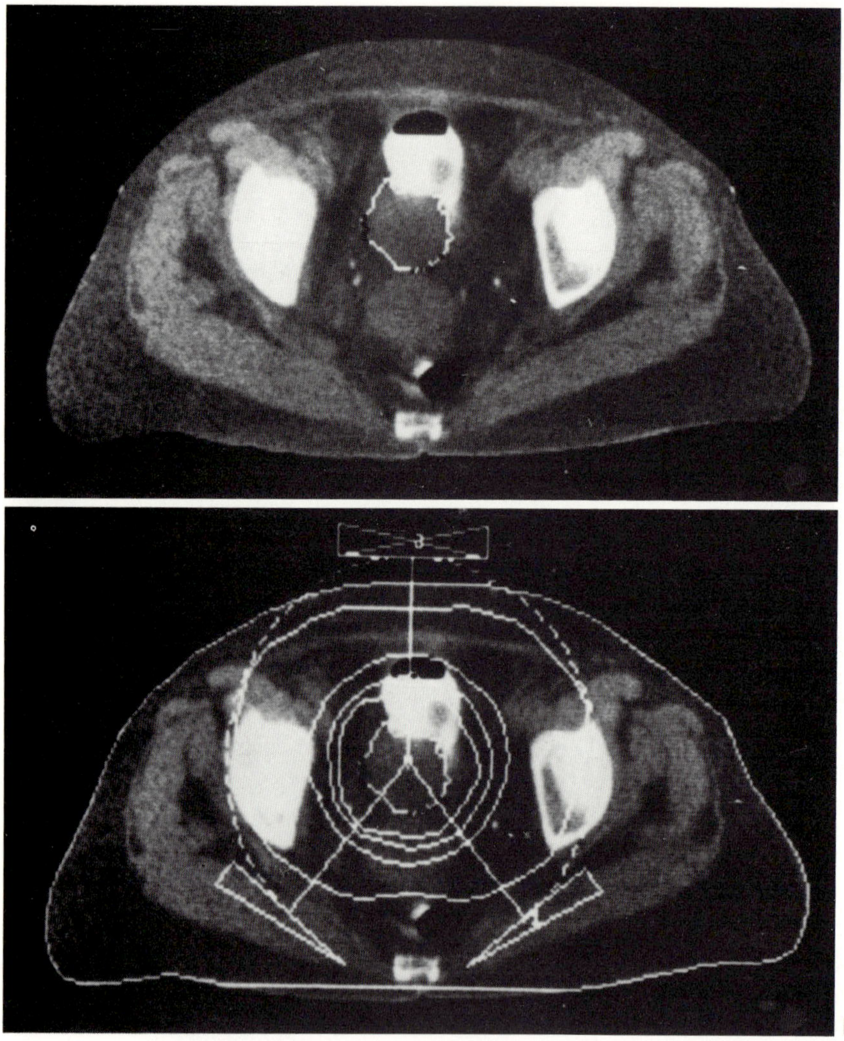

a

b

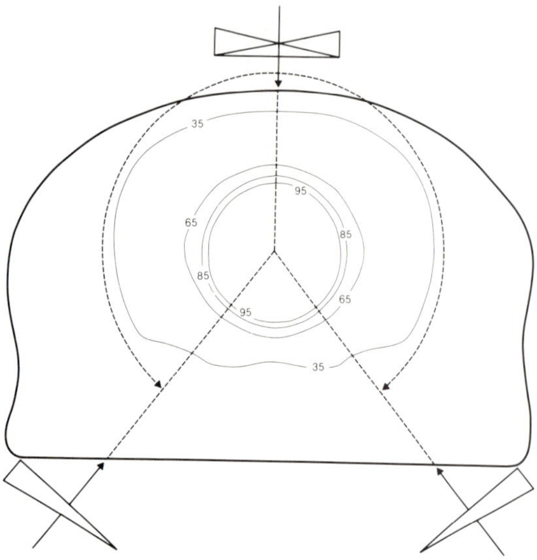

c

Fig. 12.5a–c. Rotation technique, 8-MV.

With all these techniques, the field sizes used are 50–80 cm^2. The dose delivered is 5500–5250 cGy given in 15 or 16 fractions over 21 days.

Contraindications to Radical X-ray Treatment
Specific circumstances where surgery is the preferred treatment method or where radical X-ray therapy would be hazardous are uncommon. Among them are the following:

1) *Contracted bladder*. Where there is considerable reduction in bladder capacity and the bladder is removable.
2) *Multiple tumours*. Where the bladder mucosa is clearly unstable and there are multiple tumours involving much of the organ.

3) *Involvement of the prostatic urethra.* Where there are multiple tumours in the bladder, there may be tumours involving the prostatic urethra. Cystourethrectomy is the treatment of choice.
4) *Tumour in a diverticulum.* Where there is tumour in a diverticulum, the appropriate surgical treatment is to be preferred.
5) *Previous radiotherapy to the pelvis.* Rarely bladder tumours may occur in patients who have had previous radiotherapy to the pelvis. Where the dose to the pelvis has been high, e.g. in carcinoma of the cervix, then surgery should be considered. Where the previous dose to the pelvis has been low, then radical radiotherapy to the bladder may be proceeded with, perhaps reducing the tumour dose by 5%, depending on the previous treatment.

Palliative X-ray Treatment

Advanced carcinoma of the bladder with pelvic fixation carries a poor prognosis and no significant difference in results can be shown whether the patient is treated radically or palliatively. Palliation remains the principal aim in the management of this lesion without the production of an arduous reaction. Well conducted palliative X-ray treatment will control haematuria and give satisfactory palliation in over 50% of cases. Cases for palliative treatment should be selected with care for patients in poor condition or those with grossly reduced bladder capacity will not be helped, and indeed their symptoms aggravated by any form of radiotherapy.

To achieve good palliation it is essential to plan treatment with precision. The same principles of localisation and verification as for a radical X-ray treatment are followed. The simplest form of treatment is the rotation technique previously described. Treatment is confined to the bladder, the volume subtended being in the order of $9 \times 9 \times 9$ cm, which can be treated to a dose of 3500 cGy in eight exposures over 10 days. The dose delivered should be of the order of three-quarters of the radical dose for the equivalent volume and times.

Reaction

During the course of X-ray therapy to the bladder, there may be some increase in frequency of micturition and dysuria, but this is usually not severe. Routine urine examinations should be carried out during the course of treatment but urinary infection of any note is uncommon. Some degree of rectal reaction is inevitable with any radical course of X-ray therapy to the bladder. This gives rise to tenesmus and proctitis which are reasonably tolerable and symptomatic measures only are indicated.

Follow-up

Following a course of X-ray therapy, unless there is clinical indication, review cystoscopy is carried out 4 months after the completion of treatment. Earlier review has not been found helpful in assessing the state of the bladder. Further cystoscopic review thereafter is at the discretion of the urologist and according to clinical situation presenting. Urine cytology has not been found to be of great value as a follow-up procedure. CT scanning as a review procedure has yet to prove its value. Apart from providing knowledge as to whether the patient is clinically well, out-patient follow-up is of limited value.

Recurrent Carcinoma of the Bladder

Patients with recurrent carcinoma of the bladder following irradiation should be treated by radical surgery where this is feasible. In the male this should be a cystourethrectomy, and in the female, an anterior clearance of the pelvis. Recurrent or residual superficial tumours may be controllable by endoscopic methods. The treatment of patients with recurrent carcinoma of the bladder following open surgery will be determined by the clinical situation and the nature of the previous surgery.

Complications

Complications following a radical course of X-ray therapy fall into two main groups: those affecting the bladder and those affecting the bowel.

Bladder

The two principal complications are:

1) Telangiectasia
2) Contracted bladder

Telangiectasia Some degree of telangiectasia will be seen at cystoscopy in almost all treated cases. The problem arises when there is bleeding from telangiectasia. This may be persistent and lead to a considerable degree of anaemia. There is frequently some degree of clot retention and it is essential initially that all clot be removed. It may be difficult to identify the area from which the bleeding has occurred, but if it can be, light diathermy to the area is often efficacious. Repeated attacks of haematuria from telangiectasia may be difficult to control. The instillation of various fluids into the bladder has been tried but is seldom consistently effective. When haematuria is severe, cystectomy must be considered but seldom is necessary in the absence of concomitant tumour.

Contracted Bladder Following a radical course of X-ray therapy some reduction in the bladder capacity will occur. Severe contraction with gross frequency and back pressure changes in the upper urinary tract requires urinary diversion with or without cystectomy depending on the state of the pelvis. Severe contraction is more likely to occur when there has been much previous diathermy treatment. Multiple biopsies following X-ray treatment to the bladder are to be avoided, as healing is often delayed and contraction may result.

Bowel Injuries

These fall into two main groups: lesions of the small bowel and lesions of the large bowel.

Small Bowel The terminal portion of the ileum is the common site of injury. Gross fibrosis occurs with marked stricture formation. While this may occur as a result of a loop of bowel being adherent in the pelvis as a result of previous surgery, this is not the cause in the majority of cases. The predominant symptom is that of a subacute obstruction of the bowel. Treatment is excision of the affected segment of bowel and the appropriate surgical measure. Damage to the small bowel may be asymptomatic and only found when the bowel is examined before the formation of an ileal conduit. It follows that careful examination of the ileum should be carried out before ureteric implantation is undertaken.

Large Bowel The commonest lesion is a stricture of the sigmoid colon. In some cases this may not be severe and no intervention is indicated. Where there is obvious obstruction, a colostomy will be necessary and any subsequent management will depend on the clinical situation. Injury to the rectum similar to the extrinsic rectal reaction seen following treatment of carcinoma of the cervix may rarely be seen. More commonly as a result of telangiectasia of the anterior rectal wall, persistent bleeding may occur. This is usually intermittent and not severe. Injuries of the rectum are best managed conservatively as surgical intervention may be hazardous.

The incidence of bladder and bowel complications following a radical course of X-ray treatment to the bladder is in the order of 6%.

Cystectomy Following Radiotherapy

Of patients receiving a radical course of X-ray therapy, some 9% will proceed to cystectomy, principally for recurrent tumour. No significant difference in survival has been observed between primary and salvage cystectomy, nor has the postoperative complication rate been significantly different.

Adverse factors affecting survival are:

1) Patient over 70 years of age
2) Non-function of one kidney on intravenous urogram
3) High-grade histology
4) Tumour in cystectomy specimen
5) pT3 or pT4 tumour in cystectomy specimen

The prognosis would appear to be better in women and in the younger age groups. The overall survival for salvage cystectomy is 35% at 5 years.

Results and Prognostic Factors

The policy of primary radiotherapy with surgical salvage gives corrected survival rates as shown in Table 12.1.

Table 12.1. Bladder carcinoma: survival following primary radiotherapy with surgical salvage.

Stage	Method	Corrected 5-year survival rate (%)
T_1	Interstitial	82
T_1	X-ray therapy	52
T_2	X-ray therapy	34
T_3	X-ray therapy	28
T_4	X-ray therapy	5

Prognostic factors include the following:

1) *Stage*. This is the dominant factor influencing prognosis.
2) *Age*. In all stages, the younger age groups have a better prognosis. Thus in T2 and T3 lesions treated by X-ray therapy, the younger patients have a 5-year survival rate of better than 40%.
3) *Lymph node involvement*. Lymphography (Turner et al. 1976) has demonstrated that a positive lymphogram carries a poor prognosis and is associated with a high rate of distant metastases.
4) *Obstruction*. Evidence on the intravenous urogram of obstruction of the upper urinary tract carries a poorer prognosis.

The hope that the use of high LET radiation therapy might improve the results of treatment of carcinoma of the bladder has, as yet, not materialised. A clinical trial comparing treatment by 14-MV neutrons with 8-MV photon therapy in T2 and T3 tumours has shown no significant difference in survival and complications.

The combination of chemotherapy with radiotherapy in the treatment of carcinoma of the bladder has, as yet, not been fully evaluated. This method of therapy is complicated by the fact that many of these patients are aged and do not tolerate the presently available effective agents well.

Carcinoma of the Prostate

Carcinoma of the prostate is the commonest cause of death in men from genitourinary malignancy. The majority of carcinomas of the prostate are well differentiated adenocarcinoma.

Investigation

The diagnosis is based on clinical examination, endoscopy, and biopsy. An intravenous urogram will indicate the presence of obstructive changes as well as providing a limited skeletal survey. More sophisticated forms of investigation are the use of ultrasound and CT scanning. Prostatic ultrasound has been found to be of value in assessing the local extent of the disease and is helpful in localising suspicious areas in the gland that require biopsy. Transrectal ultrasound may be of value in the subsequent assessment of local response following therapy. CT scanning has not been found to have a definitive role in the diagnosis of early carcinoma of the prostate but is of value in demonstrating extracapsular spread and involvement of the seminal vesicles, and may be used in treatment planning. Pelvic node involvement will only be found clinically, if gross. Routine lymphography has not been used. Palpation of the supraclavicular region to exclude node involvement should be part of the routine clinical examination. Pelvic node involvement may be demonstrated by both CT and abdominal ultrasound studies. As node involvement is usually associated with undetected distant metastases, it is not felt justified to subject the patient to further invasive investigation.

A bone scan should be carried out in all cases before instituting treatment, to exclude osseous metastases. Serum acid phosphatase determinations are of value in confirming gross metastatic disease. More sophisticated biochemical assays are under survey. Receptor studies for either androgens or oestrogens have, as yet, had no significant influence on treatment.

TNM Pretreatment Clinical Classification

- T Primary tumour
- Tis Pre-invasive carcinoma (carcinoma in situ)
- T0 No tumour palpable
- T1 Tumour intracapsular surrounded by palpably normal gland
- T2 Tumour confined to the gland. Smooth nodule deforming contour but lateral sulci and seminal vesicles not involved
- T3 Tumour extending beyond the capsule with or without involvement of the lateral sulci and/or seminal vesicle

T4 Tumour fixed or infiltrating neighbouring structures

The regional lymph nodes are the pelvic nodes below the bifurcation of the common iliac arteries. The juxtaregional nodes are the inguinal nodes, the common iliac nodes and the para-aortic nodes.

Management

It has been estimated that only 30% of patients with carcinoma of the prostate are potentially curable on presentation. A full appreciation of the stage of the disease is essential to the planning of the management of the patient. Where the lesion is found as an incidental finding at prostatectomy and is a small focus of well differentiated adenocarcinoma, the outlook is good and surveillance only is indicated. If, however, the lesion is larger and the histology less well differentiated, a radical course of radiotherapy is indicated.

If clinically the lesion remains localised with no evidence of metastases, a radical course of radiotherapy affords good local control with a minimum of side-effects, and is the treatment of choice. In advanced disease the principal symptoms are outflow obstruction and pain due to skeletal metastases. Palliation is the aim of treatment and the outflow obstruction is relieved by transurethral resection. Where skeletal metastases are present, endocrine therapy may be instituted or withheld until symptoms present. Conventional endocrine therapy consists of oestrogens or orchidectomy. It is estimated that 70% of patients with metastatic disease may respond to endocrine measures. Where bone pain is not responding to endocrine measures, radiotherapy either to localised sites or in the form of half-body irradiation can give useful palliation. Carcinoma of the prostate responds well to radiotherapy. The indications for its use are where the disease remains localised to the pelvis. Radical treatment is normally reserved for T_1, T_2 and T_3 lesions. Even for T_4 lesions where the tumour is fixed or infiltrating neighbouring organs, good local palliation can be achieved.

The methods available are:

(1) Interstitial irradiation

(2) Beam directed megavoltage X-ray therapy

Implantation techniques using permanent sources has been advocated but the technique is difficult and good distribution of sources is hard to achieve. With the improved sonographic methods of detection available, it may be that interstitial treatment methods should be reconsidered for well localised lesions. Beam directed megavoltage X-ray treatment affords a wider margin of safety, good local control associated with modest morbidity and remains the preferred method of treatment.

Radical X-Ray Treatment

The principle followed is to treat the primary lesion only and no attempt is made to subtend the regional lymph nodes. The treatment volume will be determined principally by the clinical extent of the disease. Ultrasound and C.T. scans may provide additional useful information.

Localisation

Cystograms are made using the technique described for bladder tumour. The majority of cases will have had a previous transurethral resection which facilitates localisation. Where the extent of the lesion is imprecise, a C.T. scan may prove useful in treatment planning.

Method

The rotation technique as described for radical X-ray treatment of carcinoma of the bladder, has been found to be the most useful treatment method. The volume subtended is normally 8×7×7 cm or 8×8×8 cm. The tumour dose delivered is 5000 cGy given in 16 fractions over 21 days (Fig. 12.6).

Reaction

The reaction from this form of treatment is mild. There may be some temporary exacerbation of urinary frequency but this settles rapidly. Similarly proctitis in the majority of cases has not been a problem.

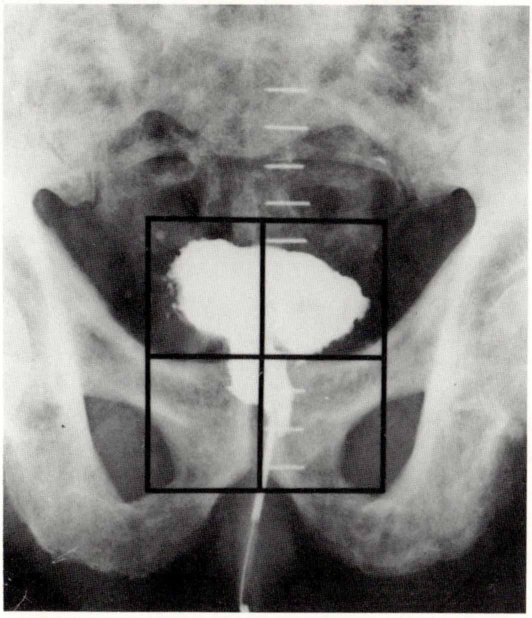

Fig. 12.6. Carcinoma of the prostate. Localisation film.

Complications

No major complications following this form of therapy have to date been seen. Occasionally there may be intermittent rectal bleeding as a result of radiation changes affecting the anterior rectal wall.

Palliative X-ray Therapy

Palliation of the primary lesion is indicated where, in the presence of known metastatic disease, the primary lesion cannot be controlled by surgical methods and is refractory to hormone manipulation. The predominant features are obstructive symptoms recurring rapidly after perurethral resection and haematuria. Involvement of the rectum with frank ulceration is seldom improved by X-ray therapy and is usually best treated by symptomatic procedures.

The technique used is the same as that employed for palliative X-ray therapy of advanced bladder cancer. A rotation treatment using megavoltage or telecobalt therapy has been found to be most efficacious. An average volume is 9×9×9 cm and the dose delivered is 3500 cGy given in eight fractions over 10 days. Simpler and shorter methods of treatment have not given good palliation and generally are not worthwhile.

Follow-up

Subsequent surveillance following a course of X-ray treatment is principally clinical with endoscopy when indicated. Ultrasound and CT scanning may be helpful. Bone scans should be repeated at 6-monthly intervals or where clinically indicated.

Recurrence

Local recurrence is dealt with by the appropriate surgical measures. Endocrine therapy may be instituted or withheld until symptoms develop.

Prognostic Factors

1) *Stage*. The most important factor is the stage of the disease on presentation.
2) *Obstruction*. Evidence on the intravenous urogram of obstruction of the upper urinary tracts carries a poor prognosis.
3) *Histology*. Undifferentiated tumours behave in a more aggressive manner and consequently tend to present in a more advanced stage and carry a poor outlook.

Results

The local control achieved by a radical course of megavoltage X-ray treatment is excellent. Unfortunately of those patients who have a negative bone scan on presentation, one third will develop skeletal metastases within 2 years of the primary treatment.

The overall survival rate is 60% at 5 years, but of those patients who present with metastases, the majority will be dead within 3 years of presentation.

Carcinoma of the Female Urethra

The mucous coat of the urethra is continued externally with that of the vulva and internally with that of the bladder. The external orifice is surrounded by the paraurethral mucous glands. The predominant form of carcinoma is a squamous cell carcinoma.

Site

From the point of view of treatment, carcinoma of the female urethra may be classified as follows:

1) Urethral orifice
2) Vulvourethral
3) Urethral

Orificial and vulvourethral lesions may be considered as accessible lesions. Tumours involving the proximal urethra are less common and usually present as a firm spindle-shaped swelling lying in the course of the urethra. This type does not ulcerate until the lesion is advanced.

Lymphatic drainage

The lymphatic drainage of the distal urethra is to the inguinal lymph nodes, and of the proximal urethra to the deep pelvic nodes, comprising the external and internal hypogastric, and occasionally a node at the promontory of the sacrum. Approximately 35% of cases present with involved nodes.

Treatment

Successful irradiation preserves normal function and is therefore preferable to radical surgery. Primary surgery, however, may be preferred for lesions unsuitable for irradiation therapy by virtue of their extent or histology.

Method

Interstitial irradiation gives good results in the treatment of early or moderately advanced lesions and remains the treatment of choice. In more advanced lesions, the mode of local spread of the disease, together with the anatomy of the part, renders satisfactory implantation difficult. Small-field beam-directed megavoltage X-ray therapy is a practical alternative to interstitial irradiation in the treatment of some extensive urethral carcinomas.

Interstitial treatments fall into two groups:

1) Permanent gold seed or grain (^{198}Au) implant
2) Radium needle (or equivalent) implant

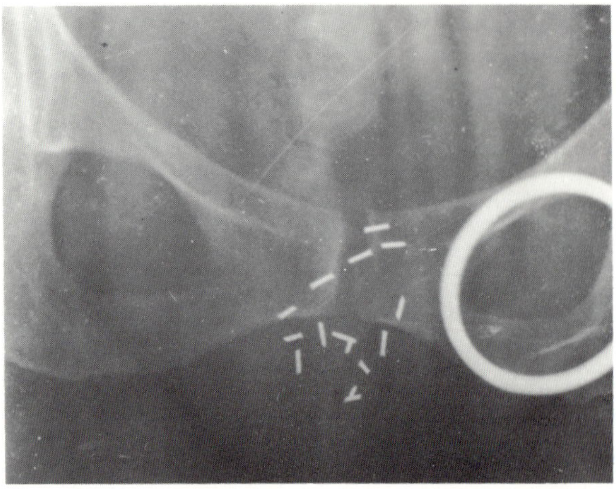

Fig. 12.7. Carcinoma of the urethra. Gold seed implant.

1) *Permanent gold seed or grain implant*. For small orificial lesions a permanent gold seed implant is a very satisfactory treatment method and is well suited to the anatomy of the region. A single-plane implant is used, aiming at a dose of 5500 cGy at 0.5 cm (Fig. 12.7).

2) *Radium needle implant*. For more extensive lesions a two-plane or volume radium needle implant is used, delivering a dose of 5250 cGy in 7 days (Fig. 12.8). Before the needles are inserted, a self-retaining catheter is introduced. Normally the needles used should not be less than 4.5 cm active length. If a volume implant is decided upon, the completion of the "ring" of needles is facilitated by sewing in the vagina a suitable piece of sorbo rubber and implanting this, thus completing the circle of peripheral needles.

Megavoltage X-ray Therapy

For lesions beyond implant and yet within a reasonable volume, a small-field beam-directed megavoltage X-ray treatment, as described for bladder carcinoma, may be used, delivering a dose of 5250 cGy over 3 weeks.

Lymph Node Metastases

Mobile involved inguinal nodes are treated by block dissection.

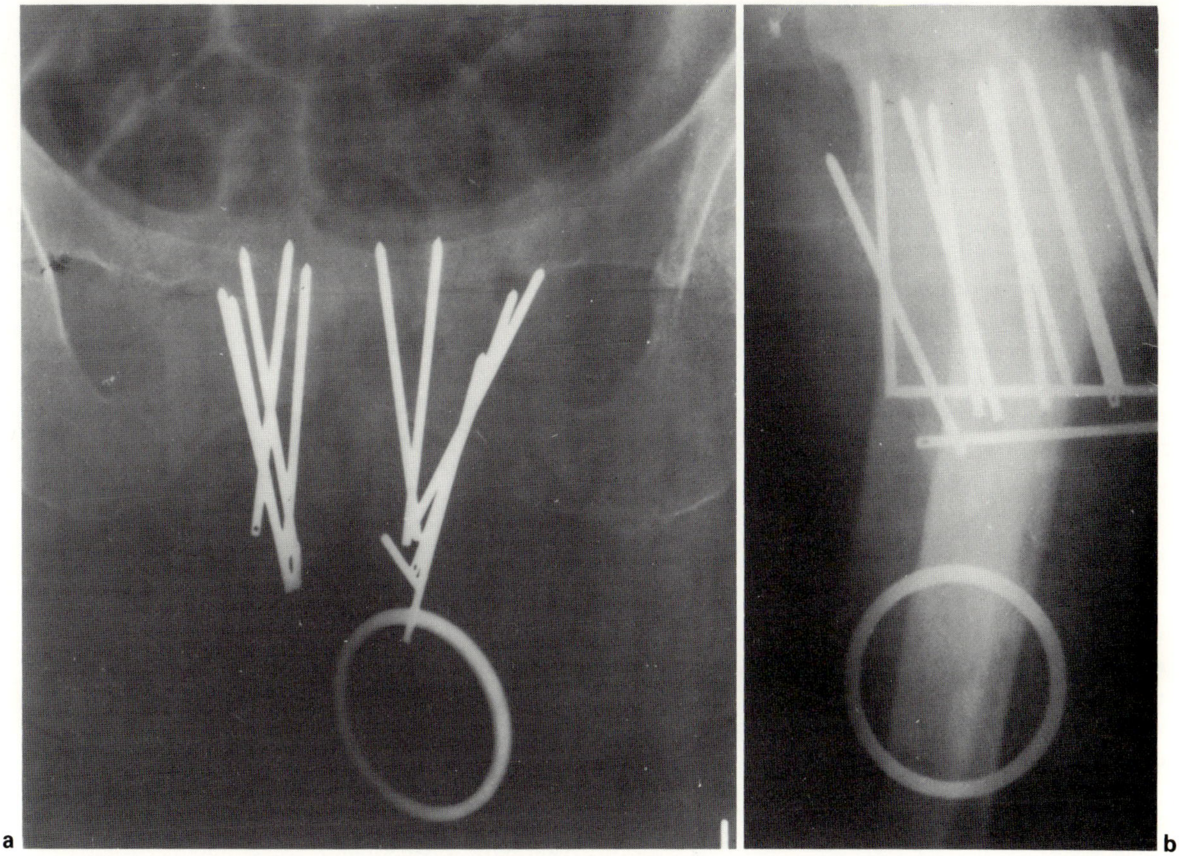

Fig. 12.8a,b. Vulvourethral carcinoma. Two-plane radium needle implant.

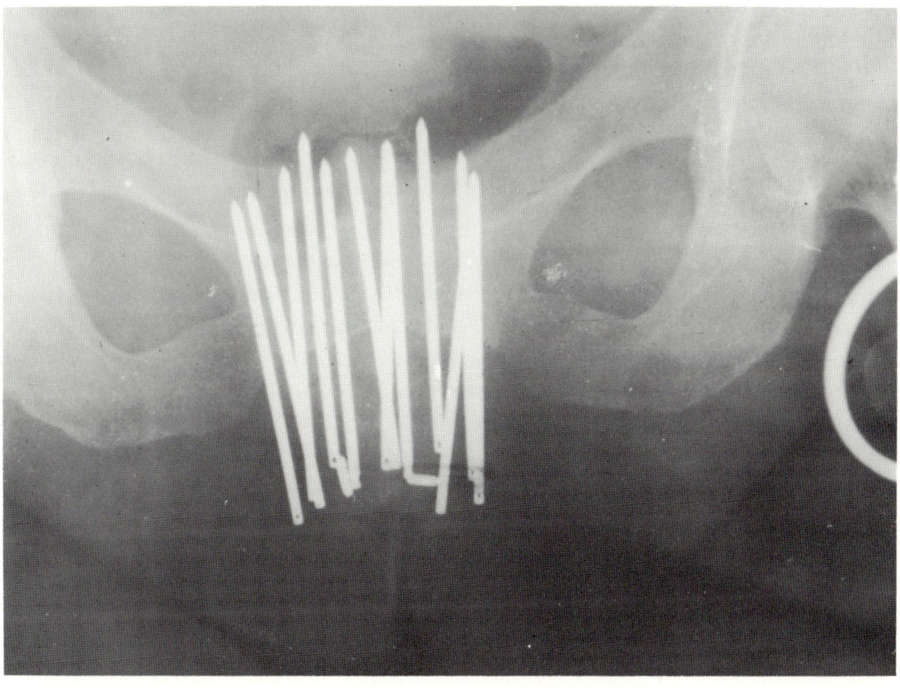

Fig. 12.9. Carcinoma of the urethra. Cylindrical radium needle implant.

Carcinoma of the Male Urethra

Primary carcinoma of the urethra is even less common in the male than the female. The onset of the disease is usually insidious and its symptoms are frequently attributed to a urethral stricture or benign lesion. When the tumour arises in the penile urethra a visible or palpable swelling may be present at a reasonably early stage. In the bulbous urethra, the presence of a urethral tumour may be overlooked or attributed to periurethral inflammation, eventually progressing to perineal abscess or fistula formation. Owing to these factors an early diagnosis is rarely made.

Treatment

Curative treatment depends on the feasibility of complete excision of the tumour. Owing to the nature of the disease, very rarely is radical radiotherapy feasible. Palliative radiotherapy seldom gives any significant benefit to the patient.

Carcinoma of the Penis

In England and Wales the incidence of carcinoma of the penis is approximately 1.5 per 100 000 males with a considerably higher incidence of the disease in aged males.

Pathological and Clinical Features

Squamous cell carcinoma of the penis arises principally from the glans penis in uncircumcised males. Less commonly, intra-epidermal carcinoma may occur of which one rare manifestation is the erythroplasia of Queyrat. The disease, as it advances, invades the corpora and in neglected cases may produce gross destruction of the penis.

Lymphatic spread is to the inguinal lymph nodes. However, as there is usually much associated sepsis, palpable inguinal nodes are invariably present and their significance may be clinically difficult to assess. Under these circumstances, the primary lesion should be dealt with and the nodes subsequently reassessed.

Treatment policy

The majority of patients with carcinoma of the penis can be treated satisfactorily by irradiation with consquent preservation of the organ and function. Contraindications to irradiation are (1) where there is obvious invasion of the corpora, amputation being then the treatment of choice, and (2) in the aged subject, when surgery affords a simple and expeditious method of treatment with minimal hospitalisation.

Treatment Methods

1) Cylindrical mould or applicator
2) 4-MV X-ray therapy
3) Interstitial irradiation

The preferred method of treatment is by means of megavoltage X-ray therapy. The advantages of this form of treatment over mould or interstitial therapy, are a high cure rate with acceptable morbidity, the reduction of significant radiation exposure to both patient and staff, and the fact that minimal technical skill is required and out-patient treatment is practicable.

Beam Direction Mould

The shaft of the organ is represented by a cylinder composed of a wooden dowel of appropriate diameter and length for the penile shaft and a wider dowel for the glans. The mould must be sufficiently long to include the organ and a minimum margin of 1.5 cm at its tip. To simulate the penis a model is assembled consisting of a brass rod upon which are fitted a wooden base dowel and two interchangeable dowels. The dimension of the shaft and glans are chosen and conjoined. The mould is constructed in two parts, connected by pairs of flanges which are clipped together, one on each side of the cylinder (Fig. 12.10b,c).

To form the mould, half the assemblage is embedded in a box of sand. The flanges are approximately 4 cm wide and are shaped over flat templates of metal or hardboard. These templates are laid along both sides of the cylinder, on the surface of the sand (Fig. 12.10d). Hot cellulose acetate sheet is moulded over the assemblage with the aid of a small thermoplastic forming machine.

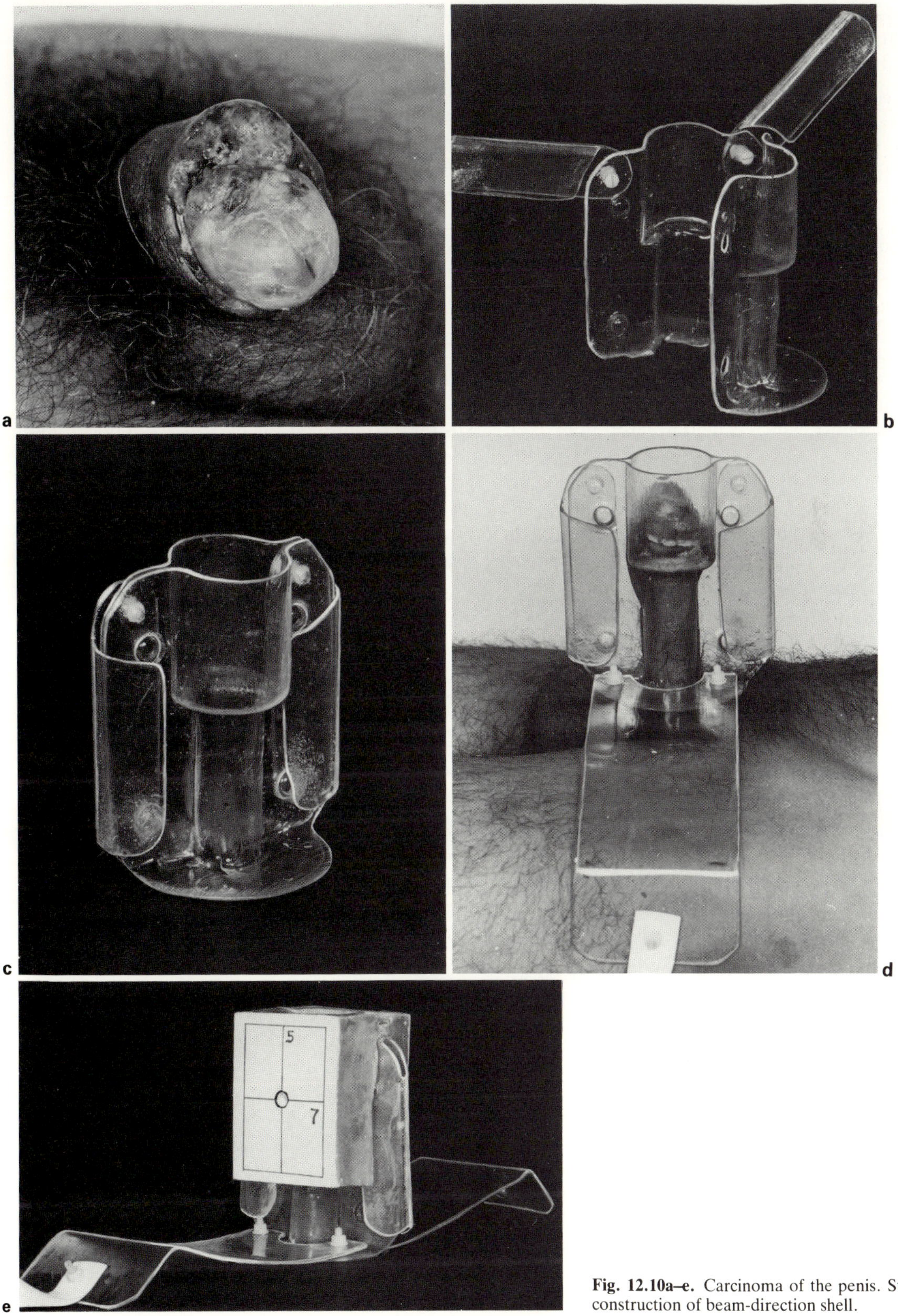

Fig. 12.10a–e. Carcinoma of the penis. Stages in construction of beam-direction shell.

The shaped plastic is trimmed to size and two large holes are drilled through each of the flanges for location purposes. The formed half of the mould is then replaced on its model and repositioned in the forming machine so that the shaped portion is embedded downwards in the sand. To avoid distortion whilst the other half of the mould is formed, the metal templates are replaced on the sand *under* the flanges. When the second half of the mould is formed, the hot CAB on its flanges sinks into the holes in their fellow flanges, producing nipples which locate the two portions together. The mould is trimmed, fitted to the patient and retained in position with two plastic clips, which hold the two flanges in contact on either side of the cylinder. The base wing is fitted to a thigh support, which is held in position by PVC straps.

The field sizes and their entrances and exits, are recorded on the plaques ready for treatment. The air-gap between the mould and the tip of the penis is packed with wet gauze bolus during treatment. A parallel pair of opposed fields is used with wax facings; these are built up with unit-density wax to ensure a minimum thickness of 1 cm. The mean interfield distance is usually of the order of 5 cm. The field sizes used to subtend the tumour with an adequate margin will vary from 5×5 cm to 8×6 cm. The dose delivered using a 4-MV linear accelerator is 5500–5250 cGy given in 16 exposures over 22 days. The ensuing radiation reaction is usually mild and settles within 4 weeks. In younger patients, satisfactory erection can be achieved, with the resumption of normal sexual relations.

Recurrence

Primary control with megavoltage is of the order of 84%. Recurrence should be treated by immediate surgery.

Necrosis

High-dose effects occur in less than 10% of cases. Necrosis of any magnitude should be treated by amputation.

Urethral Stricture

Urethral stricture at the meatus is not uncommon and can be managed by dilation. No stricture of great severity has been seen.

Secondary Inguinal Nodes

Significant mobile inguinal nodes should be treated by block dissection.

Reference

Turner AG, Hendry WF, MacDonald JS, Wallace DM (1976) The value of lymphography in the management of bladder cancer. Br J Urol 48: 579–586

13 Testis

R. Gibb and G. Read

Introduction

Despite their rarity tumours of the testis remain an important cause of mortality among young men. They rank behind only cerebral tumours and trauma as causes of death at this age. The incidence appears to be increasing world-wide. In England and Wales the Standardised Registration Ratio has risen from 2.1 to 2.8 per 100 000 males in the period from 1962 to 1972. This increase has been mainly in young men and is now the commonest neoplasm in men aged 25–34 (Table 13.1). This has also been reflected in the increased referral of patients to the Christie Hospital and Holt Radium Institute (Fig. 13.1). There is no

Table 13.1. Testicular tumours in England and Wales—rates per 100 000 in 1962 and 1972.

Age (years)	Rates		% Increase
	1962	1972	
0 –	0.4	0.6	
5 –	0.2	0	
15 –	1.8	3.1	71
25 –	4.6	7.4	62
35 –	4.0	4.9	22
45 –	2.4	2.4	0
55 –	1.4	1.6	16
65 –	1.0	1.5	
75 –	1.6	2.1	
All ages	2.1	2.8	31

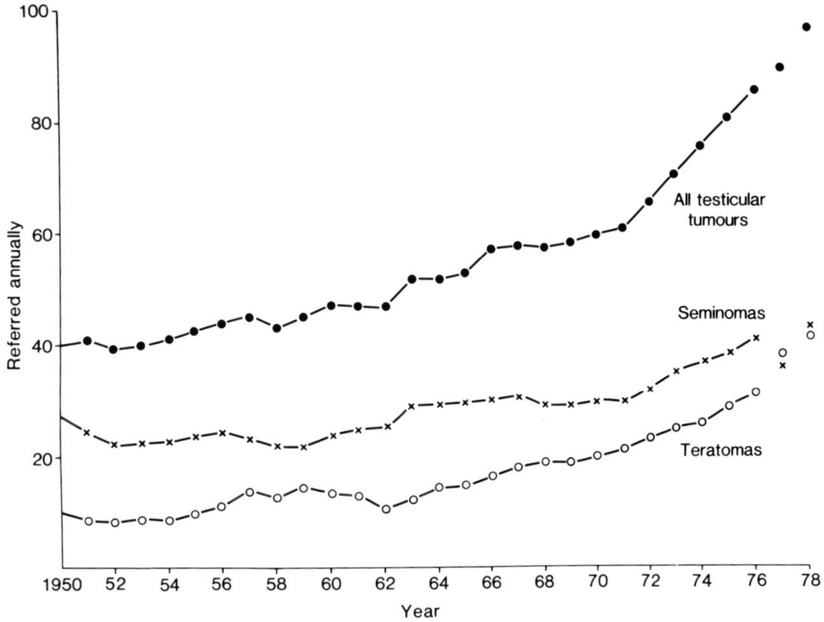

Fig. 13.1. Testicular tumours referred to the Christie Hospital 1950–1978: five-point moving average.

good explanation for these changes, the only constantly noted aetiological factor being maldescent of the testes. It has been calculated that a person with an undescended testis has roughly 50 times greater chance of developing a testicular tumour than a person with normally descended testes.

During the last 40 years there have been considerable advances in the management of these tumours. Initially, the only treatment available was orchidectomy. Subsequently, routine postoperative radiotherapy was added, and in patients adequately treated the overall 5-year survival rate rose to about 50% for all cases. Further improvement occurred when megavoltage radiation became available, and about the same time a renewed interest in the pathology of these tumours occurred in the United Kingdom sponsored by the Pathological Society of Great Britain and Ireland and the Cancer Research Campaign. A similar interest was shown in the United States by the Armed Forces Institute of Pathology. This led to more accurate histological diagnosis. The introduction of improved radiological and biochemical tests has improved the accuracy of the assessment of the spread of these tumours. Finally, the efficacy of chemotherapy has considerably increased.

Pathology

The pathological classification in general use in the United Kingdom is that of the Testicular Panel and Registry first published by Collins and Pugh in 1964 with subsequent modification in 1975. The types of tumour found in the testis, with their incidence in the Panel series, are shown in Table 13.2. The incidence of the various tumours differs with age. Teratomas are most usually found in the 20–30 age group with a mean age of 29.8 years. Seminomas are found a decade later with a mean age of 41.2 years. Tumours containing both teratomatous and seminomatous components are not uncommon. There were 13.5% "combined tumours" in the series reported by the Testicular Panel. The prognosis is that of the worst element. Malignant lymphoma of the testis is not common and is usually found in elderly men, with a peak incidence between 60 and 80 years. It is not uncommonly bilateral, whereas bilaterality occurs in other tumours in only 3%–8% of cases. The tumours are of the poorly differentiated lymphocytic or histiocytic type of non-Hodgkin's lymphoma. Apart from a few cases where the tumour is localised to the testis the prognosis is extremely poor. Their management is similar to that of extranodal lymphomas at other sites and is not described further here. Other tumours occasionally found are interstitial (Leydig) cell tumours and Sertoli cell tumours. These are usually benign and do not metastasise. In children orchioblastoma occurs and is discussed in detail in Chap. 16. The Panel's classification bears certain differences in the classification of teratomas from that of the Armed Forces Institute of Pathology generally used in the United States. The World Health Organization has attempted to produce a more universally accepted scheme. The equivalent classifications are shown in Table 13.3.

Table 13.2. Frequency of testicular tumours referred to the Testicular Tumour Panel and Registry 1958–1973. (From Pugh 1976)

	%	
Seminoma	39.5	91.4 (Seminoma to Malignant lymphoma)
Teratoma	31.7	
Combined tumours	13.5	
Malignant lymphoma	6.7	
Sertoli tumour	1.2	
Interstitial cell	1.6	
Yolk sac	1.9	
Metastasis	0.9	
Miscellaneous	0.8	
Uncertain	2.2	

Modes of Spread

A knowledge of the possible modes of spread of these tumours is vitally important in planning their investigation and treatment.

The tunica albuginea presents an effective barrier to spread. It is therefore unusual for direct extension into the scrotum to occur unless this barrier has been breached by surgical intervention. Spread may then occur to the external inguinal nodes which are normally unaffected. Usually lymphatic spread occurs via the spermatic cord through four to eight channels to the para-aortic region. The right-sided lymphatics pass principally to nodes opposite lumbar vertebrae 1–3. These

Table 13.3. Teratoma classifications compared.

TTPR 1964	TTPR 1975	AFIP 1973	WHO 1975
Teratoma differentiated	Teratoma differentiated	Teratoma mature Teratoma immature	Teratoma mature Teratoma immature
Malignant teratoma intermediate A	Malignant teratoma intermediate	Embryonal carcinoma with teratoma[a]	Teratoma with malignant transformation Embryonal carcinoma with teratoma
Malignant teratoma intermediate B Malignant teratoma anaplastic	Malignant teratoma undifferentiated	Embryonal carcinoma	Embryonal carcinoma
Malignant teratoma trophoblastic	Malignant teratoma trophoblastic	Chorioncarcinoma[a]	Chorioncarcinoma[a]
	Yolk-sac tumour	Infantile embryonal carcinoma	Yolk-sac tumour (infantile embryonal carcinoma)

[a] With other elements specified if present
TTPR—Testicular Tumour Panel and Registry
AFIP—Armed Forces Institute of Pathology
WHO—World Health Organization

nodes are situated between the aorta and the inferior vena cava and also lie anteriorly to the vena cava. The left-sided vessels pass to the left para-aortic region opposite the first and second lumbar vertebrae. Retrograde spread may occur to the common iliac nodes, but involvement of these nodes in the absence of para-aortic disease is uncommon. Similarly, spread to the contralateral nodes only may occur but is rare. Further dissemination may occur via the thoracic duct to the left supraclavicular nodes. Spread may also occur to the paravertebral and mediastinal nodes and then to both supraclavicular fossae. Haematogenous spread may occur early, particularly with undifferentiated teratomas.

Staging

Originally the Christie Hospital used a simple system of staging. Where there was no clinical evidence of residual or metastatic disease after orchidectomy, the classification was "postoperative, healed". If clinically detectable residue at the site of the primary was present, the term "postoperative, residual" was used, while "postoperative, metastatic" described the case with metastatic disease present. If the patient presented without orchidectomy the staging was either "early" or "late". However, the prognosis in testicular tumours is related not only to the extent but also the volume of the disease present. A more detailed scheme taking into account these factors is now in use (Table 13.4). This is in line with similar

Table 13.4. Staging scheme for testicular tumours as practised at the Christie Hospital.

Stage	
I	Disease confined to the testicle established by negative radiology and biochemical tumours negative or returning to normal. Tumour does not extend to cut end of cord.
IIM+	As stage I but biochemical tumour markers remain elevated.
IIA	No clinically residual or metastatic disease but abdominal nodal involvement established by investigative procedure.
IIB	Palpable abdominal nodal disease or scrotal residue.
III	Disease involves mediastinal and/or supraclavicular nodes, with or without nodal disease below the diaphragm.
IVA	Lung metastases—less than six metastases not more than 2 cm diameter.
IVB	Lung metastases—more extensive than stage IVA.
IVC	Extranodal metastases other than lung.

schemes used in other major centres. Stages I and IIA now include the patients formerly designated "early", or "postoperative, healed".

Management

Owing to the specialised nature of much of the investigation and treatment of these tumours it is generally agreed that they are best managed in regional centres with the appropriate facilities.

The majority of patients referred to a radiotherapist will already have had an orchidectomy. The operation should always be performed through a groin incision with high ligation of the cord before removal of the organ. Scrotal incisions should be avoided as this may lead to spill of tumour and the radiation reaction is more troublesome when the scrotum is included in the volume subsequently irradiated. Preliminary biopsy or frozen section is not usually advisable because of the difficulties in ensuring that a representative piece of the tumour has been obtained. Advantage should be taken while the patient is anaesthetised to palpate the abdomen for possible nodal masses. Even when distant metastases are obvious it is still desirable for the testis to be removed to allow an accurate diagnosis to be made. Biopsy of sites of suspected metastases, e.g. a supraclavicular node, may also be necessary. This may not only confirm the presence of disease at that site but may occasionally reveal that the primary tumour contains more than one pathological element.

Clinical Assessment

The radiotherapist's assessment of the patient begins with the clinical examination. A full abdominal including rectal examination is important. Residual masses in the affected side of the scrotum will more often be found to be due to haematoma than residual tumour. The presence of supraclavicular nodes must be carefully sought and any gynaecomastia noted.

Investigations

The aim of investigation is to determine the extent of the tumour and the fitness of the patient for treatment. It is not always necessary to perform all the investigations described, but only sufficient to allow proper planning of the patient's treatment. All patients, however, should have a full blood count, urine analyses, and creatinine clearance and liver function tests.

The investigations in common use are set out below:

Chest Radiography

Posteroanterior, penetrated posteroanterior, and lateral films should be taken. Only by including a penetrated film can small paravertebral nodes be seen (Figs. 13.2 and 13.3). Whole lung tomography is performed routinely in some centres, but we relied on plain films of high quality until CT scanning (see below) became available.

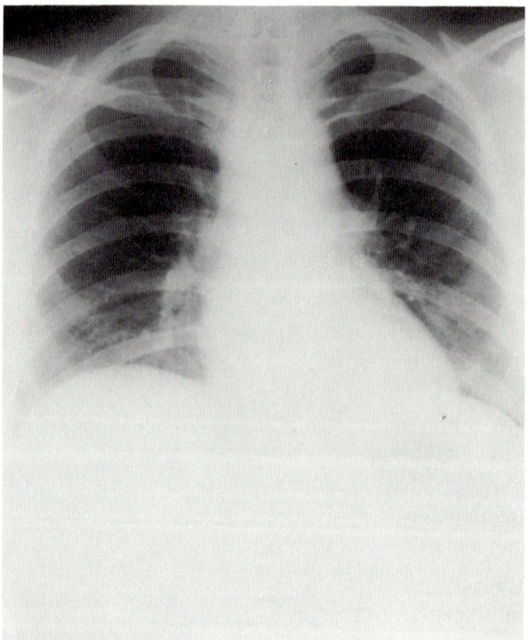

Fig. 13.2. Standard PA radiograph of chest in patient with seminoma.

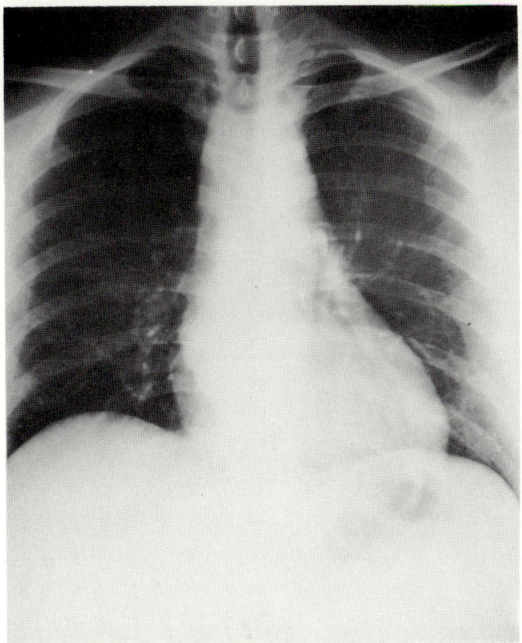

Fig. 13.3. Penetrated radiograph of same patient as in Fig. 13.2, showing paravertebral mass.

Computer Tomography (CT Scanning)

This investigation has proved to be invaluable. It is required in all cases of teratoma except those where metastases are obvious and is also necessary in cases of seminoma where an abdominal mass is suspected. Preparation of the intestinal tract is achieved with two daily doses of Isogel granules over 48 h. On the evening before and on the day of the examination 5% Gastrografin (250 ml) is given orally. Intravenous Bucospan (or Pro-Banthine) may be given to inhibit bowel movement. Intravenous iodine-containing contrast medium is also given in a dose of 50 ml in order to produce pyeloureterography. This investigation is ideally suited to assessing para-aortic and paravertebral nodes, and masses not visualised by lymphography may be demonstrated (Figs. 13.4 and 13.5). Chest metastases not visible on plain films may also be found (Figs. 13.6 and 13.7), but caution is necessary as they may appear similar to innocent "postinfective" nodules. A repeat scan after a suitable interval should be carried out where there is doubt.

Intravenous Urography

This is always required before radiotherapy to determine the position of the kidneys (see Fig. 13.8). Deviation of the ureters may be apparent due to enlarged para-aortic nodes, but this is not a reliable sign. Hydronephrosis or a non-functioning kidney is usually associated with considerable nodal involvement.

Bipedal Lymphography

Where CT scanning is not available, bipedal lymphography should be performed in teratoma patients where there is no palpable abdominal lymph node mass, but can be omitted where an obvious mass exists. In seminoma patients with no palpable abdominal mass, this investigation is omitted at the Christie Hospital because the technique used to irradiate the abdomen in such patients more than adequately covers the abdominal lymphatic pathways demonstrated by the examination (see Fig. 13.9). Apart from technical failures, about 15%–20% of patients with negative lymphograms will still have nodal metastases.

Biochemical Tumour Markers

These tests are of particular importance in teratomas, which can produce alpha-foetoprotein (AFP) and/or human chorionic gonadotrophin (HCG)—the beta subunit of the latter is the most specific (see Table 13.5). These substances are measured in serum samples. Ideally pre-orchidectomy levels should be obtained, but this is not always possible. A postoperative series of readings should be obtained to avoid confusion with previous high levels due to the primary tumour. Persistent or rising elevation is a reliable indication of residual disease. The marker levels should also be estimated at each follow-up visit. A rising titre indicates recurrent disease although it may not be clinically or radiologically demonstrable until 4–6 months later. A small proportion of seminomas produce HCG but never AFP. A raised AFP titre in a case of seminoma indicates that the primary is really a combined tumour, unless there are liver metastases.

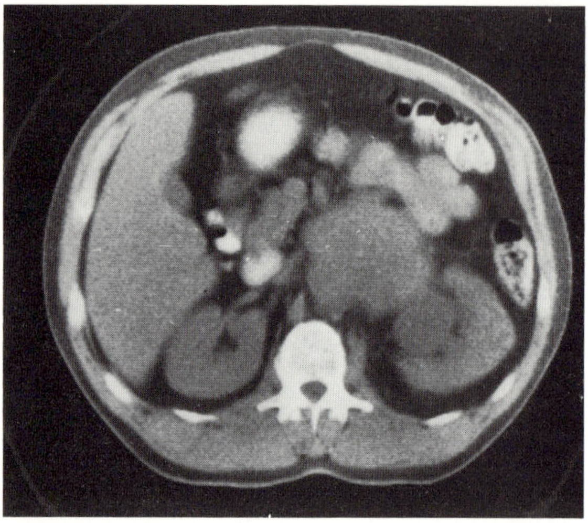

Fig. 13.4. CT scan of abdomen in a patient with seminoma showing large left para-aortic mass obstructing left kidney.

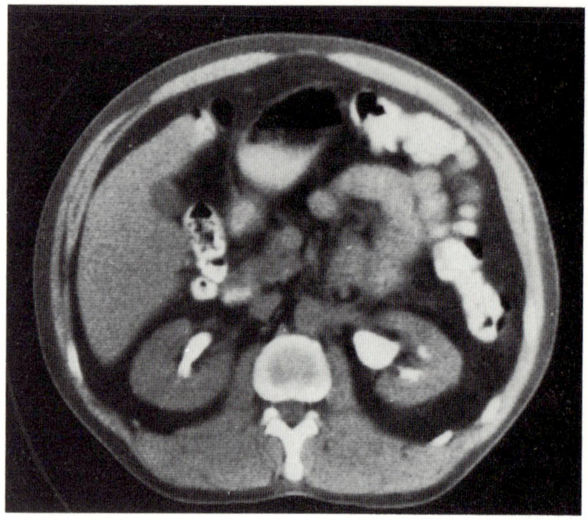

Fig. 13.5. Same patient as in Fig. 13.4, showing complete resolution of mass following radiotherapy.

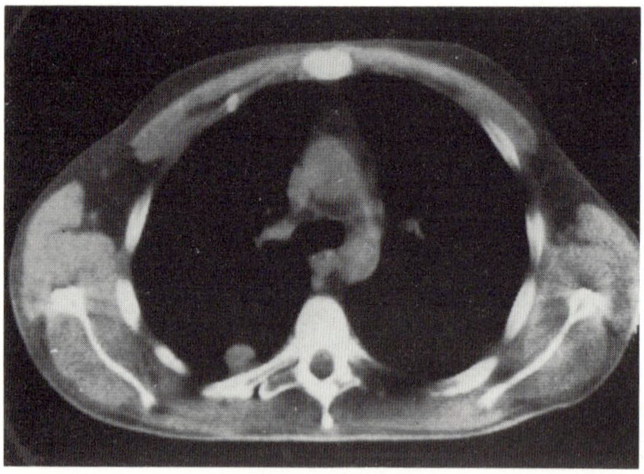

Fig. 13.6. CT scan of thorax in a patient with malignant teratoma showing subpleural metastasis.

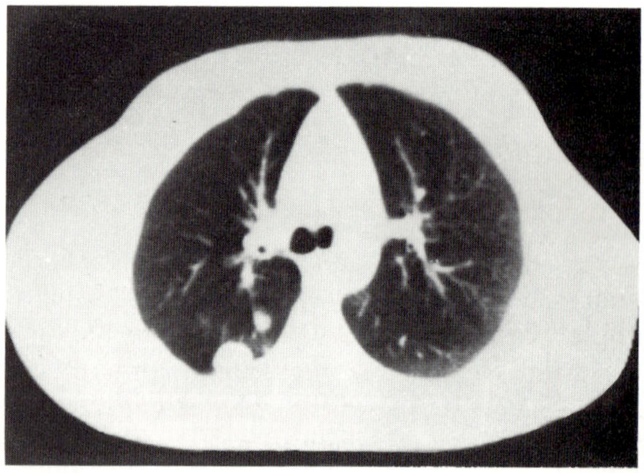

Fig. 13.7. Same patient as in Fig. 13.6: further metastasis shown by altering "window" setting.

Table 13.5. Biochemical tumour markers. (Modified from Javadpour 1979)

Units and subunits	Half-life	Cross-reactivity	Source
Alpha-foetoprotein	5 days	None	Foetal liver Teratoma of testis Hepatoma Yolk-sac tumour of ovary
HCG	24 h	FSH, TSH, LH	Placenta Seminoma/teratoma of testis
Alpha-HCG	20 min	FSH, LSH, LH	Placenta Seminoma/teratoma of testis
Beta-HCG	60 min	None	Placenta Seminoma/teratoma of testis

Isotope Scans

Isotope scans of the brain or liver are occasionally required where CT scanning is not available. Seminoma deposits, wherever situated, may be visualised using gallium-67 citrate, but the scans may be difficult to interpret. Ultrasound scanning of the liver may be helpful in identifying liver metastases.

Others

Other investigations such as inferior vena cavography and arteriography are now unnecessary since the advent of CT scanning.

Treatment

For many years the approach to treatment for both seminoma and teratoma was the same. Following a simple orchidectomy, postoperative X-ray therapy was given to the abdomen in the form of an abdominal "bath", which eventually extended from the dome of the diaphragm to the perineum. This particular technique was abandoned because of renal damage in a number of patients, and attempts were then made to shield the kidneys for part or all of the treatment time. When megavoltage irradiation became available this was comparatively easy to do and indeed a field of any desired shape was possible. It eventually became clear that higher radiation doses were required for teratoma, and to achieve this smaller volumes had to be irradiated. Lymphography and CT scanning have made it possible to tailor fields more accurately to the area of disease. In the treatment of seminoma there has been no need to alter the "bath" concept. Chemotherapy to date has been demonstrated to be of more value in teratoma than in seminoma, and in these two main groups of testicular tumours the treatment policies now show little resemblance to one another, hence the need to deal with them here under separate headings.

Treatment Policy—Seminoma

Seminoma is a very radiosensitive tumour. Large volumes of tissue can therefore be irradiated to doses which, though relatively small, are still cancerocidal. Disseminated metastases tend to occur only late in the natural history of the tumour and seminoma is therefore also eminently radiocurable.

Stage I and IIA ("Early")

Of those patients in whom there is no clinically residual disease following orchidectomy, a proportion will still have some involvement of the abdominal nodes. Although the proportion is small the difficulty of identifying these patients led to the policy of advising routine postoperative irradiation for all. The results of this decision have been so good that it has seemed unwise to change it. In particular it has not been felt necessary to advocate the more detailed assessment which is now given to patients with teratoma. All patients are therefore given large-field irradiation, with kidney shielding, to the abdominal nodes and scrotum as detailed below.

It is our policy to include the scrotum and contralateral testis in the field with consequent sterility (but not impotence). Although there is no disagreement that this should be done where there has been a scrotal incision or biopsy, some radiotherapists dispute whether it is necessary in all cases. In our series of many hundreds of patients in whom scrotal irradiation has been practised, *no true case of a second tumour has been recorded*. Second tumours, reported by other workers, may be of the same histological type as the first, or may be of the "opposite" type. Since the second tumour may prove to be fatal, its occurrence should be avoided if possible and with the availability now of sperm storage facilities for future artificial insemination, the question of sterility is of less concern to the patient. Even if an attempt is made to shield the scrotum and the lower limit of the field is at the symphysis pubis, the remaining testis will still receive a dose of scattered radiation of the order of 50–150 cGy. Whilst this may not produce azoospermia, it might well be responsible for genetic damage.

Stage IIB

In patients in this category, with palpable abdominal metastases, it may be necessary to increase the volume irradiated to include paravertebral disease in the lower thoracic region which is detected by use of penetrated X-ray films and/or CT scanning of the area. No attempt is made initially to shield the kidneys, as this might reduce the dose of radiation to involved nodes. When a midline dose of 2000 cGy has been delivered, shielding of at least one kidney (preferably both) must be introduced. Irradiation is then continued until the full dose of 3000 cGy in 20 fractions over 4 weeks is given.

It is not our practice routinely to give prophylactic irradiation of the mediastinum and supraclavicular fossae. This, however, may be considered when circumstances (such as residence of the patient abroad) will not permit careful follow-up.

Stage III

When there is involvement of the mediastinum or mediastinum and supraclavicular fossa(e) irradiation of the whole of the nodal axis from the pelvis to the supraclavicular fossae must be undertaken. This will involve the patient in two courses of radiation, separated by an interval of 4 weeks to allow recovery of the bone marrow. The chest treatment is usually given first, but if there are clamant abdominal symptoms a "holding dose" of 500 cGy can be given to the supraclavicular fossa and/or mediastinum in a single exposure and the full abdominal treatment is then given. The small single dose can be ignored when the subsequent chest treatment is given.

If there is involvement of the left supraclavicular fossa only, it is possible to irradiate this alone concurrently with the abdominal treatment. This reduces considerably the overall time the patient spends undergoing radiation treatment, but it must be accepted that about half the patients will subsequently relapse in the mediastinum and will then require further radiation.

Stage IV

There is probably no other malignant solid tumour in which it is so worthwhile to persevere with treatment even in the presence of lung metastases or other extranodal disease. Despite the radiosensitivity of the tumour, however, the prognosis at this stage is not good, but in the majority of cases an attempt must be made to irradiate systematically all sites of disease. Attention is directed first to the area causing the most clamant symptoms. If the response is satisfactory other affected areas may then be irradiated.

Consideration should be given to treatment of patients with disseminated disease by chemotherapy; although the response previously compared unfavourably with that in teratoma, newer combinations appear to be more effective. A full statement of the principles and practice of chemotherapy is given in Chap. 3 and no attempt is made to go into detail in this section.

Treatment Policy—Teratoma

Although teratoma is not as radiosensitive as seminoma, local eradication of the tumour is possible provided the volume irradiated is small enough to allow an adequate dose to be given. The tumour may, however, metastasise widely at an early stage and is therefore much less often curable by radiotherapy alone. The prognosis has improved considerably in recent years, but successful management depends upon detailed investigation of the extent of the tumour and a combination of chemotherapy, radiotherapy, and in some cases surgery.

Until recently the "postoperative, healed" or "early" cases (stages I and IIA in the present classification) were treated by prophylactic abdominal irradiation. More sophisticated methods of investigation, in particular CT scanning and biochemical tumour markers, have made it possible to differentiate accurately between stages I and IIA. In stage I cases, metastases are likely to develop in only about 20% of patients, and in about half of these lung involvement will be the first manifestation. With the advent of effective chemotherapy it is now possible to adopt an expectant policy in these cases as detailed below.

Stage I

If, after a satisfactory orchidectomy all the various detailed investigations are negative, no further treatment is given and the patient is kept on a very close follow-up. It must be strongly emphasised that this can only be safely undertaken in a specialised centre with facilities for repeating the various initial investigations. If these facilities are not available it is probably better to give prophylactic abdominal irradiation.

Stage IIA

From our previous experience of prophylactic irradiation noted above, it is to be assumed that postoperative radiotherapy alone cured some patients with minimal abdominal disease. We also know that a substantial proportion of such patients will develop further metastases, usually in the lungs. In view of this, it seems wise to give chemotherapy initially—to deal with potential metastases—and to follow this with X-ray therapy to the known disease in the abdomen. It is our experience that these treatments are better tolerated when given in this order rather than the reverse.

Stage IIB

Patients with bulky disease are not curable by radiotherapy alone. Chemotherapy is given first, and by reducing the bulk of the disease may permit the irradiation of a smaller volume to a higher dose. If the disease was very extensive, or there is an incomplete response, indicated by failure of marker levels to return to normal, the chemotherapy is extended from four to six or eight courses before the irradiation.

Stage III

Chemotherapy is given first, followed by radiotherapy to the whole nodal axis from the pelvis to the supraclavicular fossa. No prophylactic irradiation is given to the lung fields.

Stage IV

Chemotherapy is given initially, but may need to be more intensive than in patients with less extensive disease. Radiotherapy is given to sites of residual nodal disease if the response is not complete, but where the response has been good, consideration can be given to surgical excision of solitary abdominal nodes or peripheral lung metastases when these remain. These masses are frequently found to be comprised entirely of differentiated or necrotic tissue.

Radical Radiotherapy Techniques

Abdominal—Large Volume

This is used for "prophylactic" irradiation in seminoma and is described in detail. A similar method of localisation is used for the other treatment plans which follow. The technique described does not require a lymphangiogram or CT scan, but when these are available the information obtained may profitably be used to modify the plan.

An intravenous pyelogram is performed with the patient lying supine and with a wire marker across the iliac crests. The film is taken at a fixed focus-skin distance (FSD) and this allows the use of a ruler (with divisions magnified to the same extent) to be used to plan the treatment on the radiograph. The upper limit of the field is taken at the level of the upper pole of the higher kidney—usually D11. The kidneys are outlined on the film. The lateral limits of the upper portion of the field which follow the inner borders of the two kidneys are then drawn on the film. The appropriate measurements are then made using the magnified ruler (Fig. 13.8). The remainder of the planning is done on the patient using a simulator. The position of the wire marker is first drawn on the patient with gentian violet or other suitable marking material. The lines drawn on the radiograph can be transferred to the patient using a standard metric ruler. A field centred on the midline and extending laterally to the iliac crests will adequately cover the regional lymph nodes (Fig. 13.9). The operation scar is included, with adequate bolus. Using sandbags, the scrotum is displaced proximally into

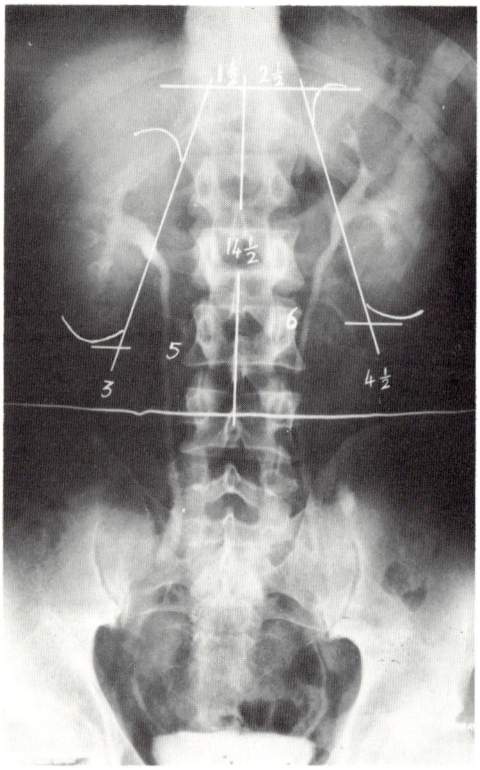

Fig. 13.8. Intravenous urogram with wire marker, upper part of field drawn with measurements.

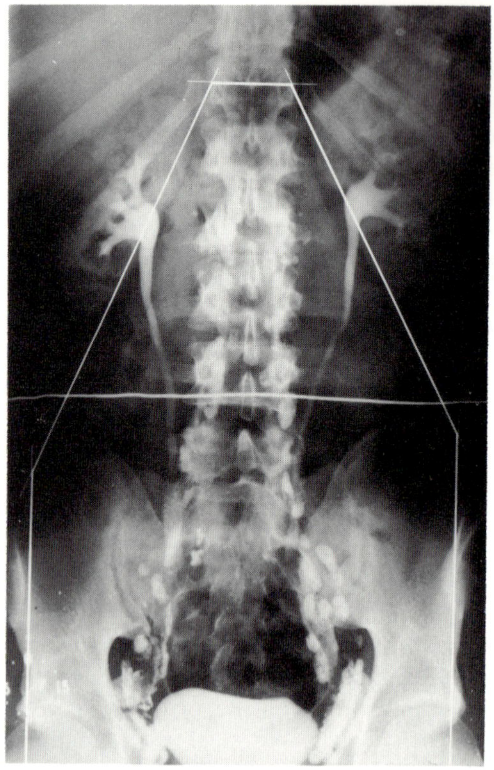

Fig. 13.9. Intravenous urogram and lymphogram showing field for prophylactic irradiation in seminoma.

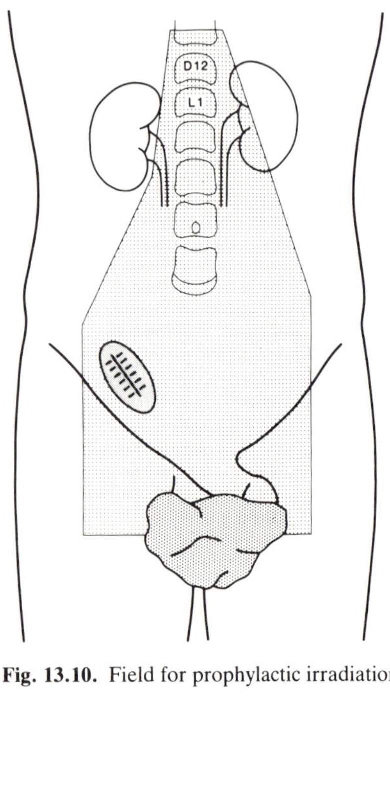

Fig. 13.10. Field for prophylactic irradiation in seminoma.

the field, thus reducing its length. The remaining lines can be drawn on the patient after the field has been "squared up", using the simulator lights. The complete field is shown in Fig. 13.10. After measuring the anteroposterior diameter, the length of the various segments of the lines is measured and recorded. The patient is turned into the prone position and the outline of the field is reproduced on the patient's back. The set-up is that of a parallel opposed pair of fields. It is important to check that the length of the posterior field is correctly positioned and includes the whole of the scrotum. The upper, lower, and lateral limits of the fields and their centres should be tattooed on the patient's skin with Indian ink, so that any future additional treatment fields, e.g. to the lung, may be accurately applied .

Because of the length of the fields involved (usually 40 cm or more) it is necessary to use an increased FSD of 140–160 cm on a 4-MV linear accelerator. Fields of this size are less easy to achieve on telecobalt machines. The mid-plane dose of 3000 cGy is delivered in 20 fractions (treating one field per day) over 4 weeks. In cases of seminoma with palpable upper abdominal disease the whole abdomen, as distinct from the volume shown in Fig. 13.10, is treated, both kidneys being included in the field. When a dose of 2000 cGy is reached in about $2\frac{1}{2}$ weeks the intravenous pyelogram is repeated, using the same marker line which was previously tattooed, and part or all of one or both kidneys is shielded to reduce the risk of subsequent radiation nephritis. The treatment is then continued to a total dose of 3000 cGy in 20 fractions in 4 weeks.

Where a patient has refused to have the remaining testis irradiated, the lower edge of the field is placed at the pubic symphysis. The scrotum is "bagged" out of the field and additional lead used at the bottom of the field. If possible, this should never be done where there has been a scrotal incision or biopsy.

The field used for "prophylactic" irradiation in teratoma is similar to that used in seminoma, except that the contralateral extent of the field is reduced, thus allowing a higher dose of 3500 cGy in 20 fractions over 4 weeks to be given (Fig. 13.11).

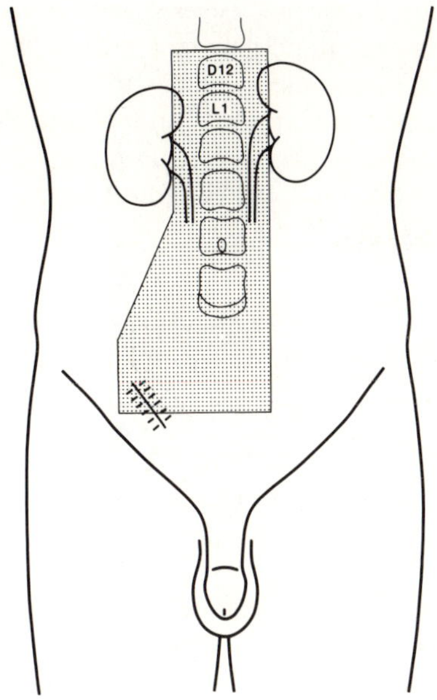

Fig. 13.12. Field for irradiation of para-aortic and ipsilateral iliac nodes in teratoma.

Abdominal—Small Volume

There is no place for the use of small fields in seminoma except for palliative treatments. Following chemotherapy in teratoma, more restricted fields are used directed to the sites of disease identified on the lymphangiogram or CT scan. The smaller volume employed allows a higher dose to be given. Figure 13.12 shows a field encompassing the para-aortic and ipsilateral iliac node areas to which a dose of 4000 cGy in 20 fractions over 4 weeks is given. If the para-aortic area only is treated, the smaller volume permits a reduction in overall time and 4000 cGy may be given in 16 fractions over 21 days (Fig. 13.13).

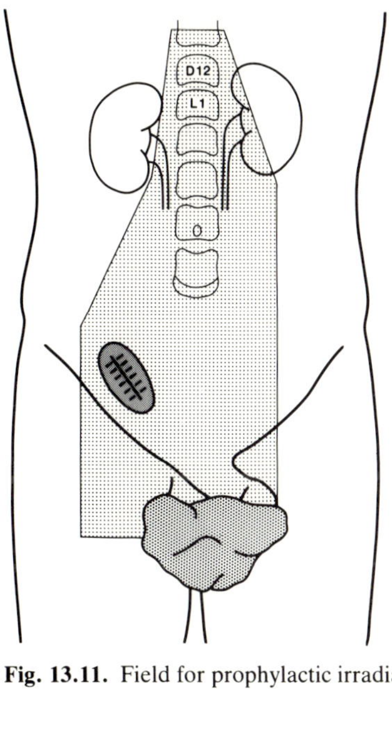

Fig. 13.11. Field for prophylactic irradiation in teratoma.

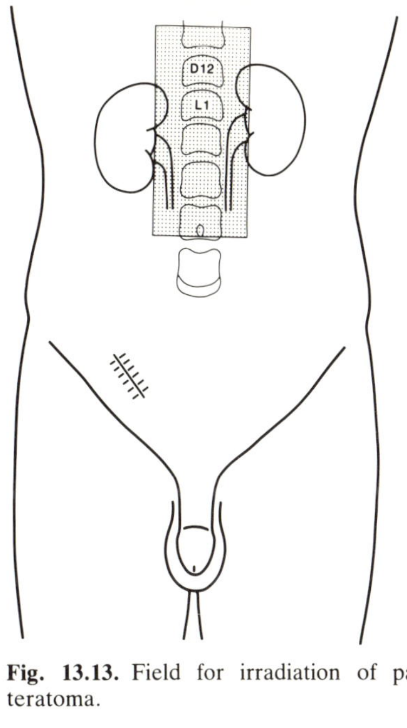

Fig. 13.13. Field for irradiation of para-aortic nodes in teratoma.

At this stage it is important to remember that following chemotherapy there may be a reduction in tissue tolerances. In particular, kidney tolerance is reduced following cis-platinum, and if much renal tissue has to be irradiated it is recommended that a dose of 1500 cGy in 3 weeks should not be exceeded.

Chest Bath

A full chest bath is rarely called for now, except in cases of seminoma with parenchymal lung metastases, although in the past complete responses were occasionally obtained in undifferentiated teratoma.

In many instances the patient will have had abdominal irradiation previously. The lower edge of the chest field may then be matched on to the tattoo marks denoting the upper edge of the abdominal field, allowing a 1-cm gap to avoid overlap at the spinal cord. Otherwise the lower edge is at the xiphisternum. As shown in Fig. 13.14, the lateral parts of the field may have to be extended downwards to ensure that the whole of the lung bases are properly included. Care must be taken to minimise the amount of radiation given to the kidneys and liver. The surface marking for the lateral border of the lungs is at the lateral border of the areola of the nipple. Superiorly the pleural reflection extends to 3 cm above the middle third of the clavicle. It is wise, however, to include both supraclavicular fossae in the field even if there is no obvious involvement. A small piece of lead is put over the larynx to minimise the reaction there. A check radiograph is taken and any necessary alterations made. The field is then reproduced on the patient's back, again taking care to ensure that the anterior and posterior fields are congruent.

Considerable inhomogeneity will result when the chest is treated by a parallel arrangement of fields because of the increased transmission of X-rays by lung tissue. A typical isodose distribution at mid-chest level is shown in Fig. 13.15. Although there will be a variation in this dose distribution at different levels in the chest, the major part of both lungs will receive 110%–120% of the central midplane dose. If no correction is made for lung transmission the maximum dose tolerable is 2500 cGy (soft tissue midplane) in 20 fractions over 4 weeks. The major part of both lungs will then receive a dose of 3000 cGy. If chemotherapy has been given previously, a reduction in dose is required and it is not safe to give more than 2000 cGy mid-plane dose in the same overall time and fractionation.

For a number of years the soft tissue midplane dose of 2500 cGy was given over 3 weeks, but a study of the patients so treated revealed that a number may have died of radiation fibrosis of the lungs without evidence of recurrent disease. This led to the increased overall time of 4 weeks quoted above.

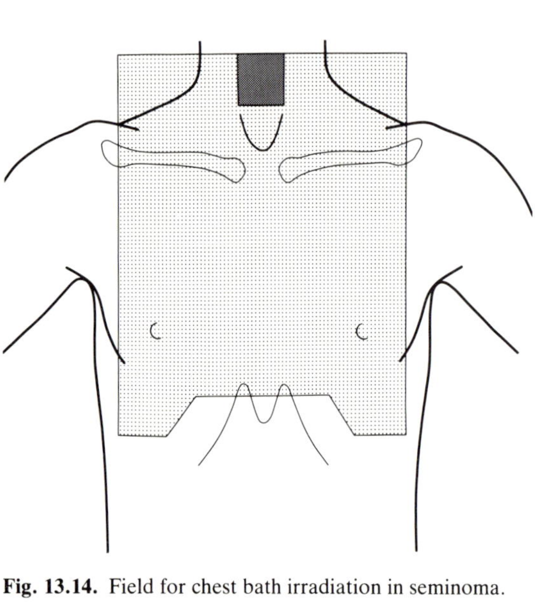

Fig. 13.14. Field for chest bath irradiation in seminoma.

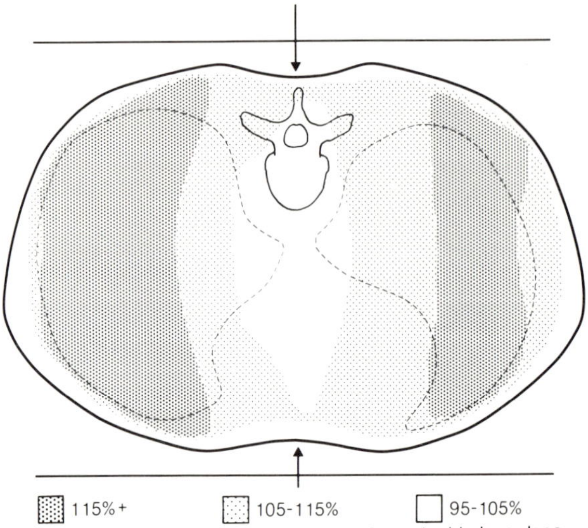

Fig. 13.15. Chest bath—isodose curves at mid chest level at 4 MV. (By permission Longman Group Ltd)

Other Chest Techniques

In the majority of cases where the mediastinum and/or supraclavicular fossa(e) are involved the whole of the mediastinum and both supraclavicular fossae will be treated by a T-shaped parallel pair of fields, as shown in Fig. 13.6. In seminoma, when only a modest dose is required, a midplane dose of 3000 cGy given over 3 weeks is satisfactory. With teratoma a higher dose is necessary and 3500 cGy is prescribed with an increase in the overall time to 4 weeks. A dose of this magnitude is likely to exceed the tolerance of the length of the spinal cord (over 15 cm) included in this volume and the cord is therefore shielded by a 2-cm-wide block of lead for half of the posterior treatments. The technique is similar to that employed in "mantle" treatments (Chap. 14) and to compensate for the loss of dose an additional 600 cGy is given to the anterior mediastinal strip.

If only the supraclavicular fossa is treated, a single megavoltage field is used, with the patient lying supine and the head straight (Fig. 13.17). Any biopsy scars will require bolus and the larynx is shielded with lead. Suitable doses are 2500 cGy in eight fractions or 3000 cGy in 16 fractions for seminoma, and 3500 in eight fractions or 4000 in 16 fractions for teratoma.

On occasions it may be necessary to treat solitary lung metastases by radical radiotherapy. Parallel-pair, three-field, or rotation techniques similar to those used in the treatment of carcinoma of the lung (Chap. 9) may be appropriate, depending upon the site and size of the lesion. Doses in the range 3500–4500 cGy in 16 fractions over 3 weeks may be given, depending upon the volume irradiated.

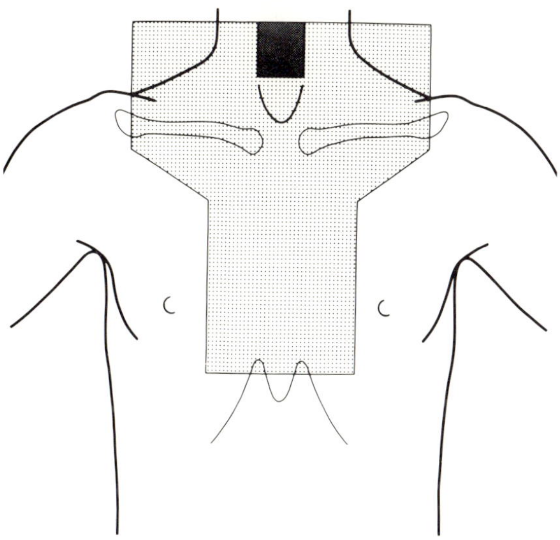

Fig. 13.16. Field for irradiation of mediastinum and supraclavicular fossae.

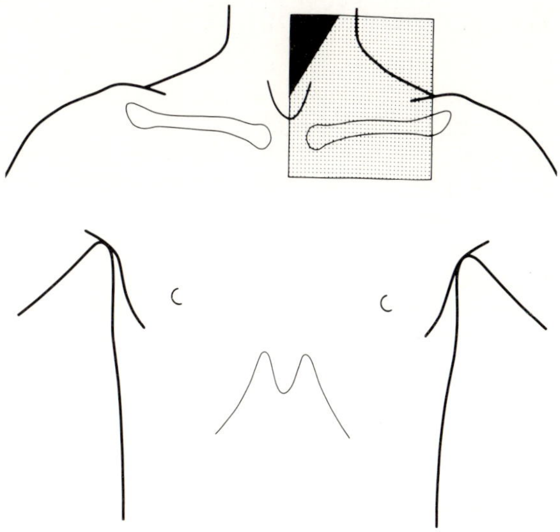

Fig. 13.17. Field for irradiation of left supraclavicular fossa.

Palliative Radiotherapy Techniques

It is seldom that an initial attempt at radical treatment by radiotherapy and/or chemotherapy cannot be made in testicular tumours. Occasionally, however, the disease is too advanced or the general condition of the patient too poor to allow a radical approach, and for such patients and for those whose disease has not been controlled initially and has become widespread, some form of palliative radiotherapy is often possible to relieve symptoms.

An extensive abdominal mass—say 20×20 cm—may be given 2000 cGy in eight fractions over 10 days using parallel opposed fields. A similar arrangement is used for chest metastases producing symptoms. In both nodal and extranodal metastases causing pain, single exposures of 1000–1500 cGy are given, depending on the field size. Cerebral metastases secondary to seminoma should be treated by whole brain irradiation, using a parallel opposed pair of fields and a midplane dose of 3000 cGy in eight fractions over 10 days.

Management During Radiotherapy

Where radiotherapy is given as the first treatment, the large volume abdominal radiation is usually well tolerated. Nausea and vomiting are mild and only experienced at the outset. If they are troublesome, the patient may be helped by pyridoxine, which is always worth trying first, or by antiemetics such as chlorpromazine or prochlorperazine. As the radiation treatment progresses some small-bowel colic and diarrhoea are experienced, but codeine phosphate in a small dose, such as 30 mg twice-daily, is usually sufficient to control this. A full blood count must be done twice weekly, or more often if the count is falling. Normally the fall in the white cell and/or platelet count is not sufficient to warrant interruption of treatment. It may, however, occasionally be necessary to suspend treatment to allow some recovery of the bone marrow. Even with megavoltage radiation, when the scrotum is included in the radiated volume, a troublesome but unavoidable skin reaction occurs, confined to the inner aspects of the upper thighs, the perineum and around the anus. Steroid creams, such as 1% hydrocortisone or betamethasone, either alone or combined with an antiseptic such as clioquinol, are helpful. When the reaction in the groin is severe the application of gentian violet (0.75% aqueous solution) gives the most relief. In patients with extensive deposits of seminoma, a rapid response to radiotherapy can occasionally result in large amounts of uric acid being released into the bloodstream. Should this occur, treatment with allopurinol will be required to prevent renal damage.

If chemotherapy has been given previously the radiation reaction may appear earlier or be more severe. Particular care must be given to regular monitoring of the blood count. If it becomes severely depressed, platelet or granulocyte transfusions may be required to support the patient until the bone marrow recovers.

Chest treatments are usually well tolerated, but the blood count must be carefully monitored if the abdomen has already been treated. Dysphagia occurring towards the end of treatment may be helped by paracetamol mucilage.

The various reactions have usually settled by 1 month after the last exposure.

After-care

Follow-up

In both seminoma and teratoma the majority of recurrences occur within 12 months of the initial treatment and 90% within 2 years. Careful and regular follow-up is of crucial importance in the management of testicular tumours. Where an expectant policy has been adopted in patients with stage I teratoma (all investigations for metastatic disease being negative) the patient should be seen at monthly intervals, or more often if there is any suggestion that the disease is recurring. After 12 months the interval can be extended to 2 months and then in the third year to 4 months. The patient is seen 6-monthly in the fourth and fifth years. For those patients with either seminoma or teratoma with early disease and who have had a radical treatment, it is satisfactory to see them 2-monthly for the first year and 3-monthly for the second year. Thereafter they are seen every 4 months in the third year and 6-monthly in the fourth and fifth years. Patients with advanced disease can be seen as the clinical situation demands.

At each visit a full clinical examination is performed, particularly with respect to the supraclavicular fossae and the abdomen. Posteroanterior, penetrated posteroanterior, and lateral chest films are done routinely. Where a lymphangiogram has been performed previously a plain abdominal film is also done to see if any change in the nodes has occurred. The AFP and HCG levels must be determined in patients with teratoma. A repeat CT scan is done 3–4 months after treatment. This is essential to determine whether or not there has been complete resolution of disease and to identify the sites of persistent tumour. The need for and mode of further treatment can then be assessed. One of the difficulties experienced with teratoma is that metastases may differentiate rather than disappear following treatment, so that a residual but inactive mass persists on the scan. Delayed resolution may also occur following chemotherapy. The appearances of the scan thus have to be interpreted with care in the light of the full clinical situation.

Treatment of Recurrent, and Metastatic Disease

Seminoma

Recurrence following abdominal irradiation is fortunately rare. Usually the supradiaphragmatic nodes or the lung fields will be involved and radical radiotherapy can then be given as described above. Radical irradiation of solitary metastases at other sites is also worthwhile, as it may occasionally be followed by long survival. If the recurrence is within the previously treated area, or the disease is disseminated, chemotherapy should be initiated. Occasionally further irradiation of an area previously treated can safely be given for localised masses, as the original dose of radiation is well within local tolerance levels.

Teratoma

Where abdominal irradiation alone has been given, the development of metastatic disease is common. Even if the metastases appear to be localised, e.g. in a supraclavicular node, the disease is usually already widespread and chemotherapy should be instituted. Further radiotherapy may be considered following the chemotherapy. Radical small-field radiotherapy is occasionally possible for solitary metastases, for example in the lungs.

With a patient in reasonable general condition the surgical treatment of metastases should be considered. This is particularly appropriate where there is a solitary lung metastasis, especially where it is peripheral in position. Surgery may also be used to deal with abdominal lymph nodes causing pain where these have recurred following radiotherapy and/or chemotherapy.

Complications

The immediate complications of radical radiotherapy have already been described.

The long-term sequelae of abdominal irradiation as given above are remarkably few. Many patients experience a slight increase in bowel frequency, but a frank malabsorption syndrome is rare. It has been reported that an increased incidence of peptic ulceration may occur, but we have no evidence to substantiate this.

All patients become sterile due to azoospermia following scrotal irradiation, but are not usually impotent. Hormonal replacement therapy can be successful if lack of potency does develop.

Renal failure is rare if by kidney shielding the dose to the kidneys has been kept below 2000 cGy in about 3 weeks, unless chemotherapy has also been given, in particular cis-platinum, which is particularly nephrotoxic.

Pulmonary fibrosis due to chest bath radiotherapy is not expected to be a problem with a dose of 2500 cGy now that the overall time has been extended from 3 to 4 weeks.

Results of Treatment

Seminoma

Five-year survival rates (age correlated) in the order of 95% for stages I and IIA, 65% for stage IIB, 40% for stage III, and 10% for stage IV may be expected.

Teratoma

Previously, with radiation alone, survival rates of 70% in stages I and IIA, 20% in IIB, and less than 10% in III and IV were obtained. With more accurate assessment and modern chemotherapy it is anticipated that survival rates in stage I should exceed 90% and in other stages will be of the order of 50%–70%.

References

Javadpour N (1979) Semin Oncol 6(1)

Pugh RCB (1976) Pathology of the testis. Blackwell, London

14 Malignant Lymphomas (including Myeloproliferative Disorders)

I. D. H. Todd (in collaboration with D. Crowther and P. M. Wilkinson)

Introduction

This chapter deals with the radiotherapy and cytotoxic chemotherapy of the malignant lymphomas. Included within this group are Hodgkin's disease, non-Hodgkin's lymphoma, mycosis fungoides, and chronic lymphatic leukaemia. A further section deals with the myeloproliferative disorders, including granulocytic leukaemia, polycythaemia vera, and primary thrombocythaemia. Excluded are myeloma and reticulum cell sarcoma of bone, which are dealt with in Chap. 15, and acute leukaemia, which is discussed in Chap. 16. With regard to Hodgkin's disease, the past 25 years have seen general recognition of the curative potential of radiotherapy, at least in the local stages, and, more recently, awareness of the ability to achieve long-term survival after combination chemotherapy in generalised or in recurrent disease. At the same time the importance of staging has become appreciated and the introduction of procedures such as lymphography, staging laparotomy, and computer tomography (CT) has enormously increased its reliability. Advances have not been so dramatic in the complex group of non-Hodgkins's lymphomas, but are still very real.

Hodgkin's Disease

Investigation and Staging

By the time the patient is referred to the oncological institute the histological diagnosis will have been made in most cases. It is essential to have the slides and preferably the tissue blocks reviewed, not only to confirm the diagnosis but to determine its appropriate histological classification (Table 14.1).

Table 14.1. Histological classification of Hodgkin's disease.

Lymphocyte predominant
Nodular sclerosing
Mixed cellularity
Lymphocyte depleted

If there is doubt, it is justifiable to have a further node removed for histological opinion. If there is a choice, the histopathologist will usually prefer a node from the neck or axilla rather than the groin. Once the diagnosis is certain, the precise extent of the disease must be determined as this will govern the subsequent treatment. At the same time this information is used to stage the disease (Table 14.2), in order that the results of treatment for a series of patients can readily be compared with those from another centre.

The length of history obtained from the patient may sometimes be of value. The presence of lymphadenopathy, especially if not showing a noticeable increase in size over several years, would suggest an indolent course with a good short-term prognosis. On the other hand, a short fulminating course would support the need for urgent treatment, possibly before full routine investigation is complete. Of most importance in the history, however, is the presence or absence of B symptoms. These are sweats and weight loss. The sweats, of course, are an indication of fever, they usually occur at night, and may be associated

Table 14.2. Staging of Hodgkin's disease (after the Ann Arbor classification).

Stage 1	Nodal involvement confined to one region
Stage 1E	Single extralymphatic organ or site
Stage 2	Nodal involvement of two or more regions on the same side of the diaphragm
Stage 2E	Localised extranodal site and nodal involvement on the same side of the diaphragm
Stage 3	Nodal disease on both sides of the diaphragm
Stage 3E	Nodal disease on both sides of the diaphragm with single site of extra-nodal extension
Stage 3S	Nodal disease on both sides of the diaphragm with splenic involvement
Stage 3ES	Nodal disease on both sides of the diaphragm with splenic and localised extranodal involvement
Stage 4	Diffuse or disseminated involvement of one or more extralymphatic organs or tissues, with or without node involvement

Systemic symptoms
B denotes the presence of otherwise unexplained pyrexia (temperature over 38°C usually with night sweats) or weight loss of more than 10% in the previous 6 months. A denotes the absence of B symptoms. Note that pruritus alone does not qualify for B classification.

with rigors. If they occur regularly and are severe enough to make the patient change his night clothes, they can be regarded as significant. There may also be confirmatory objective evidence of fever if this has been charted. If there is loss of weight to an extent of 10% of the body weight over 6 months, without an adequate alternative explanation, this too is significant.

Other symptoms may be very important although not counting as B symptoms. Pruritus is one of these and is often a feature, perhaps a dominating one, in the later stages of the disease. It is less common as a presenting symptom. Pain occurring shortly after taking a drink containing alcohol is a well-recognised feature and is particularly associated with bone involvement, either direct infiltration such as sternal involvement from mediastinal adenopathy or frank distant metastasis. "Alcohol pain" is not confined to patients with bone involvement and may occasionally be complained of at the site of a node mass, or indeed at other sites of extranodal disease. Many patients, especially those in relapse after previously successful therapy, complain of alcohol intolerance rather than pain. They have no appetite for such drinks and this may be an indication of liver infiltration.

Physical Examination

The sites and measurements of the enlarged nodes should be recorded, preferably with a diagram and with reference to adjacent bony landmarks (this is particularly important if there is a possibility that radiotherapy to sites of initially bulky disease may be in the treatment programme as a sequel to effective chemotherapy). The most commonly enlarged nodes are those in the cervical regions and there is a tendency for involvement of adjacent lymph node regions such as the axilla and infraclavicular and supraclavicular fossae. In contradistinction to the non-Hodgkin's lymphomas, epitrochlear nodes are rarely enlarged. Likewise, in Hodgkin's disease it is rare to find involvement of the structures in Waldeyer's ring. Enlargement of the liver and/or spleen must also be recorded. Rarely one finds infiltration of other organs such as the skin, breast, or salivary glands, and again, if present, this would raise the possibility of non-Hodgkin's disease rather than Hodgkin's disease.

Routine investigation will always include a peripheral blood count, chest X-ray, and liver function tests. The blood count may confirm anaemia, a feature of late disease; there may be granulocyte leucocytosis, seen especially in florid disease with fever; and rarely eosinophilia as an unexplained finding. Chest X-ray, including penetrated and lateral views, is essential to demonstrate mediastinal or hilar node enlargement with or without lung infiltration.

Marrow examination, including trephine as well as aspiration, should be carried out when there is reason to suspect marrow involvement, i.e. stages III and IV and all patients with B symptoms. When anaemia is present it may be due to marrow infiltration, but is more often the normocytic normochromic anaemia of chronic disease. Of the liver function tests, the most useful are raised alkaline phosphatase, raised serum aspartate aminotransferase (AST), and reduced albumin, but none is really specific for liver involvement and must be interpreted in the light of the physical findings. Numerous imaging techniques are available to supplement "conventional" X-rays. If there is mediastinal node enlargement, even without sternal swelling or pain, thick-plane tomography may demonstrate sternal erosion (Fig. 14.1). Of most importance, however, is the demonstration of adenopathy below the diaphragm. Para-aortic nodes have to be very large before they are palpable. Occasionally, a node mass in this region can be inferred by displacement of kidneys or ureters at intravenous pyelography, or by indentation of the inferior vena cava during vena cavography. Rather more reliable information can be obtained from scans using ultrasound, but the most reliable techniques are lymphography and CT. Lymphography requires cannulation of lymphatics on the dorsum of the foot with the subsequent instillation of an iodised oil (e.g. ultrafluid lipiodol). This takes about 2 h and the initial films are of little diagnostic worth with regard to nodes, as the detail is obscured by the full, engorged, lymphatics. Films taken at 24 h have usually cleared and allow examination of inguinofemoral, iliac, and para-aortic nodes (Fig. 14.2). Interpretation of the findings is facilitated by taking oblique or, preferably, stereoscopic views in order to separate the nodes. There may be frankly abnormal nodes showing typical lymphomatous patterns or abnormal nodes may have to be inferred because of non-filling. Lymphography can be very helpful, on occasion, but seldom opacifies all the nodes of interest and does not demonstrate the full extent of the disease. CT scanning will almost always give all the information available from lymphography and more besides. This technique will disclose nodes, such as those in the porta hepatis, at the splenic hilum, or in the retrocrural region, which are not accessible to pedal lymphography. To obtain the best results it is necessary to quieten the bowel using Pro-Banthine, or similar agent, or to use a fast scan time (say 3 s), and at the same time the small bowel

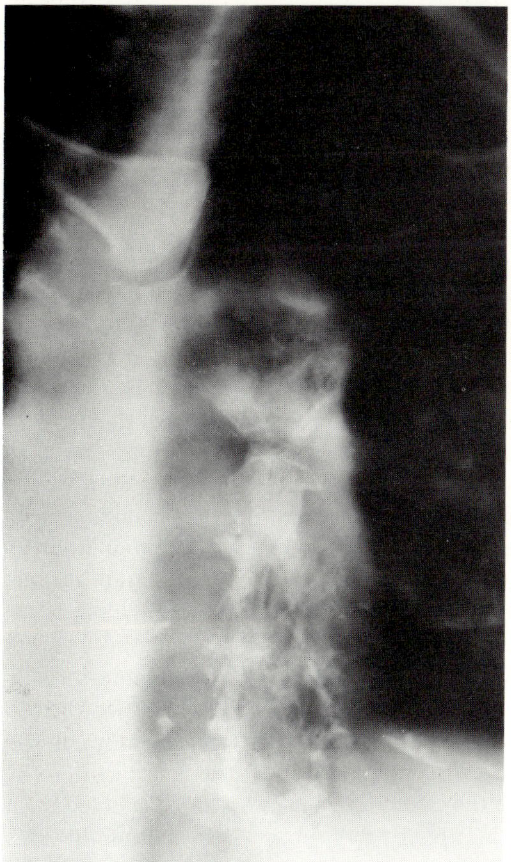

Fig. 14.1. Radiograph of the sternum to demonstrate erosion due to Hodgkin's disease.

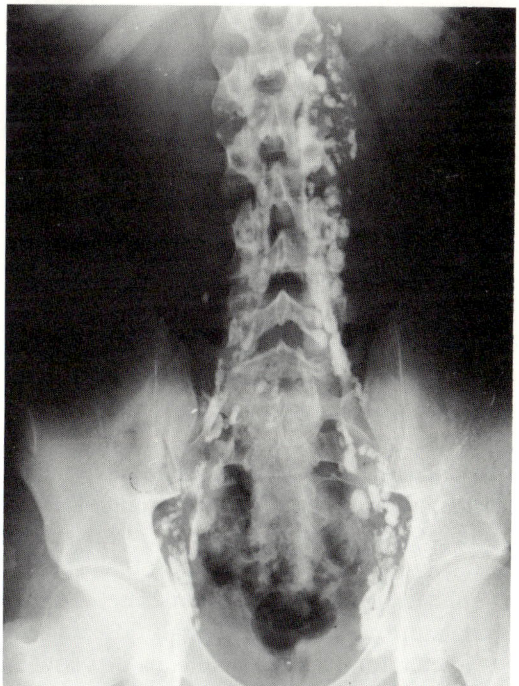

Fig. 14.2. Lymphadenogram using lipiodol to show appearance of nodes involved in Hodgkin's disease.

should be opacified (e.g. with Gastrografin) to make it more easily identifiable. Good though it is for demonstrating nodes, CT is less reliable at revealing splenic or hepatic involvement.

Where there is suspicion of liver involvement on clinical and biochemical grounds, liver biopsy should be considered, but the results are often inconclusive. In the majority of patients with apparently early supradiaphragmatic disease it will be necessary to consider staging laparotomy. This is particularly indicated to find out for certain if the liver or spleen is affected. Where there is doubt about the safety of operation from the anaesthetic point of view (e.g. suspicion of mediastinal obstruction due to node mass), this investigation should be avoided. When staging laparotomy is carried out it will include the methodical mapping of the node areas with biopsy of representative specimens and marking of these sites using radio-opaque clips, as well as liver biopsy, splenectomy, and possibly iliac crest biopsy for marrow examination.

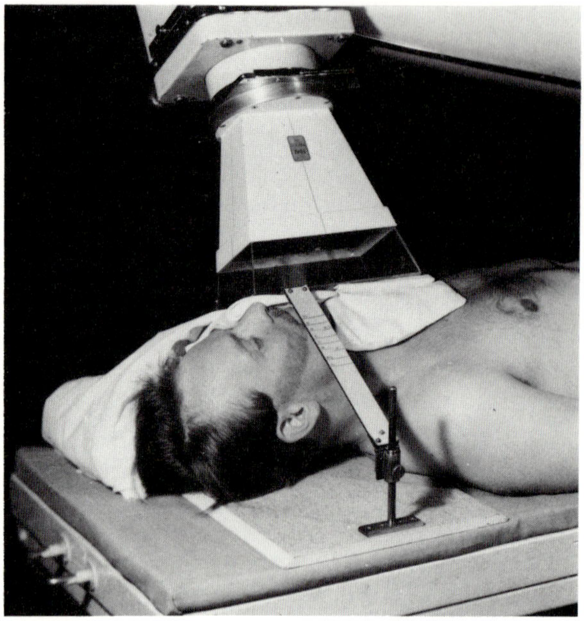

Fig. 14.3. Patient being set up using the Manchester trunk bridge.

Radiotherapy

It was appreciated at an early date that if one hoped to obtain lasting control of local disease it was necessary to take a substantial margin around the clinically identifiable tumour. Traditionally, this margin was of the order of 5 cm so that the field sizes tended to be around 20×25 cm and often a parallel pair type of field arrangement was used. With the depth doses available from kilovoltage apparatus this gave an inhomogeneous dose distribution, especially at the neck and upper thorax. The Manchester trunk bridge was developed to improve this and is shown in Fig. 14.3.

Since megavoltage radiotherapy equipment became widely available, the radical radiotherapy of this disease has been carried out exclusively on such machines. The better depth dose and absence of selective absorption in bone have led to a much more homogeneous dosage pattern, whilst the reduced scatter, giving a sharper edge to the beam, has simplified the shielding of structures such as the spinal cord and lung. The high dose rate of linear accelerators facilitates the use of longer target-skin distances and thus of larger fields, so that it becomes possible to use fields big enough to encompass adjacent, as well as involved, lymph node regions. This has led to the adoption of the mantle treatment as the standard approach for disease confined to nodes above the diaphragm.

Mantle Technique

The patient lies supine on the simulator couch with the hands placed above the head and skin marks are made on the upper pectoral region to indicate the permissible upper limit of the lung shielding. These marks will take account of the presence of infraclavicular node involvement or of the proximity of enlarged axillary nodes. Lengths of thin lead wire are attached to the skin over these marks using adhesive tape. The tube, tray, patient, and cassette are arranged as in Fig. 14.4, so that the target-to-tray distance is 80 cm, the target-to-skin distance is 140 cm, and the target-to-cassette distance is 170 cm. The position of the cassette remains constant at 30 cm below the anterior skin surface. Only exceptionally will the patient be too deep to be accommodated and even then the additional centimetre or two will not materially affect the geometry. A field size is selected such that the upper margin passes just below the eyes and the lower margin is at about the level of the xiphisternum. The centre is marked on the skin. A grid is placed on the tray to overlie the lower part

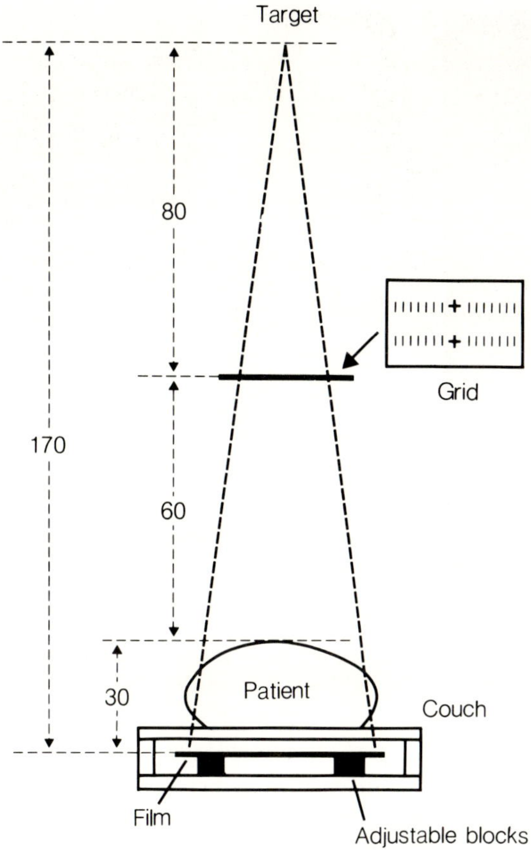

Fig. 14.4. Diagram to show relationship of target, shielding tray, patient, couch and cassette during preliminary steps when a radiograph is taken so that the extent of shielding can be decided. Note that the distance between cassette and patient can be varied in order to keep the focus to skin distance constant at 140 cm and the focus to cassette distance at 170 cm.

of the field and the shadows cast by the radio-opaque marks on to the skin are indicated with ink so that the grid can readily be replaced in the same position. The patient is asked to breathe quietly and a radiograph is taken in mid-respiration in order to approximate to the state of affairs during treatment. This radiograph is compared with a standard diagnostic film taken previously with the patient erect and in full inspiration. In the simulator film the lung fields will appear smaller and the mediastinal shadow will be broader. An estimate is made of the mediastinal coverage which is required and, taking account of this and of the marks which indicate the acceptable clearance of the infraclavicular and axillary regions, it is possible to outline on the simulator film the amount of lung which can be shielded with safety. This film (Fig. 14.5) is now placed on the illuminated panel at the base of the jig shown in Fig. 14.6. This jig has the same geometry as the treatment machine, with the target at the top and a wire attached to this. The wire has a heated section which passes through an expanded polystyrene block fixed on the tray. There is a cursor on the end of the wire which is used to outline the areas to be shielded. The heated section of course cuts out a pattern in the polystyrene blocks (Fig. 14.7) and this is used as a mould (Fig. 14.8). The alloy used for making the blocks is MCP 69 (this shielding alloy contains lead, bismuth, zinc, and cadmium; it is supplied by Mining and Chemical Products Ltd., 11 Margaret Street, Stone, Staffordshire ST15 8EQ, England). It has a melting point of 70 °C which is readily achieved in a water bath. The metal is poured into the mould in layers each a few millimetres thick. This is necessary to prevent air bubbles being left in the casting. The finished blocks (Fig. 14.9) are 6 cm thick and have absorption characteristics similar to lead (SG 9.4 compared with 11.3 for lead), i.e. for 4-MV X-rays about 6% of the incident dose will be transmitted. The accuracy of the casting is now checked by placing the patient on the simulator couch, in the treatment position, putting the grid on the tray in its previous position and placing the blocks on the grid using the original simulator film for reference. A verification film (Fig. 14.10) is taken and compared with this. Any necessary correction in position is made but only occasionally is it necessary to recast the block. The entire process is then repeated with the patient in the prone position, so that an anterior and posterior pair of blocks are made. Before the prescription is written, any areas of skin, such as a recent biopsy scar, which require the full dose to extend up to the surface, are outlined so that bolus can be placed thereon; likewise, the possibility of placing a small block of lead on the tray to shield the lips is also considered. Usually advantage is taken of the skin-sparing effect of megavoltage radiation, so that bolus is not used to create a uniform thickness of torso. In order to determine the interfield distance for the prescription the following procedure is adopted: measurements are taken, both prone and supine, of the maximum, the minimum, and of the middle of the fields, all in the midline. These six figures are averaged to give the interfield distance. Tested empirically over a wide range of body sizes this has ensured an administered tumour dose within 10% of the prescribed dose in all cases, and usually within 5%; this can be relied upon for radiation of 4 MV and upwards.

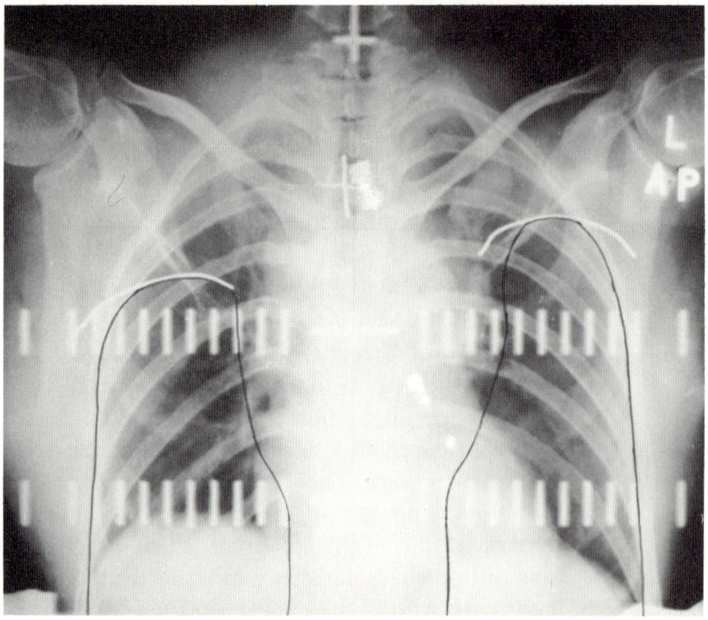

Fig. 14.5. Radiograph, taken on the simulator, on which the outline of the proposed lung shielding has been marked.

With regard to dose, the intention is to give 3500 cGy in 20 fractions over 4 weeks with 4-MV X-rays. This is probably too high a dose for the length of spinal cord which is included in the treated volume and the cord is therefore shielded for part of the treatment. For the second half of the treatment, a brass shield (Fig. 14.11) is used, its position having been checked radiographically (Fig. 14.12). This reduces the cord dose but also casts an unwelcome shadow through the mediastinum. In order to compensate for this, an additional field, 4 cm wide, and usually about 16 cm long, is placed over the sternum (Fig. 14.13) on the last day and a single exposure of 600 cGy is given. With this prescription most of the tumour volume receives 3500 cGy, the minimum dose (in the vicinity of the cord) is 2900 cGy, and no tissue receives a dose in excess of 4000 cGy. The immediate side effects of this treatment include dryness of the mouth followed by mild dysphagia and temporary epilation over the nape of the neck; later, there may occasionally be a transient radiation myelopathy. After a further year or two the reduced salivary flow associated with retraction of the gums may lead to caries around the necks of some teeth. The dysphagia is helped by paracetamol mucilage 10 ml before meals and the caries is managed conservatively.

For treatment of localised Hodgkin's disease below the diaphragm, it is usual to irradiate the coeliac, para-aortic, and inguinofemoral lymph node chains in one block. Sometimes the spleen or splenic bed is also included in the treatment volume. This type of treatment, the inverted Y, is carried out using a parallel pair of fields with appropriate shielding, and megavoltage radiation. It is necessary to make use of radiography such as lymphography, excretion urography, and CT scanning, to delineate the involved node areas and to demonstrate the kidneys, so that they can be protected. A typical volume is shown in Fig. 14.14. The dose given is 3500 cGy in 20 fractions over 4 weeks, using megavoltage radiation. Nausea and, occasionally, vomiting may be a problem, but not usually at this relatively low input rate. It is a help if the patient is advised to lie down for a couple of hours immediately after each fraction. In the uncommon event of vomiting, an antiemetic such as chlorpromazine 25–50 mg is given 30 min before the treatment and is usually sufficient to control it. During abdominal treatment of this type it is essential to monitor the marrow by way of the peripheral blood count, as a substantial proportion of the active marrow is included within the irradiated volume. If the patient has had preceding mantle radiotherapy or cytotoxic chemotherapy, this is even more important.

In some centres an attempt to shield the ovaries is made when the abdominal lymph node chains are irradiated. At the time of the staging laparotomy the ovaries are sutured behind the uterus (oophorpexy) so that they can be shielded later.

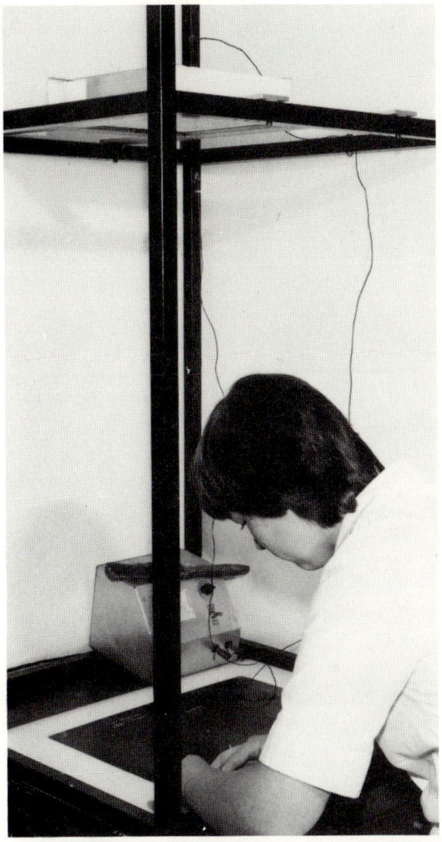

a

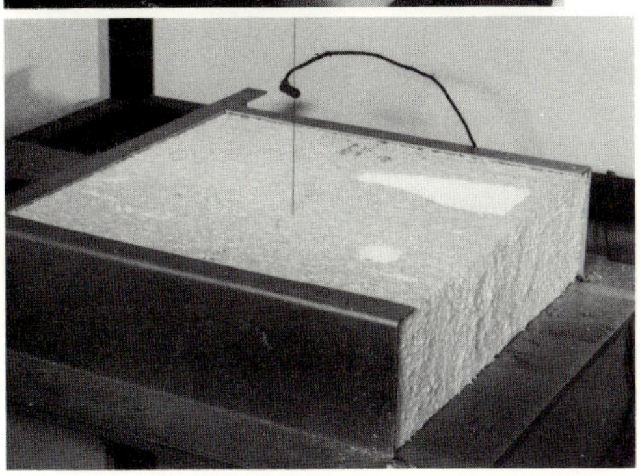

b

Fig. 14.6a,b. The jig which is used to cut the individual moulds for the lung shielding. Note that this has the same geometry as the treating machine, and that there is an electrically heated wire passing through the polystyrene block.

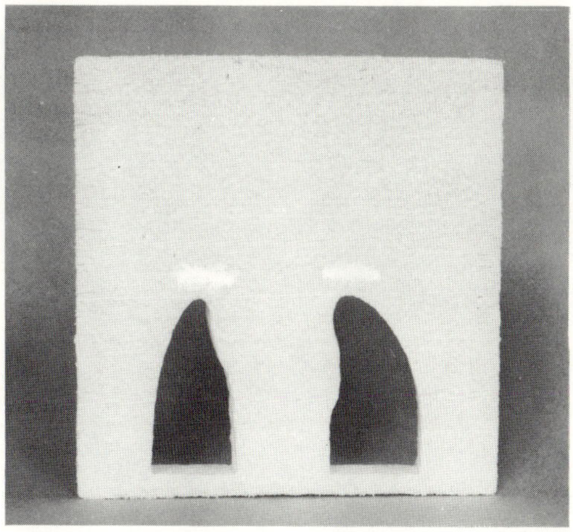

Fig. 14.7. Photograph of a polystyrene block which has been cut to make moulds for a pair of lung shields.

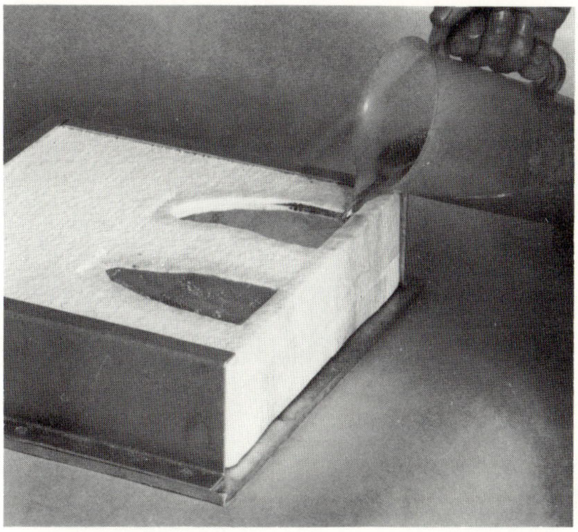

Fig. 14.8. Polystyrene mould being used for the casting of the lung shields. The low-melting-point alloy MCP89 is being used.

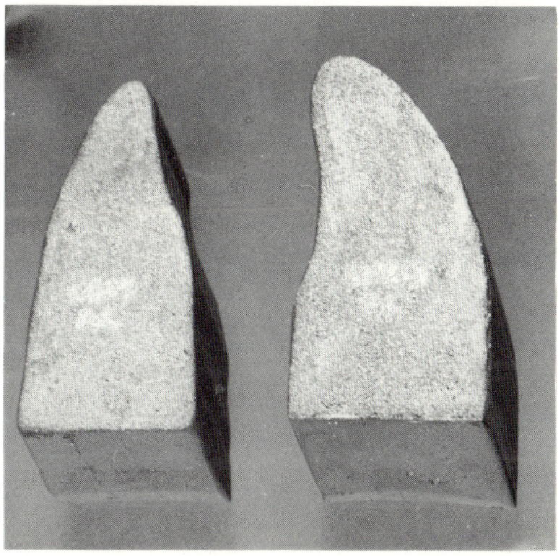

Fig. 14.9. The finished lung shields.

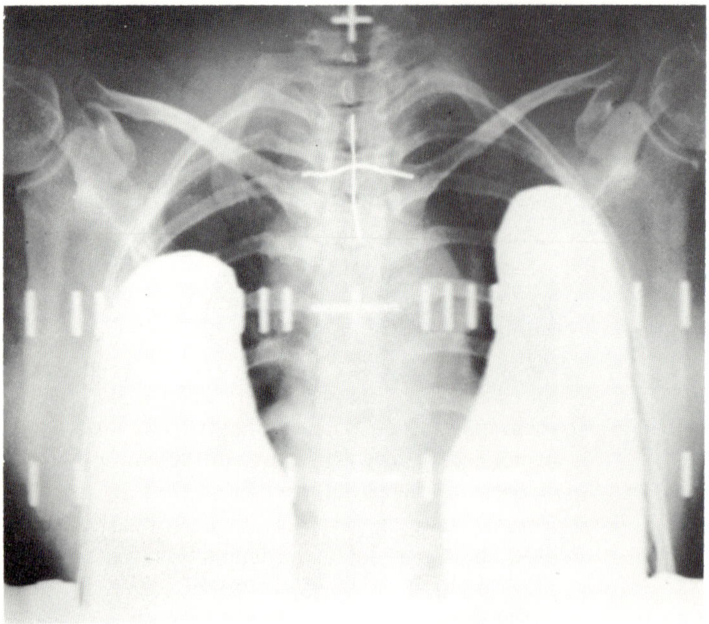

Fig. 14.10. Verification radiograph taken to confirm that the blocks have been accurately cast. Compare with the radiograph shown in Fig. 14.5.

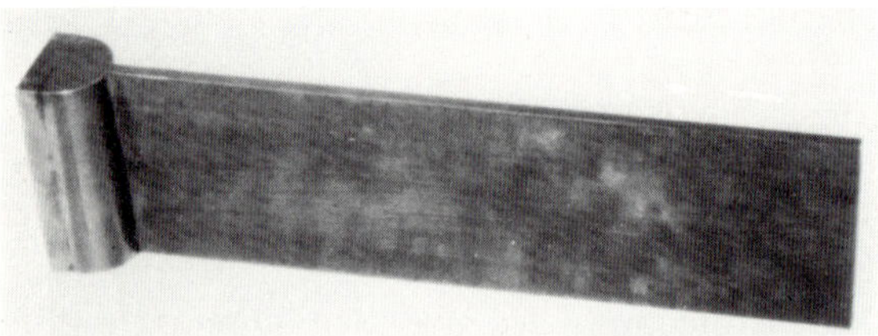

Fig. 14.11. The brass shield which is used for spinal cord shielding.

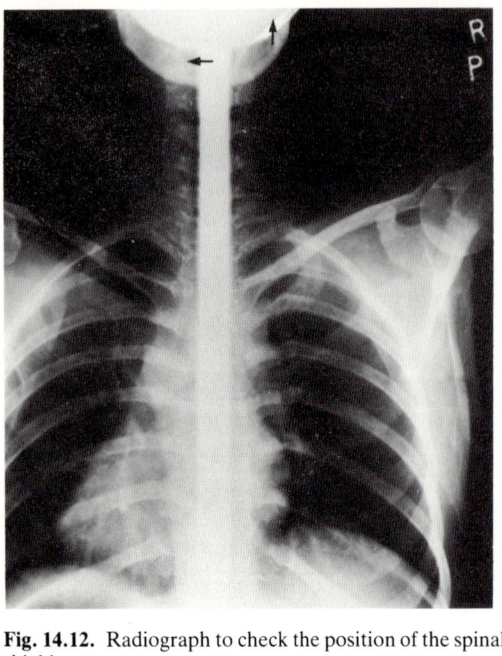

Fig. 14.12. Radiograph to check the position of the spinal cord shield.

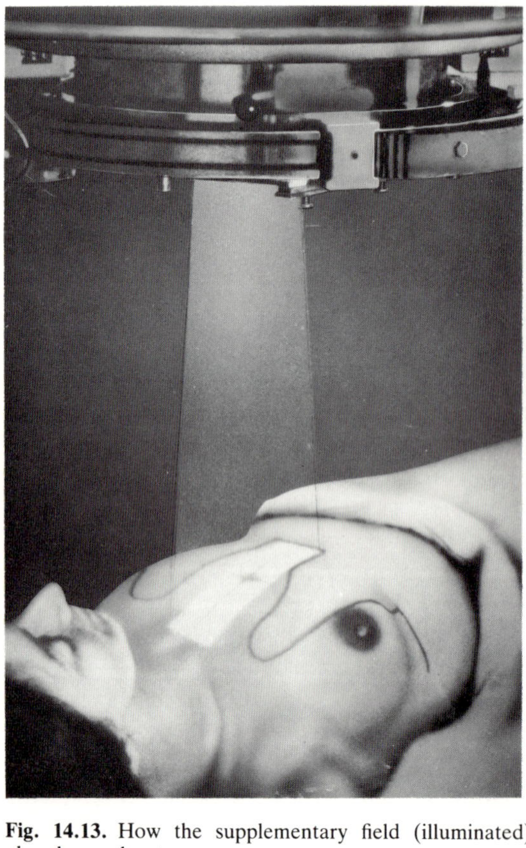

Fig. 14.13. How the supplementary field (illuminated) is placed over the sternum.

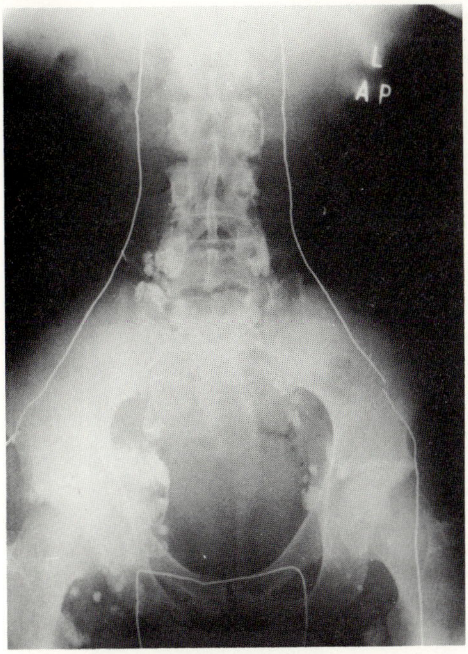

Fig. 14.14. Radiograph to show the outline of an inverted-Y field which is being used to treat disease (demonstrated by lymphography) in the para-aortic and iliac chains.

This procedure is not recommended because the combination of transmitted and scattered radiation to the ovaries will be about 10% of the tumour dose and they will therefore still receive a significant dose. Moreover, because of their proximity to the iliac nodes an attempt at shielding may, inadvertently, lead to protection of an involved node.

Sometimes, as a matter of policy, it may be decided to use adjuvant radiotherapy when employing radical chemotherapy, the rationale being that in the event of failure the disease tends to recur in sites where it was bulky at presentation. Under these circumstances "bulk sites" will be identified and clearly documented by skin marks, anatomical reference points, and/or radiologically, at the outset of treatment so that on completion of the chemotherapy appropriate radiotherapy can be prescribed. No attempt is made to use wide fields as there may not be enough marrow tolerance. Instead a much narrower margin is taken. This in turn allows a shorter course of fractionated X-ray treatment, say 2500 cGy in eight fractions over 10 days with megavoltage irradiation. Usually these bulk sites are nodal, with a minimum diameter of 5 cm, and not more than two are identified in the one patient. Care must be taken not to irradiate more than half of the active marrow.

So far, consideration has been given to the role of radiotherapy only when it is employed as a potentially curative treatment or as part of a potentially curative regime in combination with chemotherapy. When radiotherapy is used for palliation it is usual to employ simple field arrangements (single field or parallel pair), to take less margin around the known extent of the deposit, and to treat at lower dosage using fewer fractions in a shorter overall time. Suggested doses are 800 cGy single fraction, 1750 cGy in four fractions, and 2000 cGy in eight fractions. Apart from causing very little upset to the patient, these doses have the advantage of leaving tolerance for further treatment. Rather higher doses should be used for the relief of bone pain or for treating paraparesis.

Chemotherapy

The accepted chemotherapy involves the use of a four-drug regime. The most commonly used combination is MOPP—mustine, Oncovin (vincristine), procarbazine, and prednisolone—but the combination recommended here is MVPP where vinblastine is substituted for the vincristine in MOPP because it is less neurotoxic and gives rise to less alopecia.

The course of chemotherapy lasts 2 weeks and is followed by a 4-week rest period. Unlike the MOPP regime, prednisolone is given with each course. The course should not be repeated until the marrow depression from the previous course has resolved.

A typical response to MVPP is shown in Fig. 14.15, where a patient who 5 years previously had been treated using mantle radiotherapy for supradiaphragmatic Hodgkin's disease relapsed with gross adenopathy in the para-aortic region. The degree of response in the node mass after a single course is readily apparent.

A different patient with generalised adenopathy at presentation is shown in Fig. 14.16, where incomplete resolution is demonstrated after one course and complete resolution after two courses.

There have been many recommendations as to the optimum number of courses. It has been our practice to give a further six courses after remission. With the evidence of long-term complica-

Table 14.3. MVPP regime.

Mustine 6 mg/m^2 Vinblastine 6 mg/m^2	intravenously days 1 and 8
Procarbazine 50 mg three times daily Prednisolone 25 mg twice daily	by mouth days 1 to 14 inclusive

A 1-month rest period is allowed between courses, so there is a 6-week cycle.

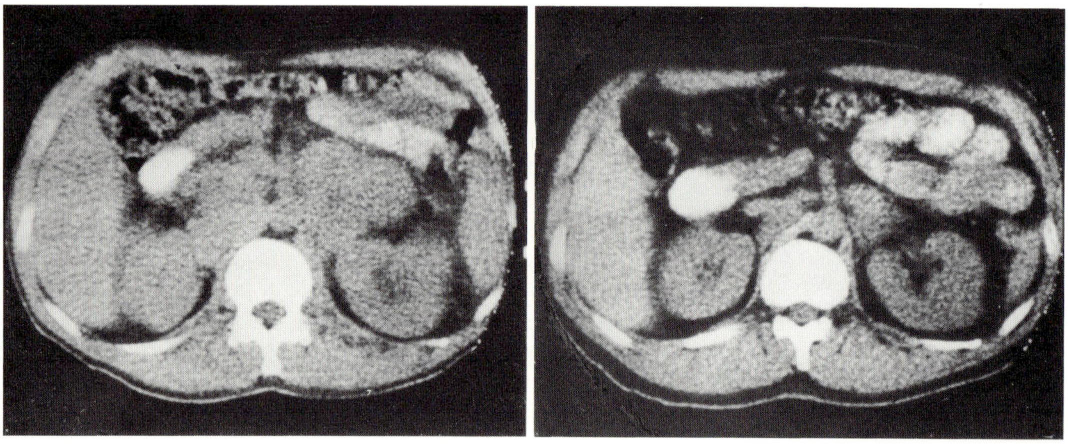

Fig. 14.15a,b. Para-aortic node mass in a patient with Hodgkin's disease, demonstrated by CT (by courtesy of Professor Isherwood): **a** before and **b** after treatment with a single course of MVPP.

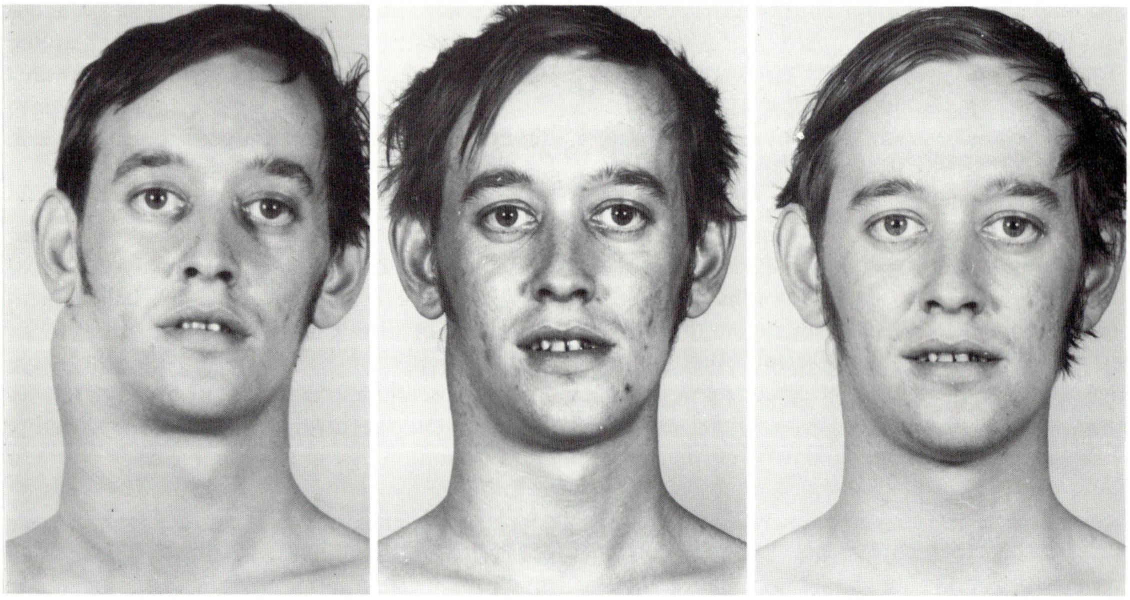

Fig. 14.16a–c. A patient with generalised lymphadenopathy, due to Hodgkin's disease, in whom response to MVPP is shown. **a** The cervical lymphadenopathy before therapy; **b** incomplete resolution after one course; **c** complete resolution after two courses.

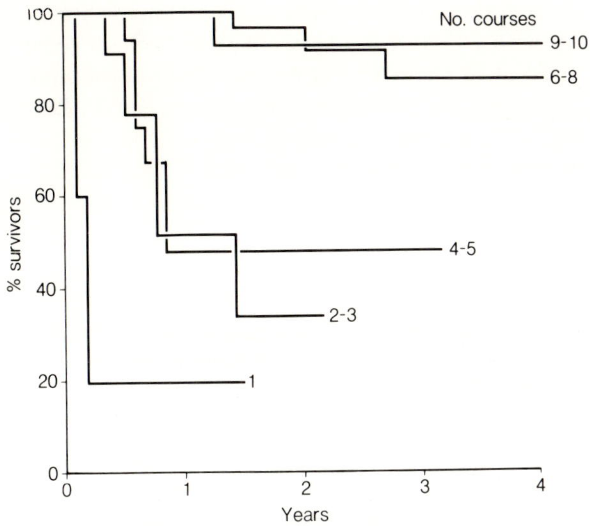

Fig. 14.17. Results of chemotherapy in the Manchester Lymphoma Group's study of the use of MVPP in stage 3B and 4 disease. The results are given with reference to the total number of courses administered. Less than six courses is followed by significantly poorer survival.

tions, such as a second malignancy, it is well to keep to the minimum effective regime. Figure 14.17 gives recent data which shows an advantage for those patients receiving a total of six courses but no clear advantage for more than that.

When patients are started on MVPP it is advisable to admit them overnight for the initial injection, but thereafter most of the treatment can be given on an outpatient basis. It is mandatory to have a peripheral blood count on the day of treatment to ensure that the white count and platelet count are normal. The mustine and vinblastine are freshly made up in separate (and labelled) syringes, and injected into a fast running saline drip. The procarbazine and the prednisolone are given in divided doses by mouth. Nausea and vomiting are almost universal in each course, and start about 1.5 h after the first injections. An intravenous dose of an antiemetic such as metoclopramide 10 mg along with the mustine and the vinblastine sometimes helps. Nausea and vomiting are much less of a problem after the second injections. Should the vomiting be insupportable, then in subsequent courses the mustine may be omitted and chlorambucil by mouth substituted, as in Table 14.4. This regime is better tolerated than MVPP and may well be as effective. Apart from nausea, the most frequent side effect is marrow depression, so that the peripheral blood count must be seen before each injection. If the count has not recovered to its normal level before the next course it is recommended that the course be postponed for, say, a week rather than reduce the doses. Because of the tendency of procarbazine to potentiate the effects of alcohol in a rather unpleasant fashion, alcohol should be eschewed during the course of MVPP and for the day before and the day after. Prednisolone may give rise to troublesome side effects. There is usually some "mooning" of the face and often fluid retention, which may be manifested by a brief diuresis when the drug is stopped abruptly. The abrupt withdrawal of the drug may also be associated with a transient feeling of depression. If this upsets the patient he should be advised to taper off the drug over a few days. More serious is the occasional psychosis which prednisolone can induce. If this is encountered the drug must be abandoned altogether. The psychosis usually responds to psychiatric treatment, but it may take many weeks for the patient to return to normal. Another feature of steroid therapy in these patients is the development of avascular necrosis in bone. This is usually found in the femoral heads, but can be seen in the humeral heads also, and does not always give rise to symptoms. When it does give symptoms this is usually in the young male. It is more frequent when combination chemotherapy and local radiotherapy are both given. When symptoms are severe it is justifiable to seek orthopaedic advice with a view to hip replacement if the prognosis from the point of view of the Hodgkin's disease is reasonably good. Prednisolone may, of course, unmask diabetes or precipitate peptic ulceration. Neither complication is an absolute bar to further prednisolone therapy, for the diabetes can be controlled and the prophylactic use of cimetidine

Table 14.4. Chlorambucil VPP.

Vinblastine 6 mg/m^2	intravenously days 1 and 8
Chlorambucil 5 mg twice daily Procarbazine 50 mg three times daily Prednisolone 25 mg twice daily	by mouth days 1 to 14 inclusive

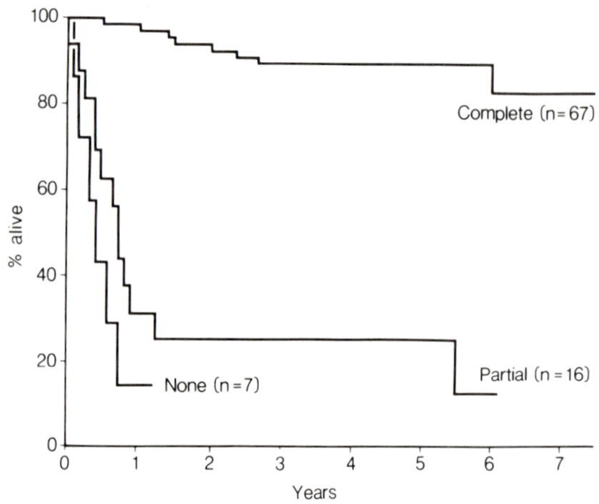

Fig. 14.18. Results of chemotherapy in the Manchester Lymphoma Group's study of MVPP in stage 3b and 4 disease. These data demonstrate how important it is to achieve complete remission if there is to be long term survival.

may prevent further peptic ulceration. However, failure to obtain a complete remission on MVPP is serious.

In this event alternative therapy must be considered. If the disease is confined to nodes and the spleen the most promising line is to change to total nodal irradiation, i.e. a combination of mantle and inverted-Y fields. But even without previous chemotherapy and a substantial interval between the two radiotherapy prescriptions there is often difficulty in administering full dosage. When the marrow has already been prejudiced by unsuccessful chemotherapy this adds to the problem and it is wise, therefore, to consider whether the fields can be trimmed in any way which will spare red marrow. If there is visceral involvement by disease then recourse will have to be made to an alternative chemotherapy regime, but at the time of writing, the most promising of these is ABVD or BCAVE (Tables 14.5 and 14.6) though neither can be recommended with confidence.

Table 14.5. ABVD regime.

Adriamycin	25 mg/m^2	i.v.	Days 1+14
Bleomycin	10 mg/m^2	i.m.	Days 1+14
Vinblastine	6 mg/m^2	i.v.	Days 1+14
DTIC	150 mg/m^2	i.v.	Days 1 to 5 incl.
	Six-week cycle		

Table 14.6. B CAVE regime.

Bleomycin	5 mg/m^2	i.m.	Days 1, 28, 35
CCNU	100 mg/m^2	p.o.	Day 1
Adriamycin	60 mg/m^2	i.v.	Day 1
Vinblastine	6 mg/m^2	i.v.	Day 1
	Six-week cycle		

Choice of Treatment

Having completed the investigations of the patient with Hodgkin's disease, the decision on treatment can be taken. In general terms, if the disease is localised, main reliance will be placed on radiotherapy, but for generalised disease chemotherapy will be the treatment of choice.

With stage 1 or stage 2 disease, above the diaphragm, mantle radiotherapy should be considered and will often be appropriate. An important exception would be the patient with a large mediastinal mass, especially if this is associated with substantial axillary or infraclavicular nodes, because it may not be possible to cover the known extent of the disease without irradiating an excessive volume of lung. In such a case, it is preferable to start with chemotherapy, a decision which may be further supported by the presence of B symptoms. These patients may indeed present a special problem when the mediastinal mass is such as to preclude a staging laparotomy, thus preventing accurate staging. For such a patient the decision will often be taken at the outset to administer radical chemotherapy, followed by radiotherapy to the mediastinum on completion of this. In our experience, if it is going to recur, the disease is likely to do so in sites where it was bulky at presentation. So far, however, it has not been possible to prove that this policy is better than chemotherapy alone (Fig. 14.19).

With stage 3 or stage 4 disease, radical chemotherapy will be the treatment of choice, but, as in the case of mediastinal involvement mentioned in the preceding paragraph, consideration should be given to the possibility of radiotherapy to the sites of initial bulky disease on completion of the chemotherapy.

In stage 1 or stage 2 disease below the diaphragm, inverted-Y radiotherapy may be appropriate but, in such cases, the investigations may not have included laparotomy, so that there may be doubt as to the accuracy of the staging, especially with regard to the liver and the spleen. If

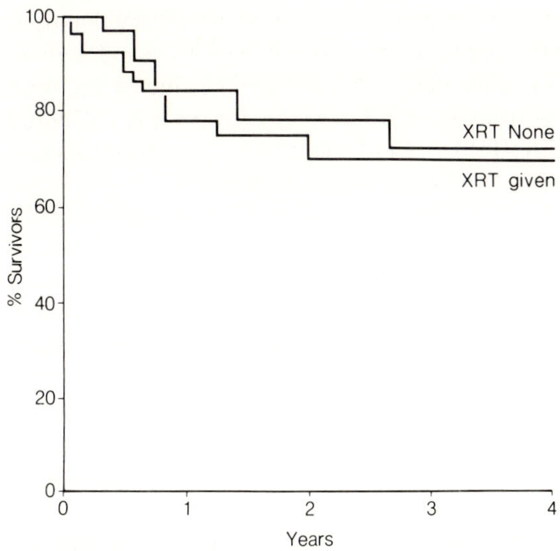

Fig. 14.19. Results of chemotherapy in the Manchester Lymphoma Group's study of MVPP in stage 3B and 4 disease. In this study some patients were given supplementary radiotherapy to sites where the disease was bulky at presentation but it is not possible to demonstrate a significant advantage. Note, however, that this was not a random trial.

the latter is the case, and laparotomy is not planned, it would then be safer to resort to radical chemotherapy. A special problem arises when a patient relapses or is unable to tolerate the first-line treatment. Relapse after apparently successful radiotherapy is a clear indication for chemotherapy, and in this situation there is a good chance of obtaining remission with subsequent long-term survival. In the case of relapse after effective chemotherapy the proper course of action is less clear. The patient should be re-staged because if the relapse is confined to nodes, it may be possible to embark on radical radiotherapy, such as total nodal irradiation (mantle plus inverted Y, but with a gap of some 6 weeks between the courses to permit the marrow to recover). If the relapse involves viscera, further chemotherapy will be indicated. If the relapse occurs 2 years or more after completion of the previous course of chemotherapy the best prospect lies with further MVPP, perhaps substituting vincristine for the vinblastine. A summary of the lines of treatment suggested is given in Table 14.7. However, there is now an increasing tendency to use chemotherapy first for all patients with demonstrable mediastinal node involvement.

Special Problems

Certain special problems arise with sufficient frequency to deserve separate consideration. These include concurrent pregnancy, the occurrence of paraparesis, and certain late sequels to treatment such as second malignancy and the depression of gonadal function.

Pregnancy

When Hodgkin's disease presents during the first trimester, or early second trimester, the immediate reaction is to suggest abortion so that one may proceed with the normal investigations and appropriate treatment. However, the patient may be quite unwilling to accept this. She may, for example, be a primagravida over the age of 30 whose fertility would be much reduced after treatment, or she may have religious objections to abortion. Under these circumstances it may be possible to modify the management of her disease without seriously impairing her prognosis, but any decisions must be taken in consultation with the obstetrician, the patient, and her husband. Apart from biopsy, a peripheral blood count and a biochemical profile, investigation and treatment can be held back until the patient is well into her second trimester, since the main risk to the foetus is during the first 10 weeks of the first trimester. It should then be safe for radiography of the chest

Table 14.7. Summary of suggested management of Hodgkin's disease.

Stage 1A through 2B	Mantle radiotherapy unless there is bulky lymphadenopathy. MVPP reserved for the patient with bulky mediastinal lymphadenopathy, or who fails to respond to radiotherapy.
Stage 3A	MVPP given to six courses beyond remission. Total nodal irradiation reserved for the patient who fails to go into remission on chemotherapy. Radiotherapy to "bulk" disease may be considered on completion of chemotherapy.
Stages 3B and 4	MVPP given to six courses beyond remission. Radiotherapy to "bulk" disease should be considered on completion of chemotherapy.

and ultrasonography of the para-aortic regions and liver. If the disease is apparently confined to regions above the diaphragm, mantle radiotherapy can begin. Doses to the abdominal wall during such therapy have been measured using thermoluminescent dosimetry. With megavoltage apparatus the beam has a sharp edge with little scatter and the dose 20 cm below the lower margin is of the order of 1.4% of the tumour dose. (If this lower margin is at the xiphisternum, the point of interest would be near the uterine fundus at term). At the umbilicus the dose is about 1% and at the symphysis pubis about 0.7% of the tumour dose. Thus, with a tumour dose of 3500 cGy these scattered doses would be respectively 50, 35, and 25 cGy. After the mantle treatment the patient should be kept under close observation so that, if there were any suggestion of activity of her Hodgkin's disease, labour could be induced as soon as the obstetrician judged it to be safe. In any case, soon after delivery investigation of the Hodgkin's disease can be resumed, including, if indicated, staging laparotomy, and further therapy can be given if necessary.

With presentation late in the second trimester every effort should be made to avoid termination as this is so distasteful for all concerned. Usually it will be possible to manage the patient on the lines stated in the previous paragraph. Even if she does have symptomatic disease, it may still be possible, using local X-ray treatment, to tide her over until the obstetrician judges that the foetus is viable and that labour can be induced or caesarian section performed before embarking on systemic therapy.

With presentation in the third trimester it will almost always be possible to wait until after delivery before fully investigating and treating.

Paraparesis

Direct involvement of the central nervous system is very rare in this disease, but spinal compression is not at all uncommon. This may arise from vertebral involvement or from extradural infiltration (this latter complication may be due to extension from paraspinal nodal deposits). It usually progresses slowly over several days or a week or two. Slow progression and an absence of sphincter disturbance are favourable prognostic features. Paraparesis is a very distressing complication and it makes such heavy demands on the nursing services that it is always worth a determined attempt at correction. Physical examination, especially if a sensory level can be found, is most useful. Plain X-rays may show vertebral infiltration or a paraspinal shadow, but myelography is usually required to demonstrate the lower limit of the deposit. Cisternal myelography may be necessary to demonstrate the upper limit. In Hodgkin's disease there is usually just a single deposit to deal with, as compared with non-Hodgkin's lymphoma where such deposits are often multiple. If the diagnosis is known and the patient has not previously received chemotherapy, then chemotherapy with radiotherapy (if the area has not previously been irradiated) is as good as, if not better than, neurosurgery. However, if it is anticipated that the response to chemotherapy and radiotherapy will be poor (in the light of previous treatment) or if the diagnosis has not been established, then urgent neurosurgery is indicated. The radiotherapy will often be a single field to the affected area, taking a margin of, say, one vertebra above and one below the known limits. The dose is, of course, limited by cord tolerance, so that the vertebral body, which is often involved, will receive a lower dose. For this reason, a multi-field arrangement as in Fig. 14.20 may be preferred to avoid the falling dose. The overall treatment time should be short—single, 4-day, or at the most 8-day fractionation. The chemotherapy should be a standard combination such as MVPP.

Apart from the specific measures, the general

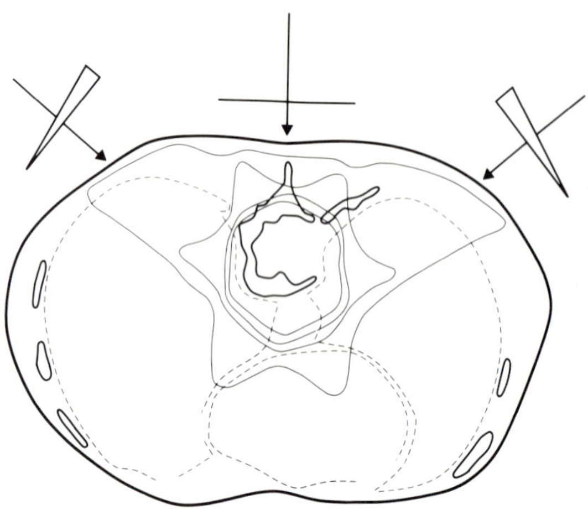

Fig. 14.20. Diagrammatic representation of a three-field arrangement (a single-plane posterior field with two postero-lateral wedged fields) used for a patient with a paraparesis due to Hodgkin's disease involving the 10th dorsal vertebra.

management of the paraparetic patient must be attended to. This will include physiotherapy and care of the bladder, especially if catheterised.

Second Malignancy

It is becoming very clear that there are serious late sequels to the treatment of Hodgkin's disease and that increasingly aggressive treatments must take due account of this if more is not to be lost than is gained. The most serious of these is the development of a second malignancy. This is most likely to be seen after the combination of total nodal irradiation with many courses of quadruple chemotherapy such as MOPP.

The most commonly seen second malignancy is an acute non-lymphoblastic leukaemia with a very poor prognosis. The incidence of second malignancies is difficult to ascertain with accuracy but is of the order of a 20-fold increase.

Progressive Multifocal Leucoencephalopathy

This is another late complication. It is a demyelinating condition which runs a relentless course over a few weeks or months as a terminal event, usually in a patient who has received extensive chemotherapy and radiotherapy for lymphoma.

Gonadal Dysfunction

A further important late complication is depression of gonadal function. In the male it is difficult to give sufficient shielding to the testes, during irradiation of the inguinal regions, to preserve fertility, since the testes are appreciably more sensitive than the ovaries. Likewise, a single course of, say, MVPP will be followed by at least temporary aspermia. The duration of the aspermia after scattered irradiation or several courses of cytotoxic drugs is not predictable but may be very long lasting. In the female the situation differs in that, although there may be temporary loss of fertility this often recovers, especially under the age of 30. Many younger women have now conceived and delivered normal babies after radical chemotherapy using six or more courses of MVPP or MOPP. As already mentioned, fertility is less likely to recover after attempts to shield the ovaries during abdominal irradiation. Apart from temporary or permanent loss of fertility, there may be other gonadal effects. Reduction of libido is frequent and there is occasional impotence in the male. One may have difficulty when assessing this latter symptom to know whether to ascribe it to the therapy, the debility associated with the disease and treatment, or to a more specific neurological complication of the use of the vinca alkaloids. The women over 30 will often experience lasting amenorrhoea. In patients with symptoms suggestive of depressed gonadal function, an endocrinologist should be asked to make a hormonal assessment and to advise if hormone replacement therapy is required.

Infections

Intercurrent infection is common in Hodgkin's disease owing to the suppression of the immune system by the disease and its treatment. Of particular note are the so-called opportunist infections. These are due to organisms which seldom under normal conditions give trouble, for example *Candida* and *Pneumocystis carinii*. Lung infections are particularly common, but one also finds conditions such as meningitis caused by yeast. It is most important to identify such causative organisms by swabs, blood culture, etc., because the patient will probably be started on treatment with a potent antibiotic before a firm diagnosis is made. Ewing stated that "tubercle follows Hodgkin's disease like a shadow". The association is not as common as it was in his day but is still seen frequently enough for the clinician to keep the possibility in mind.

Pruritus

Intractable pruritus is an occasional feature of late disease. If the disease responds to specific treatment, the pruritus is usually relieved, but the problem really arises in the patient who is no longer responding to treatment. It is worth looking for some other cause for the symptom, such as an infestation or sideropenia, but this will seldom be found.

Symptomatic measures are not very effective, but an antihistamine such as Vallergan and a local application such as crotamiton cream may help a little. Antiserotonin compounds have been used without benefit. Bleomycin at the rate of 1 mg/day injected subcutaneously has been recommended but has proved disappointing in our experience. Superficial X-rays or low-energy electrons may help with a local troublesome patch but the skin is usually too widely affected for this to be of more than occasional use. Cimetidine does, occasionally, control the pruritus.

Results of Treatment in Hodgkin's Disease

The potential long-term survival after adequate radiotherapy was recognised more than 20 years ago. Since then, the introduction of a range of active cytotoxic agents and the development of effective combination regimes coupled with improved staging methods have led to greatly improved survival rates. At the present time (Fig. 14.21) the overall 5-year survival rate is 80% while the survival rate for stages 1 and 2 is over 90%.

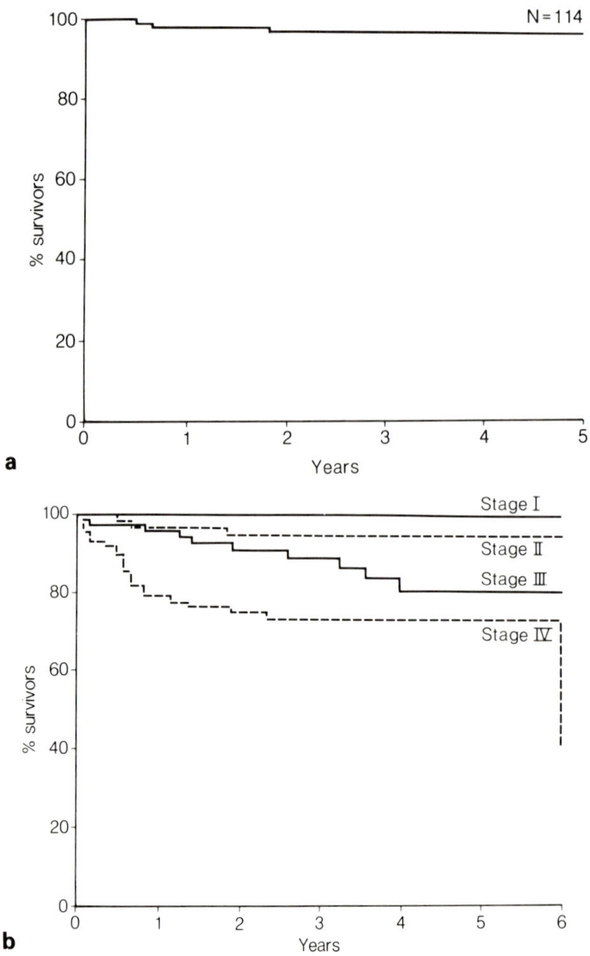

Fig. 14.21. a Actuarial survival curve for all Hodgkin's patients studied by the Manchester Lymphoma Group, 1974–1979. **b** The curve from Fig. 14.21a is broken down to show the effect of stage, at presentation, on the survival rates.

Non-Hodgkin's Lymphoma

General Features

Under this heading are included the lymphocyte-derived solid tumours. Classification of these tumours is controversial, but the classification adopted here is given in Table 14.8. This is useful for comparison with other published work but may well be superseded before long.

The various types of non-Hodgkin's lymphoma are gathered into two broad groups, grade I and grade II. This grouping refers to the short term prognosis. In the grade I group, the immediate outlook is good, but the diseases do tend to run a continually relapsing course as shown in Fig. 14.22. In the grade II group, the immediate outlook is bad, but once past the first 2–3 years there are relatively few relapses, as shown in Fig. 14.23. To be strictly accurate this applies more to the histiocytic diffuse than to the poorly differentiated diffuse lymphocytic tumour. It should be noted that the nodular histiocytic type does not fit comfortably into either group and occupies an intermediate position. Reticulum cell sarcoma of older classification approximates to diffuse histiocytic, and Brill-Symmers' disease to poorly differentiated nodular lymphocytic. Unlike Hodgkin's disease these lymphomas are frequently found to involve extranodal sites, and indeed often do so without any associated nodal disease. Extranodal sites which are rich in lymphocytes, such as tonsils and Peyer's patches, are particularly prone to involvement but almost any organ can be the site of presentation; examples are the thyroid, testis, bone, orbit, skin (excluding mycosis fungoides), and the gastrointestinal tract. Often these diseases are confined to nodes but, if so, rarely to a single region. It is much more common to find involvement of epitrochlear, mesenteric and even popliteal nodes in the non-Hodgkin's than in Hodgkin's disease.

Table 14.8. Histological classification of non-Hodgkin's lymphoma (after Rappaport).

Group	Histological type
Grade I	Well differentiated nodular lymphocytic Well differentiated diffuse lymphocytic (excluding chronic lymphatic leukaemia) Poorly differentiated nodular lymphocytic Mixed lymphocytic/histiocytic nodular
Grade II	Histiocytic nodular Poorly differentiated diffuse lymphocytic (including lymphoblastic) Mixed lymphocytic/histiocytic diffuse Histiocytic diffuse Undifferentiated diffuse

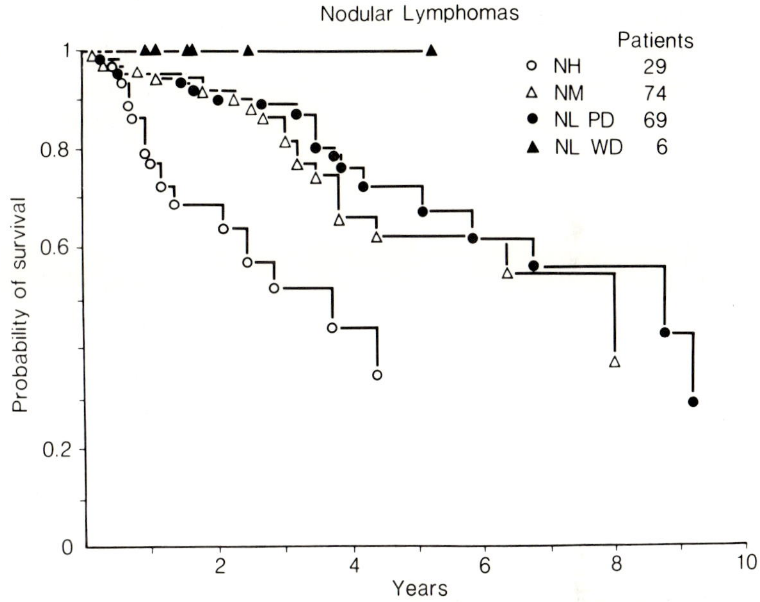

Fig. 14.22. Results of a retrospective study of "favourable" group non-Hodgkin's lymphoma. Note the pattern of continuing relapse.

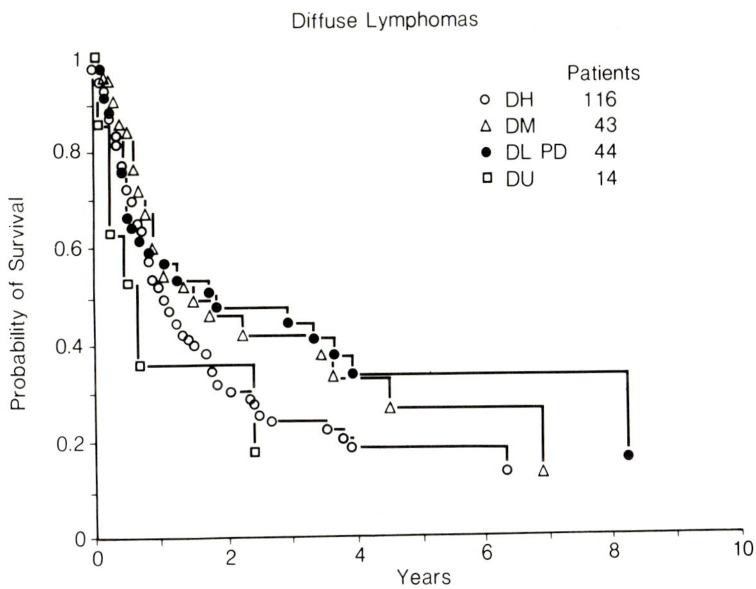

Fig. 14.23. Results of a retrospective study of "unfavourable" group non-Hodgkin's lymphoma. Note that there are relatively few relapses after the first 2 or 3 years.

Investigation of the patient will include full clinical examination, especially to assess the accessible nodal sites, peripheral blood count and conventional radiography of the chest and postnasal space. Since bone marrow is much more frequently involved than is the case in Hodgkin's disease, it should be examined in all cases, taking both aspiration and trephine specimens. In the grade I group, there may be difficulty in differentiating the solid lymphoma with secondary marrow involvement from chronic lymphatic leukaemia which has associated lymphadenopathy. Arbitrarily, chronic lymphatic leukaemia is defined by diffuse infiltration of the marrow with small lymphocytes and a total of 10 000 or more lymphocytes per cubic millimetre in the peripheral blood. Staging laparotomy is not used routinely as it is in Hodgkin's disease, because generalised disease is so much more common. More reliance is placed on marrow examination, CT of the abdomen, and liver function tests. Marrow involvement is inferred if there is infiltration with lymphoid cells exceeding 30%. If the infiltration is diffuse and consists of 30% or more of *lymphoblasts* then the patient should be considered as having acute lymphoblastic leukaemia. Liver function is more of a problem. The most reliable features are positive liver biopsy, enlargement of the organ, raised serum AST along with raised serum alkaline phosphatase, and reduced serum albumin. Liver biopsy is not advocated as a routine procedure but should be considered if liver function tests are equivocal and if the marrow is normal. (There is not much point in liver biopsy, with its attendant risks, if marrow infiltration has already placed the patient in stage 4.) As in Hodgkin's disease, CT is excellent for demonstrating nodal involvement within the abdomen, but is much less reliable for the assessment of the liver or spleen. With regard to staging, the Ann Arbor system (see Table 14.2) is used.

Radiotherapy

Radiotherapy is curative for an appreciable proportion of I E disease and to a lesser extent II E disease. The radiotherapy is similar to the radiotherapy of Hodgkin's disease, but because the spread of the disease is less predictable and since in particular there is a greater tendency for lymph node regions to be "skipped", there is less often an indication to take all the supradiaphragmatic nodes into one treatment volume. Thus, the "mantle" fields become the exception rather than the rule. Moreover, because of the high frequency of involvement of the structures in Waldeyer's ring, it is not safe to attempt to shield the lips when using anteroposterior fields. When treating disease which is localised to the cervical nodes, the fields should extend from the base of the skull to the sternal angle, and laterally should include both supraclavicular fossae. Such fields will be of the order of 25×20 cm, thus irradiating an appreciable length of the spinal cord. A safe dose would be 3000 cGy using megavoltage quality X-rays fractionated daily over 3 weeks. If there is suspicion of involvement of the postnasal space, the fields will have to extend above the eyes and these organs will therefore have to be carefully shielded, in both front and back fields, whilst allowing full dose to the postnasal space (Fig. 14.24). Where there is involvement of Waldeyer's ring, it is suggested that, on completion of the treatment from the anteroposterior fields, smaller lateral fields (arranged as a parallel pair) are added in such a way that the spinal cord, eyes, and lips are spared and an additional single dose of 500 cGy is given in the midplane. Treatment of abdominal nodes is less easy than in Hodgkin's disease because of the frequency of involvement of the mesenteric nodes. If these nodes are known to be affected, either from findings at operation or from

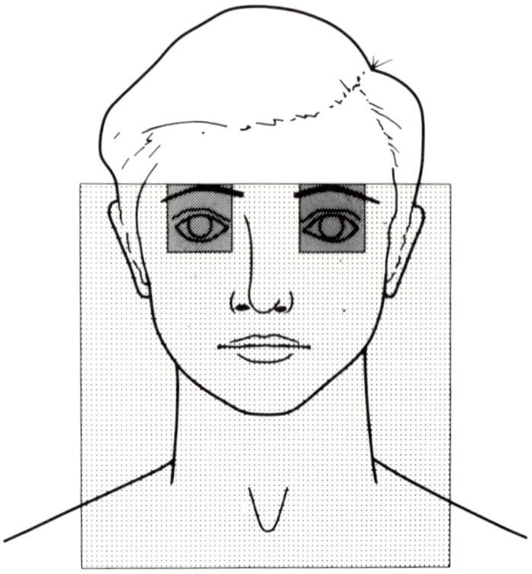

Fig. 14.24. The field arrangement, with protection of the eyes, used in treating non-Hodgkin's disease where there is involvement of Waldeyer's ring.

CT, it is best to start with large fields covering all the node regions in the abdomen and to take the dose to 1500 cGy fractionated over 10 days, accepting that the kidneys are also receiving this dose.

If treatment is then withheld for, say, 2 weeks and the abdomen reassessed by further CT, it may be found that there has been sufficient resolution of the lymphadenopathy to permit reduction of the field size with kidney shielding.

Treatment of nodes or of masses in other sites does not usually present problems, and in most cases a parallel pair of fields with a suitable margin, say 5 cm around the known extent of the disease, will be adequate. Radiotherapy to "bulk" disease is often an important part of the management of late disease, where chemotherapy is the mainstay of treatment. A decision about the desirability of this option and about the sites which are later to be irradiated must be taken before instituting chemotherapy, and details of these sites must be carefully recorded by radiographs, photographs, or anatomical measurements. Usually such "bulk" disease will take the form of node mass(es) arbitrarily of greater than 5 cm diameter. Radiotherapy to such sites should not be undertaken if it is estimated that this will entail irradiating more than half of the active marrow, and in most cases not more than two such sites will be treated. When irradiating such sites there will be complete resolution of the lymphadenopathy following chemotherapy, otherwise one is irradiating residual disease and completely different considerations apply. It will be necessary to take only a minimal margin so that the treatment volume will be relatively small, thus permitting treatment in a shorter overall time. A dose of 2500 cGy in eight fractions over 10 days is recommended.

In recent years there has been a revival of interest in whole body irradiation using small doses of X-rays from a linear accelerator. The technique is particularly suitable for the patient with widespread lymphoma but without masses of disease, especially when, perhaps because of age, he is unlikely to be fit enough to withstand demanding chemotherapy.

The treatment machine is used at an FSD of 400 cm with open jaws. The patient sits on a stool (Fig. 14.25) with his side towards the target and with his whole body subtended by the beam. A dose of 15 cGy is given. He is then turned through 180° and a similar dose given to the other side. It is estimated that the midline of the patient also receives about 15 cGy. This treatment is often prescribed twice weekly to a total dose of 150 cGy, but in practice it is safer to moderate this. Since the megakaryocytes prove to be very sensitive to this form of treatment it is recommended that the platelet count be ascertained before each fraction of the treatment. Further treatment should be withheld if it is judged that the count is falling too quickly. After the first 2 weeks it is safest to change to weekly fractionation at the same dose. This approach is often very convenient for the patient who, being frail, may find that weekly attendance as an outpatient is enough of a burden. The treatment can be most effective (Fig. 14.26) especially in the lymphoblastic or lymphocytic lymphomas. It is less good in the histiocytic lymphomas. Whole body irradiation is only palliative and may preclude late aggressive chemotherapy.

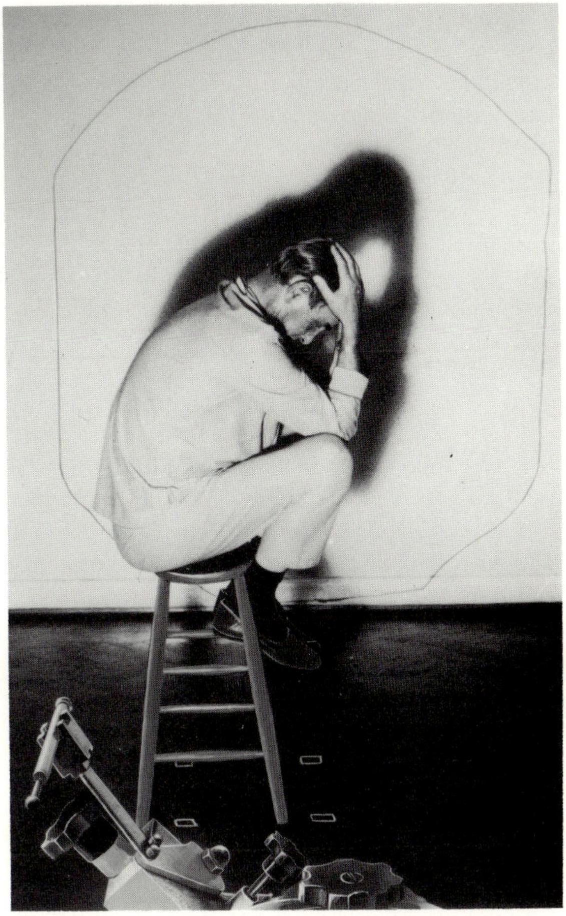

Fig. 14.25. Photograph taken whilst looking along the head of the linear accelerator when a patient is being set up for whole body irradiation.

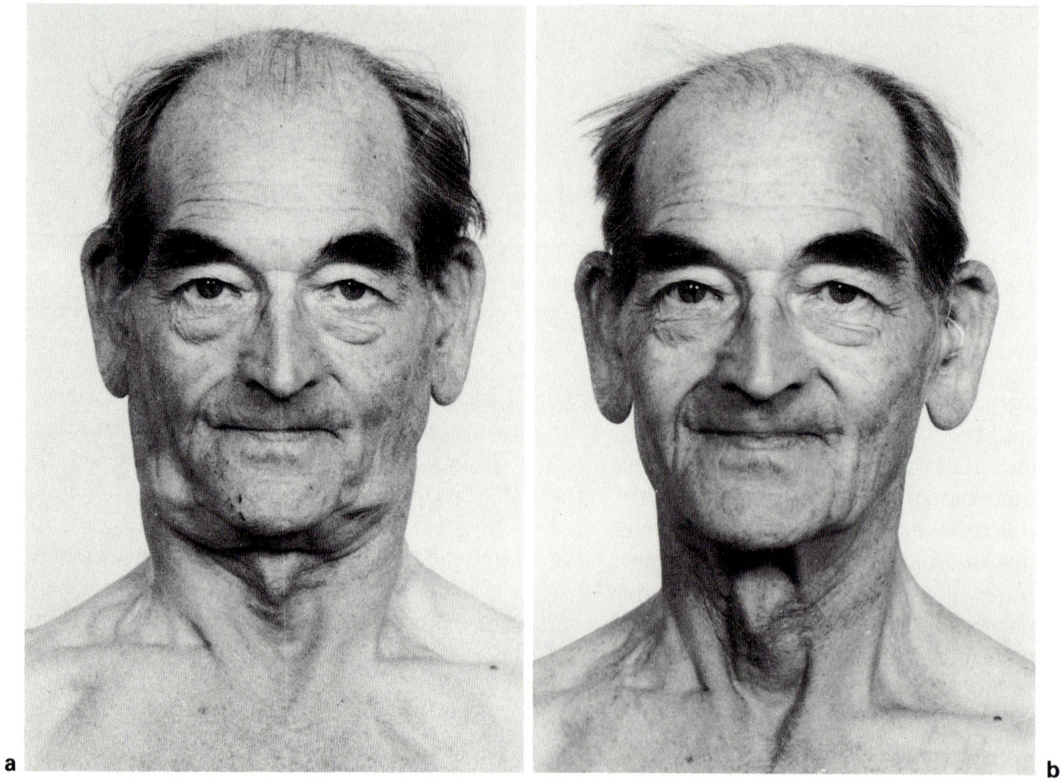

Fig. 14.26a,b. An elderly patient, with generalised lymphoblastic lymphoma, before and after whole body irradiation. Note the good, although incomplete, resolution of his cervical lymphadenopathy.

Cytotoxic Chemotherapy

Single-agent chemotherapy still has a valuable place in the management of the grade I lymphomas, but most of the radical chemotherapy is by use of combination chemotherapy. There is still no general agreement on a standard combination as there is concerning MOPP or MVPP in Hodgkin's disease. In 1971 Luce and his colleagues described the use of cyclophosphamide, vincristine, and prednisolone (CVP) in the therapy of malignant lymphoma. This particular combination (Table 14.9) is still as effective as any, as an induction regime in the grade I group. The vincristine is given as an intravenous injection on day 1, in a dose not exceeding 2 mg and is followed by oral dosage with prednisolone and cyclophosphamide for 5 days. Courses are given at 21-day intervals, usually to a total of six or more courses. There is however, no evidence that CVP is superior to chlorambucil alone for the most common grade I lymphoma—the nodular lymphocytic. Chlorambucil is given at a dose of 5 mg twice daily for 14 days, interspaced with 14-day rest periods, the dose being modified according to the peripheral blood count. For the "unfavourable" grade II groups, various combinations have found favour in the past, but because they were cyclic, relapse tended to occur between the courses. For this reason a sustained induction, on the lines of the chemotherapy used for acute leukaemia, has been tried and may be superior. This VAP regime is shown in Fig. 14.27. The prednisolone is given daily by mouth, the vincristine weekly by intravenous injection (again with a maximum dose of 2 mg each time) and the adriamycin intravenously every 2 weeks. At the end of the course the prednisolone is tailed off over a period of a few days. This induction regime may be followed by consolidation using high-dose cyclophosphamide (1 g/m^2 intravenously followed by

Table 14.9. CVP regime.

Vincristine 1.4 mg/m^2 (total not to exceed 2 mg i.v. day 1)	
Cyclophosphamide 400 mg/m^2	by mouth days 2 to 5 inclusive
Prednisolone 25 mg twice daily	

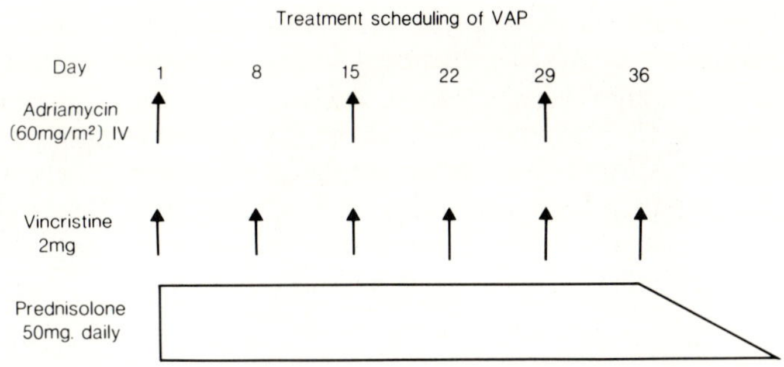

Fig. 14.27. Diagram to show the timing when the VAP regime is administered.

hydration, every 3 weeks for three doses), by radiotherapy to "bulk" disease, or both. There is no clear evidence that maintenance chemotherapy is of advantage, especially in diffuse histiocytic lymphoma, where the important thing is to achieve complete remission. In poorly differentiated diffuse lymphoma, where continuing relapse is seen, further chemotherapy may well be required. This continuing chemotherapy may take the form of the continuous regime given in Table 14.10, or an intermittent regime as, for example, in Table 14.11. This intermittent therapy is given every 3 weeks until tolerance for adriamycin is exhausted (this is the point at which, including the induction course, the total dose reaches 550 mg/m^2).

Table 14.10. Mercaptopurine/cyclophosphamide/methotrexate maintenance regime.

Mercaptopurine 50 mg/m^2 by mouth daily	
Cyclophosphamide 200 mg/m^2	by mouth weekly
Methotrexate 10 mg/m^2	by mouth weekly

Table 14.11. Adriamycin/cyclophosphamide regime.

Adriamycin	40 mg/m^2	i.v. day 1
Cyclophosphamide	200 mg/m^2	p.o. days 2 to 6 (incl.)
Four weeks between courses		

Current Policies in the Management of the Non-Hodgkin's Lymphomas

For patients with stage 1 or 2 disease of grade I type, X-ray treatment to the known disease, taking a safe margin, is adequate. So far there is no evidence that adjuvant chemotherapy either increases the relapse-free interval or improves the overall survival rate. Numerous trials are being carried out, throughout the world, in an attempt to refute this statement, but at the time of going to press it holds good.

For patients in stage 3 or 4 with grade I histology, chemotherapy is the mainstay of treatment. The CVP combination is suggested as an induction regime, not because it is highly effective but for want of something better. The use of chlorambucil, as a single agent, may be as good. Because of the tendency of the disease to relapse at sites which were bulky at presentation, consideration should be given to the possibility of radiotherapy to one or possibly two of these sites, provided the CVP induces a complete remission. If remission has not been obtained after, say, six courses, the CVP should be abandoned and alternative measures considered. Given good marrow reserve with, in particular, a normal platelet count in the peripheral blood, whole body irradiation should be tried since this is capable of inducing complete remission even, occasionally, where chemotherapy has failed. With inadequate marrow reserve it is probably best to treat troublesome deposits with simple local X-ray treatments and thereafter to keep the patient under surveillance. Before the days of effective chemotherapy, this type of radiotherapy, the so-called "chasing technique", provided the best available management and a small but significant group of these patients survived for very many years and enjoyed an excellent quality of life. For the patient who does go into complete remission, with or without radiotherapy to "bulk" disease, consideration may be given to the advisability of maintenance chemotherapy, possibly using chlorambucil as a single agent. However, as with the adjuvant chemotherapy discussed for early-stage disease in the preceding paragraph, the evidence to support this approach is not yet secure.

For patients in stage 1 or 2 with grade II pathology, local X-ray treatment will again be the first step. However, here there is a better case for adjuvant chemotherapy because the relapse rate is high, about 60%, and the chemotherapy is more effective than it is for the grade I group. Either the VAP regime or an intermittent schedule such as CMOPP (Table 14.12) may be chosen. Before committing the patient to such a course, he should be apprised of possible sequelae, such as interference with gonadal function. Certain patients in this grade II group, even in stages 1 and 2, carry a particularly bad prognosis. This includes those with massive intra-abdominal disease and gastrointestinal lymphoma beyond stage 1. Because of this, it is suggested that these patients be managed in the same way as those patients in stage 3 or 4, as described in the next paragraph.

Table 14.12. CMOPP regime.

Cyclophosphamide	650 mg/m^2	i.v.	Days 1+8
Vincristine	1.4 mg/m^2	i.v.	Days 1+8
Procarbazine	100 mg/m^2	p.o.	Days 1–14 incl.
Prednisolone	25 mg twice daily	p.o.	Days 1–14 incl.
Six-week cycle			

Patients with grade II histology who are in stage 3 or 4 have a very bad prognosis. This being so, if their general condition warrants it, they should be given initial chemotherapy, radiotherapy to "bulk" disease if appropriate, and possibly maintenance chemotherapy. The chemotherapy of choice is VAP as an induction regime, followed in due course either by the mercaptopurine/methotrexate/cyclophosphamide or by the adriamycin/cyclophosphamide regime. If elderly and unfit, and where the histology is of diffuse poorly differentiated type, whole body irradiation may be the optimum choice, but this would not be advisable if there were significant thrombocytopenia. Where the histology is of histiocytic type, VAP should be tried and continued if tolerated and if the patient is responding to it.

Complications of Treatment

Much of what has already been said about the side effects and late complications of chemotherapy in Hodgkin's disease applies with equal force to the treatment of non-Hodgkin's disease. Adriamycin is used more frequently in these lymphomas and carries the particular risk of cardiotoxicity. This can be kept to an acceptable level if the *total* dose is not permitted to exceed 550 mg/m^2. The risk to the myocardium is increased if the heart is also heavily irradiated, as may be the case with some mediastinal tumours.

Another drug which is used more freely in this group of lymphomas is cyclophosphamide. Apart from marrow depression and epilation, which it shares with other agents, the drug can also give rise to a very troublesome cystitis. This is a sterile haemorrhagic cystitis, apparently caused by excretion of the metabolite acrolein, and it may persist long after the cyclophosphamide has been withdrawn. Having once occurred, it is very likely to be provoked by subsequent challenge with the drug, suggesting that there may also be an element of sensitisation present. Adequate hydration during administration of the drug is the best way of avoiding this complication. For example, when giving the drug in a dose of 1 g/m^2 this should be given in a litre of infusion fluid and be followed by a further 2 l intravenously as a minimum. The use of the detoxifying agent mesna is currently being assessed for its value in preventing cystitis. Cardiac toxicity is also an occasional feature of cyclophosphamide therapy.

Special Problems

The situation here is much as it is in Hodgkin's disease. Again one may be faced with concurrent pregnancy and the course of action will be dictated by the attitude of the patient and her spouse as well as by obstetrical considerations and the natural history of the disease. However, in the case of "unfavourable" group disease in its later stages, it will seldom be possible to put off systemic treatment until after normal term and there will be great pressure to terminate the pregnancy or to induce early delivery. In the early stages, even in the "unfavourable" group, it will usually be possible to hold the disease with radiotherapy unless there is substantial abdominal involvement.

Central nervous system (CNS) disease is much commoner than in Hodgkin's disease and intracranial (especially meningeal) deposits are quite frequent. Because of the all-too-frequent finding of CNS involvement, particularly in the diffuse poorly differentiated group, and in those with diffuse histiocytic lymphoma, prophylactic treatment, similar to that used in acute lymphoblastic leukaemia, has been tried, but with disappointing results.

Paraparesis may occur as in Hodgkin's disease, but is much less likely to be due to an isolated deposit. There is therefore a strong indication to treat the whole CNS with a combination of irradiation (cord and spine) and intrathecal methotrexate. Unfortunately, a lasting response, even to the most vigorous and comprehensive treatment, is so rare that the management of this complication must be regarded as very palliative. Progressive multifocal leucocephalopathy will be seen occasionally as in Hodgkin's disease, where there is the predisposing combination of ill-controlled lymphoma and protracted chemotherapy. Likewise "opportunist" infections, depression of gonadal function, and second malignancy are as much a feature of the long-term management of the non-Hodgkin's as of Hodgkin's disease patients.

Mycosis Fungoides

This is the non-Hodgkin's lymphoma which predominantly affects the skin. It is usually possible to identify the responsible cells as T cells. The problem in management is to control the widespread cutaneous infiltrates. It is seldom possible to eradicate the disease completely, but the disease does tend to run a rather indolent course over several years and can be very distressing for the patient. It is a rare disease, between 60 and 70 cases being registered in England and Wales each year, but by its nature the patient needs repeated treatments and it thus assumes an importance out of proportion to its incidence. There is excellent temporary response to local radiotherapy, but the response to cytotoxic chemotherapy is poor. Electron therapy is the preferred form of radiotherapy in order to minimise the dose to deeper organs, in particular the marrow. The following "translation" technique with a 3-MV electron beam from a linear accelerator is used. The patient is positioned on a moving couch tilted at 5° (Fig. 14.28) and drawn under the beam in a series of traverses, right and left anterior when in the supine position, and right and left posterior

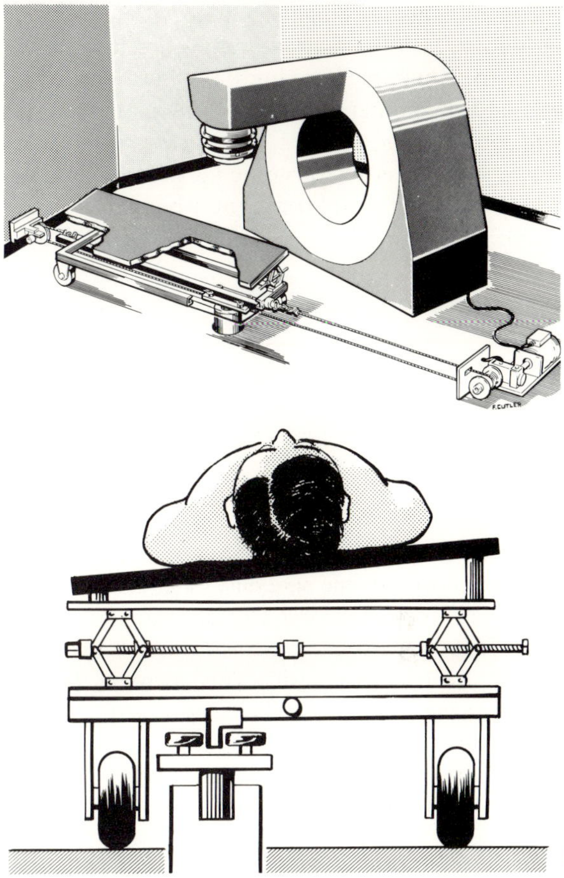

a

b

Fig. 14.28. a The arrangement of the linear accelerator and the moving couch required for the translational technique used in electron therapy of the whole body. **b** Drawing to show the 5° tilt of the couch.

when in the prone position. There is an interlock system which ensures that the couch movement and tube output are synchronised. The depth-dose curve of the 3-MV electron beam is shown in Fig. 14.29. The build-up of dose in the longitudinal axis is shown diagrammatically in Fig. 14.30. Because of this build-up it is necessary to start with the patient, or at least the area to be treated, outside the beam, to move him through the beam, and to finish with him outside the beam again. In practice he is moved through a distance 20 cm more than his length. The transverse dose distribution is shown in Fig. 14.31 and the effect of the oblique incidence, achieved by the 5° tilt, in Fig. 14.32.

Before prescribing this form of treatment, the whole skin surface must be inspected, because decisions have to be taken about areas which can be shielded and those which may require later supplementary dosage. If possible, it is wise to

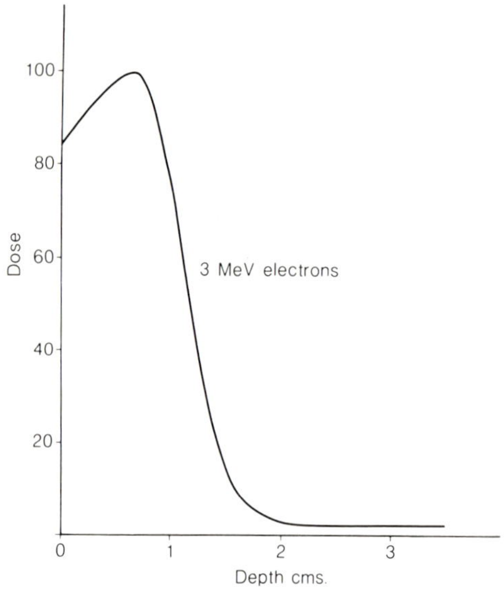

Fig. 14.29. Diagrammatic representation of the depth dose from the 3-MeV electron beam.

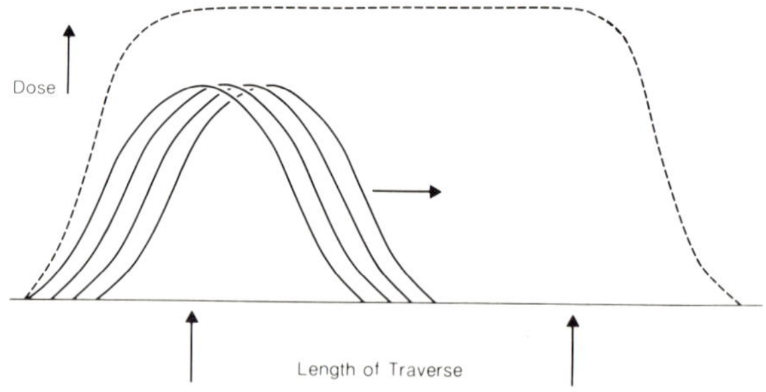

Fig. 14.31. Diagram to show the transverse dose distribution, using the 3-MeV electron beam.

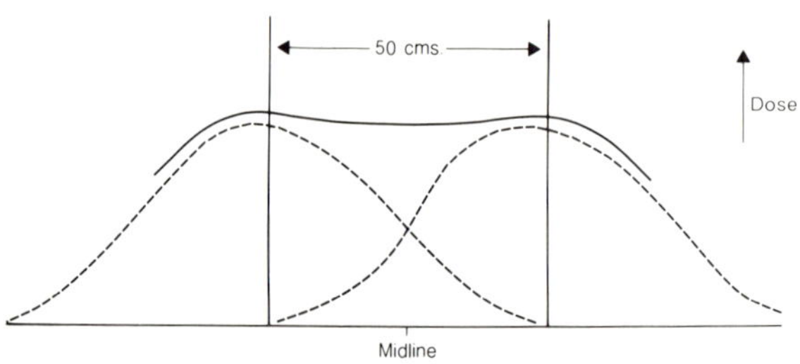

Fig. 14.30. Diagram to show the build-up of dose in the longitudinal axis when the patient is traversed, using the 3-MeV electron beam.

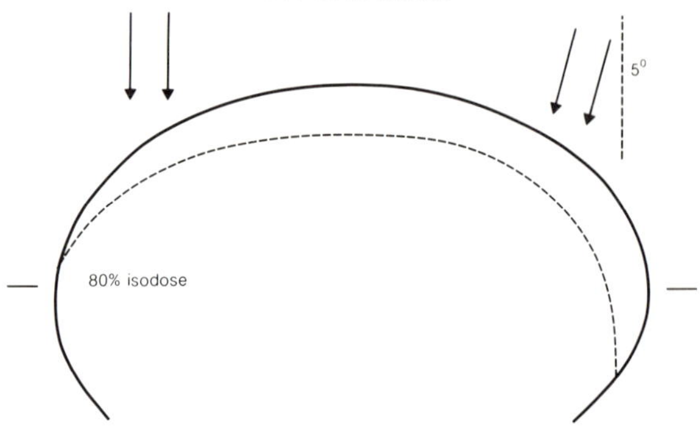

Fig. 4.32. Diagram to show the effect of the 5° tilt on the dose distribution when using the translational technique.

shield the finger and toe nails lest the radiation cause them to be shed. Even if the nails are involved by the disease, it may be wise to shield the palmar, or plantar, surface of the digits, since dose from each side will summate undesirably in the midline (see the depth-dose curve, Fig. 14.31). Such shielding may be employed for half the treatment. For shielding purposes 2.0 mm lead is sufficient. If there is no evidence of scalp involvement this area can be conveniently shielded by the use of a lead-lined tunnel (Fig. 14.33). The eyes, and of course the lids, should be shielded throughout treatment to prevent dosage to the lens and conjunctivae. This is done with a spectacle frame in which the lenses are lined with lead. If there are infiltrates around the lids it will be necessary to treat these separately by inserting an eye shield and giving a single exposure, possibly using 45-kV photons, rather than electrons, for convenience. The perineum and axillae may be relatively underdosed by this translational electron technique, so that it may later be necessary to give supplementary irradiation to these sites. Likewise, any unduly thick plaques should also be reviewed later. A patient under treatment is shown in Fig. 14.33.

With regard to dosage, treatment to one quadrant is given on one day. Each quadrant is

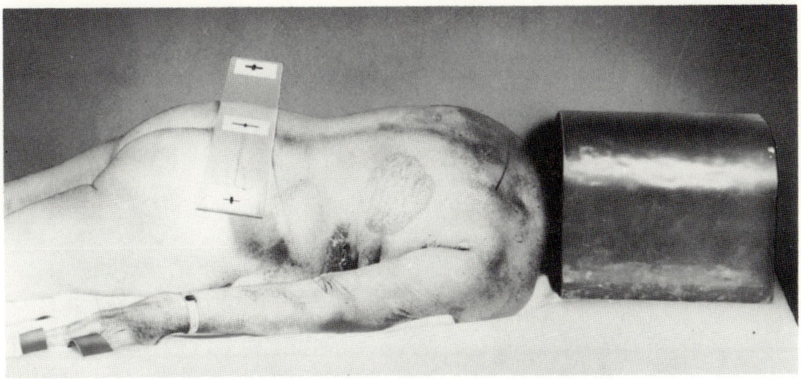

Fig. 14.33. A patient with mycosis fungoides undergoing electron beam therapy. Note that it has been possible to shield the whole head as well as the nails.

given three treatments, so that the patient will have a total of 12 treatments, usually spread over 3 weeks. At each treatment 800 cGy is given and the dose administered to the whole integument is stated as 2400 cGy. This is well tolerated and usually accompanied by no more than mild erythema, but an occasional patient does experience a more severe reaction. Doses of 3000 cGy have been given without upset. Treatment is not associated with evidence of marrow depression. There is no late skin atrophy or loss of dermal appendages. Treatment, using the above dosage, has been repeated on up to three further occasions without anxiety. This technique has been used to palliate other conditions, such as cutaneous infiltrates associated with refractory chronic granulocytic leukaemia (Fig. 14.34), and for the rare condition of myxoscleroderma (Fig. 14.35).

A case of mycosis fungoides before and after electron therapy is shown in Fig. 14.36.

If low-energy electron therapy is not available, then "patching" treatment using multiple fields with a superficial machine operating at about 45 kV must be used. The doses will be of the order of 800 cGy in single exposures. Currently there is much interest in PUVA. In this form of treatment the skin is sensitised with 8-methoxypsoralein and then irradiated with relatively long-wave ultraviolet light. It is thought that the action of the photosensitising drug along with the ultraviolet light is to inhibit DNA synthesis (much as does methotrexate). This treatment can be effective, especially for very superficial disease, but its place in overall management has yet to be defined.

Chemotherapy is of occasional value. The application of topical mustine may give some local control and systemic therapy gives worthwhile

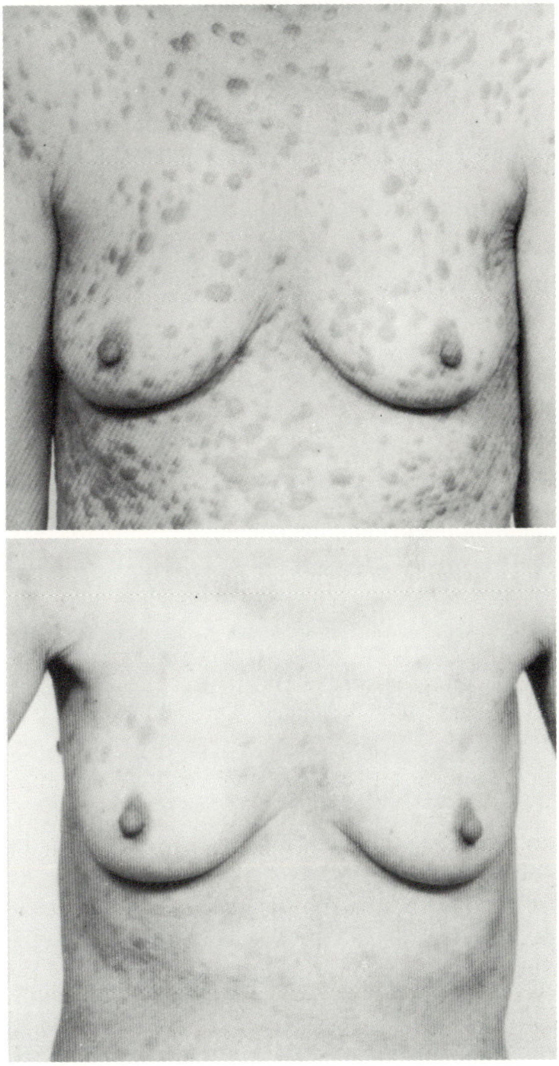

a

b

Fig. 14.34a,b. A patient in the late stages of chronic granulocytic leukaemia, who was no longer responsive to cytotoxic agents, and who had discomfort from cutaneous infiltrates is shown before and after palliation with whole body electron beam therapy.

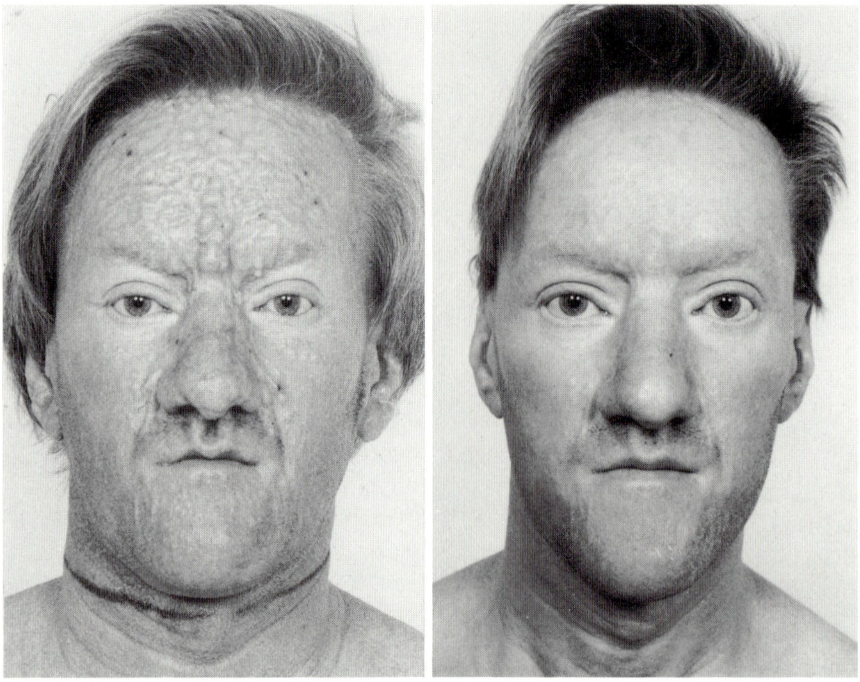

Fig. 14.35a,b. A patient with disfiguring myxoscleroderma before and after electron beam therapy. The skin was improved but unfortunately the patient later succumbed to systemic complications of his disease.

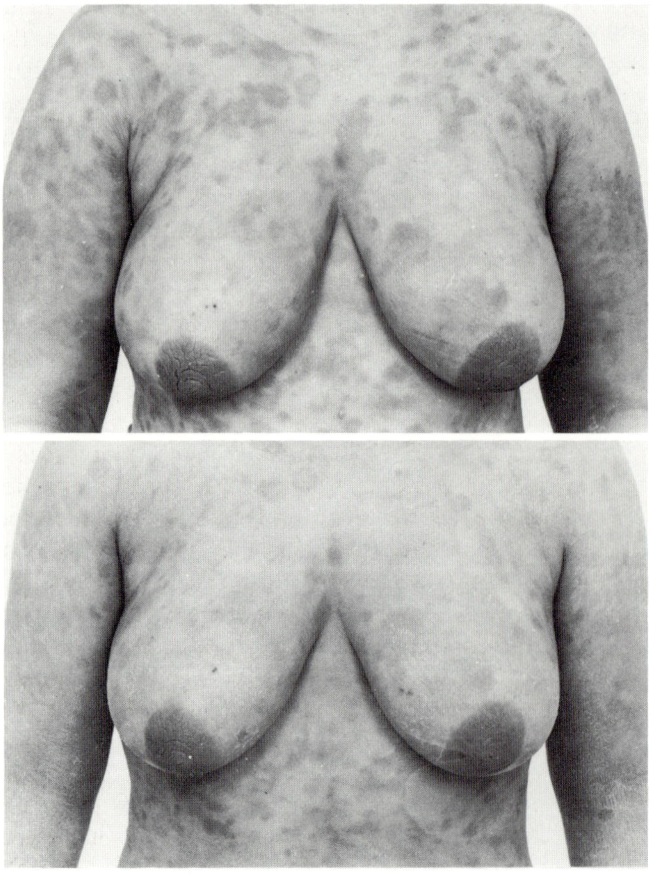

Fig. 14.36a,b. "Before" and "after" photographs of a woman (unusually young for this disease) who has undergone whole body electron therapy for mycosis fungoides.

palliation in a small number of patients—the most effective regime being VAP (see Fig. 14.27).

Sezary Syndrome

This condition is a variant of mycosis fungoides. It is a T cell disorder and is characterised by the presence of abnormal lymphoid cells which are readily seen in the peripheral blood. The clinical picture is of a chronic lymphatic leukaemia with marked erythroderma, lymphadenopathy, and hepatosplenomegaly. The formation of plaques, tumours, and ulcers is less of a feature than in mycosis fungoides. Histologically, however, the appearance of the affected skin is very similar to mycosis, but haematologically a characteristic cell is found in the peripheral blood. Treatment with cytotoxic agents such as chlorambucil may have some palliative effect. The use of electron therapy or PUVA is of less value than in mycosis fungoides. The use of leucopheresis may be considered as an alternative form of therapy. A patient with Sezary syndrome is shown in Fig. 14.37.

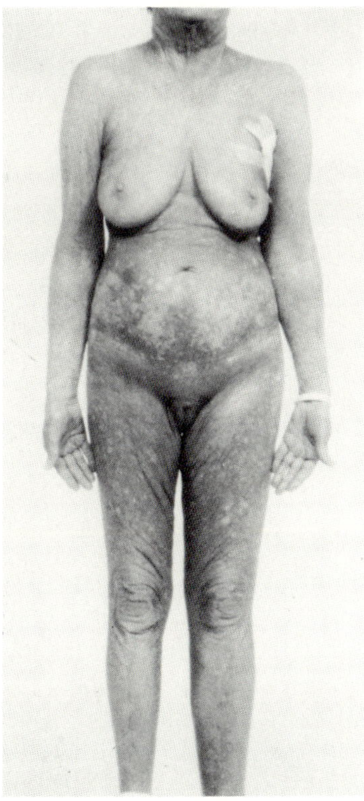

Fig. 14.37. Photograph of a patient with Sezary syndrome to show the appearance of the skin.

Chronic Lymphatic Leukaemia

This disease may occur at any age but is most common in later life. It is often not easy to differentiate from non-Hodgkin's lymphoma of well-differentiated lymphocytic type, but it is suggested that, rather arbitrarily, a peripheral count in excess of 10 000 lymphocytes per cubic millimetre along with marrow showing diffuse infiltration with small lymphocytes accounting for more than 30% of the cells should be required for the initial diagnosis. It is convenient to stage the disease as follows:

Stage 0—blood and marrow only (asymptomatic)
Stage 1—lymphadenopathy present
Stage 2—enlargement of spleen and/or liver
Stage 3—anaemia under 11 g%
Stage 4—thrombocytopenia

Often in stages 0 and 1 the patient is entirely symptom-free, the disease having been discovered as an incidental finding when the patient attends for an unrelated complaint. As the process can often be very indolent, and as there is no evidence that treatment in these early stages influences the long-term prognosis, it is usually sufficient to keep the patient under observation only, without active treatment. Should the patient be concerned about enlarged nodes, these may be treated by local irradiation with X-rays, but this is often not very effective as a single exposure, at lymphoma level of dosage, because of the recirculation of the lymphocytes.

In stage 2, the disease may also be symptom-free, as the splenomegaly may be minimal and the patient unaware of it. However, in the presence of symptomatic splenomegaly, treatment may be required. The systemic use of chlorambucil, radiophosphorus, whole body irradiation, or splenic X-ray treatment will be effective, but the last-mentioned treatment may appear to be most appropriate to the patient whose only symptom is awareness of the enlarged organ.

The patient with stage 3 disease will usually require treatment and the one selected will usually be the one most convenient for the patient, as there is no good evidence that one method is superior to the others. In practice, outpatient management using chlorambucil tends to be the first choice for this reason. There has been renewed interest in mediastinal irradiation, but we are unconvinced that this approach has any advantage over splenic irradiation (see Fig. 14.44) where the dose is "titrated" against the response.

The main therapeutic challenge is in stage 4, where thrombocytopenia may be extreme, thus limiting the possibility of cytotoxic chemotherapy or radiotherapy. Most reliance will be placed on steroids such as prednisolone, which do, of course, have a lympholytic action, as well as helping to control the haemolytic anaemia which may be a feature at this stage. Initial dosage will be high, say 50 mg daily, but this can be reduced to safer levels as response is obtained. The enteric-coated preparation, with or without cimetidine, should be used if there is any suspicion of peptic ulceration. It is possible that extracorporeal irradiation may help to kill off circulating lymphocytes without inducing further thrombocytopenia, if the technique is available (Fig. 14.38). Other supportive measures may be of value, such as transfusion, control of infection, and sometimes local irradiation for a limited node mass or area of infiltration.

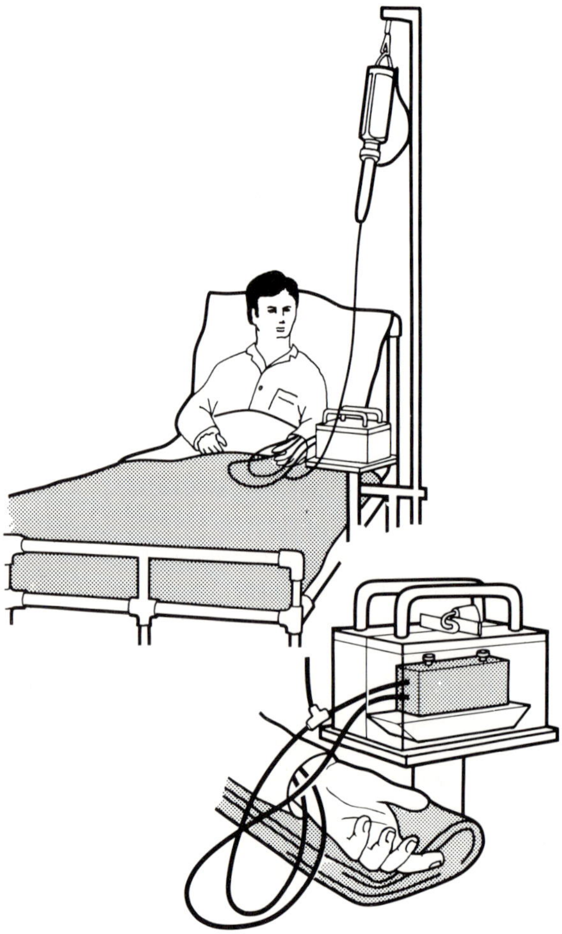

Fig. 14.38. The arrangement of patient, shunt and radioactive source used in extracorporeal irradiation of the blood.

Myeloproliferative Disorders

Polycythaemia Vera

The diagnosis of polycythaemia vera is not always easy even when the usual cardiorespiratory causes of secondary polycythaemia and renal disease have been excluded. Estimation of the red cell mass has proved to be particularly useful and is recommended in all cases when seen for the first time. This disorder can be managed effectively either by radiotherapy or by chemotherapy. In terms of survival and quality of life there is little to choose but radiotherapy does have the advantage of convenience. As the disease usually occurs in those past middle life and, as it tends to a protracted course, often over 10 years or more, it is easier for the patient to adopt a line of treatment which involves follow-up visits about once in 3 months and outpatient treatment every year or two, rather than the continuous treatment and frequent monitoring which is inseparable from chemotherapy. Current radiotherapy is with radiophosphorus (^{32}P), although other forms of radiotherapy, such as whole body irradiation using photons from kilovoltage apparatus, were used before radiophosphorus became available. As absorption of ^{32}P is erratic and incomplete when given by mouth, the intravenous route is preferred. The maximum recommended dose is 300 MBq for a man of 70 kg with a lower or higher dose in proportion to the weight of the patient as compared with the 70-kg man. In practice, one seldom exceeds 400 MBq and tends always to give rather less than the recommended maximum since it is easy to give a supplementary dose and there is not much to be done about a high dose should the patient prove unduly sensitive to it. It is wise to monitor the response carefully after the first dose, as this will give help with subsequent doses and, as with the radiophosphorus treatment of the leukaemias, the dose required to produce the same effect in a given patient remains fairly constant. This applies particularly to the effect on white cells and platelets. Usually the nadir is recorded at about 6 weeks after the injection, although of course the full effect is not seen on the red cell mass for some 4 months. The haematogram of a patient receiving radiophosphorus for polycythaemia is shown in Fig. 14.39. The long-term risk with

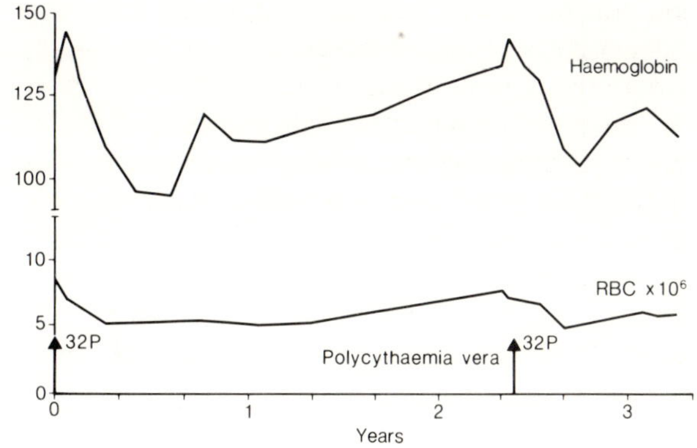

Fig. 14.39. Haematogram of patient with polycythaemia, treated with radiophosphorus.

radiotherapy is that this may increase the proportion of patients whose disease transforms into leukaemia, and it is possible that this risk is proportional to the overall dose of radiophosphorus administered. Having said this, it is still noteworthy that the survival in Halnan and Russell's series (Fig. 14.40) is at least as good in the radiotherapy as in the chemotherapy cases. Where doses of radiophosphorus are required at fairly long intervals, say every 2 years, this is perfectly acceptable, especially in the older age groups, but in the younger patients—there are some in their twenties and thirties—there is a tendency to prefer chemotherapy.

Many cytotoxic drugs have been shown to be effective in polycythaemia. Alkylating agents, especially busulphan, are popular, and folate antagonists such as pyrimethamine have also been of more than occasional use. Busulphan is the chemotherapeutic agent of choice because it is slower and more predictable in its action than pyrimethamine. Apart from the well-established risks of excessive marrow depression, amenorrhoea in menstruating women, skin pigmentation and occasional gastrointestinal toxicity, busulphan also produces rare complications including testicular atrophy, pulmonary fibrosis, and a syndrome suggesting adrenocortical insufficiency. This last syndrome consists of pigmentation, weakness, anorexia, and weight loss, but without laboratory evidence of adrenal failure.

Apart from the specific treatment of polycythaemia, which is usually slow in its effects and must be regarded as long-term, one must not forget that venesection may be required to tide the patient over a crisis. Venesection is not recom-

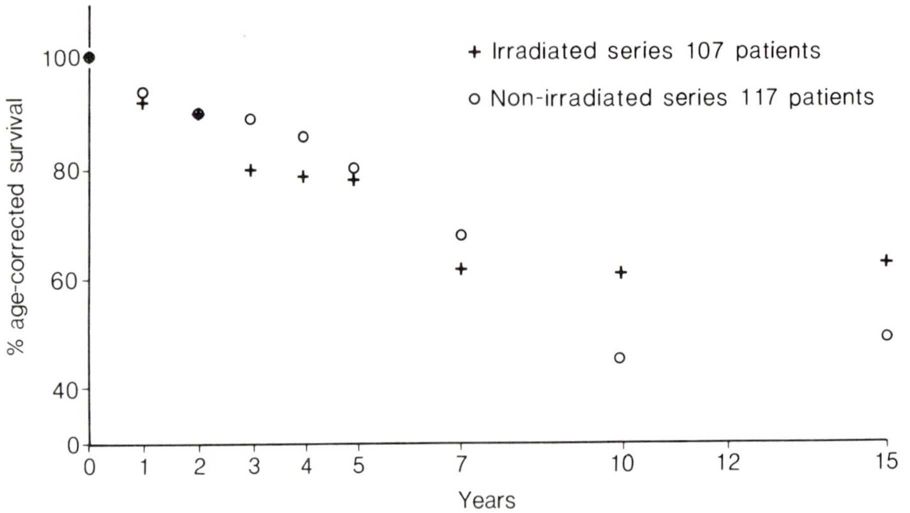

Fig. 14.40. Chart comparing survival in patients with polycythaemia treated by radiotherapy and by chemotherapy.

mended for long-term management, because it tends to provoke thrombocythaemia and iron deficiency. If hyperuricaemia is a feature then allopurinol is useful.

Essential Thrombocythaemia

This disorder is closely related to polycythaemia vera and may, with time, become indistinguishable from it. The only abnormal finding is of a grossly raised platelet count, and this may be associated with thrombotic or haemorrhagic features. This condition is usually very amenable to radiophosphorus and the practice is to give a rather lower dose than in polycythaemia—say 300 MBq maximum. The interval between doses may be quite long and is commonly several years.

Radiophosphorus

Radiophosphorus has a part to play in the management of polycythaemia vera, essential thrombocythaemia, and the chronic leukaemias. The isotope which is used is ^{32}P. This isotope has a physical half-life of 14.3 days and a biological half-life of about 11 days. It is a beta emitter with a maximum energy of 1.7 MeV and a mean energy of 0.68 MeV. The maximum range in water is 8 mm. Radiophosphorus is administered as a salt (phosphate) and is usually given intravenously, as absorption from the intestinal tract is erratic and may only amount to approximately three-quarters of the dose. The phosphorus is not evenly distributed and the following absorption ratios (tissue : normal) are typical—red marrow 1.5, testis 2.0, and lymph node 1.5–2.5. For treatment purposes radiophosphorus is presented as a sterile solution with a strength lying within the range of 400 MBq in 2–10 ml. Individual doses are commonly around 200 MBq. As there is only beta radiation to consider, protection can be achieved by the use of a transparent plastic case for the syringe (Fig. 14.41). The solution is drawn into the syringe behind a further transparent plastic sheet, and over a tray lined with blotting paper in case of accidental spillage. The operator uses surgical gloves which are discarded afterwards along with the syringe so that they can be disposed of safely. The patient does not need to take any special precautions following treatment. When used in the management of chronic granulocytic or chronic lymphatic leukaemia, Easson's method is recommended. A dose of, say, 100 MBq is given and the total white count is plotted, on a logarithmic scale, over the following 2 weeks. These counts are also plotted against the dose of radiophosphorus calculated as millibecquerels destroyed (i.e. using the 11-day biological half-life) as shown in Fig. 14.42. From this graph one can calculate the supplementary dose which is required to bring the count down to normal levels (10 000 per cubic millimetre). Once the dose has been established for the individual patient it tends to remain constant, thus simplifying subsequent treatments.

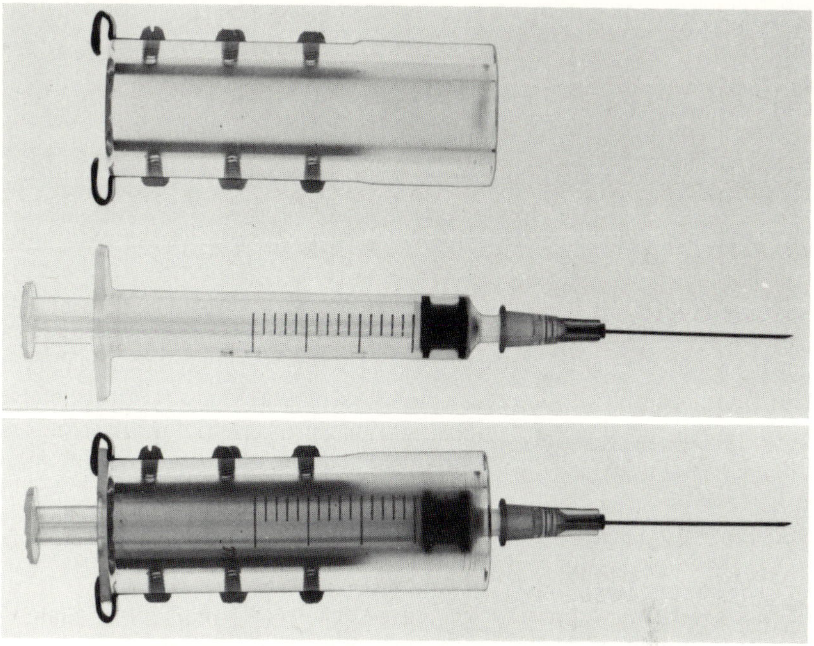

Fig. 14.41. The transparent plastic syringe guard with syringe used in the administration of radiophosphorus.

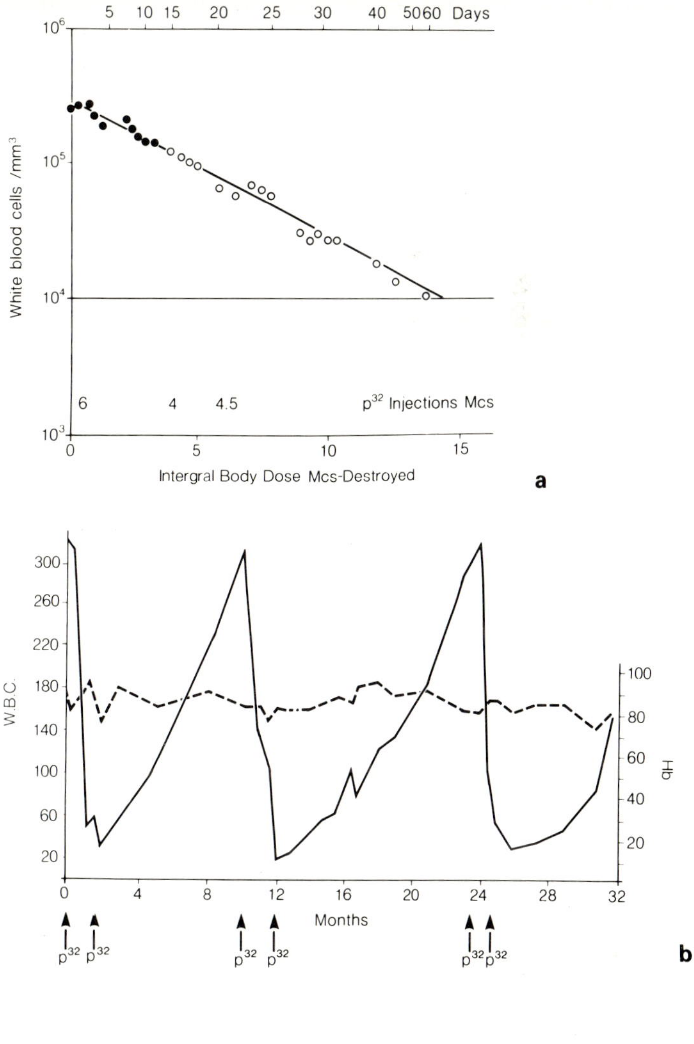

Fig. 14.42. **a** Graph to show how the total white count (shown on a logarithmic scale) can be plotted against the dose of radiophosphorus given as "millicuries destroyed". This is used after a test dose to project the total dose of radiophosphorus which will be required to bring the white count down to a normal level. **b** Haematogram to show the total white count in a patient with chronic lymphatic leukaemia being treated with radiophosporus.

Chronic Granulocytic Leukaemia

This is a relatively rare disease which can occur at any age but is most commonly found in middle life. Classically it is marked by the presence of the "Philadelphia" chromosome. The mainstay of management will be chemotherapy with cytotoxic drugs, but radiotherapy does sometimes have a useful part to play. Unfortunately, at present, all treatment must be regarded as palliative, although a partial clinical remission is usually obtained and may last for several years.

Busulphan is the cytotoxic drug of choice. It is an alkylating agent which is given by mouth. During induction therapy the dose is 4 mg daily. It is dangerous to exceed this dose because quite a precipitate fall in circulating granulocytes and also in platelets may result from marrow depression. Marrow depression of this sort may be very slow to recover. When the peripheral count is falling the dose should be dropped to, say, 2 mg daily until a normal level has been reached. Using this method it may take several months (Fig. 14.43) to achieve a complete remission. When remission has been obtained, weekly dosage with busulphan is preferred for maintenance, since this is associated with less marrow toxicity. The dose is adjusted to maintain the white blood cell count at $5–9 \times 10^9$/l. There is, therefore, something to be said for using a faster technique for induction. Splenic irradiation does this. In this technique kilovoltage apparatus is used and up to three fields are arranged, as in Fig. 14.44, to cover most of the organ. It does not matter if part of the spleen does not come within the irradiated fields. One field is treated each day and the peripheral count is noted before deciding the dose to be used. Typically one would start with 50 cGy and increase the dose by 25-cGy increments to about 150 cGy daily. This will usually bring the count down to near normal levels within 3 weeks, at which time a switch should be made to low-dose maintenance with busulphan. The "saw-tooth" pattern of the haematogram of a patient managed throughout with intermittent courses of splenic irradiation is shown in Fig. 14.45, as a contrast to the patient in Fig. 14.43 where busulphan alone was used in the first four years.

When complete remission is obtained consideration should be given to the advisability of splenectomy. It used to be thought that this procedure might delay transformation to the blastic phase, though this is uncertain. However, it does at least help with the later management as a proportion of these patients do suffer great disability from massive splenomegaly when the disease relapses. During relapse splenectomy is much more hazardous because of its size, the presence of adhesions associated with infarcts, and often an unsatisfactory blood count. In the later stages of the disease, when relapse is occurring but before it has progressed into a frankly blastic disease, thrombocythaemia may present a difficult problem in management. This feature is associated

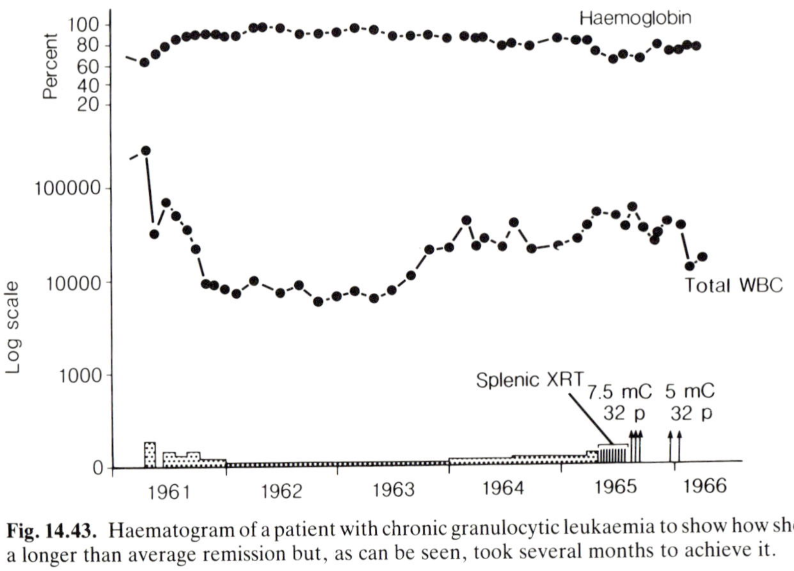

Fig. 14.43. Haematogram of a patient with chronic granulocytic leukaemia to show how she responded to Busulphan. She enjoyed a longer than average remission but, as can be seen, took several months to achieve it.

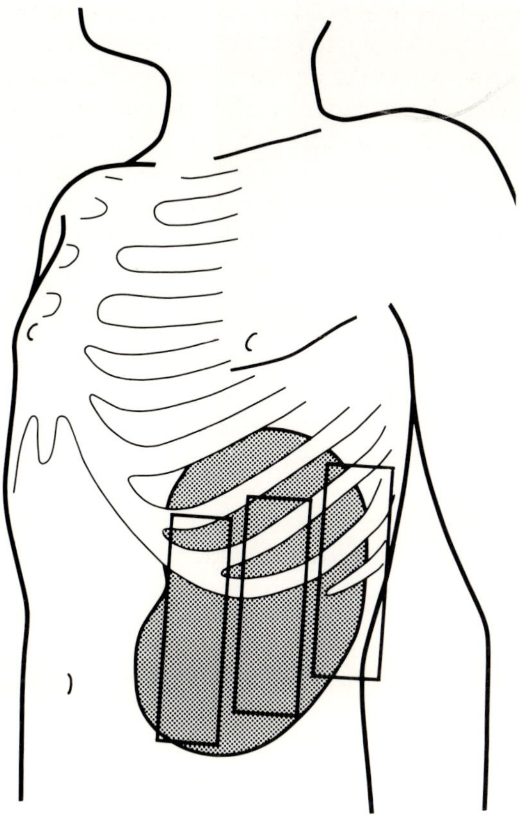

Fig. 14.44. The field arrangement for splenic irradiation in chronic leukaemia using kilovoltage apparatus. Note that it is not essential to cover the spleen completely.

with obvious risks and may be found without any other significant abnormality, the platelet count being often well over 1 million and possibly up to 5 million per cubic millimetre. This will often be controlled by using radiophosphorus. A dose of, say, 200 MBq is given intravenously and may be expected to have its full effect in about 6 weeks. During this period thioguanine (dose 40–120 mg daily) will give control. In fact, if thioguanine is well tolerated, and provided the need for frequent blood counts to monitor its dosage is not a problem, then full reliance may be placed on this agent. The thrombocythaemia is sometimes very resistant even to repeated doses of radiophosphorus, so that whole body irradiation may be tried.

Busulphan is not the only effective drug for the management of this disease in its early stages. Dibromomannitol is probably as good in the hands of those who are experienced in its use. Mercaptopurine is also effective, but the response obtained is erratic and therefore requires the patient to attend more frequently for adjustment in dosage. When busulphan is losing its effectiveness, drugs such as dibromomannitol are also unlikely to control the disease. However, although often for all too brief a period, it may be possible to bring the process back under control by the use of hydroxyurea or thioguanine. Hydroxyurea is given by mouth in a dose of 20–30 mg/kg daily. The dose of thioguanine is as given above.

Once the disease enters the blastic phase it becomes very difficult to influence its course and it

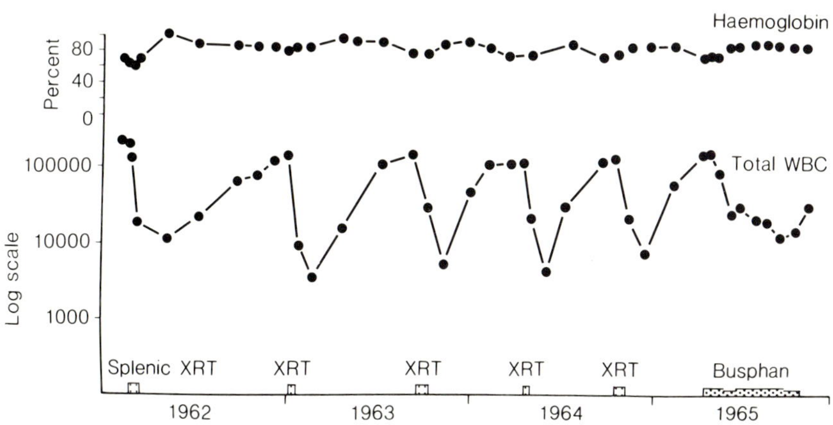

Fig. 14.45. Haematogram of a patient with chronic granulocytic leukaemia who was managed with intermittent courses of splenic irradiation. This should be compared with Fig. 14.43.

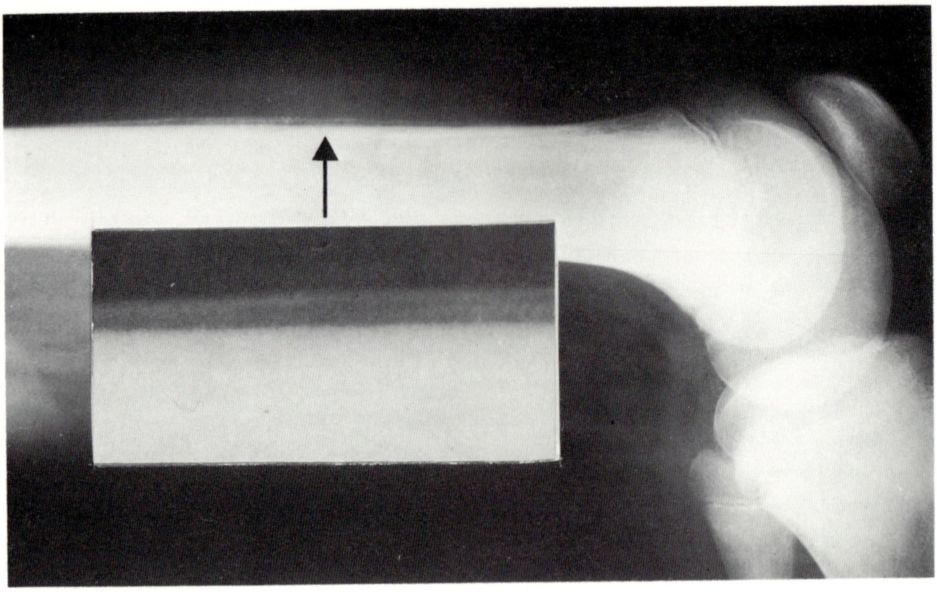

Fig. 14.46. Radiograph to show periosteal elevation causing severe pain in a patient in the later stages of chronic granulocytic leukaemia. Pain was relieved by local radiotherapy.

is probably kindest not to subject the patient to further, almost certainly ineffectual, chemotherapy. However, in about 10% of cases, the transformation is to a lymphoblastic state when treatment with vincristine and prednisolone may be of temporary benefit. Occasional patients do develop deposits of myeloid cells in unusual sites, especially in the later stages of the disease process. An example of cutaneous infiltration is illustrated in the section on electron therapy for mycosis fungoides. A more common complication is painful bone involvement, such as the periosteal elevation seen in Fig. 14.46 or painful vertebral collapse. Such features respond very well to local X-ray treatment at relatively low "lymphoma" dosage.

Recommended Further Reading

Crowther D (1979) Annual review: chemotherapy for lymphoma. In HM Pinedo (ed) Cancer chemotherapy annual

de Vita VT, Canellos GP, Chabner B, Schein P, Hubbard SP, Young RC (1975) Advanced diffuse histiocytic lymphoma, a potentially curable disease. Lancet I: 248–250

de Vita VT, Lewis BJ, Rosencweig M, Muggia FM, (1978) The chemotherapy of Hodgkin's disease. Past experience and future directions. Cancer 42: 979

Halnan KE, Russell MH (1965) Polycythaemia vera: comparison of survival and causes of death in patients managed with and without radiotherapy. Lancet II: 760

Irving M (1975) The role of surgery in the management of Hodgkin's disease. Br J Surg 62: 853–862

Johnson RE (1972) Remission induction and remission duration with primary radiotherapy in advanced lymphosarcoma. Cancer 29: 1473

Kaplan HS (1980) Hodgkin's disease. Harvard University Press, Cambridge, Mass.

Lutzner M, Edelson R, Schein P, Green I, Kirkpatrick C, Ahmed A (1975) Cutaneous T-cell lymphomas: the Sezary syndrome, mycosis fungoides and related disorders. Ann Intern Med 83: 534–552

Schein PS, Winokur SH (1975) Immunosuppressive and cytotoxic chemotherapy: long-term complications. Ann Intern Med 82: 84–95

Shalet SM (1980) Effects of chemotherapy on gonadal function of patients. Cancer Treatment Rev (1980) 7: 141–152

Smithers DW (1973) Hodgkin's disease. Churchill Livingstone, Edinburgh London

15 Soft Tissues and Bone

D. P. Deakin

Sarcomas of Soft Tissues

Soft tissue sarcomas are tumours of mesenchymal origin. They can arise in virtually any connective tissue and account for about 1% of all malignant tumours in adults. In children they are proportionately more common because of the higher incidence of embryonal rhabdomyosarcoma. This is dealt with in Chap. 16. In adults, soft tissue sarcomas are encountered in most age groups but are commonest in the fifth and sixth decades.

Aetiology

This is generally unknown but in certain instances malignant change is seen in a pre-existing benign tumour, e.g. the neurofibroma of von Recklinghausen's disease can become a neurofibrosarcoma and uterine "fibroids" can become leiomyosarcomas. Patients who survive to adult life following treatment of retinoblastoma in infancy have a high incidence of various types of second tumours; soft tissue sarcoma is one of them. Occasionally sarcomas are radiation-induced.

Pathology

Histology

The main histological types are shown in Table 15.1.

Table 15.1. Histological types of soft tissue sarcoma.

Angiosarcoma	— haemangio-endotheliosarcoma — haemangio-pericytoma
Leiomyosarcoma	
Liposarcoma	— well differentiated — myxoid — round cell — pleomorphic
Malignant fibrous histiocytoma (fibrosarcoma)	
Neurofibrosarcoma (malignant schwannoma)	
Rhabdomyosarcoma	— embryonal — alveolar — pleomorphic
Synovial cell sarcoma	— biphasic (spindle cell and epithelioid) — monomorphic (spindle cell or epithelioid)
Undifferentiated sarcoma	

All the tumours listed have their benign counterparts and, in addition, there are a bewildering number of fibromatoses, xanthomatoses, and tumour-like conditions of uncertain histogenesis which may cause diagnostic difficulty. As always, the radiotherapist must rely heavily upon the opinion of the histopathologist.

In most reported series, fibrous histiocytoma accounts for about 30% of cases, with a fairly even distribution amongst the other histological types.

Sites of Origin

About 50% of tumours occur in the extremities, the rest being divided between the trunk and head and neck.

Spread

Local

Soft tissue sarcomas are not truly encapsulated. They spread through tissue planes and along nerve sheaths and some are possibly multifocal in origin. Infiltration of skin and underlying bone is not uncommon. After simple excision or enucleation local recurrence occurs in up to 80% of cases.

Lymphatic

The lymph nodes draining the primary site may be involved but this is a relatively rare event when compared with nodal spread from epithelial tumours.

Haematogenous

Distant metastases occur at some time in the course of the disease in about 65% of cases. The common sites for metastasis are lung, liver, bone, and brain.

Clinical Features

The usual mode of presentation is an enlarging lump which is at first painless but later painful, when skin and periosteum become involved. Retroperitoneal tumours may present with bowel or ureteric obstruction. There may be regional node enlargement and oedema of a limb (Fig. 15.1). Late in the course of the disease the clinical picture is that of any widespread malignancy. Some tumours, particularly liposarcomas, do not metastasise readily, so that the terminal picture is one of vast uncontrolled local disease, amounting to many kilograms of tumour and producing toxic

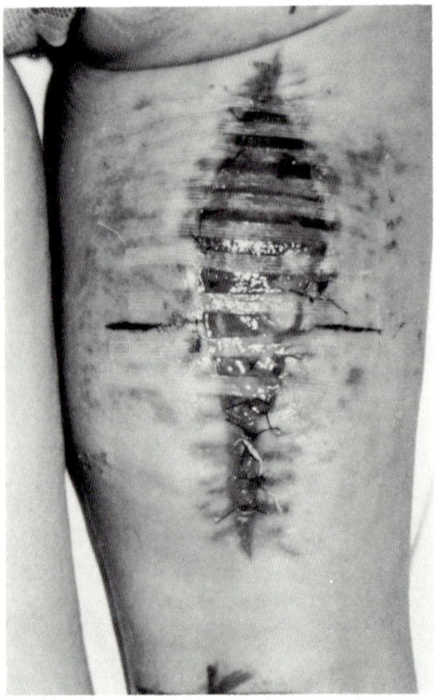

Fig 15.2.

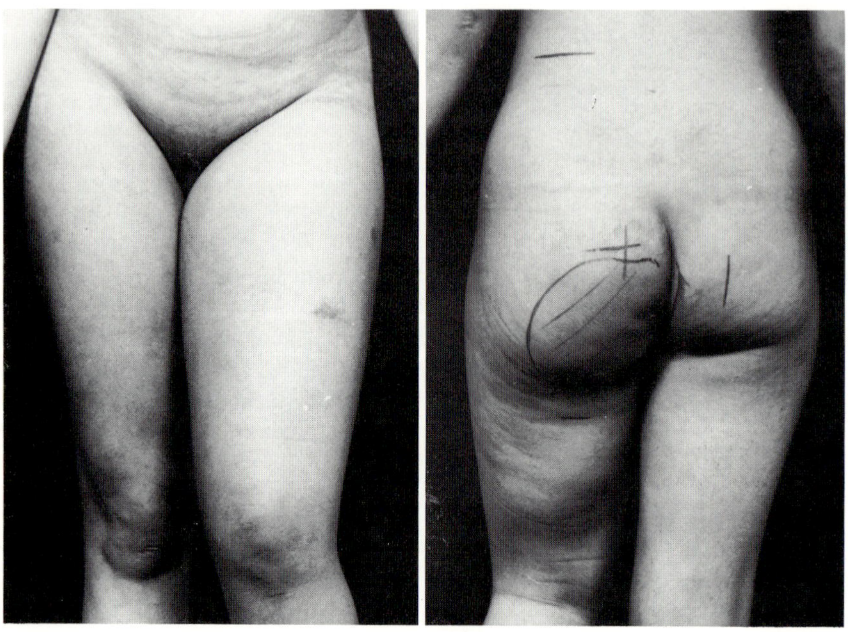

Fig 15.1.

symptoms. The growth rate of soft tissue sarcomas is very variable. Liposarcomas and some fibrous histiocytomas usually enlarge slowly over many months, whereas rhabdomyosarcomas and undifferentiated sarcomas often show explosive growth over a few weeks. The time taken for local recurrence after inadequate surgery follows a similar pattern (Fig. 15.2).

In the case of slowly growing tumours, the main differential diagnoses are benign tumours of soft tissue, ganglia, and areas of fat necrosis. A rapidly growing tumour associated with skin erythema may be mistaken for an acute abscess or a solitary vascular subcutaneous metastasis.

Management

Background

Surgery

Local recurrence after non-radical surgery occurs in 40%–80% of cases. The highest local recurrence rates are seen with large tumours and those of a high grade of malignancy. Histological type is of less importance in this respect, but fibrous histiocytomas, neurofibrosarcomas, and synovial cell sarcomas seem to have the highest risk. Not only does local recurrence require further local intervention but it is of serious import prognostically, since two-thirds of patients who develop metastases do so only concomitantly with or subsequent to local recurrence. There is also an enhanced risk of further local recurrence. More aggressive surgery involving excision with a wide margin around the tumour reduces local recurrence to 25%–30% but the best results are obtained with radical surgery involving amputation of a limb or clearance of a whole muscle compartment.

Radiotherapy

The results of treating large inoperable tumours and extensive postoperative recurrences are disappointing. Some tumours do not respond at all, some may be held in check for a time, whilst those few that regress rapidly, re-grow equally rapidly. Soft tissue sarcomas have, therefore, been labelled "radioresistant". However, there is evidence that non-radical surgery followed by high-dose radiotherapy in selected cases can reduce local recurrence rates to approximately 15%. In most cases, function of the part is retained.

Chemotherapy

Combination chemotherapy has had limited success in the treatment of recurrent and metastatic soft tissue sarcomas. There is about a 40% overall response rate, but only one third of these are complete responses. Local disease tends to respond better than metastatic disease. The duration of remission can be many months.

As with many other tumours, the place of adjuvant chemotherapy is still being investigated.

Treatment Policy

Once the diagnosis of soft tissue sarcoma has been proved by biopsy, a full assessment of the extent of spread of the disease needs to be made before a definitive treatment policy can be formulated. Many primary tumours and associated nodes can be palpated and measured quite simply. Recording their site, fixity, and dimensions on a diagram is an easy form of documentation. Deep-seated tumours, such as those of the pelvis and retroperitoneal areas, may require radiography for their delineation. A plain abdominal X-ray may reveal displacement of the normal bowel shadows by the tumour and deviation of the ureters from their normal positions may be seen on intravenous urography. The CT scanner provides an invaluable method of tumour definition. It is vital to know if metastatic disease is present or not. The commonest site of metastases is the lungs. Posteroanterior and lateral radiographs of the chest are mandatory. Some centres find whole lung tomography helful and CT scanning of the chest may increase the detection rate. The value of radioisotope imaging for detecting metastatic disease in bone and liver in asymptomatic patients is a debatable issue and the pick-up rates vary widely between centres.

In addition to the extent of the disease, the patient's age and general condition will influence the clinician's decision as to the correct form of treatment. The Karnofsky index provides a useful semi-objective measure of the patient's disability and degree of illness. Some factors contributing to a poor general condition may be easily remedied with rapid improvement in the patient's state, as, for example, correction of anaemia. A blood count and if necessary further haematological investigations should be performed. Management of the patient may also be influenced profoundly by the presence of major hepatic or renal dysfunction so that tests for these are also indicated.

Radical Treatment

Surgery

In the absence of demonstrable metastatic disease it is our policy to recommend a radical removal of the tumour if this is possible and if it is thought that the patient will tolerate it. (Age of itself is no bar to surgery but an extensive operation such as a hindquarter amputation is probably best avoided after the age of 70.) The surgery may involve wide excision of tumour with clear margins all round, compartmental resection, or amputation of a limb. If it is performed satisfactorily, postoperative radiotherapy is not necessary. The first attempt provides the best chance of cure.

Radiotherapy

There are situations in which, despite his very best endeavours, the surgeon cannot obtain a clear margin of normal tissue around the tumour. Postoperative radiotherapy is then required. If surgery had been performed on more than one occasion, either for local recurrence or for an inadequate first operation, the risks of recurrence are so increased that radiotherapy should certainly be given. Sometimes is is justifiable to treat a patient with local surgery followed by radiotherapy in an attempt to save a limb from amputation. In general, local control with this approach will be inferior to that achieved by amputation, but some patients will accept this increased risk in order to avoid ablative surgery. Close follow-up is mandatory for these patients since amputation will still be possible in the event of failure.

Large inoperable tumours are not curable by radiotherapy, but a patient with a small tumour which is inoperable because of its site may justifiably be treated radically.

Techniques For postoperative cases it is necessary to irradiate the whole of the tumour bed plus an adequate margin to a uniformly high dose. The full length of the scar must be included in the tumour volume. In the case of soft tissue sarcomas this is a counsel of perfection. The volumes involved are often large and complex, limiting the dose that can be delivered as well as its homogeneity. Where tumours arise in the trunk the close relationship of critical dose-limiting organs, such as the lung, the spinal cord, or the kidneys, may severely restrict the available ways to plan a treatment and a less than ideal dose distribution may have to be accepted. The radiotherapist needs to have the whole spectrum of techniques at his or her disposal. The general principles of treatment and some of the more commonly occurring situations will be discussed further.

X-RAY TREATMENT Megavoltage therapy is the mainstay of treatment. The advantages of megavoltage over kilovoltage—high percentage depth dose, skin-sparing, and little excess bone absorption—help the radiotherapist in the quest for a high uniform tumour dose. Scars, a common site of tumour recurrence, must be adequately covered by bolus to ensure full dosage at the surface. The tumour volume is defined from preoperative clinical measurement and radiography, and from the surgeon's description of the findings at operation. It is extremely helpful if radio-opaque clips have been used to mark the extent of the tumour. The tendency of these tumours to spread along natural soft tissue planes should be remembered when deciding upon a margin beyond tumour.

FIELD ARRANGEMENT A single field is the least satisfactory form of X-ray treatment. Not only will there be a dose gradient across the treatment volume, but the deeply penetrating megavoltage beam will irradiate a considerable amount of normal tissue beyond it. Nevertheless, on occasions more complex field arrangments may not be able to improve upon a single field.

A parallel opposed pair will produce a more or less uniformly irradiated zone between the fields. It is a useful arrangement for limb tumours, the small interfield distance ensuring good dose homogeneity. Often the irradiation can be confined to one muscle group in the limb, thus sparing a proportion of the circumference and preventing distal oedema (Fig. 15.3). In the trunk and head and neck regions the use of a parallel pair would often entail irradiation of critical organs and is, therefore, less useful. In such situations the tangent pair comes into its own. Two or three

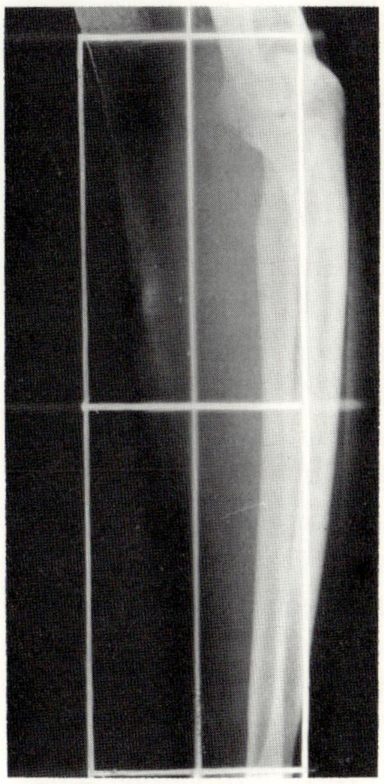

Fig 15.3.

wedge-field techniques sometimes appear to be the best methods. They have two main problems, however. Firstly, it is not technically feasible to wedge a field of more than 15 cm, as balancing becomes impossible and hot spots invariably occur. Often the tumour volume required for a sarcoma is bigger than this. Secondly, the shape of the high-dose volume produced, particularly by these wedged beams, may not be suited to the tumour volume and care must be taken not to compromise the margins. Wedge techniques may be used with or without a beam direction shell (Fig. 15.4). When irradiating limbs, problems may be encountered in the physical application of the X-ray fields. Treatment of the posterior compartment of the thigh can be difficult. With the patient supine or prone the opposite thigh interferes with the positioning of a medial field. A way around this problem is to treat the patient in a lateral position with the unaffected thigh flexed so that it is out of the field. Even this approach is not possible when the tumour volume extends onto the uppermost thigh or onto the buttock.

Another difficult situation involves a tumour volume which extends from the anterior aspect of the upper thigh across the inguinal ligament onto the lower abdominal wall. An approach to this problem is shown in Fig. 15.5. A wedged pair of fields is used but the large interfield distance means that the dose distribution is not perfect.

Irradiation of the anterior or posterior compartment of the forearm is best done with the forearm semi-pronated and parallel to the long axis of the couch. A slight variation in position can lead to a marked misalignment of radius and ulna and the use of a beam direction shell is advisable.

It is sometimes necessary to irradiate a hand or a foot. In most cases the palmar or plantar surface can be placed flat on the couch and a single megavoltage field applied. Bolus material is needed to ensure a full subcutaneous dose. More complex arrangements usually do not improve upon the dose distribution obtained by this simple method.

DOSAGE As for other tumour types the radical X-ray treatment of soft tissue sarcoma is based on 15 or 16 fractions of treatment delivered as five daily fractions per week. The upper or lower half of limb (excluding the hand or foot) will tolerate a midplane dose of 4500 cGy in 3 weeks. Similarly,

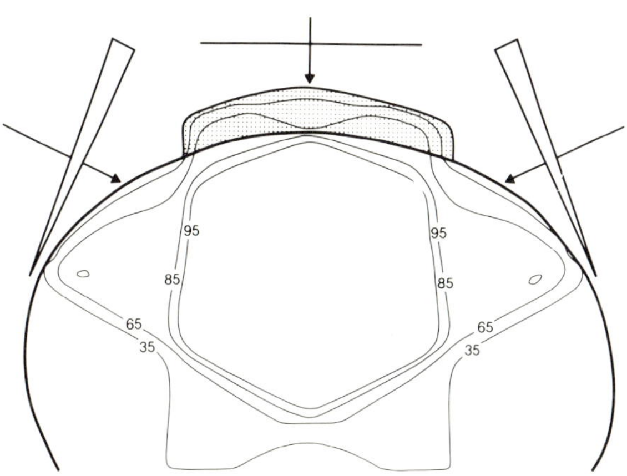

Fig 15.4.

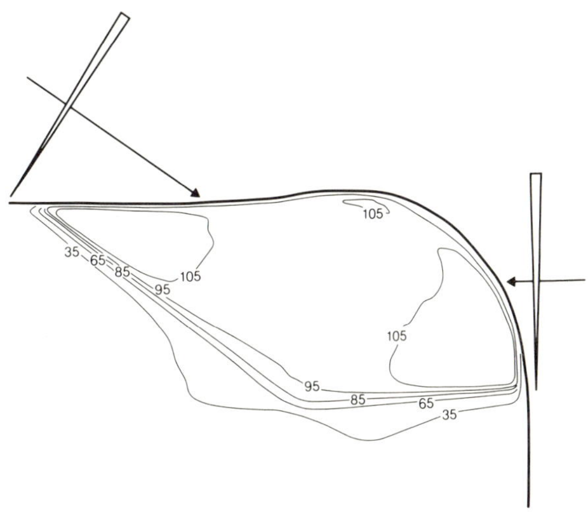

Fig 15.5.

4500 cGy in 3 weeks can be delivered to moderate volumes of the trunk if only musculoskeletal tissues are involved. In practice, however, included volumes of lung, liver, kidney, spinal cord, or bowel often limit the dose to tolerance levels for these structures. Doses to the full thickness of the hand or the foot should probably not exceed 4000 cGy in 3 weeks.

ELECTRONS The depth-dose characteristics of electron beams—a virtual high-dose plateau followed by a region of rapidly falling dose—make them suitable for treating relatively superficial lesions. A single field is used. Bolus is needed for scars, unless the applicator contains a layer of scattering material, and a generous margin should be allowed at the periphery because of the edge characteristics of the beam. (The energy of the beam should be chosen to give the required depth dose. It is easy to fail because of inadequate dose at depth.) Electron beams are not readily matched or wedged.

NEUTRONS Some early results suggest that neutron therapy might be effective in controlling large soft tissue sarcomas but a proper controlled trial has yet to be undertaken.

INTERSTITIAL IRRADIATION Interstitial irradiation is not generally used as a treatment for soft tissue sarcomas at the Christie Hospital. It has its advocates at other centres, however, where it tends to be used in two different situations. In the first, an implant is the only form of radiotherapy used, usually for a small lesion. The behaviour of these tumours necessitates irradiation of a wide margin around them and homogeneous irradiation of the required volume is very difficult to obtain with an interstitial implant. In the second situation, an implant is used to increase the dose at the centre of a volume irradiated by beam therapy. Irregular volumes can rarely be perfectly implanted and the need for this approach remains to be proved.

Radiation Reactions The acute radiation reactions occurring in various internal organs are dealt with in other sections and will not be reiterated here. Skin reactions may be quite troublesome when large volumes of the limbs are irradiated. A perifollicular erythema begins towards the end of the second week and then coalesces. The reaction usually reaches its height in the fourth week, when it may become moist in the flexures. The skin over the lateral malleolus is easily traumatised and may break down. Aqueous gentian violet, although unsightly, is still extremely useful in the treatment of areas of moist desquamation. When painted over and allowed to dry it forms a bacteria-free coagulum under which the area can heal. Cytotoxic drugs, in particular actinomycin D and adriamycin, given concurrently with the radiotherapy can produce an early and severe skin reaction necessitating the stopping of treatment. These combined radiation/drug effects are unpredictable and probably depend on the precise timing of the two therapies. Curative radiotherapy for soft tissue sarcomas requires high doses to be given—doses that are at tolerance levels for the normal tissues. If this normal tissue tolerance is reduced by drug treatment disastrously high necrosis rates will follow. Actinomycin D and adriamycin should not therefore be given during this kind of radiotherapy. It is really the late effects of radiotherapy that are the dose-limiting factors for connective tissues, particularly those of the limbs. This is discussed in more detail in the section on bone tumours.

Results of Radical Radiotherapy Of patients treated with radiotherapy according to the criteria detailed above, about half will die from metastatic disease and the best one can hope for in those cases is that there is local control until death. The evidence suggests that overall local recurrence should be kept to approximately 20%, but this will vary with site, size, histological type, and grade of tumour. Soft tissue sarcomas are a rare and heterogeneous group of conditions and it is unlikely therefore that even a large oncological centre will be able to collect enough clinical material to permit a valid analysis of prognostic factors. New treatment policies must be formulated on the basis of results of international collaborative studies.

Palliative Treatment

For gross local disease a 3-week course of X-ray treatment is often disappointing. Partial regression of the disease usually occurs but it may not be enough to relieve the patient's symptoms. Much depends upon the site. Tumour re-growth is often prevented for a time.

Once-weekly treatment delivering 300–350 cGy per fraction can be a more effective way of obtaining local control in slow-growing tumours. Radiotherapy is continued until deep pigmentation and dry desquamation of the skin occurs or until induration is encountered in the deeper tissues. This may take several months and total doses up to 7000 cGy can be given in this way. The tumour shrinks gradually and is usually controlled for several months after the end of treatment.

Current chemotherapy regimes for soft tissue sarcomas are very toxic and are not curative, so that for local disease radiotherapy should be tried first. Metastatic disease commonly occurs in the lungs, the liver, and bones. As with metastases from other tumours, a single X-ray exposure will relieve the pain of a bone metastasis in the majority of cases without undue upset for the patient. It is not generally in the patient's interest, however, to irradiate metastatic disease in the lungs and liver. The metastases are usually widely scattered, necessitating irradiation of the whole organ. The doses that can be given are thus severely limited and are certainly not enough to influence the growth of most sarcomas. If the patient's general condition permits, a trial of chemotherapy should be instituted; otherwise, the kindest treatment is opiates.

Bone Tumours

Primary bone tumours are rare and account for less than 1% of all malignancies in the United Kingdom. As with soft tissue tumours, there is a spectrum of histology from reactive to benign to locally aggressive to truly malignant. Only the last two categories will be considered here. Unlike the soft tissue sarcomas, where the different histological types can be grouped together for most clinical purposes, bone tumours must be studied separately. There is no universally accepted staging classification for bone tumours.

Osteosarcoma

Osteosarcoma accounts for 30% of all primary bone tumours. In clinical practice it is encountered in older children and teenagers, associated with the growth spurt of puberty, and in patients in middle and later life, when it often arises as a result of Paget's disease of bone.

Aetiology

Apart from the association with Paget's disease, there are other known contributing causes. Osteosarcoma is occasionally radiation-induced. It may be produced by ingestion of bone-seeking isotopes and sometimes occurs within radiotherapy fields many years after treatment. There is a high incidence of osteosarcoma in adult patients who have previously been cured of retinoblastoma in childhood. These tumours occur both within and distant from irradiated areas. There seems to be a genetic tendency for osteosarcoma in these patients, accentuated by the carcinogenic effect of radiation.

Pathology

When it arises on Paget's disease, osteosarcoma is commonest in the pelvic bones and may arise from any part of the bone. In the commoner type of tumour which affects young people, however, the disease originates in the metaphysis and the commonest sites are the lower end of the femur, the upper end of the tibia and the upper end of the humerus. It can also occur in the spine, the pelvis, the small bones of the hands and feet, and in the skull. On macroscopic examination the majority of tumours are endosteal. A tumour mass is seen spreading within the marrow cavity, destroying the cortex, breaching the periosteum and infiltrating the soft tissues. These tumours are very vascular, with areas of haemorrhage and necrosis. There are varying degrees of bone destruction and new bone formation. The parosteal sarcoma is a distinct entity which grows as a subperiosteal fleshy mass.

Histologically the picture is very varied, but osteosarcoma is basically a spindle cell tumour which produces tumour osteoid, recognised by its irregular poorly formed appearance blending with the stroma. Invasion of the thin-walled vessels is common and the blood sinusoids may actually be lined by tumour cells. In addition to direct local extension into surrounding muscle and along the medullary cavity, there may be foci of tumour within the bone separated from the main mass by seemingly normal tissue—the so-called skip lesions. Lymphatic spread is rare, but metastases are sometimes seen in the regional lymph nodes draining the primary tumour and in mediastinal nodes. Blood-borne metastases are very common, occurring mainly in the lungs. Other bones are involved in a few per cent of cases only. Occasionally osteosarcoma is truly multifocal.

Clinical Features

Almost invariably the presentation is that of a painful swelling of a bone—the end of a bone in the juvenile type. The pain may prevent full movement of the adjacent joint. The swelling is often warm and may be pulsatile. Patients with advanced local disease are often toxic with malaise, sweating, fever, and anorexia but recover very quickly after adequate treatment to the primary tumour. The clinical picture may suggest osteomyelitis, septic arthritis, or an infected bursa. Less inflammatory tumours may be confused with benign bone tumours or metastases.

Investigation and Treatment

Historical Background

In order to devise a rational policy of management, it is necessary to have a historical perspective. For many years amputation was the only effective treatment for osteosarcoma in the limbs. Some surgeons preferred a disarticulation because a few patients develop recurrences in the stump. The cure rate following amputation was around 20% and this was the universal experience. The 80% of patients who died did so, almost without exception, from lung metastases, death occurring in the vast majority in less than 2 years. Attempts to use radiotherapy to ablate the primary tumour were successful in between 10% and 30% of cases only, but some form of local control was possible in a rather greater number. It was tragic that four of every five patients subjected to amputation died fairly soon of metastatic disease and, at a time when little could be done to treat the metastases, attention was turned to reducing the rate of needless amputation. To this end the primary tumour was treated with high-dose irradiation and an elective amputation performed 6 months later provided the chest X-ray was still clear. This method had its successes but also its failures. Sometimes the radiotherapy failed to control the primary and amputation was required for advancing painful local disease. In some cases lung metastases developed shortly after the amputation and in others, where both the primary and the chest were well, patients refused the delayed surgery. The advent of chemotherapy changed the situation considerably. Metastatic disease was seen to respond partially to various single agents and combinations of them. Chemotherapy, it was argued, would be most effective where tumour cell numbers were small and its use in an adjuvant manner was begun, to deal with the subclinical lung disease which was present in 80% of cases. Chemotherapy would be less effective if the lungs were constantly being reseeded from an inadequately treated primary tumour so that amputation was preferred by most authorities. The argument against primary irradiation with chemotherapy and subsequent amputation was the fact that when patients were not cured the appearance of lung metastases was often delayed by chemotherapy, making it impossible to pick the optimum time for elective amputation. Major centres were obtaining 50%–55% 5-year survival rates with primary amputation followed by various adjuvant chemotherapy regimes. In addition, the aggressive treatment of lung metastases was producing long-term palliation and possibly some cures. This treatment usually took the form of an intensification of the chemotherapy on the appearance of lung metastases and surgical resection of these followed by further chemotherapy. There are reports of multiple lung metastases being removed at several thoracotomies.

Concomitantly with the upsurge in chemotherapy came an interest in the therapeutic benefits of prophylactic irradiation of the lungs based upon the radiobiological consideration that even inherently radioresistant tumours can be cured by modest doses of radiotherapy when the number of cells is small. Prophylactic lung irradiation gives similar results to those of most drug schedules: a 5-year survival of 40%–50%.

Current developments in the treatment of osteosarcoma include preoperative chemotherapy, which enables an assessment of the response of individual tumours in vivo, and attempts at limb preservation by *en bloc* resection of tumour with prosthetic replacement of bone. At the present time the effectiveness of most chemotherapy schedules is in doubt. Modern staging techniques, particularly CT scanning of the lungs, have almost certainly led to an apparent increased survival in the highly selected "non-metastatic" group without the aid of chemotherapy. Similarly, resection of lung metastases has prolonged survival. Only prospective randomised controlled trials will demonstrate the advantage or otherwise of chemotherapy beyond doubt. However, the complex management of this disease makes such trials difficult to perform and some would argue that it is now unethical to withhold chemotherapy.

Management Policy

From the above discussion it will be obvious that there are many ways of managing osteosarcoma and much will depend upon the local facilities which are available. When presented with a patient with the clinical picture previously described, plain radiography is the first investigation to be performed. The classical features are a metaphyseal tumour with osteolysis and new bone formation, Codman's triangle, and sun-ray spicules. This picture is by no means always seen but even when it is, it should be confirmed by biopsy. No treatment should be undertaken without histological proof of the tumour type.

Radionuclide scans and angiograms help to define the extent of the local disease. The presence or absence of metastases will affect the prognosis and the treatment and a search for metastatic disease should be made. Good quality plain radiographs of the chest with posteroanterior, lateral, and penetrated views are probably all that are required for practical purposes. CT scanning of the lungs reveals more metastases than conventional radiology, but there is a considerable problem with the demonstration of pulmonary nodules which are not metastatic. An isotope whole-body bone scan helps to show the extent of local disease, but only rarely will one find unequivocal metastases in the skeleton. As for soft tissue sarcomas, tests of hepatic, renal and marrow function are important.

Radical Treatment For patients without demonstrable metastatic disease, it has been our policy to recommend amputation if the tumour is in a limb. For tumours at other sites, radical surgery has been performed if possible. Radiotherapy is not an alternative to surgery for this tumour. Surgery has been followed by adjuvant chemotherapy and it is not within the scope of this chapter to discuss the relative merits of different chemotherapy regimes. Our current regime is shown in Table 15.2.

We have just begun to use a preoperative chemotherapy schedule, with surgery being performed after 9 weeks of drug treatment. We have not been happy to use prophylactic lung irradiation. Many of our patients have not completed their growth and radiotherapy in this situation will prevent full size of the thorax from being achieved and leave them with a reduced vital capacity. There will also be the problem of poor breast development in prepubertal girls. On balance, we feel that chemotherapy can produce at least as good a survival as lung irradiation without, as far as can yet be seen, the late sequelae. Chemotherapy is of course a potential cause of acute toxicity and death but, in experienced hands, it is now fairly safe. One would expect a long-term disease-free survival of 40%–50% with this approach.

When the primary tumour is situated in the spine or pelvis, it is often unresectable. An attempt at radical radiotherapy should be made, in the absence of metastatic disease, and adjuvant chemotherapy should be given thereafter. The radiotherapy technique employed will vary with the site and size of the lesion. Spinal tumours may be treated by a three-field wedge technique similar to that shown earlier in this chapter. The dose will, of course, be limited by the length of spinal cord in the field. Pelvic tumours are often large and have a considerable soft tissue component, making the planning of a homogeneous treatment difficult. A tangent pair with one wedged field may be possible. The amount of bowel in the field will determine what dose is possible. Unresectable osteosarcoma has a bad prognosis. The primary tumour is usually not controlled by radiotherapy alone.

Palliative Treatment Patients with metastases in the lungs at presentation are still, with the rare exception, incurable and it is usually unacceptable, therefore, to amputate a limb. In this situation it has been our policy to irradiate the tumour to tolerance dose, taking a wide margin proximal to the tumour, but not irradiating the whole bone. A parallel opposed pair of megavoltage fields is used and a midplane dose of 4500 cGy is delivered in 16 fractions over 3 weeks. This will result in a brisk erythema at the end of treatment. When a patient has known metastatic disease, it is tempting to start chemotherapy concurrently with the radiotherapy. If methotrexate or adriamycin is given in this way an extremely brisk skin reaction

Table 15.2.

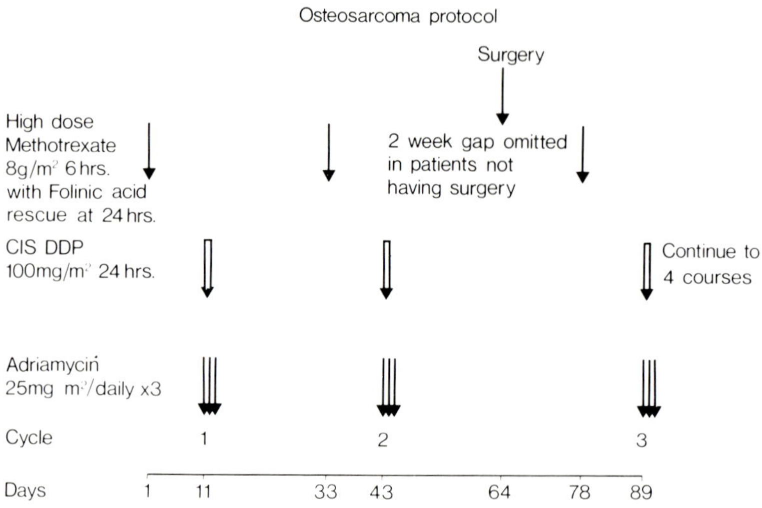

will ensue and probably progress to moist desquamation. If there is concern about advancing lung disease it is much better to give one or two courses of chemotherapy before starting the irradiation but to withhold drugs during the radiotherapy. Late radiation effects are discussed below in connection with Ewing's tumour.

Despite one's best endeavours some primary tumours will not be controlled and amputation will be necessary for pain or fungation. If the primary tumour and the lung metastases respond well the surgical removal of residual lung disease should be advised and, in the absence of further recurrence thereafter, amputation should be considered. The timing of this is difficult—too early and further lung disease may soon appear, too late and renewed activity in the primary may reseed the lungs. Most patients will never get to this stage, but will die of uncontrolled metastatic lung disease within a few months. Advancing lung metastases despite chemotherapy demand that X-ray treatment to the whole chest be considered. The whole of both lung fields will need to be treated and after chemotherapy a dose of more than 2000 cGy in 16 fractions over 3 weeks runs a high risk of producing pneumonitis. Any benefit obtained from lung irradiation given at this stage is likely to be very temporary.

The rare cases with bone metastases and multifocal tumours sometimes get pain relief from single X-ray exposures to the sites of disease.

Chondrosarcoma

Chondrosarcoma is a malignant tumour of cartilage and continues to form neoplastic cartilage. It may occur at any age from childhood onwards but is commonest in later life. Benign cartilaginous tumours may become malignant. Thus chondrosarcoma not uncommonly arises from enchondroma or from the cartilage cap of an exostosis, but it may arise de novo. It has been estimated that one in ten patients with hereditary multiple exostoses develop chondrosarcoma at some time. Most tumours arise from the trunk or the upper ends of the humerus and the femur and form firm grey lobulated masses with softer areas of myxomatous degeneration. The histology may vary from one part of the tumour to another, some areas being so well differentiated that they present the appearance of a benign chondroma. Careful search, however, will often reveal anaplastic cells which lack a regular arrangment. Mitoses are never numerous and these are slow-growing tumours. Dissemination by the bloodstream to the lungs is usually a late phenomenon.

Clinical Features

Pain at the tumour site is the usual first symptom and it may be many months before a swelling is detectable. The tumour, usually in the buttock or

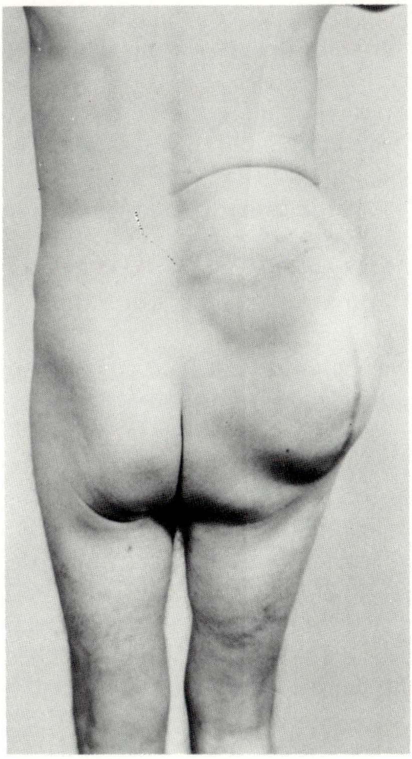

Fig 15.6.

shoulder girdle, grows slowly but inexorably and often produces considerable deformity and interference with the function of the limb (Fig. 15.6). Chronic pain and the metabolic effects of a large tumour mass may severely affect the patient's health before metastatic disease develops. Radiographs show an endosteal lytic lesion with destruction of the cortex of the bone. A large soft tissue mass which contains areas of calcification is characteristic.

Treatment

Few radiotherapists would be enthusiastic about the results of treating chondrosarcomas, although small tumours are occasionally controlled for many years. Radical surgery seems the only curative treatment. Unfortunately, probably because of the sites of origin, these tumours are often too advanced for curative surgery at presentation. A less than radical operation invites local recurrence and a case can be made for immediate postoperative radiotherapy in this situation, much as for soft tissue sarcomas. There is not sufficient information available to know if this is curative, however. One is most often faced with a patient with extensive local disease. When there is pain and interference with function a definitive 3-week course of X-ray therapy is given as the quickest way of relieving the symptoms. A parallel opposed pair of fields may be the best that can be managed and the dose is often limited to 3000–3500 cGy by the extent of the tumour volume. Nevertheless, although much reduction in tumour size is rarely achieved, pain is often controlled and tumour growth halted for a time. When the need for pain relief is less urgent a weekly type of treatment, as for advanced soft tissue sarcoma, is a satisfactory approach.

Chemotherapy has been of very limited benefit for these tumours, with a 17% overall response rate the best that can be expected.

One can expect a 50% 5-year survival for all patients with chondrosarcoma, but deaths from disease continue after this time and the 10-year survival figure is about 30%.

Fibrosarcoma

This is an uncommon bone tumour which tends to be of low-grade malignancy. Any bone may be affected and the tumour may arise from the periosteum or from the medullary cavity, eroding the cortex as it expands. The metaphysis or the diaphysis may be the site of origin. Microscopically the tumour resembles the fibrosarcoma of soft tissue and is best managed in a similar manner. Survival rates of 50% at 5 years are to be expected.

Ewing's Tumour

This is a rare bone tumour which has only fairly recently been universally recognised as a true pathological entity.

There are only about 80 new cases per year in the United Kingdom. Ewing's tumour affects children and young adults and is very rare after the age of 30. There are no obvious predisposing factors.

Pathology

The tumour most commonly arises in the femur, tibia, or humerus but also occurs in the pelvis, ribs, and vertebrae and in the other long bones.

Typically it begins in the midshaft of a bone in the medullary cavity. It invades and destroys the cortex and elevates the periosteum, causing concentric layers of reactive bone to be laid down. There is often an extensive tumour mass outside the original boundaries of the affected bone and spread along the length of the medullary cavity is common. The microscopic picture is that of a small round-cell sarcoma with the closely packed cells arranged in sheets or columns. The cells contain glycogen granules in their cytoplasm.

Metastatic spread is mainly by the bloodstream to the lungs and to other bones, but lymph node spread can occur. The secondary bone lesions are commonly in the vertebrae, skull, pelvis, and ribs and, like the primary tumour, they have a large soft tissue component. In some cases widespread bone marrow involvement occurs.

Clinical Features

Pain is the first symptom and sometimes the patient states that it is worse at rest. It may occur several months before a swelling is detected. The pain is attributed to tension on the periosteum and is sometimes relieved when the tumour breaks through this structure. Pain and swelling lead to failure to use the affected part and joint deformities may occur. Occasionally, the patient presents with a pathological fracture. Patients with locally advanced or metastatic disease are often lethargic, anorexic, and pyrexial.

Investigations and Treatment

Background

Ewing's tumour is moderately sensitive to radiation. The local recurrence rate for limb tumours following radiotherapy is 10%–20%. This is only achieved, however, by using tolerance dosage of radiotherapy. When the tumour is large, as is often the case with pelvic tumours, or when vital structures limit the radiation dose that can be given, local control rates are much less. Despite the good overall local control rate, only 10% of patients survive if local treatment alone is given, metastatic disease in lungs and bones appearing later. The treatment of overt metastatic disease with combination chemotherapy, using vincristine, actinomycin D, cyclophosphamide, and adriamycin, has produced many worthwhile remissions but few cures. However, extension of the use of cytotoxic drugs to an *adjuvant* role has been a major success with this tumour. Five-year disease-free survival should now be in the region of 45%–50%. It now seems clear that chemotherapy can eliminate microscopic metastases.

Management Policy

A child or young adult with persistent skeletal pain should be examined and investigated very carefully. Plain X-rays of the appropriate area in two planes should be taken, with due regard to the possibility that the pain may be referred from an area other than that in which it is felt. One child in the author's experience had an X-ray picture of the knee taken at another hospital because she complained of pain in the knee. The film was reported as normal. A year later the child presented again, now with an advanced tumour of the midshaft of the femur. Re-examination of the original X-ray film of the knee showed a few millimetres of periosteal elevation at the top edge of the film. A film of the whole femur would undoubtedly have shown the tumour at this earlier stage.

The classical radiographic appearance (Fig. 15.7) is of midshaft patchy cortical bone destruc-

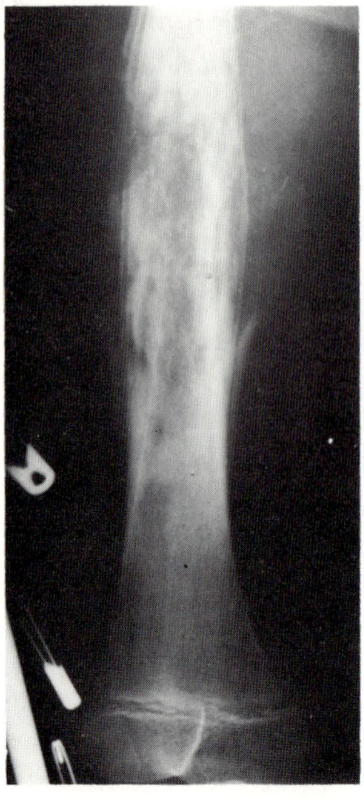

Fig 15.7.

tion and layers of subperiosteal new bone formation (the onion skin appearance). An extra-osseous tumour mass can usually be seen. The clinical and X-ray appearances can be confused with those of chronic osteomyelitis and the distinction is, of course, very important. As with all bone tumours, biopsy is mandatory. The histology of Ewing's tumour can be difficult and a good biopsy, taking full thickness of the cortex as well as a portion of the soft tissue element, is essential. If only a small biopsy, not including bone, is taken and this histologically shows no malignancy, one is still left in doubt as to whether the biopsy material has failed to include tumour. A repeat biopsy will be needed and valuable time will be lost. Once the diagnosis of Ewing's tumour is confirmed, investigations are required to show the extent of the disease and its effect, if any, on major organ systems. If the primary tumour is in a limb nothing is gained by angiography to define the extent within the bone, since the whole of the involved bone needs to be treated. Good quality plain radiographs to show the soft tissue mass are all that are required. For primary tumours of the axial skeleton, however, the extent of the soft tissue disease within the trunk needs to be assessed. The CT scan, if available, is the most elegant method of doing this, but helpful information can also be obtained from intravenous urography and the ultrasound scan.

The major sites of metastatic disease should be investigated. As for osteosarcoma, plain chest X-rays may be supplemented by whole lung tomography or CT scanning. A whole-body isotope bone scan is important because of the frequency of metastatic bone disease. A bone marrow biopsy —aspirate and trephine—is also indicated. The blood count and tests of renal and hepatic function are needed before chemotherapy is begun. The serum lactic dehydrogenase level is a prognostic factor in Ewing's tumour, an elevated one indicating a poor prognosis.

Radical Treatment Patients without overt metastases should be treated with curative intent. In addition, patients who present with metastatic disease should be given a trial of radical treatment since prolonged survival is often obtained and a small percentage will be cured.

The ability of radiotherapy to control the primary disease in the great majority of cases makes it the treatment of choice for this tumour. The dose is critical and must balance local control rate against normal tissue damage so that a functional limb results. All patients require adjuvant chemotherapy to deal with the microscopic metastatic disease which is present in about 90% of patients. There is increasing evidence for many types of tumours that cure rates are dependent upon the time at which the chemotherapy is started—the sooner the better. Chemotherapy, however, is not at its most effective when there is a large bulk of viable tumour present. The solution would seem to be to start chemotherapy immediately and at the same time give radiotherapy to destroy the primary tumour. Unfortunately, two of the most effective drugs, actinomycin D and adriamycin, reduce the normal tissue tolerance to radiation and cannot be given safely during X-ray therapy. The schedule currently in use is shown in Table 15.3. Chemotherapy with vincristine, cyclophosphamide, and adriamycin is given on the first occasion, and thereafter vincristine and cyclophosphamide are given weekly for 7 weeks. Radiotherapy is started 2 weeks after the adriamycin dose to prevent enhancement of the radiation reaction. The 2 weeks of preradiation chemotherapy does not, however, allow enough time for a significant shrinkage of the soft tissue element of the tumour to occur. Where such shrinkage would enable radiotherapy fields to be reduced and normal tissue to be spared, a more prolonged course of chemotherapy should be given before radiotherapy is begun. In practice, the need to irradiate the whole of the involved bone often precludes the usefulness of this approach. Radiotherapy techniques appropriate to Ewing's tumour almost invariably involve X-ray therapy, sometimes in combination with an electron field. For the same reasons given in the section on soft tissue sarcomas, only radiation of megavoltage quality should be used. Because of the potential involvement of the whole of the medullary cavity, the whole bone must be irradiated. The fields must, of course, contain all the extra-osseous mass. The actual technique selected will depend upon which bone is involved. Limb bones are most easily treated by a parallel opposed pair of fields applied anteriorly and posteriorly. The upper and lower margins of the fields will pass through the joints immediately above and below the affected bone. It is important to try and spare a strip of tissue at the lateral or medial side of the field as this lessens the late radiation effects. Verification by

Table 15.3.

Ewing's tumour protocol

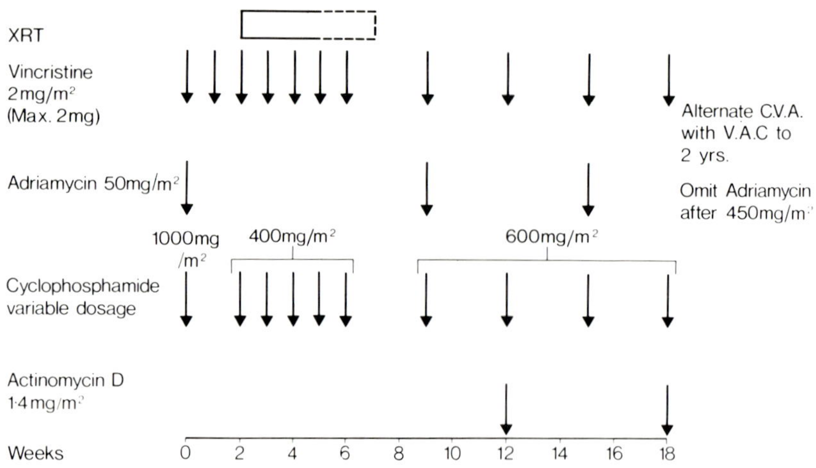

simulator screening or films is essential. It may not be possible to spare any part of the width of the limb and still treat the whole bone—this situation occurs particularly around the knee joint—in which case the need to irradiate the whole bone takes priority. The dose usually given is 4500 cGy midplane in 16 fractions over 3 weeks. Ewing's tumour primarily affecting a vertebra may be treated with a three-field wedge technique as for osteosarcoma. The field should cover an uninvolved vertebra above and below the lesion, and again due notice should be taken of the soft tissue extension.

The fields will not be less than 10 cm long and spinal cord tolerance will therefore limit the dose to 4000 cGy in 15 fractions over 3 weeks. Ewing's tumours involving the pelvis are often large and sometimes huge. Initially, a parallel pair of fields is required to cover the hemipelvis and treat it to a dose of 3000 cGy in 16 fractions over 3 weeks at the midplane. This done, it may be possible to cone down to treat the actual tumour area to a further 1500 cGy in 10 fractions over 2 weeks, using a tangent pair or a single megavoltage field. Resolution of the soft tissue mass may be slow and it is sometimes necessary to delay the application of the extra dose, in effect using a "split course" treatment. Patients with rib tumours have usually had some sort of surgical resection before being referred to the radiotherapist. In young adults this is probably a good thing, allowing tumour bulk to be removed without unacceptable deformity, but the situation is very different in the case of children, where rib resection usually leads to a progressive kyphoscoliosis. The irradiation of a whole rib necessitates irradiating a substantial proportion of one hemithorax and its contained lung. Our policy is to do this with anterior and posterior opposed fields but to limit the dose to 2500 cGy in 16 fractions over 3 weeks, that is, to lung tolerance. An additional 1500 cGy in 10 fractions over 2 weeks is then delivered with a 10-MeV electron beam to the area of the resected tumour.

Radiation reactions, as always, are usefully considered as early or late. The early skin reaction has been dealt with already in this chapter. The late effects of radiotherapy to the limbs are the ones that limit the dose which can be delivered. Patients with Ewing's tumour of a limb bone usually have pain and some degree of limitation of function. The biopsy can add to these problems, and as a result limitation of joint movement is usually present before treatment is begun. The joints most likely to be affected are the elbow and the ankle. Radiotherapy delivered to a joint in this situation may cause a virtual ankylosis. It is vital that physiotherapy is started as soon as the patient is seen and that it continues throughout the radiotherapy. Thereafter, patients should perform exercises on their own as instructed and should attend the physiotherapy department weekly for assessment of progress until normal activities have been resumed. Pain and fear of fracture may be suggested as arguments against the use of physiotherapy. Neither is valid. Pain relief usually occurs very soon after the beginning of treatment and useful physiotherapy can be given with the constraints applied by a rather weakened bone. Two to three months after the end of radiotherapy there is usually some oedema in the treated area. It is much less common to see chronic oedema distal to the treated volume. By 6–8 months the swelling has usually settled and muscle atrophy begins to become apparent. The muscles start to feel diffusely indurated. This happens to some extent in all patients but it is much worse in those who have limited joint movement and they can end up with a thin wasted segment of limb (Fig. 15.8).

By far the best functional results occur in young adults who determine that they will get back to a normal life, including playing sport, as soon as possible. The importance of rehabilitation cannot be too strongly emphasised, as there is little point in recommending radiotherapy rather than surgery if the patient ends up with a useless painful limb. Bones irradiated to the doses recommended are never quite normal. Following the successful treatment of a Ewing's tumour the extra-osseous mass shrinks and at the same time calcifies and ossifies. Progressive repair takes place within the bone. Healing continues for many months and remodelling may take years. Compared with the uniting of a simple fracture, the healing process is slow; probably it is also affected by the chemotherapy. There is a danger of fracture of weight-bearing bones. Even many years after radiotherapy, the bone texture is abnormal (Fig. 15.9).

The late effects of therapy on bone are, of course, much worse in the case of children. The irradiated bone does not grow properly and an affected limb will be shorter than its fellow. Correction of the shortening by providing a "raise" for the shoe is simple and if not done it can lead to a postural scoliosis. If the humerus or femur is irradiated before the age of epiphyseal fusion there is very likely to be slipping of the upper humeral epiphysis or of the femoral capital epiphysis with resulting pain and restriction of joint movement. Several of our children have had successful pinning of slipped femoral capital epiphysis produced by lower doses of irradiation delivered for reasons other than Ewing's tumour (for example, 3000 cGy over 3 weeks), but after

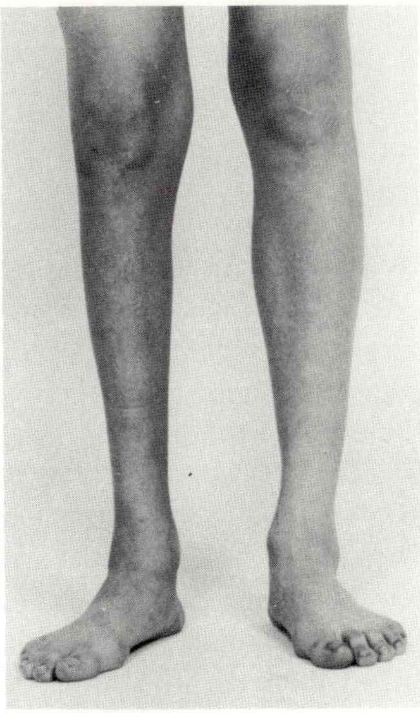

Fig 15.8.

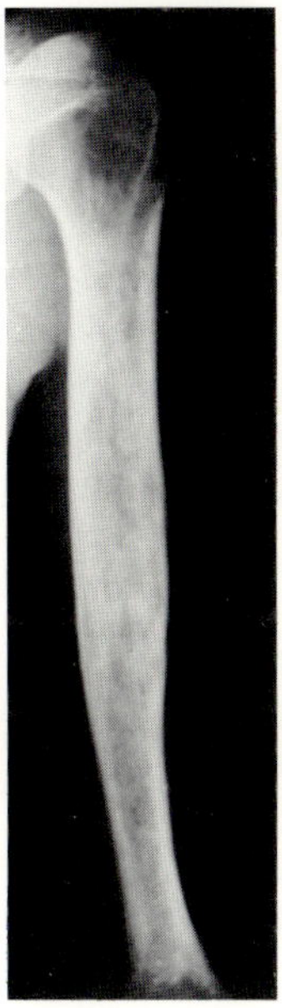

Fig 15.9.

4500 cGy over 3 weeks, the danger of precipitating an osteonecrosis must be high and we would not recommend surgical intervention.

Growth deformities of the pelvis, spine, and ribs are relatively less functionally disabling. There is, of course, a small chance of a radiation-induced tumour occurring at a later date, but we have not yet seen one following successful treatment of a Ewing's tumour at the Christie Hospital.

Further management after the radiation therapy is important, and combination chemotherapy should be continued as pulsed treatment for 2 years. With this approach a 5-year survival of about 50% should be possible. Patients with large pelvic tumours do badly, whereas those with rib tumours do well. Local recurrence in limb bones in the absence of metastases can be treated by amputation and further chemotherapy with some success.

Palliative Treatment When metastases occur they almost invariably do so in lung or bone or both. Some series contain occasional patients with brain metastases, but these are not of such a frequency as to make prophylactic cranial irradiation justifiable. Bone metastases are almost always heralded by pain and a soft tissue mass may be obvious clinically. The X-ray appearances are often subtle, with only minor alteration of bone texture in the early stages. Single X-ray exposures control the pain well but there is little hope of further control of the disease process by chemotherapy. The situation with regard to lung metastases is somewhat different. Worthwhile long-term remissions have been achieved, even after conventional doses of the most active drugs have failed, by the use of high-dose melphalan with autologous bone marrow rescue. If this specialised technique is available it should be performed before palliative lung irradiation is given, in order that the marrow in the sternum is not damaged by radiation and is available, if needed, for harvesting. Whole-lung irradiation to 2000 cGy over 3 weeks is worth doing if autologous marrow transplantation is not possible, since prolonged remissions can occur with this treatment. The surgical removal of limited lung metastases should also be considered, but if there is also bone disease, as is usually the case, it is best not done. As with all progressive malignant disease the time comes when anything more than simple symptomatic treatment is unkind. Paraplegia due to extensive spinal deposits is often a preterminal event in uncontrolled Ewing's tumour.

Reticulum Cell Sarcoma of Bone

This tumour is best regarded as a primary malignant lymphoma of bone. It is rare and the experience at any one institution is limited. It is less common than secondary bone involvement by lymphoma. The commonest age range for presentation is 30–50 years, but it can occur at any age. The pattern of bone involvement is very similar to that of Ewing's tumour, but the metaphyseal part of the bone tends to be affected first with later spread to the shaft. Macroscopically the tumour has a large soft tissue component like Ewing's tumour. Histological examination reveals "histiocytes", lymphocytes and lymphoblasts. The picture may be difficult to distinguish from Ewing's tumour, but there is an absence of intracellular glycogen and staining for reticulin demonstrates a fine framework between the cells. Spread to regional nodes is fairly common, but distant nodes, other bones, and viscera are only involved late in the course of the disease. A true multifocal variant of the disease is recognised. The clinical presentation is one of insidiously developing pain and swelling, but systemic symptoms are not usually present. The regional lymph nodes may be palpable. X-rays reveal patchy bone destruction and a soft tissue mass, but the appearances are not diagnostic. Even after biopsy has been performed there may be some doubt about the diagnosis. In practice there is not usually much difficulty in excluding secondary lymphoma, as this tends to involve bone late in the course of the disease and there will be clear evidence of general nodal or organ involvement. Differentiation of reticulum cell sarcoma of bone from Ewing's tumour may be more difficult. Due regard must be paid to the histological evidence from special staining as mentioned above and the generally young age of patients with Ewing's tumour.

Investigation of the extent of spread of the disease should be as for non-Hodgkin's lymphoma and should include a bone marrow biopsy and examination of abdominal lymph glands by lymphography or CT scanning. When there is no demonstrable spread beyond the regional nodes, radical radiotherapy is the treatment of choice. The tumour is a radiosensitive one, so that local recurrences are unusual.

The techniques employed are as for Ewing's tumour but with an extension of the fields to cover the nodes (whether or not they are palpable). A tumour of the femur, for example, would require the inguinal nodes to be irradiated in addition to the whole femur. This extension does not add much to the field size, but it means that all the lymph drainage channels from the limb are irradiated. For this reason it is necessary to reduce the dose to 4000 cGy at the midplane of a parallel opposed pair delivered in 16 fractions over 3 weeks. The management of early and late reactions is as for Ewing's tumour. With radiotherapy alone, a 50% 5-year survival rate is to be expected and even if generalised disease develops its course can be slow. A case for adjuvant chemotherapy can be made, but the tumour is so rare that adequate testing of this policy would be very difficult. The tendency is, therefore, to use radiotherapy alone in the first instance and to treat generalised disease when it occurs with combination chemotherapy.

Multiple Myeloma and Solitary Plasmacytoma

Multiple myeloma is a malignant plasma cell tumour which is most common in old people. It is such a complex disease nosologically and in its management that only the basic radiotherapeutic aspects will be discussed here. The diagnosis rests on the finding of at least two of a triad of features. These are:

1) Increased numbers and abnormal forms of plasma cells in the bone marrow
2) Lytic bone lesions seen on X-ray
3) A monoclonal gammopathy as shown by an "M band" on plasma electrophoresis

It is a generalised disease and usually relentlessly progressive. Pulsed combination chemotherapy whilst not curative can, in most cases, suppress the disease for a time and can control the paraproteinaemia with its attendant hazards such as renal failure.

The radiotherapist may be called upon to treat painful bone lesions and might have to make the diagnosis of myeloma in patients referred with lytic bone lesions. In this latter context patients are sometimes referred with lytic disease particularly in the spine and are labelled as having metastatic disease from an unknown primary tumour. The possibility of myeloma should be considered in these circumstances and further investigations performed if there is doubt. The X-ray appearances may help. Myeloma seldom affects the pedicles of vertebrae, whereas metastatic cancer commonly does so. A skull X-ray may reveal the typical round punched-out lesions of myeloma. Plasma protein electrophoresis and bone marrow examination will confirm or refute the diagnosis.

Bone pain is a common feature of myeloma. X-ray therapy can relieve the pain, prevent vertebral collapse or pathological fracture, and help to keep the patient mobile. Once patients with myeloma become bed-ridden they are much more likely to develop hypercalcaemia with its attendant vomiting, polyuria, dehydration, and renal failure. Single megavoltage fields are usually used on the spine and parallel pairs for limbs or pelvis. The fields cover the involved areas with generous margins. Single exposures are used unless the field sizes become large, when four fractions are given. A 16×7 cm spinal field may be given 1000 cGy in one exposure, and a half pelvis 1750 cGy midplane dose in four fractions. Single spinal treatments often induce vomiting if anti-emetics are not given.

A particular problem in myeloma is spinal cord compression. This may result from vertebral collapse with angulation of the spine or from extradural tumour spread. An urgent laminectomy should be performed and the cord decompressed. Instability of the spine may need to be rectified surgically and radiotherapy should be started as soon as possible. The three-field wedge technique is best in this situation as it produces a homogeneous dose distribution with a better chance of long-term disease control. A tumour dose of 3500 cGy over 8 days can be given if the fields do not exceed 15 cm in length.

Occasionally, one sees solitary plasmacytomas in soft tissues extradurally, in the nose or nasal sinuses, in the testis, or in the lung. By definition there is no bone marrow involvement, but a paraproteinaemia may be seen if the tumour bulk is large. They should be treated by radiotherapy as for extranodal non-Hodgkin's lymphomas.

Careful follow-up is needed as about half the cases develop further solitary plasmacytomas or the features of generalised myeloma.

Giant Cell Tumour of Bone

This is a rare tumour thought to arise from osteoclasts. It is very unusual to find it before the age of 20 years (although it has been described in childhood) or after the age of 40. Very occasionally it occurs in older people when it is secondary to Paget's disease, although it is much less commonly found in this situation than is osteosarcoma. Giant cell tumour affects women twice as commonly as it does men. The long bones are the ones most commonly affected, particularly the lower femur, upper tibia, and lower radius, but the tumour may also occur in the pelvis, skull, ribs, and vertebrae on rare occasions. Its origin is in the epiphysis but it may spread to the metaphysis. The gross appearance of the tumour is that of an expanded bone with the cortex reduced to a thin shell. Bony septa remain within the tumour, demarcating areas of soft tumour tissue, bone lysis and haemorrhage. Microscopically two types of cell can be recognised: plump fusiform cells and multinucleated giant cells resembling osteoclasts. The diagnosis is often difficult as reactive giant cells are found in many other conditions, particularly around areas of haemorrhage, for example in solitary or aneurysmal bone cysts, in benign chondroblastoma, and in the bone lesions of hyperparathyroidism. Review of biopsy material by an experienced tumour pathologist is essential before treatment is begun. Many lesions which were called giant cell tumours in the past would not be so diagnosed today.

Giant cell tumour of bone shows a spectrum of behaviour from totally benign to frankly malignant and metastasising. The grading system of Jaffe categorises the tumour by the appearance of the stromal cells. Grade III is a malignant tumour from the outset, whereas grade I and II tumours seldom metastasise although they may recur locally. Occasionally a tumour may change its nature and recur and metastasise despite benign-looking histology. The clinical presentation is of an insidious onset of pain near a joint, with later swelling and occasional pathological fracture. The X-ray appearance is of a lytic area in the epiphyseal region. A thin rim of cortex remains and residual bony septa may give a "soap bubble" appearance.

Management Policy

A patient who has a frankly malignant tumour but no metastatic disease should be treated by radical surgery as for osteosarcoma. If surgery is impossible an attempt at radical X-ray treatment may be feasible. Adjuvant chemotherapy is, as yet, untried in this uncommon situation. It is much more difficult to formulate a rational policy for the treatment of patients with grade I and II tumours, as one does not want to overtreat an essentially benign condition, nor does one want inadequate treatment to lead to local recurrence and perhaps a change to a more aggressive type of tumour. It is not easy to learn from past experience. The histological confusion mentioned earlier is compounded by previous use of kilovoltage irradiation with its high bone absorption. At the Christie Hospital a technique was developed for giving 2000 R (later 2000 rad) in eight fractions over 10 days and repeating this in about 2 months and again in a further 4 months. Several patients who were treated on 3 occasions developed an osteonecrosis and subsequently retreatments were reserved for tumours that failed to heal. Now that giant cell tumour is a better defined clinical entity and its potentially aggressive nature is better understood we have abandoned this approach in favour of an initial definitive treatment.

The treatment recommended will depend upon the site and a dialogue between the radiotherapist and the orthopaedic surgeon is advisable. When a giant cell tumour can be excised without undue deformity or disability, as when it occurs in the head of the fibula, this should be done. Radiotherapy is not then required. When there is a tumour of a limb bone which is not removable without severe mechanical problems, for example of the femoral condyles, then curettage and packing with bone chips is permissible if a close follow-up is maintained. If there is evidence of renewed tumour activity, a course of X-ray treatment is recommended. This will usually amount to anterior and posterior parallel opposed megavoltage fields applied to the tumour with a modest margin and delivering a midplane dose of 4000 cGy in 16 fractions over 3 weeks. The previously mentioned precautions relating to joints apply here too. Following the radiotherapy, bone resorption may continue for 2–3 months, but after this there should be X-ray evidence of healing. If this does not occur a further biopsy is indicated, and if the tumour is still active, excision with prosthetic replacement or even amputation is necessary. Lesions of the pelvis and skull are often too extensive for surgical resection. They have a bad reputation, with 50% becoming malignant at a later date if inadequately dealt with. Following a biopsy radical X-ray treatment should be given. The techniques will be the same as those used for Ewing's tumour, but it is probably wise to reduce the dose by 500 cGy for this initially benign tumour. Giant cell tumour of the spine usually presents with spinal cord compression, and surgical decompression with biopsy is a matter of urgency. Thereafter, radical X-ray treatment, with a three-field wedge technique as previously described, should be performed.

16 Paediatric Radiotherapy

D. Pearson

Introduction

Incidence

Malignant disease in childhood is extremely rare, and particularly so when the mass of malignant disease at all ages is considered. However, its rarity does not diminish its importance both to paediatrics and to oncology. In the Manchester Children's Registry there are on average 105 cases each year for a population of 1 million children between 0 and 15 years of age. The incidence figures in Table 16.1 are important in planning for the management of tumours in children for two main reasons. First, the small numbers of tumours in the different tumour sites mean that substantial experience of these patients and their management is impossible except in specialised centres. Second, the types of tumours are significantly different from those which occur in adults—only 4% are epithelial in origin, whereas in adults these are the common tumours. Even those groups of tumours which do extend into the adult age range, such as Ewing's tumour and osteosarcoma, occur mainly in young adults. Central nervous system (CNS) tumours in children differ, both in site and histology, from those occurring in adults.

Table 16.1. Manchester Children's Tumour Registry annual incidence of tumour types per million children.

Leukaemia	31
Non-leukaemia reticulo-endothelial	10
Gliomas	19
Sympathetic nervous system	8
Retinoblastoma	3
Connective tissue	12
Renal	6
Gonadal	1
Teratomas	3
Epithelial	4
Ewing's	2
Miscellaneous	4
Malignant unclassified	2
Total	105

Reproduced from Tumours in Children.

Differences in Normal Tissue Sensitivity

Many normal tissues in childhood are still growing and therefore there will be a greater effect on them by radiation, resulting in deformity and changes in the function of certain organs as the child develops. The tissues which are adversely affected are as follows:

1) *Bone* will show some lack of growth if irradiation has to be given before full bony growth is completed.
2) The *brain* is particularly sensitive in children under the age of 2 years.
3) The *lens* of the eye is more likely to develop cataract when irradiated even at quite low doses in the very young.
4) *Endocrine organs* are sensitive to radiation, particularly the gonads, the pituitary, and the thyroid.

Other normal tissues such as skin, soft tissue, and muscle do not seem to be any more sensitive than in adults, as far as both immediate and late effects are concerned.

It is important therefore that any radiotherapist

who is concerned with treating children should be aware of the differences between tumours and normal tissues in adults and children and must not base the treatment of children solely on adult experience.

Management

The management of children with tumours calls for close cooperation between surgeons, radiotherapists, and paediatricians trained in chemotherapy and oncology. In addition, the total management of these children will involve specialists in other disciplines, such as endocrinologists, to advise on the management of the unavoidable side effects of treatment.

Surgery

Surgery has an important role to play, both in terms of active treatment and in providing a histological diagnosis. Because of the many different sites at which tumours occur, the various surgical specialists who may be involved include general paediatric surgeons, neurosurgeons, ophthalmologists, and orthopaedic and thoracic surgeons. Since each will be concerned with very small numbers of appropriate cases it is important that they should all have good collaborative links with radiotherapists and paediatric oncologists.

Radiotherapy

Radiotherapy may have a locally curative role or an adjuvant role, e.g. in leukaemia, where the main treatment is chemotherapy. Because of the many sites involved, many different techniques have to be used. Some are similar to those used for treating adult tumours, whilst others are specific for those tumours which are commonest in children and young adults. It is these latter neoplasms which will be described in full in this chapter; the others will be mentioned, but a full description of the appropriate therapeutic techniques is given in other chapters.

Chemotherapy

Extensive use is now made of chemotherapy in the treatment of children with tumours, either as the main treatment, or as adjuvant treatment. It has become quite intensive and requires special expertise for its control. There is a need for the paediatricians who are responsible for this chemotherapy to cooperate with their radiotherapy colleagues and vice versa, especially since there is considerable interaction between radiation and drug effects. It is essential to have a carefully coordinated treatment programme so that the optimum use of all methods of treatment can be ensured.

Management of Individual Tumour Types

Leukaemia

The different types of leukaemia which occur in childhood are shown in Table 16.2. The main

Table 16.2. Different types of leukaemia in children—percentage of total seen in Manchester Children's Tumour Registry.

Acute lymphoblastic (ALL)	54.0
Acute stem cell (ASC)	26.9
Acute myeloid (AML)	12.9
Acute monocytic	3.0
Acute myelomonocytic	2.0
Acute erythroleukaemia	0.4
Chronic myeloid leukaemia (adult type)	0.6
Chronic myeloid leukaemia (juvenile type)	0.2

group includes those arising from the lymphocyte series of cells—the acute lymphblastic leukaemias. These children usually present with pallor and lassitude of recent onset, and on examination are found to have glandular enlargement and often hepatosplenomegaly. Investigations usually reveal some degree of anaemia, and platelets are commonly reduced. The total white cell count may be low, normal, or high, but the distribution of the different white cells is abnormal, with neutropenia and an excess of lymphocytes, many of which are lymphoblasts. Bone marrow examination confirms the diagnosis. It is now recognised that the different lymphocytes may be differentiated by cell markers; moreover these leukaemias seem to have a worse prognosis compared with the common cell type. The clinical management of children with acute lymphoblastic leukaemia has improved considerably since chemotherapy first became available and today most of these children will enter remission following induction therapy with vincristine and prednisolone. Further maintenance therapy for 2–3 years, using methotrexate, 6-mercaptopurine, rubidamycin, asparaginase, and occasionally other agents, resulted in a considerable increase in long-term survivors. It was found, however, that even though the marrow remained in remission, the disease relapsed in the central nervous system. Unfortunately, when this kind of relapse occurs it has proved well nigh impossible to achieve a cure. In view of this we now endeavour to prevent relapse by prophylactic treatment of the central nervous system with cranial radiation and intrathecal methotrexate. American workers have so far achieved the best control of these children, so that at present our cranial radiation dose is 1800 cGy in 11 exposures, treating 5 days a week, as in the most successful United States trial. The volume treated is shown in Fig. 16.1.

More recently in boys who are long-term survivors there has been a disappointing increase in testicular relapse, showing as painless swelling of the testicle. As with CNS relapse, many of these boys remain in marrow remission. It has been suggested that, as for the cranial problem, testicular prophylaxis should be undertaken. This would have to be done by irradiation and, since the dose required would be similar to that needed for cranial prophylaxis, this would be followed by testicular damage. Sterility would be certain, if not complete radiation castration with damage to the interstitial cells as well as the germ cells, resulting in hormone deficiency and lack of pubertal development. Another possible approach, which at present looks promising, is to treat only those boys who do relapse, irradiating both testes (Fig. 16.2) to a dose of 2400 cGy in 3 weeks. At the same time, the boys are re-induced with chemotherapy, and so far the result are proving satisfactory. This approach avoids the sequelae of radiation in those boys who do not develop intratesticular relapse.

The other cell types of acute leukaemia, such as myeloid, monocytic, and combined myelomonocytic leukaemia, do not as yet have the same response to intensive chemotherapy as the acute lymphoblastic disease. Nevertheless, a few long-term survivors have also developed CNS relapse,

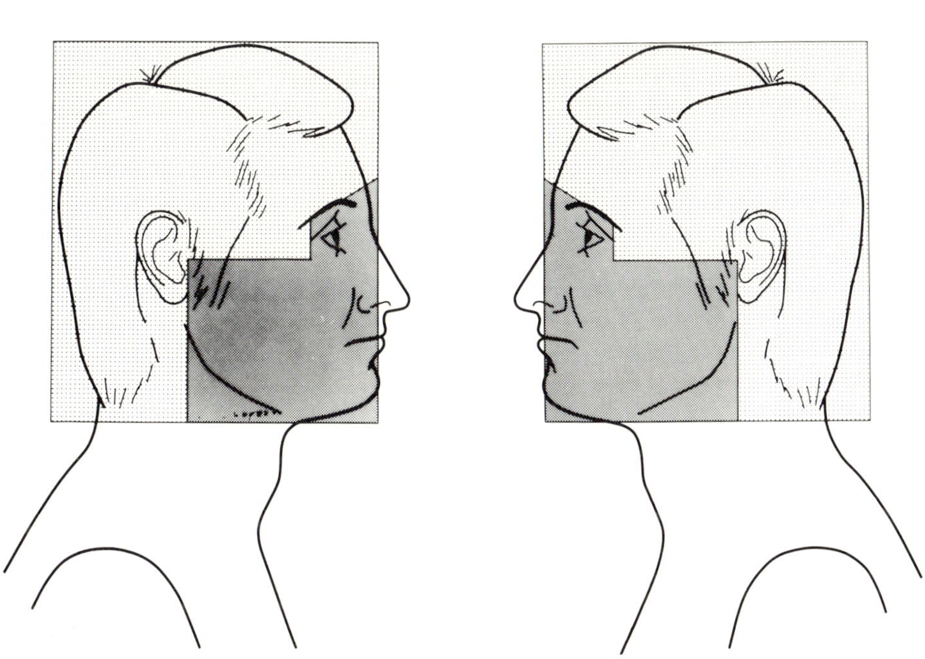

Fig. 16.1. Parallel opposed fields for prophylactic radiation of the cranium in acute lymphoblastic leukaemia.

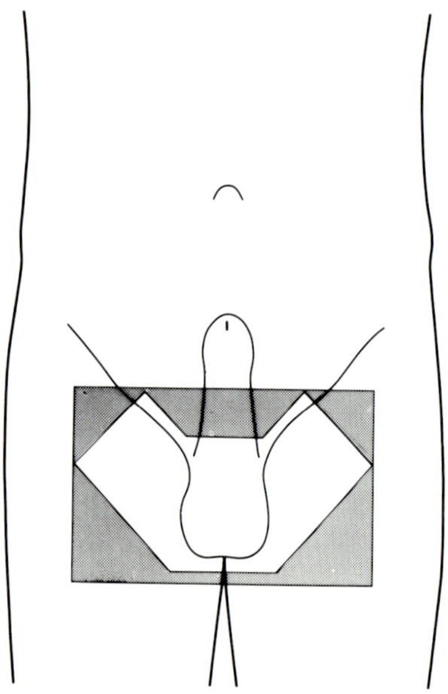

Fig. 16.2. Irradiation field to the testes in boys with acute lymphoblastic leukaemia at relapse.

so that if and when more effective treatment becomes available prophylactic radiotherapy may be needed for these patients as well. However, recent developments in bone marrow transplantation suggest that these other leukaemias may be treated successfully with transplantation, which will require the use of total body irradiation.

Non-leukaemic Reticulosis

Hodgkin's Disease

In our 15-year series there were only 50 children with Hodgkin's disease. Its presentation and behaviour were similar to those seen in adults. The incidence of the different histological types is shown in Table 16.3. Our series differs from those reported in the United States in that nodular sclerosis histology was rarer, and nearer to the European distribution. Investigation and staging are carried out as in adults, but there are more risks after splenectomy in children than adults, and for young children there is a reluctance to do a splenectomy. In all children a prophylactic antibiotic is given after splenectomy, to try to reduce the incidence of severe infections.

Table 16.3. Histological types seen in Hodgkin's disease in childhood in Manchester.

Lymphocytic predominant	40%
Nodular sclerosis	10%
Mixed cellularity	44%
Lymphocytic depleted	6%

Management

The management of Hodgkin's disease in children differs from that pursued in adults to ensure as far as possible reduction of the late effects of therapy. In stage Ia and stage IIa disease with favourable histology (i.e. lymphocyte predominant and nodular sclerotic) radiotherapy is the treatment of choice, being confined to the involved anatomical region in stage Ia and mantle therapy in stage II patients. The limited-field radiation therapy for the most common presentation in the neck is shown in Fig. 16.3. In patients with B symptoms or stage III or IV disease we rely on chemotherapy using mustine, vincristine, procarbazine and prednisolone. Radiotherapy to residual or bulk disease is also used. In patients who have relapsed after chemotherapy total nodal radiation has been used with good effect and is well tolerated by children, but we would not use it as the first line of approach, because the late sequelae, particularly in relation to growth, are bound to be greater. The mantle and inverted-Y field to the abdomen are achieved in the way described for adults in Chap. 14.

Non-Hodgkin's Lymphoma

These tumours occur throughout life, but there are differences between the disease in children and in adults. The incidence in childhood extends throughout the age range, but it is very uncommon under 2 years. After 2 years the incidence is constant until the early teens are reached. Boys are affected more than girls, in the ratio of 3.5:1. Gastrointestinal, abdominal, and anterior mediastinal presentations are commoner in children than in adults. Presentation may be nodal or in extranodal lymphatic sites and even in nonlymphatic tissues such as the CNS, orbit, etc. Clinical presentation will depend on the primary site as follows:

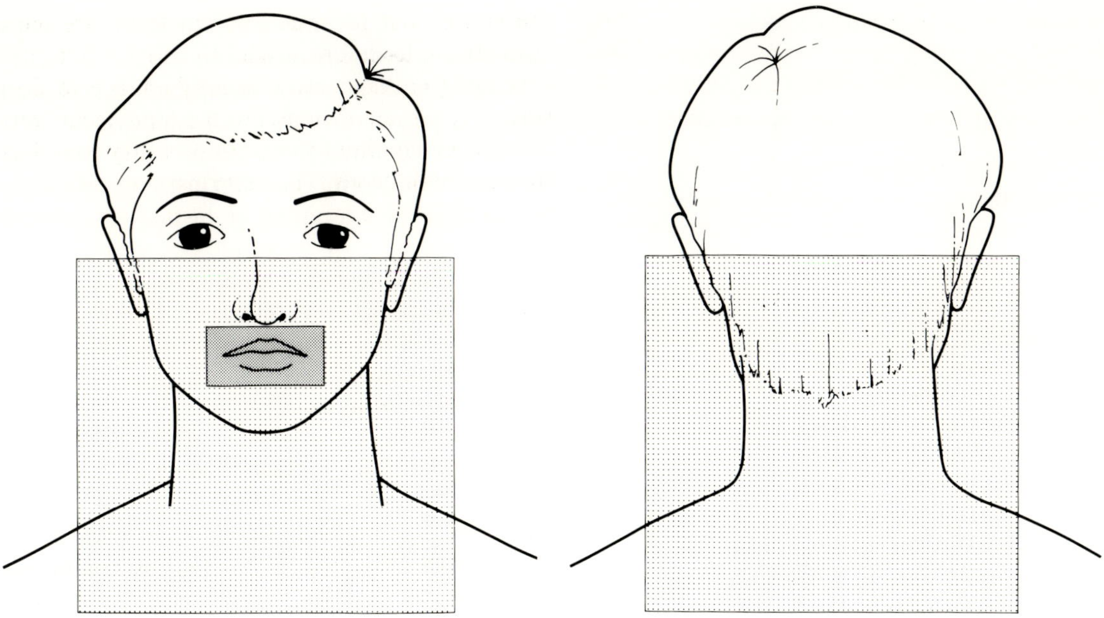

Fig. 16.3. Limited-field radiation technique for stage 1 Hodgkin's disease.

Anterior Mediastinum

A non-Hodgkin's lymphoma often presents as a medical emergency with dyspnoea and a superior vena caval obstruction. Chest X-ray reveals a large mass of nodes in the anterior mediastinum and is often associated with pleural effusions. Other nodes may be palpable in the lower neck or the axillae.

Gastrointestinal Disease

The sites most commonly affected are the terminal ileum, caecum, appendix, and ascending colon. Presentation is usually as an acute abdominal emergency, such as intussusception, and the diagnosis is usually made only at laparotomy, and frequently only after histological examination of obviously thickened bowel.

Advanced Intra-abdominal Disease

This is more common in our experience. These children present with large abdominal masses, often associated with ascites.

Nodal

Enlarged lymph nodes in the neck, axillae, and groins may be the presenting feature, usually painless, and the diagnosis is only established by node biopsy.

Pharyngeal Mass

A tonsillar or pharyngeal mass may be a presenting feature but is usually not the only abnormality, as commonly there is also bilateral cervical node enlargement.

Non-Hodgkin's lymphoma in children, as well as having many different presenting sites of involvement, becomes generalised early, and the histological types are more likely to be those of the diffuse type, with a poorer prognosis. Bone marrow infiltration is not uncommon and some cases develop blood changes consistent with acute lymphoblastic leukaemia.

Management

Before the use of multi-agent chemotherapy, when treatment was limited to radiation, the number of cures in children with non-Hodgkin's lymphoma was very small indeed. Of the 44 children treated in Manchester between 1954 and 1968, only 10 survived and all either obviously had disease localised to one lymph node group or had had very localised gastrointestinal disease. Thus, a different approach to treatment had to be developed to deal with the other more aggressively malignant disease.

The present approach can be summarised as follows:

1) In early disease, stage I, with a well-differentiated histological picture, it is known that patients can be cured by adequate radiation therapy, using extended-field techniques and a dose of 3000 cGy in 3 weeks. Even in this group, however, it is possible that the addition of multiple drug chemotherapy may increase the survival, and this is being tested in various clinical trials at present.
2) The more aggressive forms of this disease tend to become rapidly more generalised, and local treatment was always unsuccessful. These patients are now primarily treated by multiagent chemotherapy, and results are already showing that this is an improvement. The role of radiotherapy is at present unclear, and trials are taking place to assess its value in treating the site of bulk disease once remission has taken place. Radiation therapy may also contribute in T cell lymphoma and leukaemia to the prevention of CNS relapse, as in acute lymphoblastic leukaemia.

   Early results in the United Kingdom, using this approach, are already encouraging.

Histiocytosis X

This group of conditions in the Manchester Series is slightly less common than Hodgkin's disease and slightly more common than the non-Hodgkin's lymphomas. It occurs mainly in early childhood and there is no apparent sex difference. The manifestations of this disease vary from solitary to multiple bone lesions (characteristically sharply defined osteolytic areas with little new bone formation), or from minor to major soft tissue and organ involvement. The previously described spectrum of syndromes —eosinophilic granuloma of bone, Hand-Schueller-Christian disease and Letterer-Siwe disease—are now considered manifestations of the same underlying condition. The exact nature of histiocytosis X is not understood, and there are some who do not regard it as a malignant process. However, until its true nature is determined, and since the treatment used is similar to that for malignant disease, it seems appropriate to discuss it here.

A definite diagnosis is usually made following biopsy from an obvious lesion, unless the bony lesions are confined to an inaccessible part, e.g. the base of the skull. The main histological feature is a diffuse proliferation of histiocytes, though granulomas may or may not be present. Eosinophils, lymphocytes, plasma cells, and large histiocytes can be seen accumulated in the lesions.

Clinical Presentations

The disease may present as painful bone lesions or, in certain sites such as the skull, as painless swellings. Pathological fractures have been reported but seem to be rare. Lesions in soft tissues may present as rashes of a seborrhoeic type, as chronic discharging ears, and as nodules on the gums. There may be proptosis, polyuria and polydypsia associated with diabetes insipidus, either at the time of diagnosis or later as the disease progresses. The liver, spleen, and lymph nodes may enlarge and thrombocytopenia may also occur. Dyspnoea may result from pulmonary infiltration, which on X-ray appears as a fine reticulation in the lung fields.

Investigations

These should include a chest X-ray, skeletal survey (even for apparently solitary lesions, since others may be found), full blood count including platelets and bone marrow aspiration. Measurement of the urinary specific gravity and the urine and serum osmolality will confirm or exclude diabetes insipidus. It is helpful in clinical practice to record the sites of the lesions on a chart, providing a graphic historical record of events from the date of the initial diagnosis. A scanning system is used as a guide to the severity, i.e. the extent of the disease process, in each patient. A score of 1 is given for a solitary bone lesion, 2 for multiple lesions, 3 for each organ involved (liver, spleen, etc.), with a maximum score of 8 for the most widespread disease.

Treatment

Clinicians with experience of treating these children are aware that spontaneous regression can occur and that the disease may burn itself out as the child grows older. This being so, as long as the child is reasonably well, treatment should be as little as possible.

X-ray Therapy

Solitary bone lesions respond very well to a single given dose of 600 cGy. It seems likely from other reported series that doses as low as 400 cGy are successful. The pituitary hypothalamic areas may be treated by using a parallel pair of fields and delivering a midline dose of 1000 cGy in 4 days. A similar dose may be used for deposits of the disease in the ear. When treating painful bone lesions, which may be quite small, it is essential that verification films be taken to avoid "geographic misses". For slowly evolving and mainly bony disease, local radiotherapy directed to lesions as they appear may be all that is necessary. However, consideration must be given to the accumulating total body dose and to the marrow impairment which may result from this. A decision must be taken to change from radiotherapy to chemotherapy before the marrow is too impaired to permit this.

Chemotherapy

Histiocytosis X responds to a variety of agents. Steroids were the first to be used and are still the first choice. Other drugs used are vincristine, vinblastine, cyclophosphamide, chlorambucil, and 6-mercaptopurine. However, there is at present no clear indication as to what is the best drug or combination of drugs, an assessment made more complex because of the varied natural behaviour in this condition.

Other Treatment

The diabetes insipidus when confirmed requires continuous treatment for its control. It is now best controlled by the use of desmopressin which is absorbed by instillation into the nose. This provides much better control than the previously used pituitary snuff.

If lung function is impaired care must be taken to avoid chest infections which should be quickly treated. Emphysema may be a late consequence of this organic involvement.

Prognosis

This is quite good particularly for those whose score is at the low end of the Lahey scale. In the Manchester series, 27 of 45 children survive. As the Lahey score increased to 5 or more organs involved, mortality increased to 100%.

Late Effects

Diabetes insipidus is permanent and requires treatment for the rest of the child's life. In this group there may be other pituitary hormone deficiencies, especially growth hormone, and appropriate investigations are needed so that in suitable cases growth hormone therapy can be initiated. Even in those children without diabetes insipidus, growth seems to be sometimes impaired without demonstrable growth hormone deficiency, and more investigation of these children is necessary. It is unusual with the radiation doses employed to see any cessation of skeletal development.

Central Nervous System Tumours

This group of tumours is the largest of all the solid tumours in childhood, in contrast to their low incidence in adults. In children the distribution of brain tumours by site is such that two thirds of them arise below the tentorium and only one third above. The reverse is true in adults. The histological types are also different from those found in adults. The largest group are the astrocytomas which, in the Manchester series, account for 40% of all cases. In this group there are five histological types, as shown in Table 16.4. The juvenile type of

Table 16.4. Astrocytoma histological types.

Juvenile astrocytoma	62%
Adult grades III and IV	30%
Mixed juvenile and adult	4%
Gemistocytic	1%
Giant cell	3%

astrocytoma is distinct histologically from the adult types, and is characterised clinically by its often slow growth. The adult types are seen in patients of all ages and have histological variants from fairly hypocellular to very pleomorphic and anaplastic types.

The medulloblastoma accounts for 24% of all cases and occurs in children and young adults. It arises in the cerebellum and cerebellopontine angle, and is characterised by its ability to metastasise via the cerebrospinal fluid to other parts of the central nervous system. In about 7% of cases metastases occur outside the CNS, mainly to bone. The third most common group are the ependymomas, accounting for 12.5% of children with CNS tumour. They occur at all sites in the CNS. Like the medulloblastoma, the malignant type of ependymoma may metastasise throughout the CNS. Other tumours such as the oligodendroglioma and pinealoma are rare. Craniopharyngiomas account for 5% of childhood tumours. In 12.5% histological diagnosis is not possible because the site of the primary in the midbrain and third ventricle makes a biopsy dangerous or impossible. The mode of presentation of brain tumours in children is that of a space-occupying lesion within the skull. The symptoms of increased intracranial pressure are headache and vomiting, particularly in the early morning. Papilloedema is also commonly present. Localising symptoms and signs are dependent on the primary site. Incoordination—presenting as unsteadiness, broad-based walk, nystagmus, past-pointing, and positive Rhombergism—is present in posterior fossa primaries. Midbrain lesions produce many cranial nerve palsies. Supratentorial lesions may produce hemiparesis, while lesions around the pituitary and optic nerve produce defects of the field of vision. Though a VIth nerve palsy may not be a localising sign, but merely indicative of raised intracranial pressure, it can also be the first sign of a midbrain tumour.

Radiological investigation is supplemented by CT scanning, but this is not always positive, particularly with tumours in the posterior fossa and midbrain. In our experience a negative CT scan often becomes positive later and it is our belief that, if unexplained symptoms persist, other investigations should be pursued, and if necessary a posterior fossa exploration performed.

Management

Surgery

Once the diagnosis of a probable brain tumour has been made, there is in all patients an urgent need to achieve a reduction of the raised intracranial pressure. The neurosurgeon is therefore the first to be consulted in the management of these patients.

In some children, particularly those with juvenile astrocytomas of the cerebellum, the release of the increased pressure and opening up of the cerebrospinal fluid pathways is combined with the removal of all the tumour or a major part of it. This may also be all that is necessary as a first procedure in medulloblastoma. In supratentorial tumours removal of a large part of the lesion will also reduce the pressure. The midbrain tumours and cerebellar tumours which are extending forward into the midbrain are not amenable to simple removal. In these patients a shunt from the ventricles to the atrium or the peritoneum is needed before other treatment can be considered. In most patients surgery will reduce pressure and provide tumour tissue for a histological diagnosis. In those juvenile astrocytomas where complete removal has been possible, this will be the only treatment that is needed.

Radiotherapy

Apart from those patients who have had a complete surgical removal, radiotherapy has been used as primary curative treatment and will be described for each tumour type.

Juvenile Astrocytomas This tumour arises in many sites in the brain and spinal cord, but is commonest in the cerebellum and third ventricle and optic nerve (Table 16.5). In certain sites, such as the cerebellum and parts of the cerebral hemispheres, a total surgical removal is possible and for such patients no futher treatment is indicated. In the other sites total removal is dangerous and likely to leave unwelcome sequelae, and although these are

Table 16.5. Anatomical site of juvenile astrocytoma.

Cerebellum	49%
Cerebrum	10%
Brain stem	10%
Third ventricle and optic nerve	26%
Spinal cord	5%

slow-growing tumours, symptoms such as visual defects and local effects in midbrain and third ventricle demand that some other treatment be tried. Although this is a well-differentiated tumour, improvement in the clinical state of the patient often follows local radiation treatment.

The radiation treatment techniques used are dependent on the precise site involved, but all employ megavoltage radiation. The volume irradiated consists of the tumour with a margin of 1–2 cm of normal brain around it. For residual tumours in the cerebellum a wedge pair of fields to include the posterior fossa is used and the isodose distribution for such a case is shown in Fig. 16.4. For optic

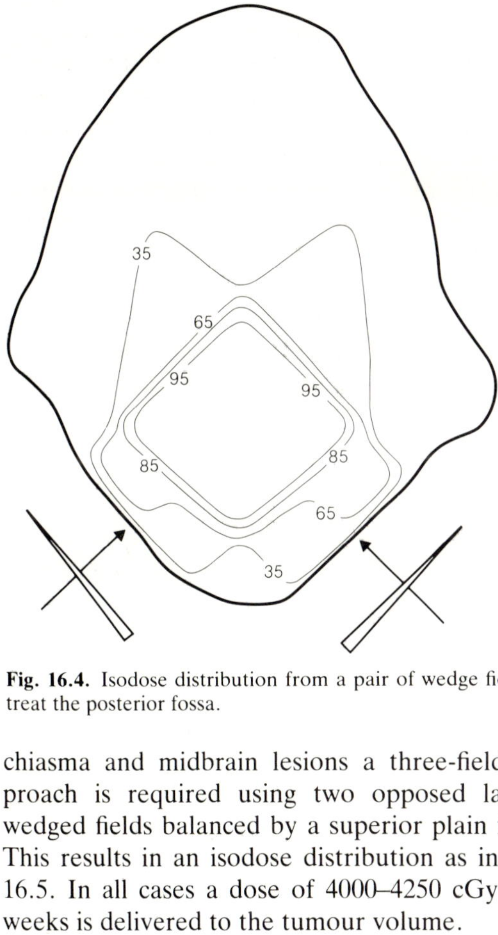

Fig. 16.4. Isodose distribution from a pair of wedge fields to treat the posterior fossa.

chiasma and midbrain lesions a three-field approach is required using two opposed lateral wedged fields balanced by a superior plain field. This results in an isodose distribution as in Fig. 16.5. In all cases a dose of 4000–4250 cGy in 3 weeks is delivered to the tumour volume.

Adult Astrocytomas These supratentorial tumours are much more extensive than the juvenile type and are often more infiltrating than they appear on scans or at operation. Because of these features, the radiation volume needs to be quite large. The result is that half to three-quarters of the whole

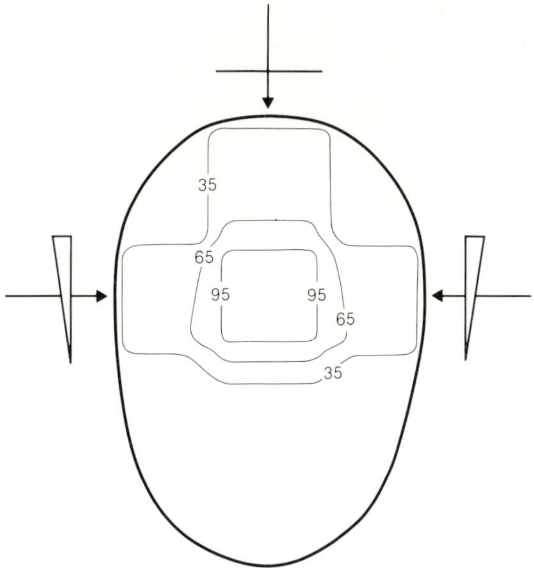

Fig. 16.5. Isodose distribution using a three-field technique for optic chiasma and midbrain tumours.

brain is irradiated—the details of this technique are described in Chap. 8—and the doses necessary for children are the same as those given to adults.

Medulloblastoma and Malignant Ependymoma Because of their cerebrospinal spread the treatment of both these tumours requires some form of therapy which can be applied to the whole CNS. Historically, it was noted that these tumours were quite sensitive to radiation, as rapid recovery occurred when the primary was irradiated. However, in all cases so treated spinal deposits manifested themselves in a short time, and although quick relief of symptoms again occurred with spinal treatment, cure could not be obtained. Radiotherapy techniques were developed which encompassed the whole of the CNS in one undivided volume. This was achieved in the early days by using a dominant 300-kV posterior field with a long FSD and subtending the whole CNS from the top of the head to 2.5 cm below S2. The spinal width was achieved by lead shielding of the lateral parts of the field. This was achieved by having the patient lying prone underneath a table which supported the lead shielding. The tumour dose in the spine was expressed as the dose at the posterior surface of the spinal bodies. In the head the dose anteriorly was increased by adding angled 500-kV fields, or later, lateral wedged megavoltage fields. The dose distribution achieved by this technique is shown in Fig. 16.6. The tumour dose was stated as the lowest dose—2700 cGy in 3 weeks—and because this was essentially a dominant posterior field, the dose rose in the posterior fossa and was highest on the skin at the back of the head. It is thought that this higher dose at the primary tumour does contribute to the success of this treatment. The small spinal deposits are apparently controlled at lower doses, as suggested by the fact that, in those patients in whom treatment is not successful, the recurrence occurs at the primary site in the majority of patients.

For many years this kilovoltage technique proved an effective method of treating patients with medulloblastoma. However, as megavoltage became more the radiation of choice, and as kilovoltage equipment was likely to become less available, we decided to change the technique, using megavoltage radiation only. The objective was to increase the degree of homogeneity of dosage throughout the CNS, while the extra dose thought to be desirable in the posterior fossa would be achieved by extra fields to this site. The whole-CNS technique now consists of a cranial and a spinal component appropriately matched to one another. The cranial component involves two lateral opposed fields which irradiate the entire cranium and also the cervical spine down to the shoulders. This is achieved by making for each patient a shell in two parts, posterior and anterior.

This posterior shell is placed in wax in a box of Perspex and the patient lies supine on the table with his head in the shell (Fig. 16.7). The anterior shell is then placed on the face and neck and the anterior half of the box is placed in position (Fig. 16.8). For treatment, the patient lies supine on a high table and the Perspex box sits on a platform on a car jack which can raise and lower the box. The height is adjusted so that the cervical spine lies

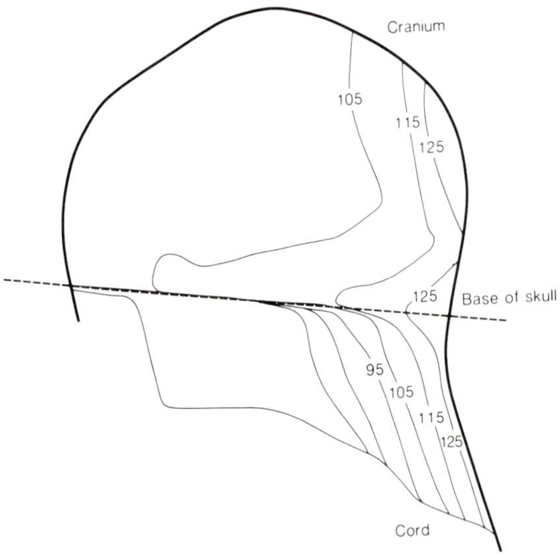

Fig. 16.6. Isodose distribution in the cranium and spinal cord for whole-CNS radiation using kilovoltage technique.

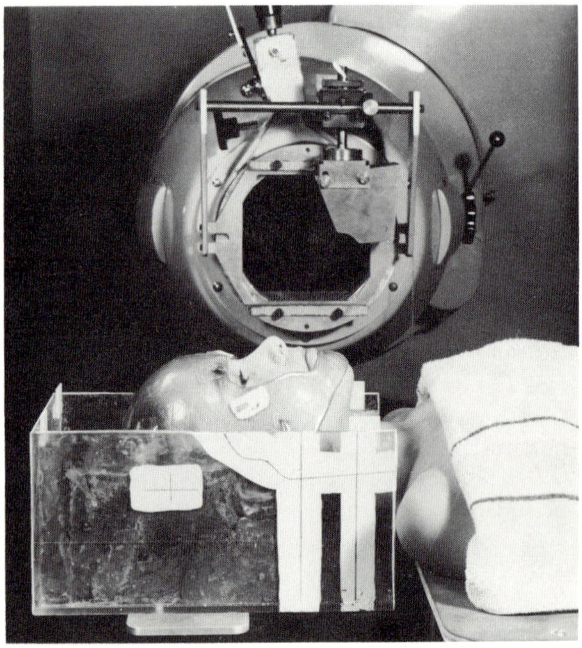

Fig. 16.7. Patient in position in the head shell in the posterior half of the box jig.

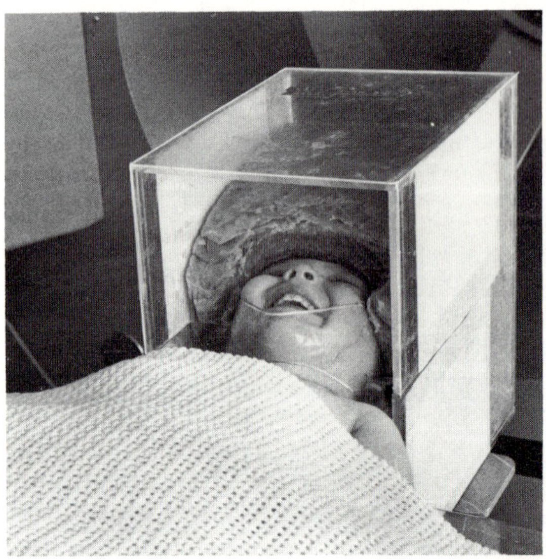

Fig. 16.8. The complete box jig with the anterior wax in place over the cranium.

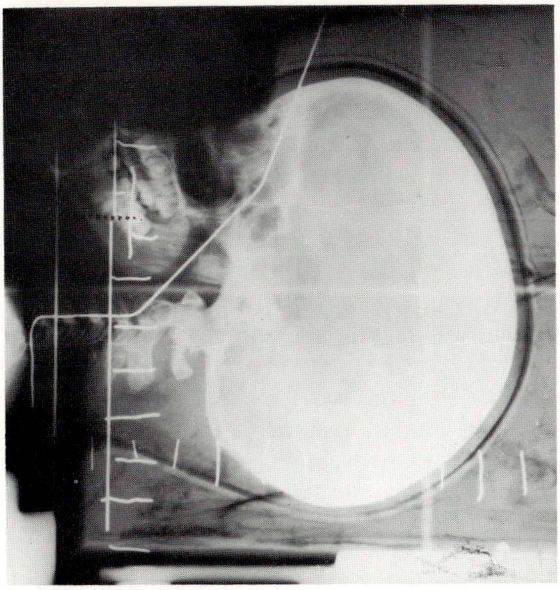

Fig. 16.9. The lateral X-ray with marker in place for the shielding of the face and anterior neck from the parallel opposed craniocervical spine fields.

horizontal (Fig. 16.9), checked by a lateral film. When this has been achieved, the shielding for the eyes, face, and anterior neck is placed on the film and, after checking, transferred to the sides of the box. The shielding block to cover this is attached to the X-ray tube (Fig. 16.10).

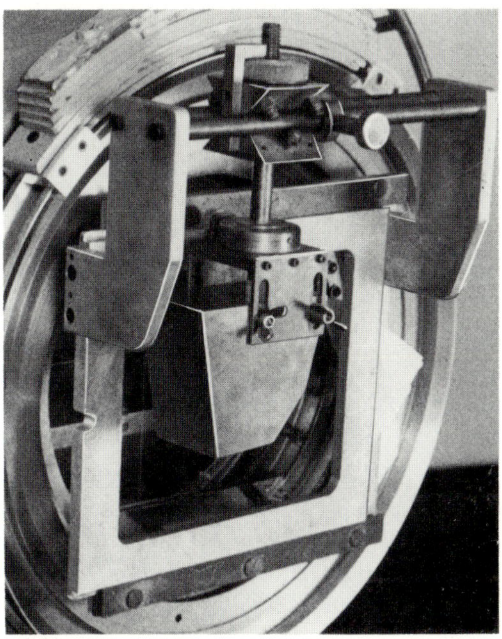

Fig. 16.10. Shielding block in place on the X-ray tube.

The spinal component is treated by pairs of wedged fields at an angle of 50° to the vertical and come in below the patient on the high table. The table has a Perspex window in which there is a central straight line. A line is drawn on the patient joining the vertebral spines, and this is lined up to coincide with the line on the table. The angled fields are each 25 cm long and 5.5 cm wide. The dose distribution is shown in (Fig. 16.11) and is so

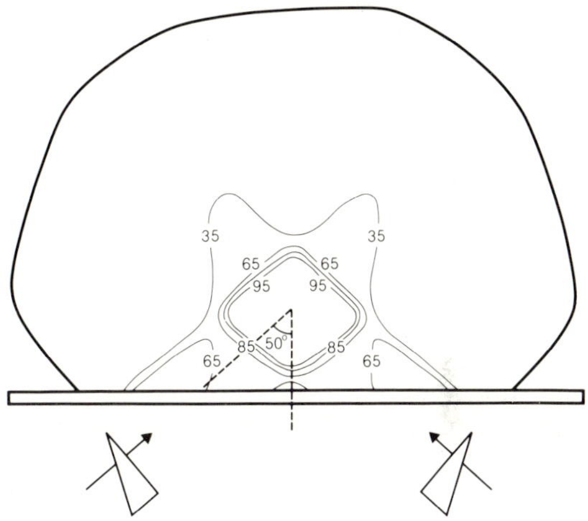

Fig. 16.11. Dose distribution from a wedge pair of spinal fields.

arranged that the high-dose volume will encompass the spinal canal throughout the lower cervical, dorsal, lumbar, and upper sacral spines. Because it is larger than needed to cover the canal, it allows for the differences in depth at the different levels. These fields are matched to the craniocervical field and to each other if more than one length is needed. The fields are slightly separated at the skin surface, but the beams meet at the spinal depth. The dose distribution across these junctions is evened out by changing the position of the patient each day. The centres of all the fields are moved by 0.5 cm each day—first caudally for 4 days, then cranially for 4 days. The unwanted lower portion of the lowest fields is blocked out by lead placed beneath the table on stilts. The dose delivered is 3000 cGy in 4 weeks. The dose to the posterior fossa is increased by using a parallel opposed pair of megavoltage fields which irradiate from the posterior clinoid to the occipital tuberosity and down to the first cervical vertebra. An extra 1500 cGy in 2 weeks is given to this, so that the primary site receives a total dose of 4500 cGy in 6 weeks and the rest of the CNS 3000 cGy in 4 weeks. In practice we do the extra posterior fossa treatment first, during which time the preparation for the whole-CNS treatment is completed.

Midbrain and Third Ventricle Tumours of Unknown Histology The absence of histology for these patients makes the planning of therapy quite difficult. If the different post-mortem histological variants in these sites are looked at, we find that varieties of astrocytoma, either juvenile or adult, are the commonest, followed by ependymoma and medulloblastoma. These patients with juvenile astrocytomas are perhaps more likely to have a longer history, indicating slower growth, and in such cases local radiotherapy (as described earlier) should be used. In patients with a shorter history the other tumour types are more likely. Since local treatment is likely to fail if given to those who may have medulloblastoma or ependymoblastoma, it seems reasonable to treat all but the juvenile astrocytomas with whole-CNS treatment as described above. This may mean that the adult type of astrocytoma is overtreated, but since this gives at least a chance of cure in other types, this is acceptable.

Sympathetic Nervous System Tumours

The three types of tumour which may arise from the sympathetic nervous system are the neuroblastoma, ganglioneuroma, and phaeochromocytoma. Of 114 such tumours in the Manchester Children's Tumour Registry, 101 were neuroblastomas, ten were benign ganglioneuromas, and there were only three phaeochromocytomas. The neuroblastomas often contained areas of differing degrees of maturation, even fully mature ganglion cells. The sites of origin were easy to determine in the ganglioneuromas and phaeochromocytomas. There were six of the former in the chest, three in the abdomen, and one in the neck. All presented as lumps in these situations and all were cured by surgical removal. The phaeochromocytomas were all in the abdomen, two suprarenal and one elsewhere along the sympathetic chain. They presented with episodes of hypertension.

The precise sites of origin of all the neuroblastomas were not as easily determined because (1) the diagnosis of these tumours can now be based on their excretion of biochemical markers (the catecholamines), so that surgical exploration has little to contribute to the management of the child, and (2) the disease is very widespread, so that at death there may be multiple tumours at different sites along the sympathetic chain. However, it seems that 77% of them arose in the abdomen, and of these, 87% arose near the kidney, probably from the adrenal. There were 16% arising in the thorax and 5% in the neck.

The metastatic spread of neuroblastomas is to the liver, bones, and lymph nodes. The typical hepatic metastasis was described by Pepper early this century, the primary tumour being thought to arise always in the right adrenal. The bone-metastasising type was described by Hutchinson —mostly cranial metastases—but it was later observed that the liver metastases tended to occur in young infants, mostly under 6 months of age, and the bone metastases in older children. There are often widespread lymph node metastases.

The presenting features of children with neuroblastoma are protean and may arise from the primary and/or from the secondary tumours. In the infant there may be a distended abdomen, neonatal jaundice, hepatomegaly, and subcutaneous tumours. In older children there may be bone metastases in the skull, causing proptosis and bruising around the eyes, or in other bones causing bone pain. These may be accompanied by a large abdominal mass, and such symptoms as anorexia and weight loss. Extra-abdominal primaries may present with a visible mass in the neck, often with an associated Horner's syndrome. Cough and dyspnoea may accompany chest primaries and the so-called dumb-bell or hourglass tumour may give rise to root pain and a paraplegia as a result of spinal cord compression. Investigations which may be helpful include bone marrow puncture to determine the presence of tumour cells, X-rays of chest and abdomen may reveal calcification, and a skeletal survey or bone scan may disclose bone metastases. Urine excretion of catecholamines is positive in the majority of cases, ranging from 77% to 96% in different series.

Neuroblastoma may be staged as follows:

- Stage I — Tumours confined to the organ or structure of origin.
- Stage II — Tumours extending in continuity beyond the organ or structure of origin but not crossing the midline. Homolateral lymph nodes may be involved.
- Stage III — Tumours extending in continuity

	beyond the midline. Bilateral regional lymph nodes may be involved.
Stage IV	Dissemination with metastases in skeleton, organs, soft tissues, distant lymph nodes, etc.
Stage IV S	Patients who would be stage I or stage II were it not for the fact that they show dissemination to liver, spleen, bone marrow (but without radiographic evidence of bone metastases), or subcutaneous tissue.

This last group are usually the young infants, and experience has shown that despite the widespread disease these children often do quite well with small amounts of treatment—or even with none at all, as in this group spontaneous regression occurs.

Management

Surgery

Where a total surgical removal of stage I and stage II disease can be easily achieved this should be done. The stage I tumours, particularly when extra-abdominal, will be cured by this means. Even for stage II tumours, the prognosis may be quite good without further treatment. Some surgeons also believe that the removal of as much as possible of very large tumours should be tried, since this might improve the effectiveness of other therapy. Other surgeons do not agree with this approach and advise only biopsy. Late surgery after shrinkage by radiotherapy and chemotherapy can be considered but neurosurgery is always needed for the dumb-bell tumour unless contraindicated by other clinical problems. In stage IV S tumours removal of the primary may help the regression or maturation of metastases in subcutaneous tissue or liver.

Radiotherapy

This should be considered for the following situations:

1) For patients with stage I and II tumours where surgery has resulted in incomplete removal, particularly in the chest where complete resection is more difficult. A dose of 2500–3000 cGy in 3–4 weeks is prescribed.
2) For patients with stage III tumours, total surgical removal is impossible. If no distant metastases are present, radiotherapy should be given to the primary site and its lymph node drainage areas. This will mean extensive field radiotherapy: for example, the whole abdomen. The dosage should be 3000 cGy in 4 weeks and at least one kidney should be shielded after 1500 cGy.
3) For patients with stage IV S tumours, removal of the primary tumour may be all that is required, particularly when the main problem is disease affecting the bone marrow or subcutaneous nodules. The very large livers in these young children preclude any operative search for the primary, and low-dose X-ray treatment to the whole liver will achieve cures. The doses should be 500–1000 cGy in 2 weeks.
4) Stage IV patients have widespread metastases and local treatment can only be used to relieve symptoms. However, X-ray therapy is a quick and easy method of relieving such unpleasant symptoms as bone pain or unsightly proptosis.

Chemotherapy

In most patients with stage III disease and in all stage IV disease, surgery and radiotherapy cannot be curative, and in view of the high percentage of these stages at presentation other treatments have been tried. The drugs which have been used are vincristine, cyclophosphamide, adriamycin, methotrexate, and actinomycin D, in a variety of combinations. Whilst in most children an initial response occurs, this is mostly of short duration and the majority relapse and die quite quickly. If systemic treatment is needed in certain stage IV S patients, gentle chemotherapy is often very successful.

Retinoblastoma

This tumour is usually detected early in life, most commonly in the first year, and the majority have declared themselves within the first 3 years of life. The tumour was bilateral in about 40% of our patients. In this series there were 17 families with multiple members with retinoblastoma, and in this group of patients there was a higher percentage of bilateral tumours. Spontaneous arrest does occur and was seen in six patients in the affected families. In patients cured of retinoblastoma there is a higher than normal incidence of second cancers, particularly osteosarcoma. Some of these occur in the radiated volume, when this treatment has been used, but others occur at distant sites and in children who have never received any irradiation. Also in the hereditary cases there is an increase in other cancers in adult life.

Treatment

Successful management of patients with a unilateral tumour can be achieved by removal of the affected eye. This is acceptable when the other eye is perfect. However, because of the bilateral tumours some other form of treatment was sought and a variety of radiation techniques have been tried. For example, external radiation has been directed to the whole *retina* of the less affected eye (the other having been removed); external radiation given to the whole *eye* using anterior fields (with inevitable cataract formation); and the whole *retina* has been irradiated by gamma radiation using special curved radium needles. The most effective radiation therapy so far devised can be described as focal radiation confined closely to the tumour and a small portion of normal retina around it. This is achieved by fixing a source of gamma radiation over the tumour on the external surface of the sclera. This was originally done by suturing a suitably sized gold tube containing a ring of radon, but specially designed cobalt-60 discs have been found to be more satisfactory.

Experience gained from treating the second eye in patients with bilateral tumours has shown reasonable preservation of sight and also a high cure rate. This being so, it is now generally agreed that all cases can be treated by irradiation and preserve some sight. As with tumours in general, the size and site of these retinal tumours will influence the precise treatment method. For patients with very small tumours (below 3 mm), focal radiation, cryosurgery, or laser coagulation will be equally successful; the choice depends on the site in the eye. For tumours of diameter 3–10 mm, focal irradiation using cobalt discs is the treatment of choice, or as an alternative, a small lateral megavoltage field. For larger tumours whole-eye irradiation is needed, as it is for multiple tumours, though preservation of sight is less important in such cases than the preservation of life by destroying the tumour. Enucleation is only necessary when there is involvement of the optic nerve, and postoperative radiotherapy is only indicated if there is evidence of tumour at the edge of the cut nerve. This approach to management results in over 80% cures and in many of these patients quite reasonable sight is preserved. Retinoblastoma is a rare tumour, a childhood population of one million yielding less than one case per year. As with most childhood neoplasms there is a clear advantage for such patients to be treated in one centre.

Embryonic Rhabdomyosarcoma

The most important soft tissue sarcoma occurring in childhood is the rhabdomyosarcoma. The only other large group of soft tissue tumours are of the fibrous tissue type—more commonly benign than malignant—and other types such as liposarcoma are rare. Moreover, these others are treated mainly by surgery and certainly radiotherapy is not of much value. In rhabdomyosarcoma, radiotherapy can be a successful treatment and today, in combination with chemotherapy, it is preferred to mutilating surgery. The histological types of rhabdomyosarcoma are shown in Table 16.6. In children the commonest is the embryonic type, which may be further divided into loose, dense, and botryoid, though all are variants of the same neoplasm. The pleomorphic rhabdomyosarcoma is the usual adult variant, while the alveolar type is quite distinct.

Table 16.6. Histological types of rhabdomyosarcoma in childhood.

Embryonic	52%
Pleomorphic	10%
Botryoid	7%
Alveolar	18%
Myoblastic	13%

Clinical Presentation

The main feature of this group of tumours is the large number of potential primary sites, which means that there can be many different presenting symptoms and a wide variety of specialists may be involved in the initial diagnosis. The different sites are listed in Table 16.7.

Table 16.7. Sites of rhabdomyosarcoma.

Orbit	9
Pharynx and mouth	11
Middle ear and pre-auricular	6
Chest and scapula	5
Abdomen	9
Genitourinary	10
Pelvis	4
Paravertebral	3
Perineum or buttock	7
Limbs	4
	68

The main presenting symptom follows the development of a primary mass. In the orbit this may cause proptosis, facilitating early detection. In other sites, nasal obstruction, epistaxis, or dysphagia may occur. The mass may present at the nares, or in the cheek, and should it originate in the middle ear it may simulate an otitis media, with discharge, often bloody, pain, and very occasionally a facial palsy. A soft tissue mass in the neck may be a primary rhabdomyosarcoma or metastases in lymph nodes from a primary elsewhere in the head and neck. In the abdomen retroperitoneal tumours may attain a large size before diagnosis, whereas those around the base of the bladder produce obstructive urinary symptoms in boys and a vaginal discharge and bleeding in girls. Others in the pelvis may also cause urinary or bowel obstruction. Pain is often a feature. Paratesticular primaries present with an obvious increasing swelling, as do tumours of the perineum. Metastases occur in regional lymph nodes and also, as blood-borne deposits, in the lung, bone, bone marrow, brain, and liver.

The age distribution for rhabdomyosarcoma shows two peaks, the first between 2 and 6 years and the second between 15 and 19 years. This latter peak is due largely to paratesticular tumours.

Management

Surgery, radiotherapy, and chemotherapy are now all established as contributing to the total management of these patients.

Surgery

Where surgical extirpation is possible without mutilation or interference with function, this is the optimum treatment for the primary, followed with few exceptions by combination chemotherapy. In all patients the surgeon's assistance is needed for an adequate biopsy, and in some of the abdominal presentations an assessment of the extent of the disease is useful. We find the following clinical grouping helpful in planning.

Group I Localised disease, completely resected

Group II Localised disease with microscopic residue

- A Grossly resected tumour with microscopic residue; no evidence of regional lymph node involvement
- B Localised disease completely resected with no known microscopic residue
- C Localised disease with involved nodes grossly resected but with evidence of microscopic residue

Group III Incomplete resection or biopsy with gross residual disease

Group IV Distant metastatic disease present at onset

This grouping can be used for comparison of different series, but this may group some patients with localised disease which has only had biopsy (e.g. of the orbit) with much more extensive disease where excision has been incomplete. Most patients for whom radiotherapy is considered to be the best treatment for the primary fall into group III.

Radiotherapy

Even before chemotherapy was used, patients with small primary tumours in the head and neck, such as the orbit, the cheek, and occasionally the middle ear, were being cured by radiation therapy. Although rhabdomyosarcoma is relatively radiosensitive and will disappear quickly with moderate doses of radiation, the tumour will recur if the volume to be irradiated is such that a high dose cannot safely be given. Successful control of the primary requires (without chemotherapy) 5000 cGy in 3 weeks. This can only be achieved with

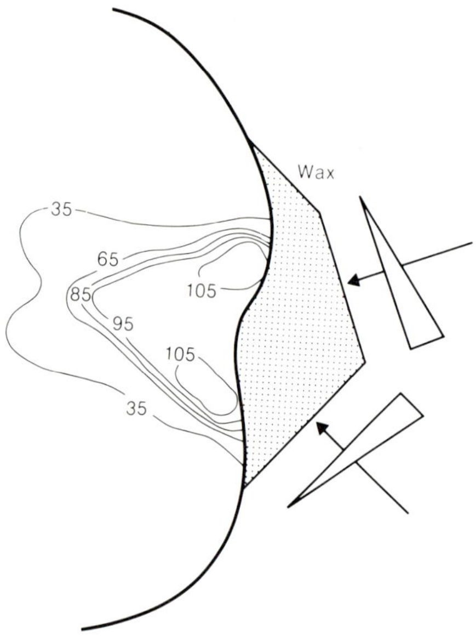

Fig. 16.12. Isodose distribution using a wedge pair of fields for treatment of an orbital rhabdomyosarcoma.

small tumours. In the head and neck this is done by using small-field beam-directed megavoltage treatment, usually a wedge pair being satisfactory. For example, the isodose distribution for an orbital treatment is shown in Fig. 16.12.

Experience with larger tumours before chemotherapy was used was universally poor in our own series. However, with appropriate adjuvant chemotherapy, successful control of the primary and of lymph node metastases seems possible with lower radiation doses. For example, lasting responses have occurred with a dose as low as 3000 cGy in 4 weeks, given for paratesticular tumours to the whole abdomen but with shielding of the kidneys (Fig. 16.13). In pelvic tumours around the base of the bladder more localised treatment has been possible and doses of 3500–4000 cGy in 3 weeks can be tolerated.

Chemotherapy

The introduction of chemotherapy into the management of these children has increased control and survival. The drugs which have been shown to have an antitumour effect, used as single agents, are actinomycin D, adriamycin, vincristine, and cyclophosphamide. Local control can be expected in more than 70% of head and neck primaries following irradiation and adjuvant combination chemotherapy. Even with some group IV patients, about 50% remain free of disease more than 5 years after diagnosis.

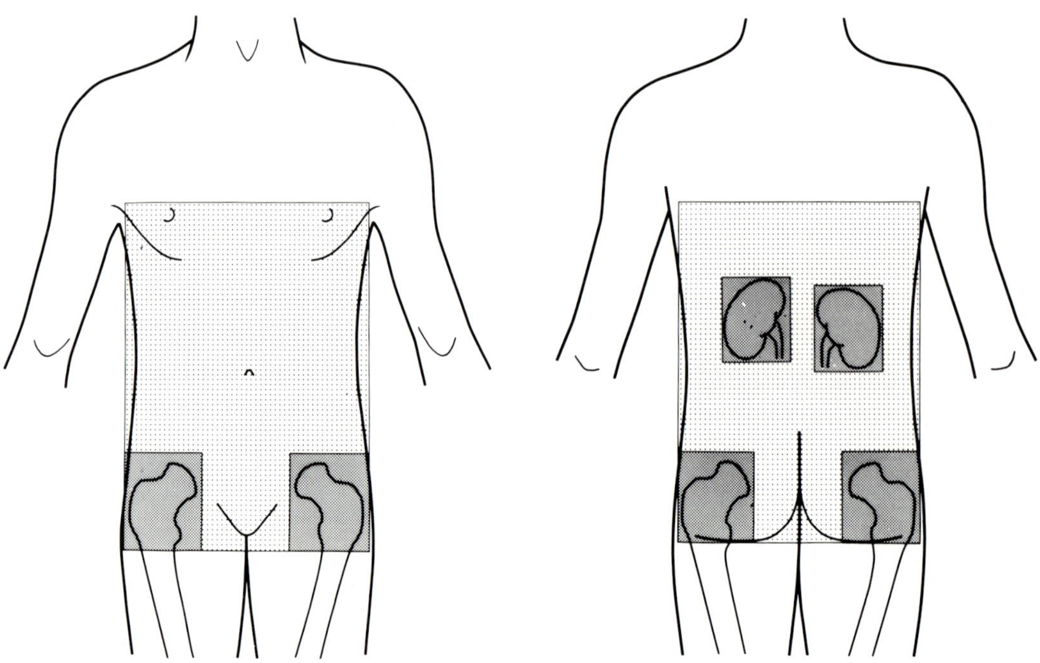

Fig. 16.13. Whole abdomen X-ray therapy for paratesticular rhabdomyosarcoma. The kidneys are shielded from posterior field throughout.

At the present time we feel it is advisable for all patients to have chemotherapy, including those with apparently localised disease at the time of diagnosis, since many of them have occult disease. For patients with very large tumours it would seem sensible to start with chemotherapy, so that if and when shrinkage occurs, a more restricted volume can be irradiated to a higher dose with a better chance of eradicating the tumour. In some cases an inoperable tumour becomes operable and second-look operations should be considered.

Nephroblastoma

This tumour, sometimes called Wilms' tumour, occurs in the kidney mainly in young children. The peak incidence is between 1 and 2 years and nearly 96% of them occur in children under 6 years of age. Very rarely they occur in adults. In the Manchester series reported by Marsden and Steward there were 38 arising in the right kidney, 41 in the left, and 3 bilateral. Sex incidence was equal. Nephroblastoma is associated with certain congenital abnormalities such as aniridia, hemihypertrophy, and urogenital malformations. As more of these patients are being cured of their nephroblastomas there are increasing reports of familial incidence occurring in siblings and different generations.

Presentation

The most common presenting feature, found in over 50% of our cases, is an abdominal swelling usually noticed by the parents. The next commonest symptom was abdominal pain (26%). Haematuria was present in only 18% of patients. Vomiting occurred in a small number of patients, as did anorexia, weight loss, and lassitude. One patient in our series presented with a scrotal swelling which was presumably the result of tumour spreading down the testicular vein. Spread usually occurs locally to lymph nodes and via the blood to the lungs, liver, and very rarely bone. Hypertension has been recorded in Wilms' tumour but is relatively uncommon.

Examination

Clinical examination will usually reveal an abdominal mass, the presence of which demands further investigation. Intravenous pyelography should be done immediately, and also radiographs of the chest. The intravenous pyelograms may show the obvious soft-tissue mass of the tumour and varying degrees of distortion of the calyceal system from minor distortion to complete lack of function on the affected side. In bilateral cases both kidneys may be abnormal.

Catecholamine excretion should be checked to exclude neuroblastoma. A full blood count including platelets should be performed and the blood pressure should be recorded. It has been our practice to include a liver scan in our investigation programme, but our assessment of its value suggests that it is not very helpful in picking up liver metastases. This may, however, be dependent on the quality of the scan that can be obtained. The value of more sophisticated X-ray techniques such as the CT scan is still being evaluated.

Staging

In children clinical staging, particularly of abdominal tumours, is difficult. We accept, therefore, a surgical system of staging, combined with pathological staging when this is available. The staging used for Wilms' tumour over many years has been as follows:

Stage I Tumour confined to the kidney and completely resected.

Stage II Tumour extending beyond the capsule of the kidney, either by local infiltration, extension along the renal vein or involvement of the para-aortic nodes, but complete macroscopic removal achieved.

Stage III Tumour extending beyond the capsule of the kidney and not completely resected or the operative field contaminated with tumour spilled at operation.

Stage IV Haematogenous deposits in liver, lung, bone, brain, or other sites.

Stage V Bilateral renal involvement either initially or subsequently. More recently this has been modified so that if lymph nodes are shown to be involved, whether removed or not, these patients now fall into stage III.

Pathology

Macroscopically the nephroblastoma has a white fleshy appearance on its cut surface. There may be haemorrhages into it. Microscopically the most notable feature is the presence of tubule formation, but this is mingled with striated muscle, and glomerular structures. The tubular differentiation appears to be related to prognosis. There is a very small group of patients whose tumours display very undifferentiated structure. Pathologists now feel that they can identify this small group, which appears also to have a much worse prognosis than the rest. This difference is now being taken into account in planning treatment.

Treatment

Once a likely diagnosis of nephroblastoma has been made, treatment should begin promptly. For patients with stage I to III disease, surgery should be undertaken as soon as possible.

Surgery

Provided that the primary is operable (inoperable patients are unusual these days) a nephrectomy should be performed through an anterior abdominal transperitoneal approach. Early ligation of the renal vessels should be done. Obviously involved lymph nodes are removed, but a complete node resection is not attempted.

Chemotherapy

There is no doubt that chemotherapy has considerably increased the cure rates in nephroblastoma. The drugs of greatest value are actinomycin D, vincristine, adriamycin, and cyclophosphamide. It is our practice to start chemotherapy on the day of the operation—this is usually the first dose of vincristine. Subsequent chemotherapy is now dependent on the stage and histological type of the tumour. For stage I patients with a favourable histology, vincristine alone is used for maintenance. For stage II patients with favourable histology, maintenance will be continued with vincristine and actinomycin D, while for stage III patients with favourable histology adriamycin is added to the other two drugs. For patients with unfavourable histology and in stage IV patients of any histological type, the prognosis is poorer and more intensive chemotherapy is used, combining all four of the drugs mentioned. The duration of the chemotherapy can in most instances be quite short. If the prognosis is good, a 6 months' course will suffice, but for poorer-risk patients treatment should continue for a year from the time of diagnosis.

Radiotherapy

Before chemotherapy became available it was generally agreed that all patients should have abdominal radiation, and this practice certainly improved the results seen from surgery alone. Radiation therapy for disease metastatic in the chest resulted in only about 14% of cures, but this was increased to 50% by adjuvant chemotherapy. Since we have been able to assess the extent of the disease more accurately, it has become apparent that when adjuvant chemotherapy is used, patients with stage I disease of favourable histology can be left without postoperative radiation. Patients with more extensive stage II disease, whilst theoretically free of disease after surgery, are more likely to have small deposits left behind than are the stage I patients, and in our opinion on present evidence postoperative radiation is needed. With stage III patients known disease is present and radiation is certainly required. Our present technique for stage II and stage III patients aims to encompass all known disease by a field which extends from the dome of the diaphragm to the sacral promontory on the affected side and across the midline to the hilum of the contralateral kidney. Using a parallel opposed pair of megavoltage fields we normally give a midplane dose of 3000 cGy in 4 weeks, in 20 exposures, treating 5 days each week. When residual disease is considered to be more widespread the whole abdomen is treated, from the dome of the diaphragm down to the pelvic floor, using parallel opposed fields. The normal kidney is shielded from the posterior field throughout treatment. Femoral heads are also shielded (Fig. 16.14). The same dose of 3000 cGy in 4 weeks is

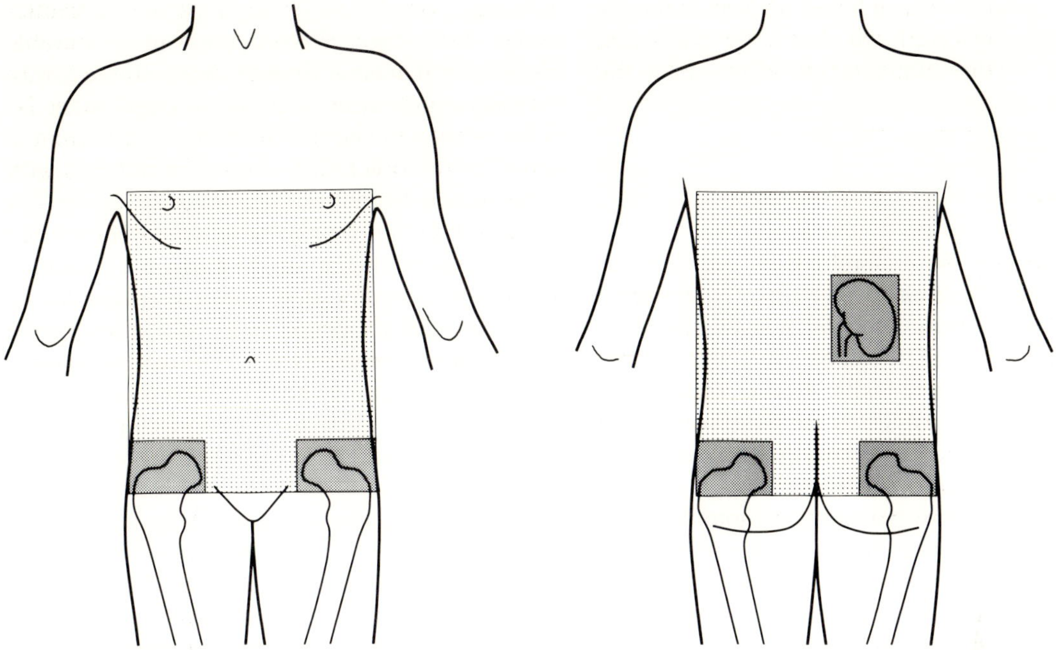

Fig. 16.14. Whole abdomen X-ray therapy for a nephroblastoma.

well tolerated. Recently, it has been suggested that lower doses could be used. Jenkins in Toronto has never used such high doses, and his results are as good as those elsewhere. It is now suggested that a dose of 2000 cGy in 2 weeks is all that is necessary. This is equivalent to 2500 cGy in 4 weeks—similar to Jenkins' dose. In stage IV patients, in addition to the radiation described above to the abdomen, radiation to the lungs is given. With the chemotherapy used in these patients doses to the whole lungs should not exceed 1200 cGy in 2 weeks. Usually the two courses can be given one after the other. If there is any doubt about whether it is safe to wait to do one region we have occasionally used a whole trunk technique, the whole being subtended by a pair of parallel megavoltage fields. A midline dose of 2000 cGy in 5–6 weeks can be achieved and is tolerated with chemotherapy, though not if adriamycin is included, because of cardiac toxicity.

Prognosis

The outlook for children with nephroblastoma is now very good indeed. With favourable histology almost 100% of stage I patients can be cured; for patients in stages II and III, 75%–80% is likely; and even for stage IV patients survival as good as 50% can be achieved. Unfavourable histology carries a much worse prognosis. The aim for the future must be to maintain the good survival rates already achieved while restricting treatment to a minimum. There is, however, still a need to find more effective treatment for those with unfavourable histology.

Bone Tumours

Osteosarcoma and Ewing's tumour occur with about equal frequency in children, the former more commonly at about the age of puberty. Younger patients are seen with Ewing's tumours. These two types of tumour have a similar presentation and clinical course in children and young adults, and the management of both should be the same. This has been described fully in Chap. 15.

Gonadal Tumours

Apart from the teratomas that arise in the gonads, gonadal tumours represent only about 1% of the total tumours seen in the Manchester Children's Tumour Registry series. Even when teratomas are included they account for no more than 3% of the total. The main groups to be discussed here are the yolk sac tumours, which occur both in the ovary and the testis, and also some of the same histological types occurring at other sites, but which are best considered as one tumour entity, and the dysgerminoma and seminoma.

Yolk Sac Tumours

These tumours have had a variety of other histological descriptions but are now recognised as one tumour type. They may arise in the testis, ovary, sacrococcygeal region, vagina, thorax, and brain, but the two largest groups are those in the testis and ovary. Previously these germ cell tumours had been thought to be epithelial in origin and both the testicular and ovarian ones had been labelled as adenocarcinoma. Later the term orchioblastoma was applied to the testicular primaries, until it was realised that they were all morphologically the same. More recently, alpha foetoprotein has been detected in increased amounts in the serum of these patients and also in the cells of the tumour. It is suggested that the protein is synthesised by the tumour cells.

The presentation of these tumours in different anatomical sites varies considerably. The testicular tumours present in boys, either as infants or very young children, as a painless swelling in the scrotum noticed by the parents. Lymph node metastases can occur, as may blood-borne secondaries to lungs. The tumour in boys is more likely to be diagnosed before spread has occurred. The ovarian yolk sac tumour occurs in older girls and young adults, the mean age being about 16 years. The history is usually short and more than a third of the patients present with an abdominal mass as a first sign. Abdominal pain is present in about a quarter. General abdominal symptoms such as anorexia, nausea, and vomiting may occur. Tumours arising in extragonadal sites produce a variety of localising signs. The big subgroup, the sacrococcygeal tumours, produce symptoms from the local tumour mass, which may be palpable externally, and may also interfere with urinary and bowel function. The age of these patients is usually similar to the testicular pattern—infants and young children. Metastases, when they occur, may involve lymph nodes, liver, lungs, and in very late cases the brain. These differences in presentation demand differences in the clinical management of the various groups of patients.

In boys, where early diagnosis of a testicular tumour is common, orchidectomy alone is probably all that is needed. If the tumour marker alpha foetoprotein returns to normal levels after orchidectomy, then no further treatment is required apart from close follow-up monitored by alpha foetoprotein estimations.

In most other patients it is common for the disease to be much more extensive before a diagnosis is made. Total surgical extirpation is therefore impossible and in all such cases further treatment is required. It has been our experience that when dealing with substantial disease, even though immediate radiosensitivity is apparent, the disease recurs very quickly after the radiotherapy is completed. Chemotherapy does seem to have some promise, although it probably needs to be very aggressive. Apparent cures have been achieved, however, using vincristine, cyclophosphamide, actinomycin D, and adriamycin and possibly bleomycin and vinblastine. The efficacy of cis-platinum—good for other teratomatous testicular tumours—is as yet impossible to judge, since too few patients with these yolk sac tumours have been available for assessment. For patients with residual ovarian, sacrococcygeal, or testicular yolk sac tumours, our present policy is to treat with an intensive regime of vincristine, cyclophosphamide, and actinomycin D, monitoring progress with the serum alpha foetoprotein. If the alpha foetoprotein falls to normal levels and remains so, chemotherapy alone is continued for 2 years. If the alpha foetoprotein level does not become normal, further surgical intervention is considered or local irradiation may be added to try to eradicate the remaining disease.

Dysgerminoma of the Ovary and Seminoma of the Testis

Both of these histologically similar tumours are rare in childhood, but the ovarian is seen more commonly in this age group than the testicular. In the Manchester series there are 12 dysgerminomas and no seminomas. The Testicular Tumour Panel for Britain found only four seminomas in children under 15 years. Dysgerminoma may also occur at any age from childhood to old age, but a greater percentage (60% in our experience) occur before the age of 20. The seminoma presents as a painless unilateral testicular swelling, while the dysgerminoma presents either as an abdominal mass or pain or both. Both may metastasise to lymph nodes and lungs. Management of seminoma testis has been described in Chap. 13 and boys under 15 should be managed in exactly the same way. Dysgerminoma is described here since the majority occur in young patients. From our experience it would appear that the correct first approach for young patients is surgical exploration and if possible a total removal of the tumour. If the tumour is confined to one ovary, postoperative radiation is not immediately needed, but a careful follow-up should be undertaken so that treatment can be initiated at the first sign of abdominal recurrence. When the disease is more extensive, or when recurrence occurs, then abdominal radiation should be given, as indeed it should to all patients over 20 years of age. The whole abdomen should be treated, the kidneys being shielded after 2000 cGy. The total dose to be delivered should be 3000 cGy in 4 weeks. This approach has resulted in 100% survival of patients with dysgerminoma under the age of 20. Over 20 this falls to about 60%, suggesting that these tumours are more aggressive in the older patient.

Care of Children During and Immediately Following Radiation Treatment

Management During Treatment

All radiation treatment needs to be applied accurately and carefully and these principles are no different in children and adults. This is obviously easier to achieve when the patient is able to cooperate and remain in the right position throughout the treatment exposure. To achieve this in children is sometimes quite difficult, especially with the very young child.

Preparation and prescribing of X-ray therapy in children may be either with mould room help (as for small-field beam-direction or whole-CNS treatments) or by the use of skin markers (as for larger field treatments using parallel opposed fields). In the mould room, making a shell for a child requires a great deal of care and patience on the part of the technician, and certainly more time needs to be set aside than in doing the same thing for an adult. Older children do not usually present any problems, but they do like an explanation of what is to happen to them. Younger children will often cooperate better if the procedure is made into a game. On occasions we have found it a great help to make a mould for a favourite toy. When preparation involves skin marks and possibly verification radiographs, the radiotherapist and radiographer also need to exercise patience and care. It is very frightening for a child to be suddenly laid on a bed and have marks applied to his body. To him any thin object could be a needle and may hurt, so that it is a good idea to draw something on, say, the back of the hand where he can see it and realise that all that is to happen is that lines will be drawn on his skin. Again, it is obviously easier with older children, but even children of three will respond to suitable explanation. It must be stressed yet again that adequate time must be devoted to this important aspect of patient care.

Having completed the prescription for the treatment, and this is often the easy part, then the actual treatment has to be carried out and the radiographer has to be sure that the child stays quite still for each exposure. In most children aged 4 years and over this is usually possible without any difficulty, especially as the child quickly learns that there is no pain with this particular form of treatment. Nearly all the children with leukaemia, who have experienced so many injections and have become very used to hospital, present no problem even when they are quite young. However, very young children are difficult to treat and may have to be restrained from moving during each treatment session. For the babies this is best achieved by using a cross-shaped padded board. The child's arms are applied to the transverse arms of the cross and the legs on the vertical part (Fig. 16.15). Soft crepe bandages are used so that no damage can occur. In slightly older children, between 1 and 3 years of age, sandbags will help to keep them fixed on the bed, and will also prevent them from rolling off. Crepe bandages are used to tie them to the bed when this is necessary. We have found that the children are often easier to handle in the therapy department if they are all brought from the children's ward at the same time. Children feel safer with other children. It is also helpful if they can help the radiographer to put some of the other children in position for treatment, and press a few buttons such as those for raising and lowering the

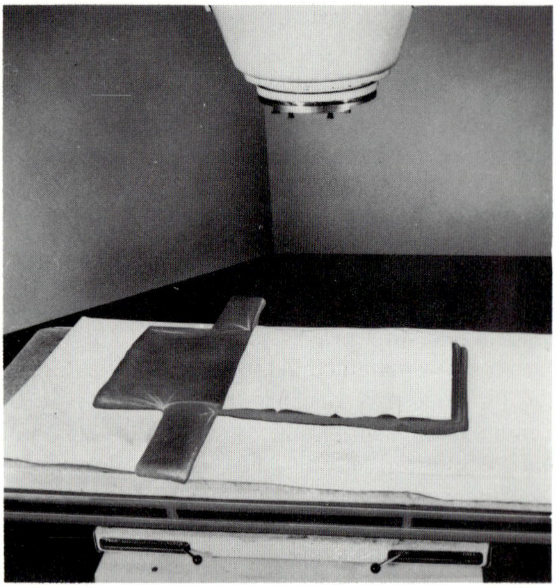

Fig. 16.15. Padded cross for keeping small children still during radiation therapy.

bed. There will, however, be occasions when this technique does not succeed, and sedation or even anaesthesia will have to be used. For sedation we have found the drug Vallergan to be the most effective, in a dose of 4 mg/kg body weight, given 30–60 min before treatment. Most children will become drowsy and once in position for treatment will fall asleep. An alternative drug is Phenergan in hypnotic doses. In infants it is also useful to plan the treatment time each day just after a feed, when the child is likely to be drowsy anyway. Quite often, after a few days' sedation during which the child becomes used to the department and the radiographers, the sedation can be discontinued. Anaesthesia may be necessary for a very fractious child; usually a simple inhalation of gas and oxygen is all that is necessary. It is important that drugs such as halothane should not be used, since daily anaesthetics have to be given. Fortunately, anaesthesia can be of very short duration and children can be up and about again very quickly afterwards. If anaesthesia has to be used, the radiation treatment should be planned early in the day so that the child does not have to be subjected to long periods of starvation, and will be able to eat normally later in the day. If sedation or anaesthesia proves to be prolonged for any reason, there may well be interference with the child's normal daily life, particularly missing feeds. Special attention may have to be given therefore to providing extra food and meals at times outside the normal for hospitals.

Acute Radiation Effects

These are essentially the same as in adults, but the effect in children may be more dangerous than in the adult.

Marrow Depression

Large-field therapy, e.g. whole-abdomen, mantle, or whole-CNS, will irradiate quite a large volume of the child and a fairly high percentage of the bone marrow, with resulting marrow depression. Twice weekly full blood counts, including total white cell count, differential, and platelet counts should be done. Should the total white cell count fall to 2500 or the platelet count to 100 000, then daily counts should be instituted so that treatment modifications can take place quickly. Treatment will need to be interrupted or modified if the white cell count falls below 2000 or the platelets below 75 000. There may be more danger if there is a rapid fall in the count than if this takes place over a period. In most uncomplicated treatments when only irradiation is being used the count is often lowest at about 3 weeks into treatment and often recovers even when treatment is continuing after this period. There may, however, be an increased effect on the marrow if cytotoxic drugs are given near to or with radiation therapy.

Skin Reactions

These are rarely a problem, except in certain small-field head and neck treatments, where the skin is deliberately irradiated to full tumour dosage. With megavoltage (the accepted radiation energy used), skin reactions, particularly for large-field treatments, rarely approach even dry desquamation, unless certain cytotoxic drugs are also being used. The enhancement and recall of skin reactions are well documented when actinomycin D is used in conjunction with radiation. The treatment of these reactions is the same as that advised for adults.

When the scalp has to be included in the radiation field, complete but temporary epilation occurs. In many instances these days this has often already occurred as a result of cytotoxic drugs used. It does not appear that the double onslaught of drugs and radiation will produce permanent hair loss and in our experience the hair has always grown again.

Mucosal Reactions

The reactions are the same as those experienced in adults, showing no difference in appearance following similar dosage. However, there may be considerable differences in the problems they create. Head and neck treatments which lead to reactions in the mouth, pharynx, and larynx may interfere with nutrition and hydration, and children need careful watching because they are more liable to become quickly dehydrated than is the case with adults. It must also be remembered that the larynx in children is considerably *narrower* and the same reaction may produce enough swelling for stridor to develop. This may be severe enough for a temporary tracheostomy to become necessary.

Another aspect of acute mucosal reaction is that in the gastrointestinal tract associated with abdominal radiation. Early in treatment post-radiation nausea or even vomiting may occur. As in adults, the degree is very variable, with some children apparently unaffected and others very sick indeed. As treatment progresses over the third and subsequent weeks a bowel reaction may develop with diarrhoea, the main effect being on the small bowel. Rectal reactions only occur when localised pelvic treatments are used at high dosage levels.

Most of these effects settle quite quickly, but again with children the risks of dehydration from vomiting and diarrhoea are greater than in adults. These effects certainly affect appetite and children having abdominal and large-field treatments lose weight throughout the treatment period. Nutrition may be maintained by the addition of high-calorie supplements to drinks as well as encouragement for the child to eat and drink as much as possible. There is some evidence that the bowel reactions and their effects may be less if the children are on a gluten-free diet during the therapy.

Whole Organ Effects

At the dose levels used in treating children with cancer it was uncommon to see any acute radiation effects on whole organs, such as the kidney, liver, lungs, or brain. However, with the addition of chemotherapy, particularly actinomycin D and vincristine, acute toxic effects have been seen in the above-mentioned organs towards the end or up to 9 weeks following the completion of the radiation. *Kidney* effects may be seen if the whole kidney is irradiated using megavoltage to a dose of 2500 cGy in 4–5 weeks. However, acute renal damage has been seen at doses of 2000 cGy and 1500 cGy when accompanied by actinomycin D. This damage is characterised by an attack of acute nephritis, which may progress to chronic nephritis. The *liver* was considered to be fairly resistant to radiation, and without chemotherapy, doses in excess of 3000 cGy in 4 weeks produced no acute effects. With this dose and para-operative actinomycin D or vincristine for nephroblastoma, when the whole liver is irradiated acute liver damage can occur. This is characterised by any or all of the following features: reduction in platelet count, changes in a liver scan showing interference with liver activity, abnormal liver function tests, enlargement of the liver, and ascites. Mild cases show only the first two, but more severe cases progress to have all five features. Rarely, death can occur. This liver damage usually settles quite quickly, but recurrence can occur if maintenance chemotherapy, particularly with actinomycin D, is used.

The sensitivity of the *lungs* is such that when the whole chest is irradiated to a dose of 2500 cGy in 4 weeks this is well tolerated. When chemotherapy with either actinomycin D or vincristine is given as well, we have found acute radiation pneumonitis occurring at the much lower dose of 2000 cGy in 5 weeks. This is characterised by acute respiratory distress, and chest X-ray shows the typical appearance of pneumonitis. This settles quite quickly with steroids and antibiotics, but again recrudescence may arise with further courses of drugs. When combined with chemotherapy, radiation to both lungs should not exceed 1500 cGy in 4 weeks if pneumonitis is to be avoided.

Brain radiation, when treating brain tumours to quite high doses (as much as 4000 cGy in 3 weeks), did not apparently have an immediate discernible effect on the brain. However, in the leukaemic children, who have a good deal of chemotherapy before their cranial prophylaxis, we find many who develop, about 6 weeks after their radiation, the "somnolence syndrome". This is characterised by a short period of extreme drowsiness, which usually recovers spontaneously.

Complications

Infections are the most serious complication in children receiving cancer therapy. The immune response of the child may be affected both by the disease (e.g. Hodgkin's) and by the treatment, both radiotherapy and chemotherapy being immune depressants. In addition, there are many local factors which may permit entry of infecting organisms. Particularly important is the development of granulocytopenia, which increases the risks of bacterial infection. Infecting organisms, however, may be bacterial, viral, mycotic, or protozoal.

Bacteria

Bacterial infections are the most frequent complication, and it is therefore important that the development of any pyrexia in a child on cancer treatment should be immediately investigated and treated. When children with low granulocyte counts, even if a focus of infection cannot be found, have a fever greater than 38.5 °C, they should be treated as though they have bacterial sepsis and treated with appropriate antibiotics.

Viruses

Viral infections of the common varieties are usually tolerated quite well, but certain viruses can have more serious effects. These are the herpes-zoster group, herpes simplex, and the cytomegalovirus. Measles may also have serious sequelae, and fatalities have occurred after inoculation with live-virus vaccines such as those for poliomyelitis, vaccinia, and measles. Many of these may be avoided by isolating the patient from possible sources of infection and by postponing vaccination in the patient until the immune depression is less of a problem. If children are exposed to chickenpox or measles then modification may be achieved by giving zoster-immune globulin in the former and measles-immune serum globulin in the latter, within 3 days of exposure. Other viral infections are less common, but the zoster infection is more commonly seen when the cancer is in remission and is commonest in patients with Hodgkin's disease. Cytomegalovirus needs to be remembered particularly in leukaemic children presenting during treatment with a fever, a rash, and a pneumonia-like illness.

Mycosis

Mycotic infections, particularly thrush of varying severity, are now a very common finding in any large population with childhood cancer, especially during intensive periods of treatment, both by radiation and chemotherapy. Local infection in the mouth can be treated by nystatin, amphotericin B, or 1% gentian violet. If systemic candidiasis or gastrointestinal lesions should develop, systemic amphotericin B is the drug of choice.

Protozoa

Protozoal infections include toxoplasmosis and *Pneumocystis carinii*. The latter causes pneumonitis and is frequently fatal in debilitated patients or where there is an immune deficiency. The illness is characterised by cough, fever, cyanosis, tachypnoea, and nasal flaring. Radiographs show diffuse bilateral infiltration typical of alveolar disease. Acute respiratory failure can occur quite quickly, and assisted mechanical ventilation may be necessary.

Treatment is with pentamidine or Septrin, the latter being preferable. It has not been possible to cover all the infectious complications in the space available, but enough have been mentioned to draw attention to this serious problem which can so often be fatal, especially if not recognised and treated at an early stage. It is also important to realise that with increasing intensity of treatment these complications are becoming more common.

Late Effects of Treatment

Children with cancer have been successfully treated since the early 1940s. For two decades the treatment methods used were surgery and radiotherapy. In that 15–20 year period the children with solid tumours who were cured have now reached adulthood and the sequelae of the treatment they received as children have been documentated. In the succeeding 20-year period more and more chemotherapy has been used and we are now able to detect the sequelae of this and also of combining radiation and chemotherapy.

Radiotherapy

The main difference in irradiating children and adults is that children present more actively growing tissues. As development proceeds the defects noted are as follows:

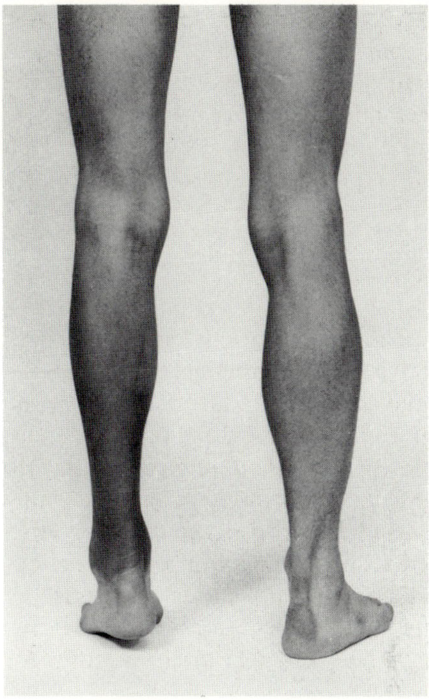

Fig. 16.16. Shortening and thinning of lower leg after radiation.

Skeletal

Irradiation of growing bone reduces the growth rate and results in early fusion of the epiphyses. This effect is best seen in the long bones of the limbs, which results in shortening of the irradiated bone and also of the whole limb (Fig. 16.16). Spinal irradiation, if symmetrical, causes shortening of the spine. For example, children who survive whole-CNS radiation have a total shortness, so that their sitting height is out of proportion to their total height. Following abdominal or chest irradiation, the spine within the field is shortened. After abdominal radiation the lower ribs and pelvis are closer together (Fig. 16.17). If, in the sagittal plane, half the spine is irradiated, then scoliosis occurs, but this should if possible be avoided by deliberately including the full width of the spine in the field even when only part of it requires to be included. Facial deformity and asymmetry can occur when the face is irradiated (Fig. 16.18). If all or part of the upper femoral epiphyses are irradiated, some years later slipping of an epiphysis may occur, characterised by sudden pain in the affected hip. X-ray appearances (Fig. 16.19) are characteristic of a slipped epiphysis. These should be treated immediately by a pinning operation, after which the prognosis

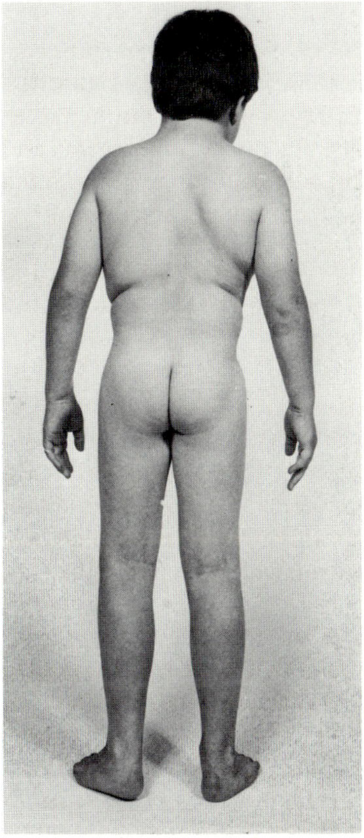

Fig. 16.17. Spinal shortening after abdominal radiation.

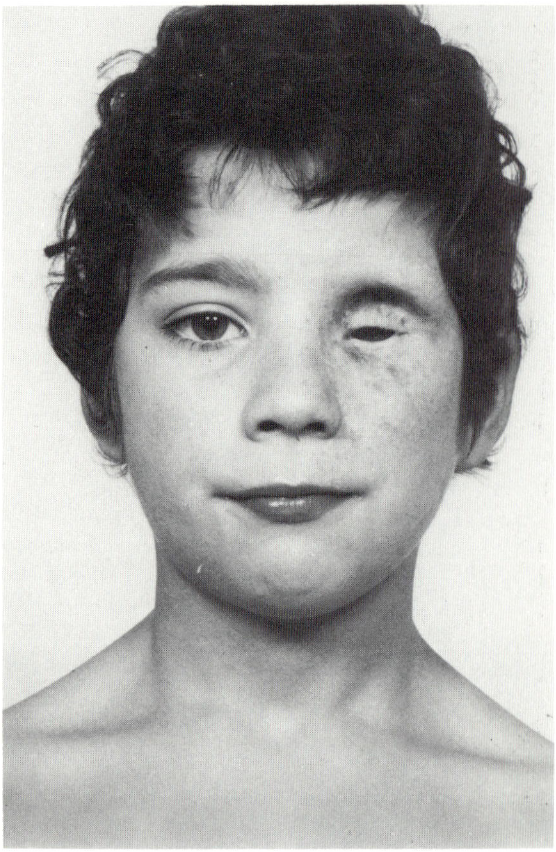

Fig. 16.18. Facial asymmetry and deformity of orbit after radiation.

seems to be good in terms of full function. We have also noted the development of benign osteomas (Fig. 16.20) which, if they remain quiescent, can be left alone. If there is any increase in size, however, it is better that they be excised. Many of these skeletal abnormalities have been found quite by chance and it seems reasonable to X-ray irradiated bones from time to time.

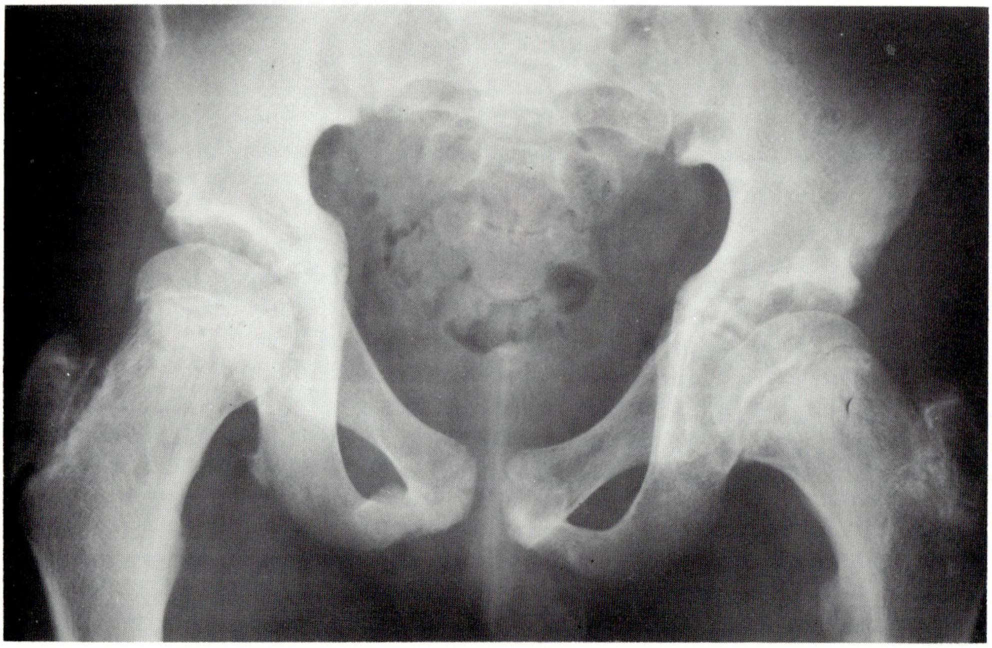

Fig. 16.19. Slipped (R) femoral epiphysis.

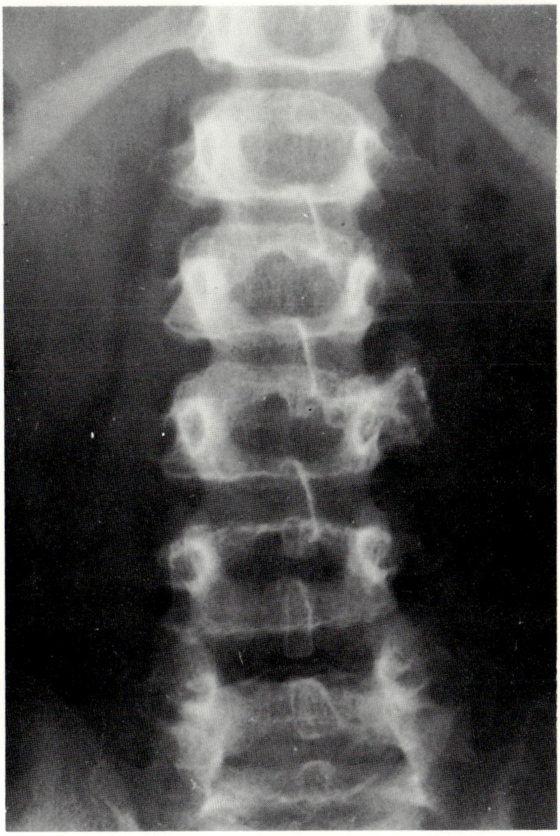

Fig. 16.20. Osteoma of a vertebra, post-radiation.

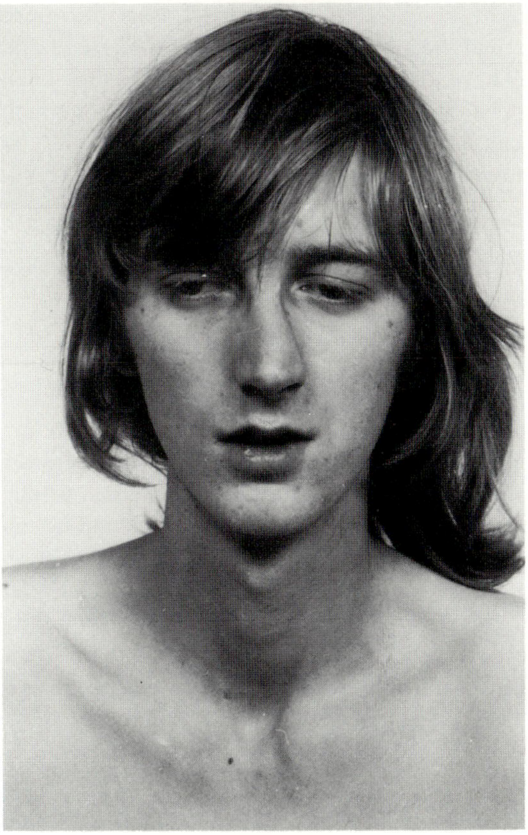

Fig. 16.21. Thinning of neck after whole neck irradiation.

Soft Tissue Effects

These changes are not confined to children but, in association with skeletal effects, they may be more obvious and more of a problem. The most obvious changes, following the use of kilovoltage radiation, are the skin changes associated with high dosage. These consist of varying degrees of skin atrophy and telangiectasis, and in hair-bearing areas some degree of hair thinning. These sequelae are now rarely seen, since megavoltage radiation has been used, unless there were clinical reasons which required the tumour dose to include the related skin. More commonly now there is thinning of the subcutaneous tissues, especially fat. The effect of this following head and neck treatment for lymphomas is shown in Fig. 16.21. It is also observed in patients treated by abdominal radiation, or to one limb (Fig. 16.22). When the eye has to be included in the radiation field a cataract will develop within 2–3 years. As time

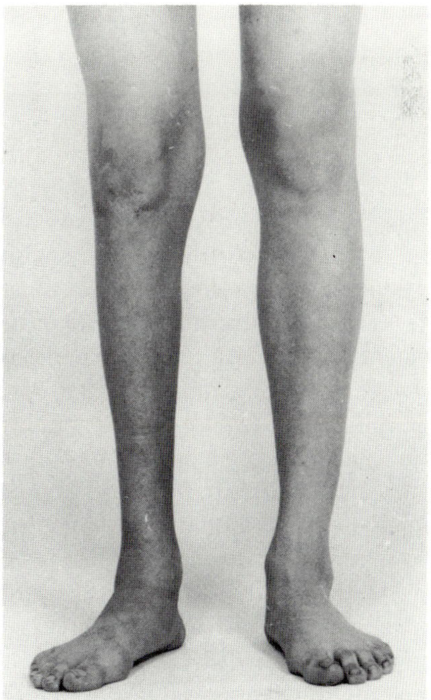

Fig. 16.22. Thinning of lower limb.

goes by, however, following high dosage the entire eye may become useless and uncomfortable and may have to be removed. If the dose has only been high enough for cataract formation but not enough to cause other damage, the cataract can often be removed when it is fully developed (see Fig. 16.18).

Endocrine Organ Effects

Pituitary

When the long-term survivors from brain tumours were assessed, we found that many were shorter than average, and that this was not totally explained by spinal irradiation. This led to an investigation of their growth hormone function and the evidence we have collected from that group and from children treated subsequently shows that a dose over 2900 cGy to the pituitary hypothalamic axis in 4 weeks is likely to produce growth hormone deficiency.

Gonads

The children treated in the early years for Wilms' tumour and neuroblastoma had irradiation to the whole abdomen, so that all the girls' ovaries received the total dose of radiation given. Some of the boys with testicular tumours had the other testis also fully irradiated, while in others the testis was outside the treatment field but received scattered radiation. The gonadal function of both the girls and boys has been assessed as regards hormone defects, and, when old enough, the boys have also been assessed for sterility. In girls with the ovaries receiving the full radiation dose, most have complete ovarian failure and require hormone replacement for pubertal development to take place. However, in a small number of patients treated early in childhood, development at puberty has occurred, including menstruation. One patient has been pregnant twice, but for other reasons (bicornuate uterus) did not go to term.

In boys who received full tumour dose to the testis complete testicular failure occurred, and again hormone replacement is needed for pubertal development. When only scattered radiation has been received by the testis, pubertal development is normal, but most of these boys are sterile, as shown by zero or low sperm counts.

Thyroid

Thyroid function has been investigated in all those children surviving for long periods after radiation therapy for early Hodgkin's and non-Hodgkin's lymphoma, neuroblastoma in the neck, and postnasal carcinoma or lympho-epithelioma. In all of these children the thyroid gland was within the radiation field. Many patients investigated have shown a compensated thyroid dysfunction with raised thyroid stimulating hormone, but usually normal T3 and T4. It is important to repeat these tests regularly at yearly intervals because thyroid deficiency may occur. This occurred in one boy 15 years after his radiation. The biochemical deficiency may pre-date clinical hypothyroidism, but thyroid replacement is better started at an early stage. Three of our children developed a single thyroid nodule, the growth of which necessitated its removal. All three were benign, and we have only seen one case of thyroid carcinoma developing in this group. All required thyroid hormone replacement after surgery, and to date all remain well.

Second Primary Neoplasms

Whatever the complex mechanism may be, there is no doubt that ionising radiations are potentially carcinogenic. Children and young adults who have had radiation therapy and have been cured of their primary neoplasm, have a naturally longer life span than patients similarly treated in later life. These children might well be expected therefore to show a higher incidence of radiation-induced second primaries than do adults. The second primary neoplasms that we have encountered are listed in Table 16.8. When these are investigated, however, we find that not all these patients have second primaries directly related to their previous radiation, and indeed some have not had any radiation. It is obvious that some are part of a particular diathesis, such as the patient with the basal-naevoid or Gorlin's syndrome, who presented with his brain tumour—a medulloblastoma — and later developed the other features of this syndrome, namely jaw cysts and basal cell carcinoma. It is interesting that these were present all over his body, but thicker on the irradiated skin, especially at the edges of the spinal field (Fig. 16.23). His family history was positive, his father

Table 16.8. Second primary neoplasms.

Neoplasm I	Neoplasm II	Time interval (years)
Posterior fossa astrocytoma	Sarcoma in loin	10
Medulloblastoma	Basal cell naevi	7
Hodgkin's disease	Lieomyosarcoma	9
Fibrosarcoma	Osteogenic sarcoma	10
Retinoblastoma	Osteogenic sarcoma	12
Teratoma	Carcinoma of breast	14
Nephroblastoma	Acute myeloid leukaemia	13
Medulloblastoma	Osteogenic sarcoma	5
Medulloblastoma	Carcinoma of colon	11
Medulloblastoma	Neurofibrosarcoma	25

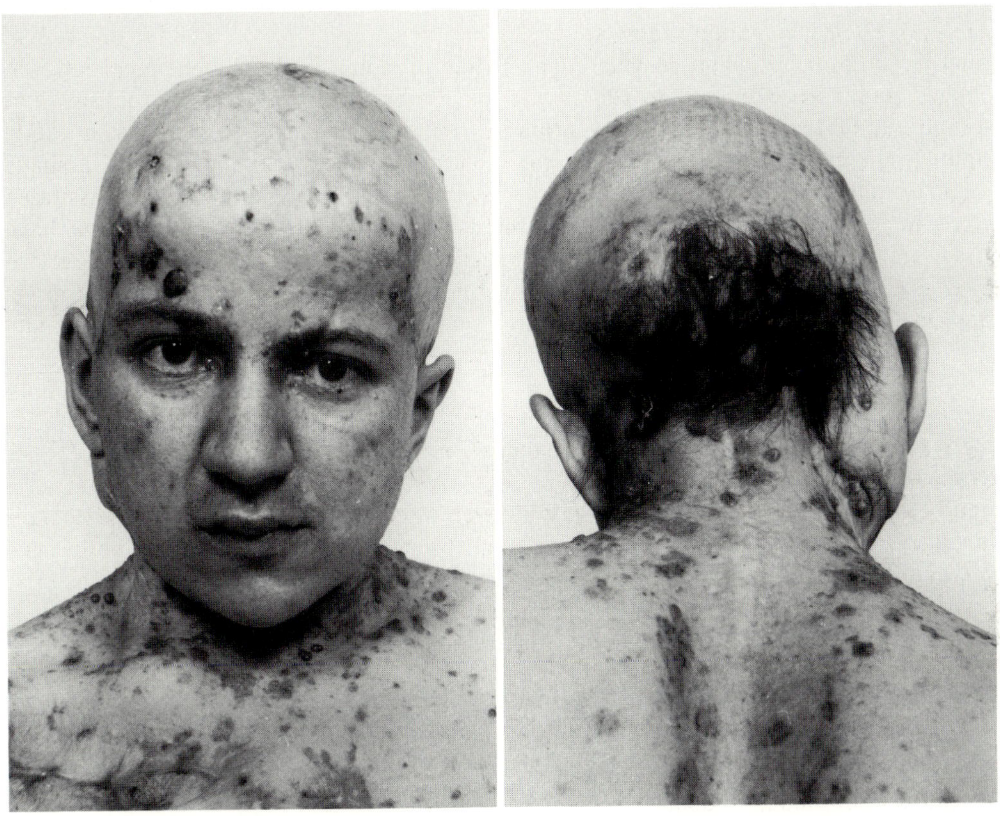

Fig. 16.23. Basal cell carcinomas in a patient with basal naevoid syndrome after irradiation for a medulloblastoma.

having had a single basal cell carcinoma and later dying of a brain tumour.

In other groups of children there is an increased risk of a second primary without radiation as a causal factor. For example, retinoblastoma has an association with the subsequent development of osteosarcomas, both in irradiated and non-irradiated bones. It therefore seems likely that these children have some defect which makes them more likely to produce second cancers and that in some instances the radiation may only dictate the site at which these will occur.

Neurological Deficit

Many of the children with brain tumours may have a variety of neurological problems. In some instances these are obviously the residual defects which arose because of the effects on brain and nerve tissue of the primary tumour or of increased intracranial pressure. An example of this is the persisting blindness as a result of papilloedema and subsequent optic atrophy after very high and prolonged intracranial pressure. Other defects after brain tumours are often more difficult to quantify, but there are some children, particularly those treated in early childhood, who are mentally retarded. It is not possible to know how much is attributable to the tumour, increased pressure, surgery, or radiotherapy. However, it is important to recognise its existence so that the children may be provided with the educational facilities appropriate to their individual needs.

In addition to obvious physical neurological deficits there may be considerable psychological problems as the children grow and develop. Since many of them are physically different from their peers, they may, unless they are handled sympathetically with a good deal of explanation, develop additional psychological problems. Sometimes such problems may also be created by the over-protective attitude of the family and acquaintances. Whatever their nature and cause, all these factors can certainly interfere with the full development of the child, and with its ability to integrate into the normal adult world.

Chemotherapy

Since the children who have received large amounts of cytotoxic drugs have been more recently treated, less is known about the late effects of chemotherapy. However, evidence is now accumulating that there are going to be effects on the gonads. Sterility in boys successfully treated with combination chemotherapy for Hodgkin's disease and leukaemia is, on present evidence, likely to occur in most patients. However, Leydig cell activity, as with low-dose radiation, seems to be less affected, so that pubertal development does take place. It had been thought that some of these changes might be reversible, but this does not appear to be the case at present.

The development of second malignancies is also beginning to be documented, but these tend to be of the reticulo-endothelial type and they occur in all immune-depressed patients, not only those with malignant disease.

Combination Radiotherapy and Chemotherapy

In view of the immediate enhancement of radiation by certain of the cytotoxic agents it might be expected that there will be greater late effects. At present, there is only limited evidence of this, though some effects do seem to be more likely with combined treatment.

Most of the late changes in combined treatment are those seen from the cranial prophylaxis of the patients with acute lymphoblastic leukaemia. Several late effects have been described. These are:

1) Children who have had CNS prophylaxis which includes cranial radiation, develop a specific learning defect. This has particularly to do with immediate memory and thus poses less of a problem with older children, although all have some learning difficulties.
2) Intracranial calcification has been noted in children who have received both cranial radiation and higher doses of systemic methotrexate. It has also occurred with higher doses of methotrexate without cranial irradiation, but so far only in the leukaemic children. This may be related to other chemotherapy.
3) Leucoencephalopathy has been found in children who have died, while CT scan changes showing reduction in brain volume may be associated with mental deterioration. However, most of these children had received, as well as irradiation, long-term treatment with intrathecal methotrexate.
4) Growth hormone deficiency has occurred in some children who received 2400 cGy in 2.5 weeks. It is interesting that in some children in whom 250-kV radiation was used, with changes in dose to allow for RBE, no cases of growth hormone deficiency occurred. This presumably is because the greater bone absorption reduced the radiation dose received by the pituitary-hypothalamic axis.
5) Second malignancies might be expected to increase and to occur with smaller radiation doses because of the enhancement effect. So far, however, patients with Wilms' tumours treated with actinomycin D and radiation seem to show a lower incidence of second malignancy than those treated with radiation alone.

17 Gastrointestinal Tract

R. D. James and R. C. S. Pointon

Introduction

At the time of writing, radiotherapy is of only minor use in the management of adenocarcinoma of the gastrointestinal tract, for a number of reasons. First, an exploratory laparotomy is generally needed for diagnosis, and if possible the tumour is resected or by-passed. Second, radiotherapy planning in the upper abdomen is complicated by the proximity of small bowel, kidneys, and spinal cord. Third, it has been assumed that these tumours cause death largely as a result of distant metastases, so that local radiotherapy, even if effective, would contribute little to survival.

The continued interest in radiotherapy for this group of tumours arises out of the poor survival rates following surgery, which have not changed for many years, and the morbidity associated with their resection (Table 17.1). It was hoped that the addition of cytotoxic agents to radical surgery would improve survival rates in carcinoma of the stomach and intraperitoneal colon. Despite a large number of well-organised prospective trials, using a variety of cytotoxic drugs, there is so far no evidence that the addition of chemotherapy to radical surgery improves survival for either tumour site. We are therefore faced with a group of tumours which are not only common, but commonly fatal (Table 17.2) and many surgeons would accept that a new approach using modern radiotherapy techniques may well be justified. There is evidence that this movement is already taking place for carcinoma of the rectum, and the indications for radiotherapy in this condition will be dealt with below. Before considering these it is worth dwelling briefly on recent changes in surgical and radiological practices which, if they fulfil expectations, might allow radiotherapy to be used for carcinoma of the colon, stomach, and pancreas as it is now used for rectal cancer.

Table 17.1. Operative mortality and morbidity for common carcinomas of the gastrointestinal tract.

	Survival %	Operative mortality	Morbidity
Oesophagus	10	5	Dysphagia
Pancreas	2	20	Diabetes
Stomach	10	5	Dumping
Colon	40	5	—
Rectum	50	5	Colostomy

Table 17.2. Frequency (%) of new tumours by site in the North West Region.

Bronchus	18
Colon and rectum	12
Breast	10
Skin	10
Stomach	7

Non-invasive Assessment

The first of these developments is the ability to obtain a biopsy from previously inaccessible areas of the gastrointestinal tract using fibre-optic endoscopy, so that a formal laparotomy is unnecessary for diagnosis. Second is the recognition that tumours can be "staged" preoperatively using examination under anaesthesia combined with modern radiological techniques such as isotope liver scanning, ultrasound imaging, and CT, so that more incurable cases are spared an "open and close" laparotomy. The introduction of some sort of staging system which is independent of surgery will require the assessment of tumour volume and infiltration of surrounding organs which is so important to the radiotherapist. We recognise that advanced tumours in sites as diverse as the head and neck and the pelvis are incurable by radiotherapy alone, and at the moment this is all that can be said of radiotherapy in the gastrointestinal tract. The results of radiotherapy for a series of early carcinomas of the stomach or colon have yet to be published and until that time the true radioresistance of these tumours will remain unknown. It is, however, well established that the cure rates of early adenocarcinomas of the rectum by radiotherapy are as good as those obtained by radical surgery.

The proportion of "late" or advanced tumours is unlikely to change, however, and it is this late presentation of tumours in the abdomen which determines the poor survival figures following surgery, a situation unlikely to change following radiotherapy.

A third development, emphasising that advanced gastrointestinal tumours frequently infiltrate surrounding organs, has been the demonstration of local recurrence in the operation bed following radical resection of carcinoma of the stomach and rectum. Accurate information on this phenomenon has been obtained by the policy of "second-look" laparotomy on asymptomatic patients following radical surgery. Up to 50% of patients in published series had re-growth of tumour in surrounding organs which were presumably penetrated by the primary tumour before the original operation. Although second-look laparotomy has now been abandoned, CT scanning can demonstrate tumour deposits almost as accurately and merely confirms the surgical findings (Fig. 17.1).

Finally, the introduction of high-energy radiotherapy beams has had the effect of reducing the volume of normal tissue which is needlessly irradiated. There now exists a large amount of information on normal tissue tolerance for various volumes and field sizes in the abdomen as a result of the treatment of lymphoma, testicular tumours, and embryonal tumours of childhood.

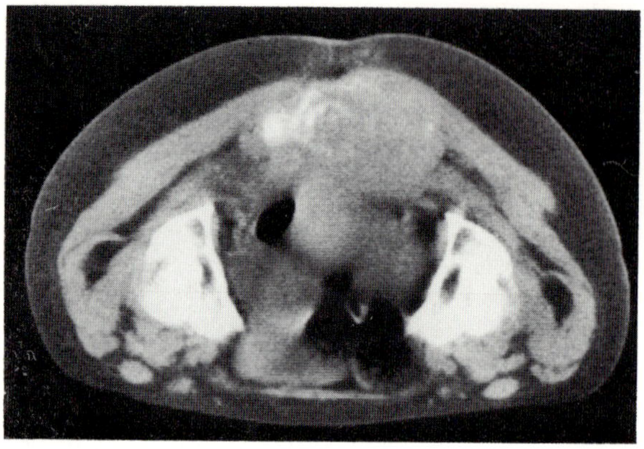

Fig. 17.1. CT scan of the pelvis showing extensive local recurrence following abdomino-perineal excision.

Carcinoma of Stomach, Colon, and Pancreas

The general comments made above regarding the difficulty of treating and assessing these tumours are particularly important for carcinoma of the pancreas and intraperitoneal colon. Both are rarely diagnosed without a laparotomy and indeed a firm diagnosis of carcinoma of the pancreas is often difficult for a histopathologist to make without clinical information. Surgery of some sort is generally needed for both, because of obstructive features. Finally, in both, local problems are frequently overshadowed by the development of liver metastases. Since radical pancreatectomy presents such a formidable surgical and postoperative challenge, radiotherapy has been considered as an alternative following decompression of the biliary tract. However, the true value of such treatment is difficult to assess, since objective tumour measurements are not made and the patient's main subjective complaint has often been relieved by surgery. The frequency of liver metastases following radical surgery for carcinoma of the colon in most published series exceeds 50%, and it has been suggested that adjuvant radiotherapy of the liver following surgery should be tested in a formal clinical study.

In carcinoma of the stomach there is good evidence that local recurrence frequently occurs and trials are now in progress to assess the value of adding local radiotherapy to the operation bed following gastrectomy. It should be remembered, however, that patients eligible for this type of study constitute only a small proportion of patients who present with stomach cancer, so that even if the policy is successful, overall improvements in survival will be unimpressive.

Carcinoma of the Rectum

In many ways carcinoma of the true rectum below the peritoneal reflection can be considered a pelvic rather than a gastrointestinal tumour. It can be examined fairly well without an anaesthetic, particularly in the female, and critical normal tissues such as spinal cord and small bowel are not dose-limiting. Radiotherapy may be justified in three situations: first, in the management of local recurrence following radical surgery; second, at the time of surgery for advanced or inoperable tumours; and third, as a radical alternative to surgery in certain specified cases.

Local Recurrence

Patients generally present with sacral pain following the abdominoperineal operation due to a mass of tumour on the anterior surface of the sacrum (see Fig. 17.1). There may be associated neurological signs due to involvement of the lower roots of the sacral plexus and these may include a neurogenic bladder. Urinary symptoms should be investigated radiologically and any hydronephrosis relieved by catheter drainage before radiotherapy. Perineal nodules and vaginal bleeding are less frequent and are usually associated with an undiagnosed presacral recurrence. Rectal bleeding and discharge are seen following anterior resection but again there is usually an associated extrarectal mass.

Patients are conveniently treated prone using a rotation or three-field wedge technique on an isocentric megavoltage machine (Fig. 17.2). Sophisticated beam direction is not indicated for what is basically a palliative situation. Our measurements using CT scanning have shown that the majority of these recurrences are included in a cylinder which lies in the sacral hollow 10 cm in diameter and 12 cm long with a central axis 6–7 cm below the natal cleft. A simulator should be used to centre the field at the level of recurrence, generally more central

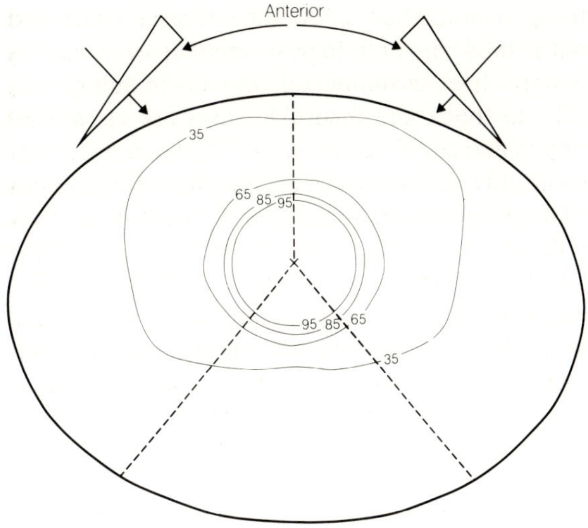

Fig. 17.2. Dose distribution for wedge-filter rotation therapy in the pelvis designed to treat rectal cancer.

and caudal following anterior than abdominoperineal resection. The field can be extended to include perineal nodules provided adequate bolus is applied to the natal cleft.

The dose and fractionation depend on a number of factors, but are generally the maximum tolerated by this volume. Prognosis is poor in patients with metastases in chest and liver, in those whose tumour has recurred within 2 years of surgery, and in those with bulky tumours (Fig. 17.3). Pain relief may be achieved by radiotherapy, but it is short-lived and patients return quickly with further

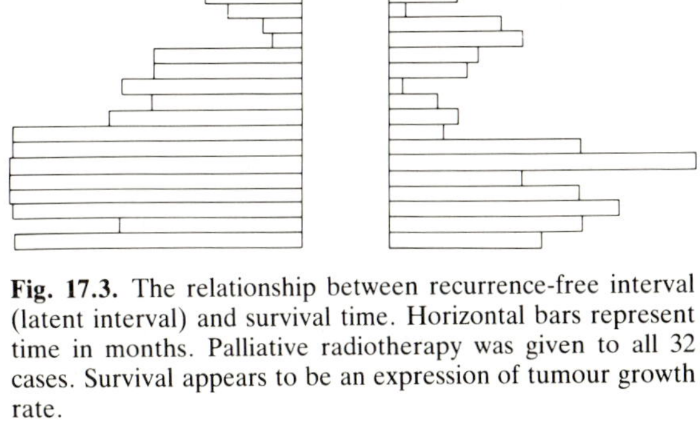

Fig. 17.3. The relationship between recurrence-free interval (latent interval) and survival time. Horizontal bars represent time in months. Palliative radiotherapy was given to all 32 cases. Survival appears to be an expression of tumour growth rate.

local disease and distant metastases. A 4-day dose of 3000 cGy should be reduced by 20% if the rectum is included in the volume. If the patient is young and fit, chemotherapy should be considered in addition.

At the other extreme are patients with long intervals between surgery and recurrence. It is important to exclude a second primary carcinoma or an unassociated benign condition, and CT scanning is particularly useful for this. Radiotherapy, if given, should be aggressive, since some of these patients survive for a number of years. A dose of 4500–5000 cGy in 16 days is possible provided the treatment volume is small (8–10 cm). Further surgery is occasionally justified in these patients, but is difficult following radiotherapy. Thoracotomy may be justified for isolated, slowly growing pulmonary metastases.

Adjuvant Radiotherapy

The probability of local recurrence following radical surgery for rectal cancer increases with tumour size and progressive invasion of surrounding structures in the pelvis. The definition of operability is subjective, since it depends on how many surrounding organs the surgeon is prepared to sacrifice in order to give the patient a chance of cure. In general a compromise is necessary and it is then perfectly clear which sites are at high risk of local recurrence. Most surgeons would claim to be able to recognise patients of borderline operability before surgery. There is now good evidence from intraoperative biopsies and CT scanning that fixity or tethering to surrounding pelvic structures in a sense constitutes inoperability if one of the standard radical operations is to be performed (Fig. 17.4). Furthermore, the introduction of the stapling device has led to a reluctance to offer patients a permanent colostomy. Some surgeons believe that when they are disinclined to perform the necessary radical operation the deficiency might be covered by local radiotherapy. At the time of writing there is no clear evidence that either pre- or postoperative radiotherapy reduces the overall risk of tumour re-growth following resection of advanced rectal carcinoma. This may well be because published controlled trials to date have used subradical doses with surprisingly large fields. Alternatively any local advantage from radiotherapy could be masked by death from distant metastases, which are common in this type of advanced tumour.

Close cooperation between surgeon and radiotherapist is required if misunderstandings are to be avoided. We believe the optimal approach is to organise a joint examination under anaesthetic when the planned operation is discussed and the tumour is marked with gold seeds. Anterior resection is unwise if part of the anastomosis is to be irradiated; it is also technically difficult for very

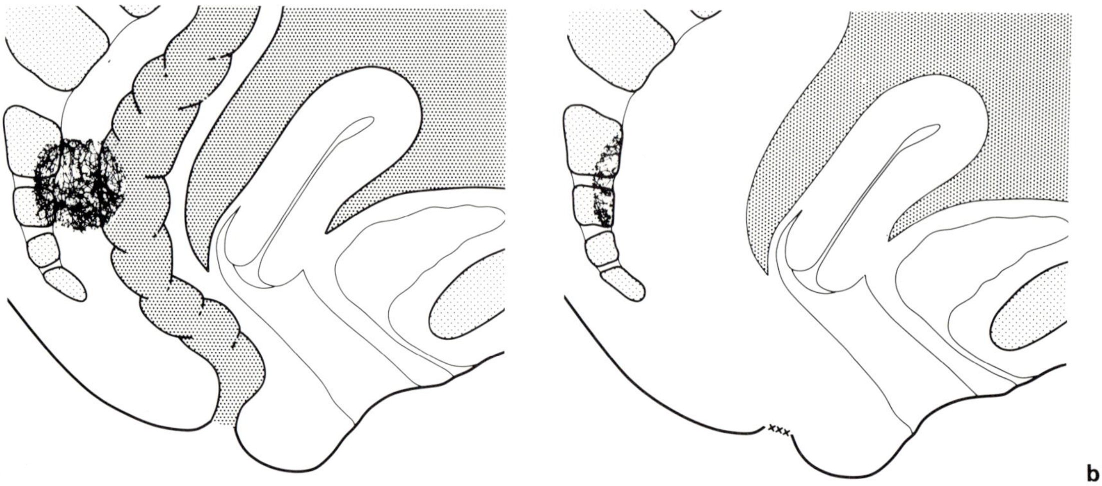

a b

Fig. 17.4. a Rectal cancer through the bowel wall onto the sacrum. **b** Following abdominoperineal resection residual tumour remains and can regrow to give a sacral recurrence.

advanced tumours. In our experience, reduction in the volume of the tumour is not generally marked even after high radiation doses, and the surgeon should expect a difficult dissection of the area of extrarectal spread. CT scanning is invaluable to the radiotherapist in confirming examination findings and allowing a reduction in the volume to be irradiated. Alternatively, high-dose postoperative radiotherapy can be given, provided areas of extrarectal spread have been marked by radio-opaque clips and the pelvis has been re-peritonealised to exclude small bowel. If a tumour is completely inoperable by one surgeon's standards it is unlikely, in our experience, that radiotherapy will alter the situation. The patient with advanced rectal cancer is best served by surgical resection, but radiotherapy may improve his fate after that operation. A palliative colostomy should always be considered in truly inoperable rectal cancer. As a rough guide, if a patient is unfit for this manoeuvre he is likely to be unfit for radiotherapy and relief of symptoms is best achieved using opiates.

Radical Radiotherapy for Operable Rectal Cancer

Patients with operable tumours occasionally refuse or are medically unfit for radical resection. The particular problem of radical beam-directed radiotherapy for small rectal cancer lies in the accurate localisation of the tumour, which is generally invisible on CT scanning, and in the management of the rectal reaction. Professor Jean Papillon has overcome both problems by using contact therapy under direct vision through a large proctoscope. Patients are treated without anaesthetic and receive three fractions of 5000 R at 2-weekly intervals. The technique is not difficult to master, but some patients are unable to tolerate the knee-chest position. It could conceivably be modified to an orthovoltage, interstitial or electron technique. However, as Professor Papillon points out, it is limited to tumours within 10 cm of the anal verge, and his 5-year survival rate of 78% in 122 patients is likely to fall if larger tumours are included. Its two main advantages over diathermy are the lack of anaesthetic and the absence of scarring, so that recurrence is picked up early. These advantages, too, might disappear if larger tumours are treated. It has been argued that regional lymph nodes should be included in a radical volume of this type. This would be logical if surgical removal of involved lymph nodes had been shown to be advantageous. In fact, surgical results clearly indicate that removal of metastatic regional lymph nodes conveys no survival benefit since it is these patients who invariably die of recurrent disease. As indicated above, this problem is likely to increase as fewer permanent colostomies are contemplated for rectal cancer. Provided a reliable radical technique is devised it would be ethically justified to consider radiotherapy as an alternative to permanent colostomy for tumours of the lower third of the rectum, since recurrence is easily detected and dealt with.

Carcinoma of the Anus

Introduction

In comparison with carcinoma of the rectum, carcinoma of the anus is uncommon.

Carcinoma of the anus arises both in the modified squamous epithelium of the anal margin and lower anal canal below the pectinate line and also in the cuboidal epithelium lining the canal between the pectinate line and the anorectal ring. This latter tissue may also be modified squamous epithelium. The vast majority of lesions will be squamous cell carcinoma, and the occasional basiloid carcinoma occurs.

Site

It is usual to consider carcinoma of the anus as arising in either the anal canal proper or at the anal orifice. In the more extensive lesions admixtures will occur.

Regional Lymph Nodes

The lymphatic drainage of the anal margin and canal is predominantly to the superficial inguinal lymph nodes; some of the upper lymphatics of the canal drain directly to the perirectal nodes and the nodes distal to the origin of the inferior mesenteric artery.

Staging

The UICC classification (1978) is summarised as follows:

Anal canal

T1 < $\frac{1}{3}$ circumference or length/external sphincter not infiltrated
T2 > $\frac{1}{3}$ circumference or length/external sphincter infiltrated
T3 Extension to rectum/skin
T4 Extension to neighbouring structures
N1 Regional

Anal orifice

T1 < 2 cm/superficial
T2 > 2.5 cm/minimal infiltration
T3 > 5 cm/deep infiltration
T4 Extension to muscle/bone
N1 Unilateral/movable
N2 Bilateral/movable
N3 Fixed

Treatment Policy

Carcinoma of the anus may be treated successfully by surgery or by radiotherapy.

Surgery, while of potentially high curative value, will in most cases necessitate a permanent colostomy, whereas successful irradiation will preserve normal bowel function. Moreover, surgery can be held in reserve in case of failure of radiation therapy. The degree of success which may be achieved with irradiation depends largely on the size of the lesion and in particular on (1) the extent of the lesion up the anal canal and (2) infiltration laterally into the perineal tissues.

Squamous cell carcinoma of the anus of small or moderate size is curable by irradiation. It is, however, a tumour of limited sensitivity, and this fact, coupled with the poor tolerance of the tissues of the perineal region, means that great care must be taken in treatment planning. In this situation, whenever possible the specified ranges of dosage should not be exceeded.

Treatment Method

The tolerance of the perineal region is such that it is very difficult to treat carcinoma of the anus with external irradiation without provoking very severe reactions and consequent morbidity. Interstitial irradiation is the treatment of choice. While radium needle implantation as practised at the Christie Hospital will be described, equivalent implants using iridium-192 are obviously practical. Preliminary colostomy is not necessary.

The patient should be admitted 3–4 days before the implant is to be carried out. The bowel is cleared and the patient maintained on a low-residue diet. Opiates may be given to maintain constipation during the period the needles are in position.

It is essential to have sources of an adequate active length available; in practice they should not be less than 4.5 cm active length.

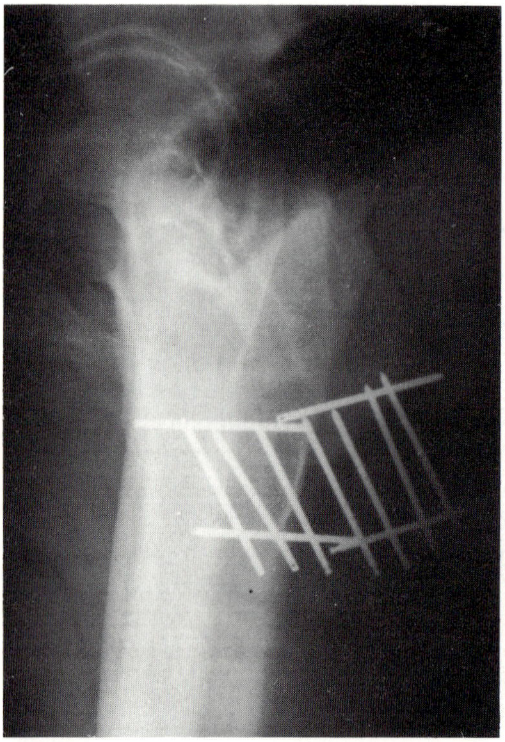

Fig. 17.5. Single-plane radium needle implant.

Calculation
Anus. Single-plane implant.
Implanted area=18.2 cm^2
Dose required=5500 cGy
Approximate treatment time=168 h
mg h/1000 cGy=372
mg radium required=12.18 mg
Needles used 6×2 mg active length 3.0 cm
5×1 mg active length 3.0 cm
mg radium used=16.66 mg (including filtration correction)
Final treatment time=123 h

The types of implant used are single-plane and two-plane implants. The single-plane implant (Fig. 17.5) is used for unilateral lesions not exceeding 1 cm in thickness. A series of parallel needles are inserted under the tumour and the mucosa of the canal. Great care should be taken to ensure that an adequate margin is taken around the lesion. The needles must be kept superficial, running just deep to the skin or mucosa. A finger in the anal canal is of great value in confirming this and also the parallelism of the plane of the needles. The use of needles of adequate active length obviates the need for an inner crossing but, if considered necessary, this may be obtained by the use of "Indian club" needles. The outer end of the implant is crossed by a needle or needles running at right angles to the main plane. Each needle should be stitched in individually. The dose to be given should be 5250–5500 cGy in 7 days.

When, however, the lesion is circumferential, then a two-plane implant should be used. The implant is carried out with the patient in the lithotomy position. The two planes are inserted as shown in Fig. 17.6, parallel to one other. The permissible separation between the planes is not great and preferably should not exceed 2 cm. The dose delivered is expressed as that received 0.5 cm from the inner aspect of each plane. In carrying out the implant, allowance should be made for the effect of restoring the patient to the supine position in which he will be nursed. The dose to be given should be 5250 cGy at 0.5 cm from each plane in 7 days.

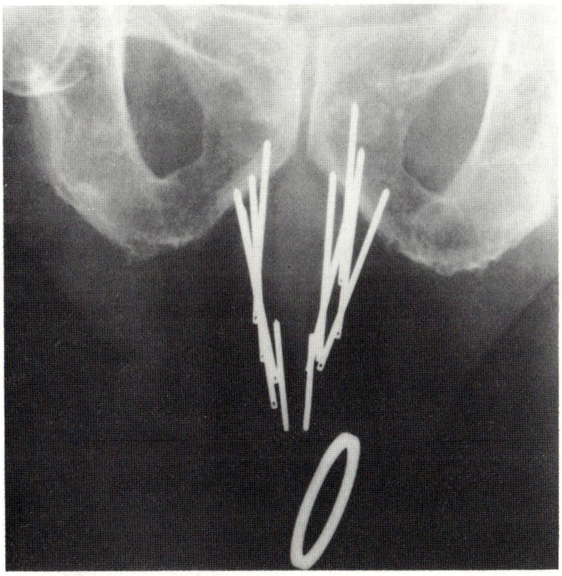

Fig. 17.6. Two-plane radium needle implant.

Calculation
Anus. Two-plane implant.
Implanted area=19.7 cm^2
Dose required=5250 cGy
Approximate treatment time=168 h
mg h/1000 cGy=393
2-Plane separation factor=1.55
mg radium required=19.04 mg
Needles used 3×3 mg active length 4.5 cm
3×1.5 mg active length 4.5 cm
mg radium used=26.19 mg (including filtration correction)
Final treatment time=122 h

On removing the needles, normal bowel action is resumed with the aid of a mild aperient. The patient should be advised on the importance of regular bowel action. Usually there should be no great problem in the control of defecation. Residual or recurrent tumour should be treated by the appropriate surgery.

Complications

Local tissue necrosis may occur. This usually responds to nursing, but occasionally light diathermy may be required. Persistent or severe necrosis should be treated by excision. Anal stricture of any moment is rare.

Palliation

Radiotherapy with palliative intent is rarely of benefit in cases of advanced anal carcinoma.

Inguinal lymph nodes

Significant mobile inguinal nodes should be treated by block dissection. The results of radiotherapy for involved inguinal nodes are extremely poor. Where it is feasible, the best palliation is obtained by the use of growth-restraint X-ray therapy, i.e. 400 cGy given once weekly until local tolerance is reached or the disease is no longer controlled. Chemotherapy of involved inguinal nodes is at present of no significant benefit.

18 Clinical Trial Methods

M. K. Palmer

Introduction

This chapter describes some of the statistical methods which the radiotherapist and oncologist are likely to need in order to evaluate critically the effectiveness of treatment for cancer. One of the oldest and greatest errors in medicine is the assumption that treatment is necessarily beneficial. The correct scientific attitude ought to be one of scepticism: a new drug or a new X-ray machine is not always better than its predecessors and may in fact be harmful. Well-established as well as new methods of treatment throughout medicine need to be continually evaluated for both efficacy and safety.

The first randomised clinical trial in the field of cancer was started at this hospital in 1947. At that time trials were criticised as potentially unethical. Attitudes have gradually changed so that today it is generally agreed that it may well be unethical not to carry out a clinical trial before introducing a new treatment. It is very important therefore to understand the statistical pitfalls and the merits and limitation of clinical trials. Hence this chapter concentrates on trials and no attempt is made to cover basic statistical methods such as frequency distributions, summarising statistics (mean, standard deviation, etc.), correlation, significance tests, and so on. The reader who is not familiar with the basic concepts of statistical analysis will still find the chapter useful, particularly the section on the design and conduct of clinical trials. The tests described under "Significance Tests" below may be difficult to follow without an understanding of the concept of statistical significance. Suffice it to say in this context, however, that the first step in carrying out a test of statistical significance is to adopt a *null hypothesis*. This is a hypothesis of doubt, for example that a new treatment is no better and no worse than an old treatment. A certain amount of evidence is then required before this hypothesis can be rejected, and its opposite, that the two treatments in fact differ, can be accepted. The p-value is a measure of the weight of evidence against the null hypothesis: the *smaller* the p-value the less likely it is to be true. Some arbitrary value, usually $p=0.05$, is chosen and if the weight of evidence against the null hypothesis is so great that the p-value is less than 0.05 the null hypothesis can be rejected. Tests of statistical significance are therefore a useful way of making decisions, albeit at the price of occasionally being wrong, when interpretation of the data is not clear-cut. Readers who wish to find out more about significance tests and other statistical methods are referred to the recommended reading list at the end of the chapter.

Clinical Trials

Introduction

With any life-threatening disease, such as cancer, evaluation of the results of treatment is crucial. Only after careful monitoring is it possible to measure accurately the success or otherwise of a certain treatment policy applied to a group of cancer patients. The application of appropriate techniques of evaluation may lead to the discovery of some features of the disease, or characteristics of the patients, which confer a better or worse chance of success. A careful comparison of the results from two (or occasionally more) groups of patients in a randomised clinical trial can be used to find the better of two alternative modes of treatment. A clinical trial therefore constitutes a special case of evaluation in oncology. The aim is to compare treatments in a scientifically valid and at the same time ethically acceptable way by allocating treatments in a random manner to patients with a specific illness. Clinical trials are difficult to design, requiring many hours of discussion involving radiotherapists, chemotherapists, surgeons, pathologists, radiologists, etc., as well as statisticians, epidemiologists, computer programmers, and data managers. The immediate aim is to decide on a *protocol*. This is a written document which spells out the questions the trial asks and how they will be answered.

The Clinical Trial Protocol

What is the Background to the Trial and Why is it being Done?

Descriptions should be included of the presently accepted treatment for the condition under investigation, what other relevant research has been done, and why a new approach is being tried. The reader must be convinced that there is a real need for carrying out the trial and that a medically important question is being asked. He or she should be satisfied that the time and expense of carrying out a trial over many years is justified and that there is enough interest in the question to sustain the cooperation of the investigators and ensure their continued collaboration to the end of the trial.

What are the General Objectives of the Trial?

The objectives, which should be stated as clearly as possible, will usually be in terms of specific end points, for example remission rate, survival time, duration of remission, disease-free time, time to primary recurrence, etc. Of all the possible end points, one in particular may be of greater interest, in which case this should be stated. For example in comparing two different induction regimes for leukaemia, special interest would be focused on remission rates, while in comparing two types of treatment for breast cancer, it might be times to local recurrence. Two treatments which have different effects on one end point, for example remission duration, may not differ in respect of some other end point such as survival time.

How are the Patients Defined?

The patients to be entered into the trial must be defined as carefully and as unambiguously as possible. Selection criteria might include:

1) The site, extent and histological type of disease
2) The patient's sex and age
3) Whether previous relevant treatment has been given and its type and extent
4) How the diagnosis was obtained, and whether all the required investigations have been done
5) The patient's status as regards haematological, renal, hepatic, and endocrine values

It is advisable also to have specific exclusion criteria which might include:

1) Pregnancy
2) Mental disability
3) Presence of other serious illnesses, in particular previous malignancy

Selection and exclusion criteria should be stated as clearly as possible and adhered to strictly, since it is important to have a well-defined sample of patients if the results of the trial are to be generalised to a population of patients with the same disease. Once the criteria have been made absolutely clear, it is obviously equally important to make sure that *all* eligible patients at an institute are entered into the trial.

What Treatments are to be Used?

The details of each treatment should be documented precisely so that each clinician knows exactly what to do. This applies not only to the treatments to be compared directly but also to any prior treatment, such as surgery, and supportive care. Treatments which are strictly forbidden must also be stated. Treatment modification or delay may be allowed, e.g. in the event of an abnormal blood picture, but details of the procedure to be followed must be included in the protocol. In trials of chemotherapeutic agents, it is useful to list the most common features of toxicity which are encountered as well as a grading scheme for assessing their severity. Dose reductions or delays can then be based in a rational way on the maximum toxicity observed. The reason why treatment modifications may be built into the design of a clinical trial is that usually it is more relevant to compare two treatment *policies* rather than two rigidly specified treatments. The former is nearer to the everyday clinical situation and the results of the trial are therefore more likely to have general applicability.

Further treatment is invariably given to patients who relapse or have a recurrence following their initial treatment and rather than leave this to each clinician's individual judgement, it might be better to incorporate it into the trial protocol as part of each treatment policy. There are indeed occasions when it is medically important to design trials comparing two treatments, or treatment policies, specifically for patients who fail after receiving some other form of treatment.

When and How are Patients to be Randomised?

The purpose of randomisation is to produce two groups of patients similar in every respect except for the treatment allocated. Randomisation is therefore the only way of ensuring that a comparison between groups of patients treated in different ways is free from bias. Randomisation should take place as late as possible in the course of each patient's management to make sure that no intervening event, such as death, occurs before the randomly allocated treatment is actually given. Moreover, the patient must be equally suitable to receive either treatment at the time of randomisation. For example, in a trial to compare two maintenance regimes for patients in remission following treatment for non-Hodgkin's lymphoma, randomisation would take place only when remission had been achieved and the patient was ready to start maintenance therapy.

Every clinician should understand the procedures for entering patients into clinical trials and for obtaining the randomised treatment allocation. A telephone call to a central office is the best way of doing this, for the following reasons:

1) To ensure that randomisation was carried out correctly, because any other system, such as numbered envelopes, is open to abuse, and even if used correctly a critical reader may not be convinced

2) So that the participants always know exactly how many patients have been randomised, both in total and in each treatment arm, as well as the names or hospital numbers of the patients

3) So that the trials office can later request overdue forms

Before the trial starts, the trials office will have prepared a list of treatments in random order using a table of random numbers. Randomisation lists should be *balanced*, so that when entry to the trial stops, there are the same, or very nearly the same, numbers of patients in each treatment group. The easiest way to ensure balance is to choose a number such as four to be the *block size*. In the first four patients, two would receive treatment A, and two would receive treatment B, similarly with the next four patients, and so on. The random order within each block is achieved by writing down all the possible combinations of two A's and two B's (AABB, ABAB, ABBA, BBAA, BABA, and BAAB) and numbering them from one to six. Numbers between one and six are then drawn from a table of random numbers. For example if the first random number from the table was five, this would determine the treatments (B, A, B, and A) given to the first four patients. The block size does not have to be four of course, but preparation of the randomisation list is easier if it is not too large.

Sometimes it is of interest to know how many patients with a particular type of cancer were not eligible for the trial, so that those who were eligible can be seen in context. To do this one might require clinicians to register ineligible patients as well. If there is a prolonged interval before randomisation takes place it is often useful to register patients by telephone call at the time of diagnosis. This is to help make sure that all patients who eventually satisfy the inclusion criteria are eventually randomised, and to find out how many patients failed to meet the criteria.

Is a Stratified Randomisation Necessary?

If patients entered into a trial are of two types, let us say with "good" and "bad" pathology, it may happen by chance, particularly in a small clinical trial, that proportionately more of the good-pathology patients fall into treatment group A than B, giving group A patients a better prognosis even if the two treatments were equally effective. A randomisation *stratified* by pathology would avoid such an imbalance by having separate randomisations for each pathology, thus ensuring that equal numbers of patients with good pathology receive each treatment, and likewise for patients with bad pathology. The final treatment groups A and B would therefore include the same, or very nearly the same proportions of good-pathology patients, and the comparison of the two treatments would be free from bias of this kind. If sex were also an important prognostic factor and the randomisation was stratified for this as well, there would then be $2\times2=4$ individual strata, with a balanced random list for each. With more prognostic factors stratification would be cumbersome, so that if used at all it should be restricted to only the most important prognostic factors. In multi-centre trials, randomisation should always be stratified by institution to allow each centre to treat equal numbers of patients with each treatment and also to make sure that differences between institutions do not bias the comparison between treatments. However, in single-centre trials with an accrual of more than say a hundred patients, a simple randomisation can usually be relied upon to produce two groups of patients virtually identical in so far as prognostic factors are concerned. Stratification is rarely necessary in such trials, particularly since the effect of any imbalance between the groups can be corrected by using methods to be described later. On the other hand there are those who argue that the slightly greater complexity in using a randomisation stratified by an important prognostic factor is a small price to pay for reducing the risk of imbalance between treatment groups even in large single-centre clinical trials. Besides, a trial that was intended to be large may terminate earlier than expected for various reasons and end as a trial with small numbers of patients and an appreciable imbalance.

What Should be the Frequency and Duration of Follow-up and what Further Investigations Need to be Done?

Many of the pretreatment clinical and laboratory examinations will need to be repeated after patients have been entered into the trial to assess their progress. Which examinations, and the frequency with which they are to be carried out, should be clearly stated and should be the same for all patients. The same clinical and laboratory methods should be used throughout and the maximum length of follow-up will also need to be specified.

How is Response to Treatment Assessed?

End points used in assessing the response to each treatment must be clearly defined. In patients with "early" cancer, starting points and end points for terms such as length of survival, time to local recurrence, time to metastatic spread, and disease free time must be decided, and for patients with "advanced" cancer the assessment of response may include some of these as well as tumour response and remission status. Any subjective element in assessing tumour response and remission status must be minimised by adopting objective criteria based on measurable characteristics whenever possible.

What Special Forms should be Used and When, How, and by Whom should they be Completed?

It is vital to the success of a clinical trial to have well-designed forms on which the important data can be recorded easily, since otherwise a proper analysis of the results is impossible. Several forms will be required to cover different aspects of each patient's treatment and progress. These might be:

1) An initial entry form, giving patient identification details, and results of clinical examinations, diagnostic investigations, laboratory tests, etc. This form can also be used to check that the entry criteria have been met.

2) A treatment form, giving details of all treatments carried out including those assigned by random allocation, and the date of randomisation. Doses of drugs and X-rays must be recorded,

together with any adverse reactions encountered and whether these were severe enough to cause treatment to be modified or abandoned.

3) A follow-up form, on which can be recorded the results of regular examinations and tests.

4) A relapse and death form, giving the site or sites of recurrence, the date on which each occurred, the date of death, and death details.

These forms should be as simple as possible and may be designed with "boxes" so that the data, as numbers, can be input to a computer directly without the need for transcribing onto other forms. The forms should be sent to a central office for review by the trial organisers and any missing or inconsistent information acted upon promptly. The trials office can also remind clinicians about overdue forms and prepare simple statistical information on the progress of the trial to help retain the interest and cooperation of all those involved.

What is the Sensitivity of the Clinical Trial?

In practice the duration of a clinical trial is limited to only a few years since if it lasts any longer it might be overtaken by the results of similar trials carried out elsewhere. If that happens the clinicians concerned might be unwilling for ethical reasons to continue entering their patients knowing that half of them would receive what was probably an inferior treatment. From the planned duration of the trial the total number of patients who will be eligible from start to finish can be estimated. (For some reason these estimates have an annoying habit of being too optimistic, probably because most trial organisers fail to realise how restrictive are the eligibility criteria they define.) A statistically significant difference in an end point (death or recurrence, for example) between the two treatment groups is usually a desirable outcome for the trial, because positive findings, that two treatments differ, are more interesting than negative ones. This is particularly true when it is remembered that "not statistically significant" can mean either that the two treatments are virtually identical in their effects or that they are different but there is not enough evidence to be sure. Unfortunately there is no way of guaranteeing that a clinical trial will produce the desired statistically significant result even if the two treatments are known to differ markedly, since the operation of chance may overwhelm the treatment difference, particularly if the numbers of patients are small. However, if we can think of a plausible figure for the size of the treatment difference (as a difference between 5-year survival percentages for example) we can then calculate the *probability* that the trial will produce a positive answer with the numbers of patients available. This probability is the *sensitivity* of the trial and we would certainly want it to be as high as possible.

For example, let us assume that 40 patients a year with a certain type of cancer are eligible for a trial lasting 3 years. Existing forms of treatment can offer only a 25% 5-year survival rate but it is expected that a new treatment could achieve 50%. Using a method devised by George and Desu, the probability of reaching a statistically significant difference (at the 5% level of significance) turns out to be 0.8. The sensitivity of the above trial would be high enough to ensure its viability from the statistical point of view.

Sensitivity calculations should always be carried out by a statistician before the start of a clinical trial. This is because, for well-established biological reasons, the maximum treatment difference which exists is often small. For example, in breast cancer the difference in 5-year survival rates for two types of mastectomy would probably be less than 10%. Differences of this magnitude can be detected as statistically significant only by very large clinical trials with at least 500 patients in each treatment group. For some cancers, for example those affecting children, the incidence is low, and the required sensitivity can be achieved only by accruing patients from several centres for many years. Table 18.1 shows how sensitivity depends on the treatment difference which the trial is designed to detect and the numbers of patients available. For a trial to be viable from the statistical point of view, it is suggested that sensitivity should be at least 0.7.

Sometimes the sensitivity of a clinical trial is low even when the most optimistic estimates are used of the likely treatment difference, the numbers of patients available, and the overall duration of the trial. In this case the investigators must decide whether to commit resources of time, money, and effort for many years to the trial or whether to devote their skills to a different area where there are perhaps better prospects of improved control of cancer and increased length of survival.

Table 18.1. Numbers of patients required in each treatment group.

Smaller 5-year survival %	Assumed difference in survival	No. of patients with full 5-year follow-up in each group for sensitivity:			
		0.5	0.75	0.9	0.95
20%	5%	550	1000	1300	1500
	10%	150	250	370	401
	20%	39	70	100	110
	30%	17	30	50	52
40%	5%	750	1400	2000	2110
	10%	190	350	500	533
	20%	45	80	125	134
	30%	19	35	55	67
60%	5%	700	1200	1900	2030
	10%	175	320	480	490
	15%	70	130	200	208
	20%	37	70	100	110
70%	5%	550	1100	1600	1720
	10%	145	275	390	401
	15%	55	100	160	163
	20%	28	50	75	81
80%	5%	450	900	1100	1250
	10%	100	180	250	270
	15%	35	60	85	95
85%	5%	350	600	900	940
	10%	70	100	160	180
90%	5%	200	400	500	550
92.5%	5%	183	300	400	450

Statistical Methods for Clinical Trials and Other Studies Requiring Prolonged Patient Follow-up

Measures of Response

Since the life expectancy of a patient with cancer left untreated would in general be much less than normal, the aim of treatment is to confer an expectation of life as near as possible to that of a comparable person of the same age and sex drawn from the general population. The most important measure of effectiveness of treatment is, therefore, the length of time lived by each individual patient—the patient's *survival time*. This must be measured from a definite and identifiable starting point, which may be the onset of symptoms, but many patients are very vague about the time of onset, and doctors vary in the skill with which they take a medical history. Some symptoms are immediately alarming while others may be insidious in their development, so that the date of onset of symptoms is too vague to serve as the starting point from which survival time may be measured. The date of diagnosis is sometimes used but often this too is imprecise. In practice the date of the start of treatment is almost always preferred, and since treatment for cancer is invariably definitive, this date is almost always known. The measurement of survival from the date treatment started has the further advantage that survival can be correlated with many clinical features, such as the stage of disease, blood picture, liver function tests etc., which are usually recorded at the same time. For patients entering a clinical trial, the date of randomisation offers a convenient starting point from which survival time may be measured. This may also avoid a potentially serious form of bias which would arise in the comparison of two treatments one of which involved delay to permit further tests and investigations.

Other measures of response may also be considered, for example disease-free interval, time to recurrence of disease in the primary site, and time to occurrence of metastases. In many studies, particularly those in which intensive chemotherapy is used, the type of remission achieved (complete, partial, or none) and the length of time in remission are important. The latter is measured as the interval from the date on which remission was established to the date of relapse. Remission and relapse need careful definition, and would usually be expressed in terms of a conjunction of physical signs and symptoms of disease as well as blood, urine, bone marrow, radiological, and other values. What is common to all these time-based measures of response is the concept of a *failure time*, that is, a time to a particular type of failure. One difficulty which might arise for failures other than death is in determining precisely the date of failure; similar difficulty might also be found, when the measure of response is remission duration, in determining exactly when remission started. Leaving aside these practical problems of definition, it is fortunate that the statistical methods for the analysis of failure times are the same whether applied to survival times, disease-free survival times, remission durations, times to primary recurrence, or any other type of failure time. One more important point must be made. If a patient has been observed to suffer a particular type of failure then his failure time is said to be *exact*. On the other hand, if the failure has not yet occurred during the period of observation it is said to be *censored*. Clearly, if we could observe a patient with a censored failure time for a longer period, a failure might then occur; thus we can say that, for patients with censored failure times, the unknown failure times must of necessity be longer than the observed censored times. For each patient, therefore, the information we have will usually consist of (1) failure times, some of which might be censored; (2) personal characteristics, such as age, sex, and marital status; (3) features of the disease such as site, stage, and histology; (4) other relevant medical details such as previous treatment, menopausal status, total white cell count, haemoglobin etc.; finally, (5) we would usually also have details of the treatment carried out, including doses of radiation and chemotherapeutic agents as well as surgical procedures.

Survival Curves

Crude Percentage of Survivors

The conventional way of describing the pattern of failure times observed in a group of patients is by means of a life table curve. This tells us the percentage of patients not yet experiencing failure at various times (say each day or month or year) up to several years after treatment. For ease of description of the various methods of calculation it will be assumed that death is the type of failure observed, and therefore instead of failure times we shall talk about survival times. The methods are the same, however, whatever the type of failure.

Suppose we wish to find the percentage of patients still alive at each year up to 5 years after treatment. If all patients were treated more than 5 years ago and none had been lost to follow-up then the exact percentages (sometimes called crude survival rates) can be found simply and directly using the equation:

$$\%\text{ survivors at } t \text{ years} = \frac{\text{Number of patients alive at } t \text{ years}}{\text{Number of patients in the group initially}} \times 100\%$$

However, if some patients have censored survival times less than 5 years (because they were lost to follow-up or were treated less than 5 years ago) then there is no way of knowing whether they would eventually survive to 5 years and therefore no simple way of calculating exact survival percentages. However, we can provide very good *estimates* of the exact percentages using what are called *life table methods*. (Sometimes the methods are called *actuarial*.) Two methods are in general use. One is called the *Kaplan-Meier* (or *product limit*) method and the other the *Berkson-Gage* method.

The Kaplan-Meier Method

If you only wish to use this method in a cookbook fashion without understanding why the calculations are carried out then you should skip the remainder of this subsection and turn straight to the example.

The key to understanding how it is possible to derive estimates of survival percentages using incomplete follow-up information lies in the very obvious statement that in order to survive, say, a whole year, a patient has to survive each of the 365 individual days comprising it. The chance of surviving 1 year is therefore

$$S_{365} = C_1 \times C_2 \times C_3 \times \ldots \times C_{364} \times C_{365}$$

where C_1 is the chance of surviving the first day,

C_2 is the chance of surviving the second day having already survived day 1,

C_3 is the chance of surviving the third day having already survived days 1 and 2, and so on to . . .

C_{364} is the chance of surviving day 364 having already survived days 1 to 363, and

C_{365} is the chance of surviving day 365 having already survived days 1 to 364.

The quantities C_1, C_2 etc. are unknown but we can estimate each one by calculating what proportion of patients at risk on a given day actually survived it. For example on day 100 let P_{100} be the proportion and consider all those patients who were alive on day 99 and were treated more than 100 days ago. (This is necessary so that we have a chance to observe their fate on day 100.) P_{100} is then the proportion of these patients who survived day 100. If no one in fact died on that day then $P_{100}=1$. Probably most of the individual Ps would be 1, but nevertheless the quantity obtained by multiplying them together provides mathematically the best possible estimate of S_{365} the life table chance of surviving 1 year. It should be noted that if we have already estimated S_{365}, then the estimate of S_{366} is just P_{366} times it. In practice we do not need to bother about the days on which no deaths occurred because on those days $P=1$ and the estimate of S will be unchanged, as will be seen from the following simple example.

Example Suppose six patients were treated for cancer and on the day of analysis four had already died (with exact survival times from treatment of 152 days, 515 days, 811 days, and 1777 days) and two were still alive (with censored survival times 1440 days and 2520 days). What are the life table estimates of the chances of surviving various lengths of time following treatment for this type of cancer?

The first step is to cast the data into the form of Table 18.2, in which survival times are listed in order from the shortest to longest. If several patients have the same survival time then the patients with exact times should be put first.

Next, write "dead" or "alive" against each survival time and in column 3 record the number of deaths observed, d, on each day T. Column 4 is the number of patients, r, at risk on each day, that is the number with survival times greater than or equal to T. The proportion dying on day T is then just d/r, the ratio of the number dying to the number at risk on day T, and then the proportion, P, surviving day T is just one minus this, i.e. $1-d/r$. Finally, the life table estimates are found by the multiplication of successive Ps, i.e. $0.833=5/6$, $0.667=5/6\times4/5$, etc. Two points are important: first, days for which there are no survival times do not need to appear in the table; and second, the life table probability estimates go down only at times at which deaths were observed: between these times the estimates remain constant.

Life table estimates of the probabilities of surviving various lengths of time are so often used in evaluating the results of cancer treatment and are so useful that the reader should work through the above example (or some data of his own) to make sure that the method is thoroughly understood.

Usually life table probabilities are converted to percentages by multiplying by 100 and then the values obtained can be thought of as estimates of the percentages of patients surviving to various times, after allowance has been made for incomplete follow-up.

A graph or table of these percentages against time is known as a *survival curve*, in spite of the fact that the graph is not a curve at all but a series of horizontal and vertical lines. Figure 18.1 shows survival curves for two groups of patients, 29 men

Table 18.2. Ordered survival times and steps in the calculation of life table survival estimates.

Survival time T	Status	$d=$ No. of deaths on day T	$r=$ No. at risk on day T	$P=$ Proportion surviving day T	$S=$ Estimated probability of surviving to day T
152	Dead	1	6	5/6	0.833
515	Dead	1	5	4/5	0.667
811	Dead	1	4	3/4	0.500
1440	Alive	0	3	1	0.500
1777	Dead	1	2	1/2	0.250
2520	Alive	0	1	1	0.250

r=number of patients with survival times T or more
$P=1-d/r$

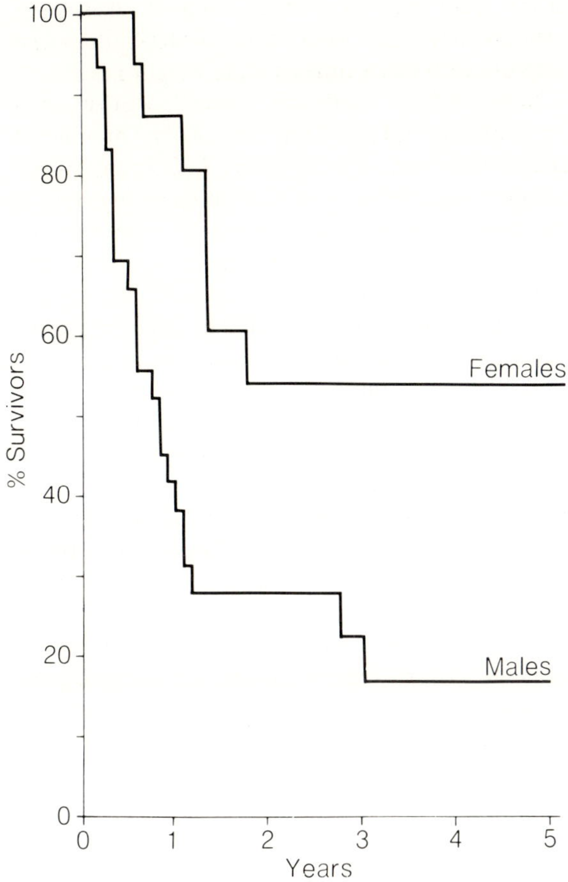

Fig. 18.1. Survival curves for 29 men and 15 women with stage 3 cancer of the mouth treated at the Christie Hospital and Holt Radium Institute, 1966–1970.

and 15 women, with stage 3 cancer of the mouth treated at the Christie Hospital and Holt Radium Institute between 1966 and 1970. Note how these survival curves were drawn. For females, the first death occurred 7 months after treatment and the percentage of survivors is 100% up to that time, while at 7 months the curve drops down to 93% where it remains constant until the next death a month later. One male patient died less than a month after treatment, and since times were calculated in months, his (exact) survival time was zero. The survival curve for males therefore starts at a value less than 100%. The patterns for the two curves are the same: the curves are horizontal *between* death times and vertical *at* death times. If groups of patients do in fact differ in their survival experience (and Fig. 18.1 suggests a substantial difference between the sexes here) then the most sensitive and effective method of showing it is by means of life table probabilities or survival curves.

The Berkson-Gage Method

Until a few years ago, a different method was almost always used. In this the time scale is split up into intervals, of 1 year for example, and the number of deaths and censored survival times counted in each. A survival percentage is then calculated at the start of each interval and the curve is drawn as a series of straight lines connecting points on a graph. The method is to form a life table such as Table 18.3. Column 1 contains the intervals: 1-year intervals have been chosen here, but if survival times are particularly short, as would be the case for gastric or colon cancer, shorter intervals would be more appropriate, while for long-term follow-up of a group of patients with a cancer carrying a good prognosis, such as early cancer of the uterine cervix, intervals of 2, 3, or even 5 years could be chosen. The intervals do not need to be equal: there may be some advantage in choosing shorter intervals for the first few years when mortality is usually greatest.

The numbers of patients, d_x, dying each interval x to $x+1$ are counted and entered in the second column. The next column is for the number of patients W_x, with censored survival times. This includes patients alive on the day of the statistical analysis or the day last seen, and patients known alive previously and lost to follow-up. These are often called *withdrawn alive* patients. Whatever the causes, the numbers of such patients in each interval are counted and entered in the table.

The first entry in column four is the total number of patients entering the study, N_0. By definition all these patients were alive at the start of the first interval. The entry below N_0 in this column is the number of patients alive at the start of the next interval and this must be numerically equal to the number entering the study minus the numbers dying and withdrawn alive during the first interval. The remaining N_x values in this column are obtained in a similar way and the last figure should equal the sum of the final d_x and W_x. Thus, in the example, 47 patients were alive at 10 years, of whom 21 subsequently died and 26 were withdrawn alive.

This is the way the data are set out, and the remaining columns are used to calculate the survival percentages.

Column 5 is for the adjusted number at risk in an interval. This is $N'_x = N_x - W_x/2$. The adjustment is

Table 18.3. Life-table calculations using the Berkson-Gage method.

1 Interval in years X to $X+1$	2 Died d_x	3 With-drawn W_x	4 Alive at start of interval N_x	5 Adjusted number at risk N'_x	6 Estimated probability of death q_x	7 Estimated probability of survival P_x	8 Estimated % survivors at start of interval S_x
0<1	90	0	374	374.0	0.241	0.759	100.0%
1<2	76	0	284	284.0	0.268	0.732	75.9%
2<3	51	0	208	208.0	0.245	0.755	55.6%
3<4	25	12	157	151.0	0.166	0.834	42.0%
4<5	20	5	120	117.5	0.170	0.830	35.0%
5<6	7	9	95	90.5	0.077	0.923	29.1%
6<7	4	9	79	74.5	0.054	0.946	26.8%
7<8	1	3	66	64.5	0.016	0.984	25.4%
8<9	3	5	62	59.5	0.050	0.950	25.0%
9<10	2	5	54	51.5	0.039	0.961	23.7%
10–	21	26	47				22.8%

necessary because the W_x patients withdrawn alive during the interval are, by definition, not at risk of dying for the whole interval. The precise times at which they were withdrawn may be known, but it is generally satisfactory to assume that, on average, the patients were at risk for half the interval. This is equivalent to assuming that half of them were at risk for the entire interval, and hence the adjustment to N_x in the equation. $q_x = d_x/N'_x$ is then the probability of dying in the interval x to $x+1$, and this is recorded in column 6.

An alternative argument which leads to the same value for q_x is that if the W_x patients had not been withdrawn and if we can assume that they were subject to the same probability of dying as other patients, there would have been about $\frac{1}{2}q_x W_x$ more deaths. The total number of deaths would then have been $d_x + \frac{1}{2}q_x W_x$, and therefore

$$q_x = \frac{d_x + \frac{1}{2}q_x W_x}{N_x}$$

Rearranging the equation gives

$$q_x = \frac{d_x}{N_x - W_x/2} \quad \text{as before}$$

If q_x is the probability of dying during the interval x to $x+1$, the probability of surviving the interval is $P_x = 1 - q_x$ (column 7).

The probability S_x of surviving to the end of a certain interval is then obtained by the successive multiplication of P_x values: $S_x = P_0 \times P_1 \times \ldots \times P_{x-1}$.

For example, the probability of surviving 3 years is $S_3 = P_0 \times P_1 \times P_2 = 0.759 \times 0.732 \times 0.755 = 0.420$.

Again it is usual to multiply this by 100% and call it the percentage of survivors at 3 years, or the *3-year survival rate*. These survival percentages may be plotted graphically and the survival curve is drawn as straight lines joining the points on the graph.

Terminology

Unfortunately confusion can be created by the lack of an agreed terminology. The consensus of opinion seems to be that the term *crude survival* refers to the situation when all patients have complete follow-up, while a *life-table* or *actuarial* method must be used when follow-up is incomplete for some patients. The methods available for calculating life-table or actuarial survival percentages are probably best referred to as the *Kaplan-Meier* method, and the *Berkson-Gage* method. In the first we have seen that the percentage of survivors is recalculated at each death time so that when plotted the curve takes on a characteristic appearance of horizontal and vertical lines, while in the second method the time scale is divided into intervals and the percentage of survivors is calculated at the start of each interval. The survival curve is then a series of straight lines joining points on a graph. Figure 18.2 shows survival curves calculated by each method using the same data, namely the survival times of 90 patients undergoing block dissection for metastatic malignant melanoma. Yearly intervals were chosen for the Berkson-Gage survival curve and it is seen that the two methods give very similar estimates at exact

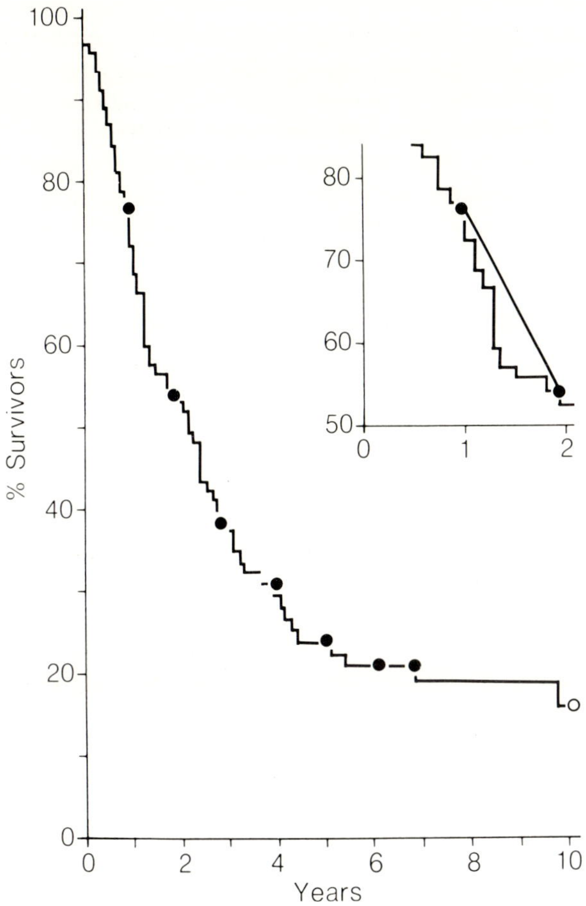

Fig. 18.2. Life-table survival curves calculated using the Kaplan-Meier and Berkson-Gage methods. Ninety patients with metastatic malignant melanoma undergoing block dissection.

years of follow-up, while at other times the curves may differ by, at most, about 10%. (For greater clarity in the figure, the points calculated by the Berkson-Gage method have not been joined with straight lines, except in the enlarged inset portion of the graph.)

With large numbers of patients, the disadvantage of the Kaplan-Meier method was that the calculations were very tedious, but now that computers are available in so many hospitals this is no longer important. For small numbers of patients the Kaplan-Meier method is always preferable since the precise times at which deaths occurred can be seen and the small number of steps in the survival curve reminds the reader of the paucity of the data.

Standard Errors of Survival Percentages

The percentages in the life table are subject to sampling variation, and if the number of patients is small this variation can be appreciable. Also, if a life-table method is used, the sampling variation becomes progressively larger as the survival percentages at later times are based on fewer and fewer patients. A knowledge of the sampling variation is important, since it is a measure of the range of survival percentages which we would be likely to encounter if the study could be repeated under identical circumstances with different groups of patients.

The standard error of a crude survival percentage S_t is just

$$\sqrt{\frac{S_t\,(100-S_t)}{N}}$$

where N is the number of patients in the group.

For a survival percentage S_t calculated using the Kaplan-Meier method, the standard error is the square root of the variance, which is found from the expression

$$(S_t)^2 \sum \frac{d_i}{r_i\,(r_i-d_i)}$$

where the summation is over times at which deaths occurred prior to time t, and d_i and r_i are as defined previously. A computationally simpler quantity is:

$$\frac{(S_t)^2\,(100-S_t)}{100\,N}$$

This is usually bigger than the correct variance but the difference is often slight.

If the Berkson-Gage method has been employed, the variance is

$$(S_t)^2 \sum \frac{d_i}{N_i\,(N_i-d_i)}$$

where the summation is over time intervals less than t, and d_i and N_i are as defined previously.

Mistakes in Interpreting Survival Curves

It is a mistake to try to read too much into the fine detail of a survival curve; in fact its general shape gives a better description of the survival experienced by a group of patients. Particular care must be exercised in interpreting the right hand end of curves: if the number of patients at risk is small then the curve will either plateau or show dramatic drops and these should not be interpreted as demonstrating either cure or sudden increase in mortality at a particular time. It is sometimes instructive to write somewhere on the graph the numbers of patients at risk at several different times so that the reader has an impression of the reliability of the estimates of the survival percentages. Alternatively, if standard errors have been calculated, they may be shown as error bars or confidence limits on the graph.

Corrections for Deaths from Unrelated Causes

The average age of all patients treated at the Christie Hospital and Holt Radium Institute is about 60 years, and a quarter of all patients are aged 70 or more. This inevitably means that some deaths will be from causes completely unrelated to the cancer for which treatment was given, and the survival curve for a group of patients may therefore give too pessimistic an estimate of mortality from that type of cancer. Fortunately methods are available which make an adjustment for the effects of intercurrent deaths.

It is well known that death certificates are not always accurate, but if patients have been subjected to regular, frequent, and careful clinical follow-up it is often possible to distinguish between related and unrelated deaths. The first method of correction is to modify the life-table method by giving censored rather than exact survival times to those patients who died from unrelated causes. The assumption underlying this change is that a patient who died of a completely unrelated cause, say $7\frac{1}{2}$ years after treatment, would have been available for further follow-up and would therefore have continued to be at risk of dying from cancer if it had not been for his unrelated intercurrent death. Effectively, therefore, as far as the statistical analysis is concerned, he is the same as a person treated $7\frac{1}{2}$ years ago who was alive with no follow-up.

This method of correction should be used only when detailed information concerning the cause of death is available for all patients in the study. Moreover one must be sure that censored rather than exact survival times are given only to those patients for whom the cause of death was completely unrelated to the cancer for which treatment was given. If there is any doubt about the cause of death (for example whether disease in the lung was a metastasis or a new primary) then the safer course is to assume that death was from the cancer for which treatment was given, so that censored survival times are reserved only for those deaths, such as accidents, which were unambiguously from unrelated causes. Adequate though cumbersome terms for this method of correction would seem to be: *percentages of survivors corrected for observed intercurrent deaths,* or *percentages of survivors (patients dying of unrelated causes counted as survivors).*

Age correction is an alternative procedure which has the advantage that causes of death do not need to be known. The first step is to calculate the proportions of the initial group of patients expected to survive various lengths of time after treatment if each patient had been subject only to the mortality (from all causes) which was normal for his or her age and sex. Fortunately these probabilities for the population as a whole have been calculated from death records and published, and a short extract appears in Table 18.4. The remaining calculations are easy as a simple example will show.

Example Ten men were treated for cancer in the period 1951–1955; their ages were 61, 62, 62, 64, 66, 67, 69, 73, 73, and 77 years. What proportion

Table 18.4. Probabilities of surviving 5 years, by age for males, England and Wales, 1951–1955 (derived from Case et al. 1970).

Age group (years)	Probability of surviving 5 years
0–4	0.9672
5–9	0.9973
10–14	0.9976
15–19	0.9957
20–24	0.9938
25–29	0.9937
30–34	0.9925
35–39	0.9895
40–44	0.9839
45–49	0.9718
50–54	0.9490
55–59	0.9163
60–64	0.8668
65–69	0.7990
70–74	0.7084
75–79	0.5759
80–84	0.4238
85–89	0.2976
90–94	0.1454
95–	0.0385

Table 18.5.

Age group (years)	No. of men, n_x	Probability of surviving 5 years, P_x	Expected number of 5-year survivors, ${}_5e_x$
60–64	4	0.8668	3.4672
65–69	3	0.7990	2.3970
70–74	2	0.7084	1.4168
75–79	1	0.5759	0.5759

${}_5e_x = n_x \cdot {}_5P_x$

would we expect to survive (1) 5 years, (2) 10 years, and (3) 15 years, if they were subject only to normal mortality for their age and sex prevailing in that period?

First of all the numbers of patients in each 5-year age group are tabulated as in Table 18.5. Expected survival probabilities are extracted from Table 18.4 and the numbers in the final column of Table 18.5 are found by multiplying the entries in columns 2 and 3. These are then the expected numbers of 5-year survivors in each age group, so the total expected number is the sum of these. If there were females in the group, expected numbers of survivors in each age group would be found in exactly the same way using normal survival probabilities for females, and added into the total expected number of survivors. In the example, the total expected number of 5-year survivors is 7.8569 and the expected proportion is therefore this number divided by 10, the total number of patients. The answer is therefore 0.78569, or roughly 0.79. The proportions of patients expected to survive 10 years and 15 years are found in exactly the same way except that we now use ${}_{10}P_x$ and ${}_{15}P_x$ normal probabilities instead of the ${}_5P_x$ values. These new probabilities can be derived from the tabulated ${}_5P_x$ values when it is realised that the probability of surviving 10 years from age x equals the probability of surviving 5 years from age x times the probability of surviving a *further* 5 years. This second probability is obtained from the tabulated probabilities for the *next* 5-year period and should be the value for the *next* 5-year age group, since a patient aged, say, 45 at the time of treatment will be aged 50 five years later. Fifteen-year survival probabilities are obtained by successive multiplications of *three* ${}_5P_x$ values, each time advancing one quinquennium and one age group. Table 18.6 shows how the next few steps in the calculations are carried out. Finally by totalling the e_x values we find the expected numbers of 10-year and 15-year survivors are 5.57755 and 3.412; and thus the expected proportions are approximately 0.56 and 0.34 respectively.

The *relative survival rate at n years* is defined as the ratio:

$$\frac{\text{crude or actuarial percentage of survivors at } n \text{ years}}{\text{expected proportion of survivors at } n \text{ years}}$$

This is often called the *age-corrected survival rate*. If only three out of ten men were actually alive 5 years after treatment, the crude survival rate would be 30% but the relative survival rate would be 30/0.79=38%. Likewise, if only two men survived 10 years and only one 15 years the relative survival rates at these times would be 20/0.56=36% and 10/0.34=29% respectively.

Valuable though this method of age correction is, it has several disadvantages. Patients with cancer in a specific site may have a higher risk of dying from some other cause. For example, in patients with laryngeal cancer there is some evidence to suggest that mortality from lung cancer

Table 18.6.

Age group (years)	No. of men, n_x	Probability of surviving 10 years, ${}_{10}P_x$	Expected 10-year survivors, ${}_{10}e_x$	Probability of surviving 15 years, ${}_{15}P_x$	Expected 15-year survivors, ${}_{15}e_x$
60–64	4	0.6962	2.7848	0.4937	1.9748
65–69	3	0.5679	1.7037	0.3339	1.0017
70–74	2	0.4184	0.8368	0.1852	0.3704
75–79	1	0.2502	0.2502	0.0651	0.0651

${}_{10}e_x = n_x \cdot {}_{10}P_x$

${}_{15}e_x = n_x \cdot {}_{15}P_x$

may be higher. Cancer patients are also likely to be drawn from a specific region and the $_5P_x$ for the whole of England and Wales may not be entirely suitable. This author has calculated correction factors which reflect the increased mortality which is known to exist at most ages in the North-West of England, the area from which patients treated at the Christie Hospital and Holt Radium Institute are drawn.

In the case of occupationally induced cancers, patients may tend to come from an even more specific geographic location where the normal survival probabilities may be appreciably different. Finally, some patients, such as those with cancer of the breast or uterine cervix, have a social class distribution different from the rest of the population, and it is well known that both overall mortality and specific causes of death vary between social classes. Unfortunately the $_5P_x$ values available at the present time lack these refinements, nevertheless the effort of calculating expected proportions of survivors is often worthwhile. It should be noted, however, that it is not generally considered useful to correct the survival of two groups obtained by random allocation (as for example in a clinical trial) in order to refine a treatment comparison, since we would expect the groups to have very similar age and sex distributions, and therefore very similar expected survival proportions.

The Concept of Cure

In evaluating the results of cancer treatments, it has long been conventional to pay special attention to 5-year survival percentages. For most types of cancer, mortality is greatest in the first year after treatment but declines continuously thereafter, so that the situation 5 years after treatment has always seemed a convenient yardstick for assessing therapeutic effectiveness. However, survival does not imply cure and undoubtedly some deaths do occur later than 5 years and survival curves generally continue downwards up to 15 years or more following treatment. Can we then ever speak of the cure of cancer in the same way that we can speak of the cure of other diseases? The answer is that we can, providing cure is defined in a statistically valid way. In the words of the late Marion Russell, formerly statistician at the Christie Hospital and Holt Radium Institute, "We may speak of the cure of a disease when there remains a group of survivors whose annual death rate from all causes is similar to that of a normal population group of the same sex and age distribution."

This eminently sensible and realistic definition thus relates cure to the normal life expectancy of the general population. To demonstrate curability, or otherwise, two curves are constructed: one showing the *actual* percentages of survivors and the other showing the *expected* percentages. Comparison between death rates in the two groups can be made most easily by plotting the curves on the same graph with a logarithmic vertical scale, since in this case when the rates are the same the curves become parallel. Now we can say that the group of patients who were still alive at the time at which parallelism was achieved were cured of their malignant disease, by virtue of our definition, while the point on the vertical scale at which the observed survival curve starts to run parallel to the expected curve indicates the *level* of definitive cure.

In the section on methods of correction for intercurrent deaths, it was shown how to estimate the percentages or proportions of a group who would be expected to survive 5, 10, and 15 years. In assessing curability, however, the expected curve must be calculated in a different way because the question now is whether a group of survivors, say patients who are still alive 5 years after treatment, have the same chance of surviving a *further* 5 years as an identical group from the normal population. If the 5-year survivors cannot be considered cured, perhaps the 10-year survivors will meet the stringent requirements of our definition of cure.

This question is answered by first calculating, in the way that has already been described, the proportion of the entire group who would be expected to survive 5 years. Denote this value by P_1. The next step is to take the age and sex distributions of the *5-year survivors* and by carrying out the same calculations determine the proportion of these who would survive a further 5 years, remembering to advance each individual to the next age group and 5-year period. Denote this value by P_2. Similarly P_3 is the proportion of the 10-year survivors expected to survive a further 5 years.

The expected survival curve then has the following values: $100 \times P_1$ at 5 years; $100 \times P_1 \times P_2$ at 10 years; and $100 \times P_1 \times P_2 \times P_3$ at 15 years.

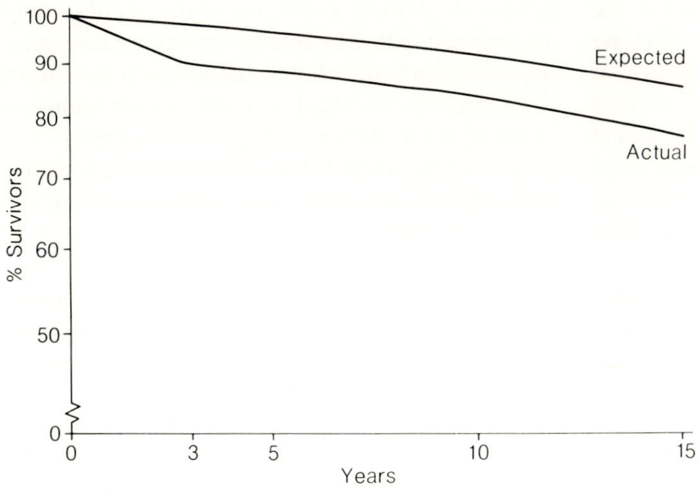

Fig. 18.3. One hundred and twenty-one (121) men with seminoma of the testis, treated at the Christie Hospital and Holt Radium Institute, 1956–1962, following orchidectomy elsewhere. Comparison of actual (*lower*) and expected (*upper*) survival curves.

Example Between 1956 and 1962, 121 men with seminoma of the testis were referred to the Christie Hospital following orchidectomy elsewhere. They were regarded as postoperatively free from malignancy and received a course of X-ray treatment to the abdomen. Since all were treated more than 15 years ago and none had been lost to follow-up, crude percentages of survivors were calculated at 3, 5, 10, and 15 years and plotted as the lower curve in Fig. 18.3. The proportions expected to survive a further 5 years were calculated for the initial group, for the 5-year survivors, and for the 10-year survivors in the way described earlier. The expected curve was found by multiplying these proportions and is shown in Fig. 18.3.

It is clear by comparing the curves that parallelism is reached by the third year after treatment and there appears to be no divergence from parallelism in the follow-up period considered. Thus we can say, according to our definition, that the 90% of men alive 3 years after treatment were cured of their cancer.

Tests of Statistical Significance

A Test between two Survival Percentages at a Fixed Point in Time

Suppose among N_1 patients the percentage of survivors (crude or relative) is $P_1\%$, and among a different group of N_2 patients it is $P_2\%$. Providing N_1 and N_2 are both greater than 30, calculate:

$$z = \frac{P_1 - P_2}{\sqrt{\dfrac{P_1\,(100-P_1)}{N_1} + \dfrac{P_2\,(100-P_2)}{N_2}}}$$

If z is negative, ignore the sign. For z between zero and 1.96 the difference between P_1 and P_2 is not statistically significant ($p>0.05$) while if z is greater than 1.96 the difference is statistically significant ($p<0.05$). Sometimes the actual value of p may be preferred; this may be found from tables in most text-books of statistics.

If either N_1 or N_2 is less than 30, then instead calculate:

$$t = \frac{P_1 - P_2}{\sqrt{P\,(100-P)\left(\dfrac{1}{N_1} + \dfrac{1}{N_2}\right)}}$$

where $P = \dfrac{N_1 P_1 + N_2 P_2}{N_1 + N_2}$ and also $\mathrm{df} = N_1 + N_2 - 2$

Again, the sign of t should be ignored if it is negative. The value of p can be obtained from a table of Student's t-distribution which may be found in any statistics textbook.

If P_1 and P_2 are calculated using an actuarial method, then the same equations can be used to calculate z or t except that N_1 and N_2 should be the numbers of patients at risk at the fixed point in time rather than the numbers of patients in the groups at the start.

It should be noted that these tests of statistical significance are valid only if the point in time, say 3 years or 5 years, is chosen *before* the survival percentages are calculated. This is to avoid any suggestion that a particular time has been chosen in order to maximise (or minimise) the difference in survival between the two groups. Furthermore, only one time should be chosen, since comparisons at a large number of times, say each year up to 15 years after treatment, vastly increase the chance that at least one of them will be misleadingly significant.

Although these tests are not *efficient* in the statistical sense, since only one point on each survival curve is selected and the remainder ignored, they are simple; the appropriate significance test should always be carried out whenever survival percentages are compared.

Tests between Survival Curves

The logrank test overcomes one of the disadvantages of the tests already described by comparing entire survival curves rather than survival percentages at just one time. Apart from its efficiency in using all the data which go to make up the survival curves, it is also in many cases the most powerful test statistically in the sense that if there really is a difference in survival between groups, the logrank test is more likely than any other test to yield a statistically significant result. This test is therefore recommended and should be carried out whenever possible. It is not the author's intention to provide a detailed account of the calculations required since a very good description (with examples) appears in Peto et al. (1976, 1977). (The reader is urged to read the two parts of this publication carefully since they also cover some of the material in this chapter.)

The logrank test and the other tests of statistical significance already described have other useful features which arise when three or more groups are being compared, since it is then possible to obtain separate p-values for *heterogeneity* and *trend*. The p-value for heterogeneity is the probability (on the null hypothesis of no real difference in survival between the groups) that the observed differences are due to chance alone. However, if the groups are ordered—for example the groups might consist of patients with different stages of disease—then it is preferable to make use of the ordering by examining the data for a *trend* in prognosis. The trend test reveals not only whether there is a difference but whether the difference is a meaningful one in which the middle groups have average prognosis and the outer groups have different prognosis in opposite directions. This test takes into account the natural ordering of the groups and answers the question whether there is a trend for prognosis to worsen (or improve) as we move from the first to the last group. Whenever more than two groups are being compared, and they have a natural order, the trend test is both more sensitive and the more medically relevant test to use.

The other useful feature of these tests is that the p-value for a comparison may be refined by making an adjustment for the concomitant effect of one or more other prognostic features such as stage or age. For example, in a group of 447 patients with mouth cancer treated at the Christie Hospital and Holt Radium Institute between 1968 and 1971 the influence on survival of the site of cancer within the oral cavity was examined. Five sites were defined—cheek, alveolus, hard palate, floor of mouth, and anterior two-thirds of the tongue—and the variation in survival between patients with these sites was not statistically significant (logrank test, $p=0.5$). It was found, however, that patients with cancer arising in the anterior tongue tended to be slightly younger and to have somewhat less extensive disease than patients with cancer of other parts of the mouth, and patients with alveolar cancer tended to have more extensive disease. Since the stage of the disease had a very marked effect on survival, whatever the site, and younger patients fared significantly better, patients with cancer of the anterior tongue were already in a more favourable category. If they had been similar to patients with other sites of cancer in respect of age and stage of disease their survival would have been somewhat worse. In addition, if the patients with alveolar cancer had had the same proportions of patients in each stage as the other patients with mouth cancer, their survival experience would have been better. Suitable adjustments were made to the survival percentages to take into account the dissimilarities between the groups in age and stage distributions, and the adjusted p-value, 0.0001, indicated a statistically highly significant difference. It was concluded that cancer of the cheek carries a relatively good prognosis and cancer of the anterior tongue a relatively bad prognosis compared with cancers of the alveolus, floor, and hard palate, and that this had been concealed by the simultaneous influence of other prognostic features.

Concluding Remarks

The prognosis of a patient with cancer undoubtedly depends on a number of factors, some of which are obvious to the clinician, for example stage and age, while other more subtle effects may be revealed only by detailed statistical analysis of data from a large number of patients. Knowledge of prognostic factors is important in differentiating between those patients with a favourable outcome, who might be spared hazardous or toxic procedures, and those patients with a poor outcome, in whom novel treatments might be attempted. New treatments, or new combinations of existing treatments, must, of course, be subjected to rigorous evaluation in randomised controlled clinical trials. Statisticians have developed over recent years a number of powerful statistical methods, including the necessary computer programs, for the design and analysis of clinical trials. Most oncologists have been convinced for many years by the ethical and scientific arguments for carrying out such trials and it is hoped that the continued collaboration of statisticians, oncologists, and other scientists will result in substantial improvements during the next decade in the treatment of patients with cancer.

References

Statistical Methods

Armitage P (1971) Statistical methods in medical research. Blackwell Scientific, Oxford and Edinburgh

Castle W (1972) Statistics in small doses. Churchill Livingstone, Edinburgh and London

Clinical Trial Design

Peto R et al. (1976) Design and analysis of randomised clinical trials requiring prolonged observation of each patient, Part I Br J Cancer 34: 585–612

Peto R et al. (1977) Design and analysis of randomised clinical trials requiring prolonged observation of each patient, Part II. Br J Cancer 35: 1–38

Life Tables

Case RAM, Coghill C, Hartley JL, Peason JT (1970) The Chester Beatty Research Institute serial abridged life tables, England and Wales 1841–1870. Chester Beatty Research Institute

Appendix 1
Physical Data

Rules for Planar Mould Treatments

The amount of activity to be used is determined from Table 1. In the following the treating distance is represented by h, while d represents the diameter of a circular mould and l the length of the side of a square mould. The dose is stated at the treated surface.

Circles

Arrange sources uniformly round the circumference; the space between the active ends of each source must not exceed h. The minimum number of sources is 6.

1) When $d \leq 3h$ all the activity should be placed on the circumference of the circle.
2) When the ratio d/h is greater than 3 and less than 6, 5% of the total activity should be placed at the centre of the circle.
3) For larger areas use two concentric circles and a centre spot as follows:
   a) Put 3% of the total activity at the centre.
   b) Use percentages of the total activity on the circumference as below:

d/h	6	$7\frac{1}{2}$	10
Percentage of activity in circumference	80	75	70

   c) Distribute the remainder of the activity on a circle of diameter $d/2$.

Squares

Arrange sources in lines round the periphery with uniform linear density (mg/cm); the space between the active ends of each source must not exceed h.

1) When l is not greater than $2h$ no additional lines are required.
2) Additional lines should be added when necessary to divide the area into strips of width not greater than $2h$.
   a) For 1 added line use linear density one-half of that of the periphery
   b) For 2 or more added lines use linear density two-thirds of that of the periphery

Elongated Areas

1) If the area is rectangular, proceed as for a square but any added lines must be parallel to the longer sides.
2) If the area is elliptical, proceed as for a circle using a diameter which is the average of the two axes of the ellipse.
3) Elongation correction. The milligram-hours per 1000 cGy table (Table 1) applies only to circles and squares. For elongated areas a correction must be made to increase the milligram-hours as follows:

Ratio of sides of rectangle or of axes of ellipse	2:1	3:1	4.1
Percentage to be added	5	9	12

Curved Surfaces

For curvatures up to a degree corresponding to a hemisphere or semicylinder, the above rules may be applied with the following proviso:

1) *Convex areas*. The amount of activity required should be calculated for the area treated, but distributed over the corresponding larger area on the applicator.
2) *Concave areas*. The amount of activity should be calculated using the area of the applicator.

Gold Seed Moulds

The above rules are used for distribution of the activity. The treatment time is continuous for 7 days, and in order to determine the amount of activity required, it has been calculated that 1 "Equivalent MBq" of gold-198 is then equivalent to 0.6 mg h of radium filtered by 0.5 mm platinum. Using this factor Table 1 may be used in the usual way.

Rules for Implant Treatments

Planar Implants

The amount of activity to be used for a single-plane implant is determined from Table 1 using a treating distance of 0.5 cm. The dose is stated at this distance.

1) Use fractions of the total activity on the periphery, as follows:

Area (cm^2)	<25	>25 and <100	>100
Fraction of activity on periphery	2/3	1/2	1/3

   Distribute the remainder of the activity evenly over the area.
2) Needles should be arranged in parallel lines, with the active ends crossed using needles placed at right angles to these. For calculation purposes for each uncrossed end deduct percentages from the area as follows:

Linear density of centre needles compared with periphery needles	1/2	2/3	1
Percentage to be deducted	7	10	15

3) The spacing between adjacent needles should be not more than 1 cm.
4) An elongation correction should be employed as under "Elongated Areas" in the rules for planar mould treatments above.
5) Two-plane implants.
   a) The activity on each plane should be distributed as above, increasing the total activity required by a factor which depends on the separation of the two planes. The dose is stated at 0.5 cm from the plane of the needles on the inside.

Separation of planes (cm)	1.5	2.0	2.5
Factor	1.25	1.4	1.5

   b) If the two planes differ in area, the area to be used for calculation purposes is the average of the two, and the activity distributed pro rata to each plane.
   c) For the largest of these separations, especially for smaller areas, the dose in the midplane will be significantly less than the stated dose.

Volume Implants (Cylinders)

The amount of activity to be used is determined using Table 2.

1) Total activity is distributed as:

Outer ring	4 parts
Core	2 parts
Each end	1 part

2) The outer ring (belt) should consist of not less than eight needles, and not less than four needles should be distributed evenly through the volume (to form the core).
3) If it is impossible to cross one or both ends, the volume used for calculation purposes must be reduced by $7\frac{1}{2}\%$ for each open end. The activity is then distributed as:
   Belt 4 parts, core 2 parts, end 1 part
   or
   Belt 4 parts, core 2 parts
4) Where the crossing needles are placed at the level of the tips of the needles, instead of at the level of the active ends as assumed above, and only one end is crossed, the distribution of activity is:
   Belt 4 parts, core 2 parts, end 2 parts

If both ends are crossed at the tips the distribution is:

Belt 4 parts, core 2 parts, each end 2 parts

5) *Elongation correction.* Table 2 applies only where all dimensions are equal, and for irregularly shaped volumes a correction must be made to increase the milligram-hours as follows:

Ratio of largest to smallest dimensions	1.5:1	2:1	2.5:1	3:1
Percentage to be added	3	6	10	15

Gold Seed Implants

The planar implant rules may be used together with Table 1. The implant is permanent, and in order to determine the amount of activity required, it has been calculated that 1 "equivalent MBq" of gold-198 is then equivalent to 0.72 mg-h of radium filtered by 0.5 mm platinum. The spacing between individual seeds should not exceed 1 cm.

Table 1. Planar implant and mould table. Milligram-hours per 1000 cGy: radium with 0.5 mm platinum filtration

Area	Treating distance *h* (cm)					
(cm^2)	0.5	1.0	1.5	2.0	2.5	3.0
0	32	129	289	514	804	1157
1	73	185	353	585	874	1230
2	105	230	405	646	934	1293
3	130	267	454	702	993	1353
4	152	300	499	754	1048	1409
5	174	331	540	801	1101	1465
6	191	360	579	845	1151	1517
7	207	388	614	885	1200	1570
8	222	415	647	923	1247	1620
9	239	441	677	960	1290	1668
10	254	468	707	997	1334	1717
11	268	493	737	1033	1375	1762
12	282	518	767	1069	1417	1807
13	296	542	795	1103	1456	1850
14	311	566	825	1137	1497	1893
15	326	589	852	1170	1537	1935
16	340	611	879	1202	1577	1976
17	354	632	905	1232	1611	2016
18	369	653	932	1264	1647	2057
19	383	673	957	1293	1681	2097
20	397	692	983	1323	1715	2137
22	424	728	1037	1382	1782	2213
24	450	764	1089	1442	1849	2286
26	477	796	1140	1499	1909	2363
28	503	828	1188	1553	1972	2434
30	529	859	1233	1606	2030	2506
32	554	889	1280	1660	2091	2570
34	580	922	1324	1714	2151	2637
36	603	949	1369	1769	2212	2702
38	627	982	1413	1820	2268	2767
40	651	1009	1454	1871	2324	2830
42	674	1039	1495	1922	2379	2891
44	696	1069	1534	1971	2435	2952
46	718	1096	1574	2020	2489	3011
48	740	1126	1609	2068	2542	3070
50	761	1158	1644	2115	2594	3129

Table 2. Volume implant table.

Volume (cm^3)	mg h per 1000 cGy
2	58
4	93
6	122
8	147
10	171
12	193
14	214
16	234
18	253
20	271
22	289
24	306
26	323
28	340
30	356
32	371
34	387
36	402
38	416
40	431
42	445
44	459
46	473
48	486
50	500
52	513
54	526
56	539
58	552
60	564
62	577
64	589
66	601
68	614
70	626
72	637
74	649
76	661
78	672
80	684
82	695
84	706
86	718
88	729
90	740
92	751
94	761
96	772
98	783
100	793

Table 3. Gold-198 single-plane moulds (7 days).

Diameter (cm)	Circumference (cm)	Area (cm^2)	MBq of Au-198 to deliver, dose at 0.5 cm (cGy)				MBq of Au-198 to deliver, dose at 1.0 cm (cGy)			
			5000	5250	5500	5750	5000	5250	5500	5750
1.0	3.1	0.8	540	560	590	620	1440	1510	1590	1660
1.5	4.7	1.8	810	850	890	930	1830	1920	2010	2100
2.0	6.3	3.1	1110	1160	1220	1280	2260	2380	2490	2600
2.5	7.9	4.9	1430	1510	1580	1650	2730	2870	3010	3150
3.0	9.4	7.1	1730	1820	1910	1990	3250	3410	3570	3740
3.5	11.0	9.6	2070	2170	2280	2380	3820	4010	4200	4390
4.0	12.6	12.6	2420	2540	2660	2780	4430	4650	4870	5090
4.5	14.1	15.9	2820	2960	3100	3250	5070	5330	5580	5840
5.0	15.7	19.6	3270	3430	3590	3760	5710	5990	6280	6570
5.5	17.3	23.8	3720	3910	4100	4280	6330	6650	6960	7280

Table 4. Mould distribution rules (%).

Diameter (cm) for mould at 0.5 cm	<1.5	1.5 to <3	3	4	5
Diameter (cm) for mould at 1.0 cm	<3	3.0 to <6	6	7.5	10
Preferred: Centre spot	0	5	3	3	3
Preferred: Inner ring	0	0	17	22	27
Preferred: Periphery	100	95	80	75	70

1 MBq Au-198 for 7 days is equivalent to 0.6 mg h (radium).
Half-life of Au-198 is 2.70 days.

Table 5. Gold-198 permanent implant table.

Diameter (cm)	Circumference (cm)	Area (cm^2)	MBq of Au-198 to deliver, dose at 0.5 cm (cGy)			
			5000	5250	5500	5750
1.0	3.1	0.8	450	470	490	510
1.5	4.7	1.8	680	710	750	780
2.0	6.3	3.1	920	970	1020	1060
2.5	7.9	4.9	1190	1250	1310	1370
3.0	9.4	7.1	1440	1520	1590	1660
3.5	11.0	9.6	1720	1810	1900	1980
4.0	12.6	12.6	2010	2110	2210	2320
4.5	14.1	15.9	2350	2470	2590	2700
5.0	15.7	19.6	2720	2860	2990	3130
5.5	17.3	23.8	3100	3260	3410	3570

1) For circles of diameter not greater than 5.5 cm, distribute $\frac{2}{3}$ of the activity round the periphery and $\frac{1}{3}$ uniformly over the area.
2) For ellipses of elongation less than 2:1 use circle whose diameter is the mean of the two axes.
3) Half-life of Au-198 is 2.70 days.
4) 1 MBq Au-198 to complete decay delivers a dose equivalent to 0.72 mg h (radium).

Appendix 2
Clinical Staging

Clinical Staging as practised at the Christie Hospital and Holt Radium Institute

The method of clinical staging as currently practised is given for each major disease group. The TNM classification is also given where this is felt to be appropriate. Where no defined staging is given an approximate division into "early" and "late" should be used. "Early" indicates a lesion confined to the area of origin and of "reasonable" size. "Late" indicates an extensive tumour or one where metastasis has occurred. For some disease groups, e.g. brain, no staging classification is recommended.

Notes on the recording of diagnosis for statistical purposes are also given.

Diagnosis

This refers to the status at the time of registration.

State

- ☐ Site of origin—e.g. mouth.
- ☐ Division of site of origin, where appropriate, e.g. mouth, floor.
- ☐ Right, left or bilateral.
- ☐ Histological type.
- ☐ Whether "new" or "postoperative".
  This refers to a definitive "cancer operation". Where a biopsy or in some cases a biopsy/excision only has been performed the disease should still be classified as "new".
- ☐ Whether "healed", "residual", or "recurrent". "Healed" indicates no clinically residual tumour (this does not refer to the state of the scar). The term healed may still be used if subclinical residue is suspected.
- ☐ Whether metastatic.

Code

- ☐ Insert K where the patient knows the diagnosis.

  Add benign if appropriate.

The designation "post-CT" should refer to a definitive course.

Bladder

Diagnosis

The term "postoperative" is to refer only to those cases where an open (per abdomen) resection has been carried out. Endoscopic resection or diathermy are to be recorded as "new".

Staging

The clinical staging is determined from the clinical examination, cystoscopy, bimanual pelvic examination and X-ray findings. It cannot be altered in the light of subsequent operative findings. Biopsy findings when indicating depth of penetration of the bladder wall shall be considered an operative finding.

Stage 1
Tumour limited to mucosa and submucosa. (No palpable mass on bimanual examination after resection of the tumour.)

Stage II
Tumour has extended into but not through the muscle layer. (Thickening in the bladder wall may be palpable on bimanual examination.)

Stage III
Tumour has penetrated into the extravesical tissue. (A mobile mass is palpable on bimanual examination.)

Stage IV
Tumour fixed to neighbouring organs or pelvic wall. (A fixed mass palpable on bimanual examination.) Distant metastases.

Breast

Diagnosis
The term "postoperative" is to refer only to a mastectomy (whether local, extended, or radical). Where an excision biopsy (or tylectomy) has been performed this is still to be recorded as "new".

Where a simple mastectomy has been performed for a stage III tumour this must be recorded as "residual".

The axilla, supraclavicular, infraclavicular, and parasternal node areas are to be recorded with the primary tumour and not as metastatic where they are involved.

Staging
With M0, classification by T and N gives stages as follows:—

Stage I	T1N0	T2N0
Stage II	T1N1	T2N1
Stage III	T1N2	T2N2
	T1N3	T2N3
	T3N0	T4N0
	T3N1	T4N1
	T3N2	T4N2
	T3N3	T4N3

With M1 stage must be IV.

TNM Classification of Breast (UICC 1968)

T Primary tumour.
T0 No evidence of primary tumour.
T1 Tumour 2 cm or less in greatest dimension.
Skin not involved, except in the case of Paget's disease confined to nipple.
No retraction of nipple.
No pectoral muscle fixation.
No chest wall fixation.
T2 Tumour more than 2 cm but not more than 5 cm in greatest dimension, *or* incomplete skin fixation (tethered or dimpled), *or* nipple retraction (in subareolar tumours), *or* Paget's disease extending beyond the nipple.
No pectoral muscle fixation.
No chest wall fixation.
T3 Tumour more than 5 cm but not more than 10 cm in greatest dimension, *or* skin fixation complete (infiltrated or ulcerated), *or peau d'orange* in tumour area, *or* pectoral muscle fixation* (incomplete or complete).
No chest wall fixation.

*Note: Incomplete pectoral muscle fixation indicates that contraction of the muscle limits tumour mobility. Complete pectoral muscle fixation indicates that contraction of the muscle abolishes tumour mobility.

T4 Tumour more than 10 cm in greatest dimension, *or* skin involvement *or peau d'orange* wide of tumour but not beyond breast area *or* chest wall* fixation.

*Note: The chest wall includes the ribs, intercostal muscles and serratus anterior muscle but not the pectoral muscle.

N Regional lymph nodes.
The clinician may record whether palpable nodes are considered to contain growth or not.
N0 No palpable homolateral axillary nodes.
N1 Movable homolateral axillary nodes.
N1a. Nodes not considered to contain growth.
N1b. Nodes considered to contain growth.
N2 Homolateral axillary nodes fixed to one another or to other structures.
N3 Homolateral supra- or infra-clavicular nodes movable or fixed *or* oedema of the arm.*

*Note: Oedema of the arm may be caused by lymphatic obstruction; lymph nodes may not then be palpable.

M Distant metastases.
M0 No evidence of distant metastases.
M1 Distant metastases present.
M1a. Skin involvement wide of breast.
M1b. Involvement of contralateral nodes or contralateral breast.
M1c. Clinical or radiographic evidence of metastases to lungs, pleural cavity, skeleton, liver, etc.

Larynx

Divisions	Sites
1. Supraglottis	
(i) Epilarynx (including marginal zone)	Posterior surface of suprahyoid epiglottis (including the tip) Aryepiglottic fold Arytenoid
(ii) Supraglottis, excluding epilarynx	Infrahyoid epiglottis Ventricular bands (false cords) Ventricular cavities
2. Glottis	Vocal cords Anterior commissure Posterior commissure
3. Subglottis	

TNM Classification (UICC 1974)

T Primary Tumour

1. Supraglottis

TIS Preinvasive carcinomas (carcinoma *in situ*).
T1 Tumour limited to the region with normal mobility.
T1a. Tumour confined to the laryngeal surface of the epiglottis or to an aryepiglottic fold or to a ventricular cavity or to a ventricular band.
T1b. Tumour involving the epiglottis and extending to the ventricular cavities or bands.
T2 Tumour of the epiglottis and/or ventricles or ventricular bands, and extending to the vocal cords, without fixation.
T3 Tumour limited to the larynx with fixation and/or destruction or other evidence of deep invasion.
T4 Tumour with direct extension beyond the larynx, i.e. to the pyriform sinus, or the postcricoid region or the vallecula or the base of tongue.

2. Glottis

TIS Preinvasive carcinoma (carcinoma *in situ*).
T1 Tumour limited to the region with normal mobility.
T1a. Tumour confined to one cord.
T1b. Tumour involving both cords.
T2 Tumour extending to either the subglottic or the supraglottic regions (i.e. to the ventricular bands or the ventricles), with normal or impaired mobility.
T3 Tumour limited to the larynx with fixation of one or both cords.
T4 Tumour extending beyond the larynx, i.e. into cartilage of the pyriform sinus or the postcricoid region or the skin.

3. Subglottis

TIS Preinvasive carcinoma (carcinoma *in situ*).
T1 Tumour limited to the region with normal mobility.
T1a. Tumour limited to one side of the subglottic region and not involving the under surface of the cord.
T1b. Tumour extending to both sides of the subglottic region and not involving the under surface of the cords.
T2 Tumour involving the subglottic region and extending to one or both cords.
T3 Tumour limited to the larynx with fixation of one or both cords.
T4 Tumour extending beyond the larynx, i.e. to the postcricoid region or the trachea or the skin.

N Regional Lymph Nodes

N0 Regional lymph nodes not palpable.
N1 Movable homolateral nodes.
N1a. Nodes not considered to contain growth.
N1b. Nodes considered to contain growth.
N2 Movable contralateral or bilateral nodes.
N2a. Nodes not considered to contain growth.
N2b. Nodes considered to contain growth.
N3 Fixed nodes.

M Distant Metastases

M0 No evidence of distant metastases.
M1 Distant metastases present.

Lip

Divisions
Upper
Lower
Commissure

Note: If the growth arises from the skin of the lip as opposed to the vermilion border this should be recorded as skin lip.

Stage I
Growth not spread beyond site of origin and less than 2 cm maximum diameter.

Stage II
More extensive tumour but has maximum diameter of less than 4 cm.

Stage III
Primary growth as stages I and II.
Mobile unilateral nodes considered to contain growth.

Stage IV
Primary growth more extensive than stage II.
Bilateral or fixed nodes.
Distant metastases present.

Lung

Divisions
Bronchus
Pleura

Staging of primary carcinoma of bronchus
Stage as "early" or "late".

Early—A primary carcinoma of lung not more than 5 cm diameter confined to the lung.

Late—Any tumour which is bigger than 5 cm diameter, and has spread outside the lung, e.g. to chest wall, hilar or mediastinal nodes, or beyond.

Lymphoma

The Ann Arbor Classification

Stage	Extent
I	Nodal involvement within one region.
IE	Single extralymphatic organ or site.
II	Nodal involvement within two or more regions, limited by the diaphragm.
IIE	Localised extranodal site and nodal involvement within one or more regions limited by the diaphragm.
III	Nodal involvement of regions above and below the diaphragm.
IIIE	Nodal involvement of regions above and below the diaphragm with localised extralymphatic site.
IIIS	Nodal involvement of regions above and below the diaphragm with spleen involvement.
IIIES	Nodal involvement of regions above and below the diaphragm with localised extralymphatic site and spleen involvement.
IV	Diffuse or disseminated involvement of one or more extralymphatic organs or tissues, with or without node involvement.

Systemic Symptoms
A or B denotes the absence or presence, respectively, of documented unexplained fever above 38 °C, night sweats, or unexplained weight loss of more than 10% in 6 months. NB: pruritus alone no longer qualifies for B classification.

Mouth

Divisions
Cheek
Floor
Tongue (anterior $\frac{2}{3}$)
Hard palate
Upper alveolus
Lower alveolus

Note the tonsils, faucial pillars, posterior $\frac{1}{3}$ of tongue, and soft palate are included under "pharynx".

TNM Classification (UICC 1974)

Primary tumour

TIS Carcinoma *in situ*.

T1 Tumour 2 cm or less in its greatest dimension.

T2 Tumour more than 2 cm but less than 4 cm in its greatest dimension.

T3 Tumour more than 4 cm in its greatest dimension.

Regional lymph nodes

N0 Regional lymph nodes not palpable.

N1 Movable homolateral nodes.

- N1a. Nodes not considered to contain growth.
- N1b. Nodes considered to contain growth.

N2 Movable contralateral or bilateral nodes.

- N2a. Nodes not considered to contain growth.
- N2b. Nodes considered to contain growth.

N3 Fixed nodes.

Distant metastases

M0 No evidence of distant metastases.

M1 Distant metastases present.

Staging

Stage I	T1	N0 N1 or	N2a	M0
Stage II	T2	N0 N1a or	N2a	M0
Stage III	T1	or T2	N1b	
Stage IV	T3	N2b or N3		M0 or M1

Ovary

Record as postoperative—healed, residual
—recurrent or metastatic

(new cases will usually be metastatic)

No staging classification is recommended.

Pharynx

Divisions

Nasopharynx	the whole of the postnasal space
Tonsillar fossa	between the pillars of the fauces
Fauces	region of the anterior pillar of fauces
Vallecula	anterior surface of epiglottis and trough of the vallecula
Posterior wall	posterior wall of any part of the pharynx other than nasopharynx
Pyriform fossa	including both medial and lateral walls thereof
Postcricoid	the retrocricoid arytenoid area
Tongue	posterior third only
Soft palate	

Staging

Stage I

Growth confined to site of origin.
No lymph node involvement.

Stage II

More extensive growth involving two or more sites.
No lymph node involvement.

Stage III

Primary growth as stage I or II.
Mobile unilateral nodes considered to contain growth.

Stage IV

Extensive growth extending beyond pharynx.
Bilateral or fixed nodes.
Distant metastases present.

Skin
(Also applicable to Anus, Penis, Vulva)

Stage I

Freely movable growth not exceeding 3 cm maximum diameter.
No palpable lymph nodes.

Stage II

Growth larger than 3 cm maximum diameter but still freely movable on underlying structures. (With exception of fixation to cartilages of the ala nasi, or of the pinna.)
No palpable lymph nodes.

Stage III

Primary growth as in stages I and II.
Mobile homolateral nodes considered to contain growth.

Stage IV
Growth fixed to underlying structures.
or
Bilateral or fixed lymph nodes.
or
Distant metastases.

Multiple lesions to be staged as that of the most advanced lesion.

Testicular Tumours

Diagnosis
The statement "postoperative healed" refers to cases where there is no clinically residual or metastatic disease following orchidectomy, but does not take into account lymphographic or other means of assessing abdominal nodal disease.

Staging

I Post orchidectomy. No clinically residual or metastatic disease. Lymphogram, CT scan or other investigations for abdominal nodal disease negative.
IIa Post orchidectomy. No clinical residual or metastatic disease. Abdominal nodal involvement indicated by investigative procedure.
IIb Post orchidectomy. Palpable abdominal nodal disease, or scrotal residue.
III Post orchidectomy with or without nodal disease below the diaphragm and with disease in mediastinal and/or supraclavicular nodes.
IV Metastases other than those noted above.

"New" cases (not orchidectomy) would usually be metastatic and should be staged according to the extent of the metastases (usually stage III or stage IV).

Thyroid Cancer

This includes tumours arising in the thyroid gland that may be of lymphoreticular origin.

The regional nodes are the cervical and supraclavicular nodes.

Stage I Technically operable
Mobile primary
No nodes

Stage II
IIa Technically operable
Mobile primary
Mobile unilateral or bilateral nodes
IIb Inoperable or small residue. **Primary and/or nodes not exceeding 5 cm.**
Small fixed primary
or Small residue of primary
No nodes
or Mobile or fixed nodes
or Residue of nodes

Stage III Inoperable. **Primary ± nodes exceeding 5 cm.**
IIIa Fixed primary and/or nodes, or large residue following operation.
IIIb Extension of primary and/or nodes into upper mediastinum.

Stage IV Distant metastases present.

Uterus

Diagnosis
Divisions Cervix
Body

Where a cone biopsy or amputation of the cervix has been performed this is still to be recorded as new when applied to invasive carcinoma. Carcinoma *in situ* may be recorded as postoperative healed only if the line of incision is clear of dysplasia.

Staging of carcinoma of cervix uterus

Stage 0
Carcinoma *in situ*.

Stage I
Carcinoma strictly confined to the cervix.
Ia. Microinvasive with normal looking cervix.
Ib. All the rest of stage I.

Stage II
Carcinoma extends beyond the cervix but does not reach the pelvic wall.
Carcinoma involves the vagina but not the lower third.
IIa. Minimal parametrial involvement only.
IIb. All the rest of stage II.

Stage III
The carcinoma has reached the pelvic wall. (On rectal examination there is no space between the tumour and the pelvic wall.)
The carcinoma involves the lower third of the vagina.
All cases with a hydronephrosis or non-functioning kidney.

Stage IV
The carcinoma involves the bladder or rectum and has extended beyond the limits previously described.
Involvement of groin nodes.
Distant metastases.

Staging of carcinoma of body of uterus
Stage as early or late.
The early cases must conform to the definition: Uterus mobile. No vaginal deposits. Cervix not involved.

Vagina

Staging

I Tumour limited to vaginal mucosa and occupying less than one third of the vagina.
II Tumour has spread into the parametrium but has not reached the pelvic side wall. Less than two-thirds of the vagina is involved.
III Tumour has reached the pelvic side wall or the whole length of the vagina is involved.
IV Spread beyond the pelvis.
Distant metastases.

Subject Index